A Lange Medical Book

CRITICAL CARE ON CALL

Edited by

Alan T. Lefor, MD, MPH, FACS
Director, Surgical Education and Academic Affairs
Director, Division of Surgical Oncology
Cedars-Sinai Medical Center
Los Angeles, California

Professor of Clinical Surgery
Department of Surgery
University of California, Los Angeles
Los Angeles, California

Lange Medical Books/McGraw-Hill
Medical Publishing Division

New York   Chicago   San Francisco   Lisbon   London   Madrid
Mexico City   Milan   New Delhi   San Juan   Seoul   Singapore
Sydney   Toronto

McGraw-Hill

A Division of The McGraw·Hill Companies

Critical Care on Call, First Edition

34567890 DOC/DOC 0987654

ISBN: 0-07-137345-4 (Domestic)

Notice

Medicine is an ever-changing science. As new research and clinical experience broaden our knowledge, changes in treatment and drug therapy are required. The authors and the publisher of this work have checked with sources believed to be reliable in their efforts to provide information that is complete and generally in accord with the standards accepted at the time of publication. However, in view of the possibility of human error or changes in medical sciences, neither the authors nor the publisher nor any other party who has been involved in the preparation or publication of this work warrants that the information contained herein is in every respect accurate or complete, and they disclaim all responsibility for any errors or omissions or for the results obtained from use of the information contained in this work. Readers are encouraged to confirm the information contained herein with other sources. For example and in particular, readers are advised to check the product information sheet included in the package of each drug they plan to administer to be certain that the information contained in this work is accurate and that changes have not been made in the recommended dose or in the contraindications for administration. This recommendation is of particular importance in connection with new or infrequently used drugs.

The book was set in Helvetica by Pine Tree Composition, Inc.
The editors were Janet Foltin, Harriet Lebowitz, and Regina Y. Brown.
The production supervisor was Richard Ruzycka.
The index was prepared by Katherine Pitcoff.
The art manager was Charissa Baker.

R.R. Donnelley & Sons Company was the printer and binder.

This book was printed on acid-free paper.

INTERNATIONAL EDITION ISBN 0-07-121227-2

To Sheila and Maarten

Contents

Editors

Consulting Editor
Leonard G. Gomella, MD, FACS
Bernard Goodwin Professor of Urology
Thomas Jefferson University School of Medicine
Philadelphia, Pennsylvania

Associate Editor for Anesthesiology
David L. Bogdonoff, MD
Associate Professor of Anesthesiology and Surgery
Vice Chair for Clinical Affairs, Department of Anesthesiology
Medical Director, Operating Rooms
University of Virginia Health System
Charlottesville, Virginia

Associate Editor for Surgery
Douglas Geehan, MD, FACS
Assistant Professor
Department of Surgery
University of Missouri-Kansas City
Kansas City, Missouri

Associate Editor for Internal Medicine
Lawrence Maldonado, MD
Director, Medical Intensive Care Unit
Cedars-Sinai Medical Center
Los Angeles, California

Associate Professor of Medicine
UCLA School of Medicine
Los Angeles, California

Contributors

Itzhak Avital, MD
Senior Resident in Surgery
Department of Surgery
Cedars-Sinai Medical Center
Los Angeles, California

David L. Bogdonoff, MD
Associate Professor of Anesthesiology and Surgery
Vice Chair for Clinical Affairs, Department of Anesthesiology
Medical Director, Operating Rooms
University of Virginia Health System
Charlottesville, Virginia

Pauline Chen, MD
Assistant Professor of Surgery
The Dumont-UCLA Transplant Center
The Dumont-UCLA Liver Cancer Center
Department of Surgery
University of California, Los Angeles
Los Angeles, California

Jason Cohen, MD
Fellow in Surgical Oncology
Cedars-Sinai Medical Center
Los Angeles, California

Joseph Eby, MD
Chief Resident in Surgery
Department of Surgery
Cedars-Sinai Medical Center
Los Angeles, California

Douglas Geehan, MD, FACS
Assistant Professor
Department of Surgery
University of Missouri-Kansas City
Kansas City, Missouri

Leonard G. Gomella, MD, FACS
Bernard Goodwin Professor of Urology
Thomas Jefferson University School of Medicine
Philadelphia, Pennsylvania

Scott Karlan, MD
Attending Surgeon
Department of Surgery
Cedars-Sinai Medical Center
Los Angeles, California

Theodore Khalili, MD
Attending Surgeon
Cedars-Sinai Medical Center
Los Angeles, California

Mia Kim, PharmD
Pharmacist
Department of Hospital Pharmacy
Cedars-Sinai Medical Center
Los Angeles, California

Wega Koss, MD
Fellow in Surgical Critical Care
Department of Surgery
Cedars-Sinai Medical Center
Los Angeles, California

Alan T. Lefor, MD, MPH FACS
Director, Surgical Education and Academic Affairs
Director, Division of Surgical Oncology
Cedars-Sinai Medical Center
Los Angeles, California

Jerome H. Liu, MD
Resident
Department of Surgery
University of California, Los Angeles
Los Angeles, California

Lawrence Maldonado, MD
Director, Medical Intensive Care Unit
Cedars-Sinai Medical Center
Los Angeles, California
ASsociate Professor of Medicine
UCLA School of Medicine
Los Angeles, California

Nick Pavona, MD
Department of Surgery
Benjamin Franklin University
Sewell, New Jersey

Bryan Weidner, MD
Fellow in Intensive Care Medicine
Duke University Medical Center
Durham, North Carolina

Contributors to On-Call Problems

Clavio Mario Ascari, MD
Resident in Anesthesiology
University of Virginia Health System
Charlottesville, Virginia

Stanley M. Augustin, M.D.
Assistant Professor, Department of Surgery
University of Missouri-Kansas City
Kansas City, Missouri

Kevin P. Bauer, MD
Resident in Anesthesiology
University of Virginia Health System
Charlottesville, Virginia

Ryan Chang, MD
Fellow in Pulmonary and Critical Care Medicine
Cedars-Sinai Medical Center
Los Angeles, California

Scott Ellison, MD
Chief Resident in General Surgery
University of Missouri-Kansas City
Kansas City, Missouri

Kerri J. George, MD
Resident in Anesthesiology
University of Virginia Health System
Charlottesville, Virginia

Cara Hahs, MD
Senior Resident in General Surgery
University of Missouri-Kansas City
Kansas City, Missouri

Christian Hinrichs, MD
Chief Resident in General Surgery
University of Missouri-Kansas City
Kansas City, Missouri

Matthew D. Holland, MD
Resident in Anesthesiology
University of Virginia Health System
Charlottesville, Virginia

Nader Kamengar, MD
Fellow in Pulmonary and Critical Care Medicine
Cedars-Sinai Medical Center
Los Angeles, California

Nevin S. Kreisler, MD
Assistant Professor of Anesthesiology
Department of Anesthesiology
Emory University School of Medicine
Emory University Hospital
Atlanta, Georgia

Rebecca R. Kuehn, MD
Resident in Anesthesiology
University of Virginia Health System
Charlottesville, Virginia

Hoang Le, MD
Fellow in Pulmonary and Critical Care Medicine
Cedars-Sinai Medical Center
Los Angeles, California

John Mah, MD
Resident in General Surgery
University of Missouri-Kansas City
Kansas City, Missouri

Holland M. Mason, MD
Resident in Anesthesiology
University of Virginia Health System
Charlottesville, Virginia

Daniel Maxfield, MD
Resident in General Surgery
University of Missouri-Kansas City
Kansas City, Missouri

Craig McClain, MD
Resident in Anesthesiology
University of Virginia Health System
Charlottesville, Virginia

B. Todd Moore, MD
Senior Resident in General Surgery
University of Missouri-Kansas City
Kansas City, Missouri

A. Butch Parker, MD
Resident in Anesthesiology
University of Virginia Health System
Charlottesville, Virginia

Gavin L. Roth, MD
Resident in Anesthesiology
University of Virginia Health System
Charlottesville, Virginia

C. Andrew Schroeder, MD
Resident in Internal Medicine
Cedars-Sinai Medical Center
Los Angeles, California

Troy Spilde, MD
Resident in General Surgery
University of Missouri-Kansas City
Surgery Research Fellow, Children's Mercy Hospital
Kansas City, Missouri

Lisa M. Sullivan, MD
Resident in Anesthesiology
University of Virginia Health System
Charlottesville, Virginia

Preface

The field of critical care has undergone a revolution in the last twenty-five years. It is now defined by contributions from surgery, internal medicine, and anesthesiology. This new text is designed to help the people "in the trenches" of critical care and has been written with contributors from each of these three disciplines. Many of the contributors are residents and fellows in critical care who work daily in this field.

It is my hope that you will carry this book with you daily and refer to it often. It is intended as a practical reference to help deal with the problems that commonly occur in the Critical Care Unit while you are "on call." Although it is often said that the best way to avoid errors is to have experience, and the only way to get experience is to make errors, this book is intended to give you a framework for evaluating the problems that arise in the course of caring for critically ill patients. Once you have seen the patient and performed an evaluation, it may be necessary to seek more experienced advice. The information in this book will provide you with a way to think about a problem and its initial evaluation.

The continued support of the editorial staff at McGraw-Hill is gratefully acknowledged. This book and others in the On-Call series could not have been created without the unflagging efforts of Ms. Janet Foltin. I also wish to acknowledge the significant efforts of all three associate editors, Drs. David L. Bogdonoff, Douglas Geehan, and Lawrence Maldonado, without whose attention to detail this book would lack the balance so important among the three disciplines represented. Lastly, and most importantly, I want to thank the families and friends of all the authors, who support us, yet allow us to devote our time, perhaps our most precious resource, to academic pursuits.

Most of all, I hope that this information will improve the care that our patients receive in critical care units.

Alan T. Lefor, MD, MPH, FACS

Los Angeles, California
April 2002

I.   On-Call Problems

1. ABDOMINAL PAIN

I. **Problem.** Seven days after a 40% burn, the patient, a 60-year-old man, complains of pain in the right upper quadrant.

II. **Immediate Questions**

    A. What are the vital signs? Fever indicates an inflammatory process. Hypotension and tachycardia may indicate shock owing to sepsis or hemorrhage. Fever may be absent in elderly patients or in those patients receiving immunosuppressive or antipyretic medications.

    B. Where is the pain located? This is only a general guide to the diagnosis of abdominal pain, because early in the course of the illness, pain may be "shifted" away from the actual site of disease, and late in the course, pain may become generalized. The classic example is appendicitis, where discomfort is initially periumbilical or epigastric and is later localized in the right lower quadrant. When the process goes unchecked, generalized abdominal pain (peritonitis) may result. Pain referred to the groin can be seen with ureteral colic, and pain referred to the back can be observed in patients with pancreatitis or a ruptured abdominal aortic aneurysm (Figs I–1 and I–2).

    C. When did it start? Acute, explosive pain is typical of a perforated viscus, ruptured aneurysm, abscess, or ectopic pregnancy. Pain intensifying for 1–2 h is typical of acute cholecystitis, acute pancreatitis, strangulated bowel, mesenteric thrombosis, proximal small-bowel obstruction, or renal or ureteral colic. Vague pain that increases for several hours is most often seen in patients with acute appendicitis, distal small-bowel and large-bowel obstructions, uncomplicated peptic ulcer disease, and various gynecologic and genitourinary conditions (see Fig I–2).

    D. What is the quality of the pain (dull, sharp, intermittent, constant, "worst ever," burning)? Classically described patterns include "burning" (eg, peptic ulcer disease), "searing" (eg, ruptured aortic aneurysm), "intermittent" (eg, renal or ureteral colic) (see Fig I–2). Have the patient scale the severity of the pain from 1 (least painful) to 10 (most painful). This gives a guide to follow the course more objectively.

    E. What efforts or activities make the pain better or worse? Pain that increases with deep inspiration is associated with diaphragmatic irritation (eg, pleurisy or inflammatory lesions of upper abdomen). Food often *relieves* the pain of peptic ulcer disease. Narcotics relieve colic but offer little relief for patients with pain caused by strangulated bowel or mesenteric thrombosis. Bending forward often relieves the pain of pancreatitis.

1

Referred Pain

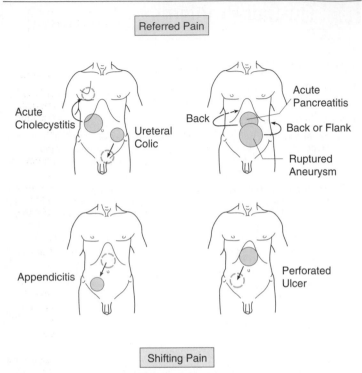

Shifting Pain

Figure I–1. Referred and shifting pain in the acute abdomen. Solid circles indicate the site of maximum pain, and dashed circles show the sites of lesser pain. *(Reproduced, with permission, from Boey JH: Acute Abdomen. In Way LW (editor): Current Surgical Diagnosis & Treatment, 10th ed. Originally published by Appleton & Lange. Copyright © 1994 by The McGraw-Hill Companies, Inc.)*

    F. What are the associated symptoms, if any? Vomiting with the onset of pain is seen in peritoneal irritation or perforation of a hollow viscus and is a prominent feature of upper abdominal diseases, such as Boerhaave's syndrome, acute gastritis, or pancreatitis. In distal small-bowel or large-bowel obstruction, nausea is usually present long before vomiting begins. Hematemesis suggests upper GI bleeding (ulcer disease, Mallory-Weiss syndrome). Diarrhea, when severe and associated with abdominal pain, suggests infectious gastroenteritis, and when bloody, may represent ischemic colitis, ulcerative colitis, Crohn's disease, or amebic dysentery. Constipation alternat-

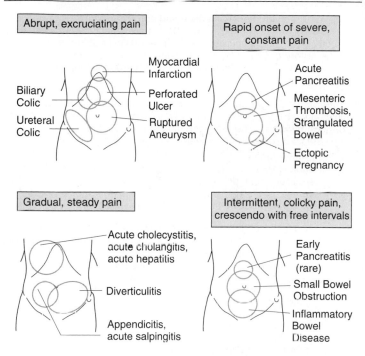

Figure I–2. The location and character of the pain are useful in the differential diagnosis of the acute abdomen. *(Reproduced, with permission, from Boey JH: Acute Abdomen. In Way LW (editor): Current Surgical Diagnosis & Treatment, 10th ed. Originally published by Appleton & Lange. Copyright © 1994 by The McGraw-Hill Companies, Inc.)*

ing with diarrhea may be seen with diverticular disease. Although constipation is often nonspecific, obstipation (absence of passage of both stool and flatus) is strongly suggestive of mechanical bowel obstruction. Hematuria suggests a genitourinary cause.

G. What are the characteristics of the vomitus?

H. When did the patient eat last? This question allows an assessment of the time course of the illness and is particularly important when anesthesia is planned.

I. What is a female patient's menstrual history? A missed or late period may suggest an ectopic pregnancy. Mittelschmerz is pain caused by a ruptured ovarian follicle, occurring at midcycle.

    J. What is the patient's medical and surgical history? Knowledge of a history of ulcers, gallstones, alcohol abuse, or previous operations along with a list of current medications aids in establishing the cause. A history of blunt abdominal trauma 1–3 d before the onset of the pain may signify subcapsular hemorrhage of the liver, spleen, pancreas, or kidney.

III. Differential Diagnosis. Abdominal pain has both intra-abdominal and extra-abdominal sources and can be associated with both medical and surgical diseases. The list is too long to reproduce in its entirety here, but listed are some of the more frequently encountered causes.

    A. Intra-abdominal

        1. Hollow viscera. Hollow viscera can perforate in the face of obstruction, and perforation represents an acute surgical emergency.

            a. Upper abdominal: esophagitis, gastritis, peptic ulcer disease, cholecystitis.

            b. Mid gut: small bowel obstruction or infarction. Obstruction may be a result of adhesions (benign and malignant), hernias (internal and external), or volvulus.

            c. Lower abdominal: inflammatory bowel disease, appendicitis, mesenteric lymphadenitis, obstruction.

            d. Gastroenteritis, colitis.

        2. Solid organs.

            a. Liver: Hepatitis.

            b. Pancreas: Pancreatitis.

            c. Spleen: Splenic infarction.

            d. Kidney: Stones, pyelonephritis, abscess.

        3. Pelvic.

            a. Pelvic inflammatory disease.

            b. Ectopic pregnancy (rupture is a surgical emergency).

            c. Other: Fibroid torsion, cysts, endometriosis.

        4. Vascular. Vascular catastrophes are surgical emergencies.

            a. Ruptured aneurysm.

            b. Dissecting aneurysm.

            c. Mesenteric thrombosis or embolism.

            d. Splenic or hepatic rupture. Usually posttraumatic.

    B. Extra-abdominal. Disease in extra-abdominal conditions may rarely be manifest as referred abdominal pain. The most important causes to remember are sickle cell crisis, pneumonia (especially lower lobe), myocardial infarction, and rarely, diabetic ketoacidosis. Remember that pain on one side of the diaphragm may be caused by disease on the other side (eg, upper-abdominal pain from pneumonia).

    C. Other

        1. Trauma patients. Blunt trauma may cause injuries to solid viscera (spleen, liver, kidney, pancreas) or to fixed structures, such as the duodenum. Penetrating trauma may injure any intra-abdominal structure.

2. **Postoperative.** Postoperative abdominal pain usually improves significantly in uncomplicated cases during the first 2–3 postoperative days. Persistent pain may indicate a problem, such as obstruction or abscess formation. Uncomplicated postoperative pain is derived from both visceral afferent fibers (because of surgical injury to peritoneal surfaces) and to somatic fibers innervating the abdominal wall.

3. **Critically ill patients.** Patients suffering severe stress from such serious insults as multiple trauma or burns, often complicated by sepsis, may suffer from potentially life-threatening intra-abdominal events.
   a. Acute stress gastritis (usually manifested as massive upper GI bleeding).
   b. Curling's ulcer with or without perforation (after burn).
   c. Acalculous cholecystitis and cholestasis from chronic use of total parenteral nutrition.

IV. Database

A. Physical Exam Key Points

1. **Overall appearance.** A patient writhing in agony is typical of colic, whereas a motionless patient is suggestive of peritoneal irritation.

2. **Lungs.** Listen for basilar rales or rhonchi indicating possible pneumonia. Dullness to percussion may represent pleural effusion or consolidation.

3. **Heart.** Look for evidence of cardiac decompensation (distended neck veins, S3 gallop, peripheral edema), especially in the patient with preexisting coronary disease. Such evidence may direct attention toward a myocardial infarction or atrial fibrillation, which can suggest emboli.

4. **Abdomen.**
   a. **Inspection:** Note presence of distention (obstruction, ileus, ascites), scaphoid (perforated ulcer), flank ecchymoses (hemorrhagic pancreatitis), caput medusae (portal hypertension), or surgical scars (adhesions, tumor).
   b. **Auscultation:** Listen for bowel sounds (absent or an occasional tinkle with obstruction or ileus; listen for hyperperistaltic sounds accompanying gastroenteritis and for rushes with small bowel obstruction).
   c. **Percussion:** Tympany is associated with distended loops of bowel; dullness and a fluid wave with ascites; loss of liver dullness is associated with free air.
   d. **Palpation:** Guarding, rigidity, and rebound tenderness are hallmarks of peritonitis. Localized tenderness is often seen with cholecystitis, appendicitis, salpingitis, and diverticulitis.

Costovertebral angle tenderness is common with pyelonephritis. Murphy's sign is present when the patient has an inspiratory arrest when the gallbladder is palpated in acute cholecystitis. Pain with active hip flexion (psoas sign) can represent an inflamed retrocecal appendix or psoas abscess. The obturator sign (pain on internal and external rotation of the flexed thigh) can be found with a retrocecal appendix or obturator hernia. Masses may also be detected.

5. **Rectal exam.** An intraluminal mass suggests a rectal carcinoma, a fissure may indicate Crohn's disease; unilateral tenderness suggests appendicitis (usually retrocecal) or an abscess. When stool is present, evaluate for occult blood.

6. **Pelvic exam.** Examine for cervical motion tenderness and purulent cervical discharge that suggests pelvic inflammatory disease (salpingitis, tuboovarian abscess). Other masses may be felt (ectopic pregnancy, ovarian cyst, or neoplasm).

7. **Extremities.** Evaluate for asymmetric pedal pulses, pain, pallor, and paresthesia for evidence of ischemia that may be associated with embolic phenomenon.

8. **Skin.** Look for jaundice and spider angiomata seen with liver disease. Cool and clammy skin from peripheral vasoconstriction is an ominous sign of severe hypotension.

B. **Laboratory Data**

1. **Hemogram.** Anemia may indicate hemorrhage from an ulcer, colon cancer, or leaking aneurysm. Leukocytosis indicates presence of inflammation. A low white count is more typical of viral infections, such as gastroenteritis or mesenteric adenitis.

2. **Serum electrolytes, BUN, creatinine.** Bowel obstruction with vomiting can cause hypokalemia, dehydration, or both (BUN/creatinine ratio > 20:1).

3. **Bilirubin, AST, ALT, alkaline phosphatase.** Hepatitis, cholecystitis and other liver diseases may be diagnosed through these tests.

4. **Amylase.** Markedly elevated levels are associated with pancreatitis. Amylase can also be elevated with perforated ulcer and small bowel obstruction; occasionally, a pseudocyst or hemorrhagic pancreatitis may result in a normal amylase level.

5. **Arterial blood gases.** Hypoxia is often an early sign of sepsis. Acidosis may be present in ischemic bowel.

6. **Pregnancy test.** Premenopausal women should be tested to rule out an ectopic pregnancy, independent of whether they use birth control.

7. **Urinalysis.** Hematuria may indicate urolithiasis; pyuria and hematuria can be present in urinary tract infections or rarely in appendicitis.

8. **Cervical culture.** Send specimen specifically for gonorrhea (anaerobic) when pelvic inflammatory disease is suspected.

C. Radiographic and Other Studies

1. **Flat and upright abdominal films.** When the patient is debilitated, a left lateral decubitus film may be substituted for the upright. Observe for the following key elements: gas pattern, bowel dilatation, air-fluid levels, presence of air in rectum, pancreatic calcifications, loss of psoas margin, displacement of hollow viscera, gall and renal stones, portal vein air, or aortic calcifications.

2. **Chest radiograph.** May reveal pneumonia, widened mediastinum (dissecting aneurysm), pleural effusion, or elevation of a hemidiaphragm (subdiaphragmatic inflammatory process). Free air under the diaphragm suggests a perforated viscus and is best seen on an upright chest film.

3. **Ultrasound.** May reveal gallstones, ectopic pregnancy, or other disease.

4. **Electrocardiogram.** Rule out myocardial infarction as a cause of upper abdominal distress and nausea.

5. **Other studies as clinically indicated:**
   a. IVP (excretory urogram is helpful in the workup of urolithiasis).
   b. Abdominal CT scan.
   c. Biliary scintigraphy.
   d. **Contrast bowel studies:** Upper GI swallow and enemas (barium, dilute barium, gastrografin).
   e. **Endoscopic studies:** Esophagogastroduodenoscopy (EGD), colonoscopy, endoscopic retrograde cholangiopancreatography (ERCP).
   f. Arteriography.
   g. Peritoneal lavage (page 348) or paracentesis (page 344).

V. Plan. Abdominal pain in any patient can present a diagnostic dilemma, but even more so for elderly patients or for those unable to communicate. The surgeon's goal is to determine when abdominal pain requires surgical treatment to prevent further morbidity. Generally, pain that is present 6 or more hours and does not improve usually has a cause requiring surgical intervention. Many cases of abdominal pain have no definite diagnosis before laparotomy. A brief period of observation may ultimately point to the cause, but operation is safer in most cases. The use of analgesics remains controversial, but most clinicians now believe moderate doses of pain medicine will not mask symptoms and will make the patient more comfortable. Specific types of therapy and operations for each possible diagnosis cannot be described here but can be found in surgical and medical textbooks. It is essential to recognize that certain conditions are life threatening and, thus, require urgent operation.

A. Observation. With the exception of catastrophes that require urgent surgical exploration, most cases of abdominal pain require close observation, medical management, and occasionally analgesics. In the case of postoperative abdominal pain, analgesics are used most frequently.

1. Keep patient NPO and consider nasogastric suction, especially when vomiting is present.
2. Administer intravenous hydration (see Chapter IV), with careful attention to intake and output.
3. Use parenteral analgesics carefully to avoid masking disease processes.
4. Serial physical exams by the same examiner are very useful in determining progression of symptoms and aid in securing the diagnosis. Be sure to accurately document these examinations.

B. **Operation.** Vascular catastrophes, perforated viscus, most causes of bowel obstruction, many splenic and hepatic injuries, ruptured ectopic pregnancies, and appendicitis require emergency operative intervention.

2. ACIDOSIS: METABOLIC

(See Appendix 2: Basic Approach to the Diagnosis of Acid/Base Disorders)

I. **Problem.** A 68-year-old man with a history of hypertension, type II diabetes mellitus, and chronic renal insufficiency is noted to be obtunded with a BP of 70/30. He is intubated and transferred to the ICU. Laboratory values are obtained showing a pH of 7.10, PCO_2 of 20, and a PaO_2 of 70, with an Na^+ of 145, HCO_3 of 8, and chloride of 110.

II. **Immediate Questions**

A. **Why is the patient in shock?** The first priority is to identify and treat the cause of shock. Cardiogenic shock (after a myocardial infarction or arrhythmia) is common in such a patient; look for and treat arrhythmias expeditiously.

B. **What is the volume status?** All forms of shock (cardiogenic, hypovolemic, septic and neurogenic) lead to lactic acidosis. Hypovolemia is the easiest to correct.

C. **Is the patient adequately ventilated?** Check the circuitry and the exhaled volume; verify the position of the endotracheal tube and the ventilator settings.

III. **Differential Diagnosis.** Metabolic acidosis may be associated with a normal or an increased anion gap. This division greatly facilitates diagnosis. In general, increased anion-gap metabolic acidosis (normally called **anion-gap metabolic acidosis**) is more likely to be seen in the ICU setting and is more likely to be life-threatening.

A. **Definitions**

1. **Defect:** Increased acid accumulation or decreased extracellular HCO_3.

2. **Laboratory manifestation:** Decreased pH, decreased plasma HCO_3.

3. **Compensation:** Increasing the rate of ventilation decreases Pco_2; cells exchange extracellular H^+ for intracellular Na^+ and K^+. The kidneys gradually compensate by excreting H^+ and generating bicarbonate. The degree of **respiratory compensation** can be estimated by the following formula:

$$Pco_2 = 1.5 (HCO_3) + 8 \pm 2$$

4. **Classification: Anion-gap (AG) metabolic acidosis** occurs with increased endogenous production of acid, as in lactic acidosis or diabetic ketoacidosis. The AG can be estimated with the following formula:

$$(AG = Na^+) - ([Cl^-] + [HCO_3])$$

The normal anion gap is 11 ± 4, although there are several exceptions. An AG acidosis can exist even with a normal AG in patients who are severely hypoalbuminemic or have pathologic paraproteinemias. For every 1 g/dL that albumin drops, the AG decreases by 2.5 to 3 mmol. Pathologic paraproteinemias lower the AG, because immunoglobulins are largely cationic. The AG may not reflect an underlying acidosis in a patient with a significant alkalemia (pH > 7.5). In these circumstances, albumin is more negatively charged, which increases unmeasured anions.

   a. **Specific Differential Diagnosis:** Lactic acidosis (tissue hypoxia, shock, cardiac arrest, overwhelming sepsis, hematologic emergencies); ketoacidosis (diabetes, alcohol induced, and starvation); renal failure (uremia metabolic acidosis); and toxins (salicylates, methanol, and ethylene glycol).

5. **Normal anion gap metabolic acidosis** is usually the result of bicarbonate loss from the bowel or kidney but can occur from treatment with exogenous acids (eg, hydrochloric acid). Normal AG acidoses are subcategorized on the basis of potassium level. Hypokalemia (>3.5 mmol/L) is associated with diarrhea, ureteral diversion, proximal renal tubular acidosis (RTA), type I RTA and hyperalimentation. Hyperkalemia (>4.5 mmol/L) can be found in hypoaldosterone states, ammonium chloride administration, and type IV distal RTA.

   a. **Specific Differential Diagnosis:** GI loss of HCO_3 (from diarrhea, an ileostomy, a proximal colostomy, or a ureteral conduit); renal loss of HCO_3 (proximal RTA, carbonic anhydrase inhibitor); renal tubular disease (ATN, chronic tubulointerstitial disease, distal RTA type-I and IV, hypoaldosteronism, and aldosterone inhibitors); and medications (ammonium chloride, HCl, hyperalimentation, and dilutional acidosis).

IV. Database

A. Physical Exam Key Points. The clinical features of metabolic acidosis depend primarily on the underlying disorder.

1. **General exam.** Mottled, cool or clammy skin may indicate sepsis, a common cause of metabolic acidosis in the ICU. Fever is also typically present.

2. **Pulmonary.** There may be rapid, deep respirations (Kussmaul's breathing) from the low pH or hypoventilation from profound shock. Rales may indicate CHF.

3. **Cardiovascular.** Hypotension and tachycardia are seen with most forms of shock. There may also be changes in systemic or pulmonary vascular resistance. Cardiogenic shock may cause acidosis; acidosis may cause arrhythmias, reduced myocardial contractility, and decreased responsiveness to catecholamines.

4. **HEENT.** Tracheal shift indicates tension pneumothorax; jugular venous distention is seen with tension pneumothorax or cardiac tamponade. *Fetor hepaticus* (halitosis of fruity odor) may suggest hepatic failure or diabetic ketoacidosis.

5. **Abdomen.** Any abnormal finding (distention, pain, peritoneal signs, etc) may be significant.

B. Laboratory Data

1. **Hemogram.** Leukocytosis may indicate sepsis. A high Hct is seen with dehydration; anemia suggests bleeding, although it may be normal with renal failure.

2. **Electrolytes, BUN, and creatinine.** Calculate the anion gap, the chloride and potassium (in non-anion gap metabolic acidosis). Look for evidence of renal failure.

3. **Lactate.** Increases with anaerobic metabolism, in all forms of shock.

4. **Glucose and Ketones.** Increases may indicate diabetic ketoacidosis.

C. Radiographic and Other Studies

1. **Chest radiograph.** Look for pulmonary edema, infiltrates, CHF, and ET-tube position.

2. **ECG and rhythm strip.** Evaluate for arrhythmias.

3. **EMG.** May be helpful when considering CNS causes.

V. Plan

A. Diagnose and treat the underlying disorder

1. Treat non-AG metabolic acidosis by replacing volume losses. Use an IV solution with low chloride and bicarbonate.

2. There are specific treatments for most causes of AG metabolic acidosis (ie, insulin for diabetic ketoacidosis, dialysis for renal failure, etc).

3. Use of sodium bicarbonate for lactic acidosis has become controversial. It has not improved survival rates when used to treat this

disorder. There are studies suggesting that bicarbonate improves cardiovascular responsiveness when the pH < 7.1. On the other hand, myocardial performance is often normal in a patient with metabolic acidosis. In addition, bicarbonate administration worsens myocardial performance in a patient with cardiogenic shock.

4. Potential complications of bicarbonate administration include volume overload, paradoxical CSF or intracellular acidosis, respiratory acidosis, impaired oxygen delivery (tissue hypoxia), hypokalemia, hypocalcemia, hypernatremia, hyperosmolarity, and overshoot alkalemia.

5. **Bicarbonate replacement:** The following formula for the amount of a needed bicarbonate replacement can be used:

$$\text{Body weight (kg)} \times 0.40 \times (24 - [HCO_3]) = \text{Total mEq of } HCO_3$$

Give 50% of this amount in the first 12 h as a mixture of bicarbonate with D_5W.

3. ACIDOSIS: RESPIRATORY

I. **Problem.** A 75-year-old man is admitted to the medical service with shortness of breath caused by long-standing COPD and new-onset tracheobronchitis. He also has a lumbar compression fracture from metastatic prostate cancer. His arterial blood gas levels are pH, 7.10); $P_{CO} \text{ } END_2$, 110, P_{O_2}, 50; and bicarbonate, 39 mEq/L (on 6 L/min of oxygen).

II. **Immediate Questions**

A. **What are the patient's vital signs? Is this a near-arrest situation, and should a code be called?**

B. This patient has neurologic impairment, respiratory depression, and acidosis. **Is one of these problems responsible for the others? Which should be addressed first?**

C. **What is the patient's respiratory rate? How are his breath sounds?**

D. **Is the acidosis respiratory, metabolic or mixed, primary, or compensatory?**
   1. **Defect:** Respiratory acidosis is caused by inadequate alveolar ventilation (from medications that depress respiration, with neuromuscular disorders, or increased CO_2 production), or by ineffective gas exchange (from airway obstruction, bronchoconstriction, or alveolar disease).
   2. **Laboratory Manifestation:** Increased P_{CO_2}, decreased pH.
   3. **Compensation:** The normal respiratory response to hypercapnia is to increase alveolar ventilation. In addition to buffers (primarily intracellular proteins), renal compensatory mechanisms (bicarbonate reabsorption) are present for 24 to 36 h.

    E. What medications has the patient received? Narcotics are the most common cause of respiratory depression.

III. Differential Diagnosis. In acutely ill patients, metabolic and respiratory acidosis commonly coexist. There are many possible causes for respiratory acidosis including airway obstruction (foreign bodies, tongue displacement, laryngospasm, obstructed endotracheal tubes, severe bronchospasm, late stages of acute asthma), respiratory center depression (general anesthesia, sedatives, narcotics, cerebral injury or ischemia, drugs or toxins, electrolyte disorders), increased CO_2 production (sepsis; seizures; malignant hyperthermia; shivering; hyper-metabolic states; overfeeding with TPN, particularly, with high carbohydrate diets), neuromuscular disorders (spinal cord injury, Guillain-Barré syndrome, myasthenia gravis, polymyositis), intrinsic pulmonary disease (obstructive and restrictive conditions, acute lung injury, acute respiratory distress syndrome [ARDS], pulmonary edema), extrinsic pulmonary disease (hemothorax, pneumothorax, flail chest, large effusions, obesity, hypoventilation syndrome), and issues related to mechanical ventilation (inadequate ventilatory support, inadvertent hypoventilation, permissive hypercapnia).

IV. Database. The clinical manifestations of acute respiratory acidosis and acute ventilatory failure are the same. They depend on the absolute increase in P_{CO_2}, the rate of P_{CO_2} rise, and the severity of associated hypoxemia.

    A. Physical Exam Key Points
        1. Vital signs. Is there tachycardia, hypertension, supraventricular or ventricular arrhythmias, or peripheral vasodilation? Check the ventilator settings.
        2. Central Nervous System. There may be somnolence or obtundation, anxiety or confusion, psychosis, tremors, myoclonus or asterixis, headache or papilledema.
        3. Pulmonary. Listen for decreased breath sounds, stridor, rales, or wheezes.

    B. Laboratory Data
        ABG. Follow serial values to assess the effects of treatment and to identify the need for intubation.

V. Plan. Support the patient with mechanical ventilation as needed. In a dire situation, administration of bicarbonate may be necessary, in addition to intubating and hyperventilating the patient. Appropriate treatment depends on correctly identifying the underlying cause for respiratory acidosis. When the patient is oversedated with narcotics, benzodiazepines, or paralytic agents, consider administering specific reversal agents. Electrolyte abnormalities, such as hypokalemia, hypophosphatemia, and hypocalcemia, should be corrected. $NaHCO_3$ should not be used in most patients with acute respiratory acidosis.

Avoid creating a posthypercapnic alkalosis. This condition occurs when a patient with compensated chronic respiratory acidosis is hyper-ventilated to a normal or near-normal P_{CO_2}. Some patients with COPD will not breathe without a high P_{CO_2} (they have a blunted response to hypoxia). Their primary respiratory acidosis is balanced by a secondary metabolic alkalosis from renal compensation (bicarbonate retention). Rapidly correcting their hypercapnia eliminates the respiratory acidosis, leaves the metabolic alkalosis, and eliminates the patient's respiratory drive. Proper ventilator management should be based on the patient's P_{CO_2}, in comparison with their baseline P_{CO_2} and current pH.

4. ACUTE LIVER FAILURE

I. **Problem.** A 28-year-old woman is admitted to the psychiatric service after attempting suicide. Three days later, she develops acute jaundice, stupor, coagulopathy, and aminotransferase levels greater than 1500 IU/L.

II. **Immediate Questions**

   A. **Does the patient have preexisting liver disease?**

   B. **Did she ingest anything (acetaminophen, oral hypoglycemics, alcohol, etc) at the time of her suicide attempt?**

   C. **What medications were given afterward, and how much?**

   D. **What are her vital signs?** This will direct her initial treatment. Her mental status, coagulation profile, and renal function will indicate the severity of her condition.

III. **Differential Diagnosis**

Acute liver failure (ALF) is also known as **fulminant hepatic failure.** It is a clinical syndrome characterized by an acute onset of hepatic dysfunction associated with jaundice, coagulopathy, and encephalopathy, in a patient without previous evidence of liver disease. There are many possible causes; acetaminophen toxicity/overdose, viral hepatitis and drug reactions are the most common in the United States. ALF is classified into the following 4 grades.

Grade 1: Patients are arousable and coherent, but their mood is altered and there are impairments of intellect, concentration, and psychomotor function.
Grade 2: Patients are drowsy (although arousable and coherent) and confused with inappropriate behavior.
Grade 3: Patients are stuporous (although arousable), often agitated and aggressive.
Grade 4: Patients are comatose and unresponsive to painful stimuli.

IV. Database. Symptoms can vary depending on the cause of ALF.

    A. Physical Exam Key Points. Patients with ALF generally lack the stigmata of chronic liver disease or signs of portal hypertension.

        1. Vital signs. Look for signs of sepsis. Patients with ALF tend to become septic, most commonly from urinary tract infections, pneumonia, and bacteremia of unknown cause. Sepsis leads to circulatory collapse, with hypotension, decreased systemic vascular resistance, and systemic vasodilatation. Cerebral edema is common in ALF, although the cause is not well understood. In contrast to sepsis, cerebral edema leads to hypertension, bradycardia, and hyperventilation.

        2. Neurologic exam. Look for signs of hepatic encephalopathy or cerebral edema. These include fatigue, malaise, and altered mental status. Decerebrate posturing, abnormal papillary reflexes, and brain stem respiratory patterns or apnea may be noted.

        3. Abdominal exam. Liver swelling causes right upper quadrant pain and tenderness.

        4. Musculocutaneous. There may be jaundice or signs of coagulopathy (bruising, petechiae, bleeding from IV sites).

        5. Gastrointestinal. Inquire about nausea, vomiting, and light-colored stools.

        6. Genitourinary. Dark urine precedes the presenting symptoms.

    B. Laboratory Data

        1. Hemogram. Leukocytosis suggests infection.

        2. Liver function tests. Serum aminotransferase concentrations (SGOT and SGPT) are typically elevated to 1000–3000 IU/L (and occasionally reach 10,000 IU/L). PT, INR, and bilirubin levels are increased, whereas glucose, phosphorus, and magnesium are decreased.

        3. Electrolytes, BUN and creatinine. Renal failure (from prerenal azotemia, ATN, hepatorenal syndrome, or drug-induced nephrotoxicity) occurs frequently and is associated with a poor prognosis.

        4. Urinalysis and electrolytes. Look for evidence of urinary tract infection and renal failure.

V. Plan. ALF has two outcomes: death and survival. For some patients, the only option is liver transplantation. Because ALF carries such a poor prognosis, a decision regarding transplantation should be made early in the course of this disease. Other than transplantation, there are few specific treatments. The main focus of ICU care is to support the patient.

    A. When ALF has been caused by toxins or medications, antidotes should be given when available (eg, N-acetylcysteine for acetaminophen toxicity).

    B. For patients with cerebral edema, cerebral perfusion pressure (MAP-ICP) should be assessed with a subdural ICP transducer. ICP should be kept less than 25 mm Hg. Hyperventilation (to a Pco$_2$ of 25–35) will transiently lower the ICP. Mannitol is also used in doses of 0.5–1.0 mg/kg (but not to exceed 100 g) given IV over 5 min.

C. Lactulose, although indicated in the treatment of encephalopathy secondary to chronic liver disease, has no role in ALF.

D. Coagulopathy is not normally corrected unless the patient needs an invasive procedure or begins to bleed. Fresh frozen plasma is used to correct a prolonged PT/INR.

For hypotension and renal failure, volume repletion is mandatory, and colloids, such as albumin and FFP, are commonly used. Renal dose dopamine (2–5 µg/kg/min) and loop diuretics (eg, furosemide) are occasionally tried in an attempt to prevent oliguric renal failure. Add pressors (eg, norepinephrine) to support blood pressure when fluid repletion is not effective. Dialysis (continuous arteriovenous hemoperfusion or hemofiltration) may be needed to correct severe metabolic acidosis or critical hyperkalemia. When hepatorenal syndrome develops, urgent liver transplantation is warranted.

E. Bioartificial Liver. Consider the bioartificial liver support trial, available at certain institutions.

F. Transplantation. The decision to transplant is usually based on the transplant team's clinical experience and the following King's College Hospital criteria:

1. **Toxicity not induced by acetaminophen:** (either/or) Transplant for (1) PT > 100 s, (INR > 6.5) or (2) of any 3 of the following: age < 10 or > 40 years; cause: non-A/non-B hepatitis, drug or toxin induced, duration of jaundice more than 1 week before encephalopathy, PT > 50 s (INR > 3.5), serum bilirubin > 18 mg/dL.
2. **Toxicity induced by acetaminophen:** (either/or) Transplant for (1) pH < 7.3 or (2) PT > 100 s (INR > 6.5) and serum creatinine > 3.4 mg/dL with stage 3/4 encephalopathy.

5. ACUTE LOSS OF PULSE IN AN EXTREMITY

Immediate actions. Loss of extremity pulses requires emergent assessment by the responsible physician. When the patient has recently had a vascular reconstruction, the bypass is in jeopardy. Limited time is available before the bypass becomes unsalvageable. Reexploration and operative angiography provide the best chance for salvaging the limb.

I. Problem. A 64-year-old man, previously admitted and intubated for community-acquired pneumonia, is found to have no pulses in his right lower extremity.

II. Immediate Questions

A. Did the patient have pulses at the time of admission? If he did not, the current finding may be of little significance. Unfortunately, many patients do not have a vascular examination documented at the time of admission. Patients and their families may be able to say whether the leg has changed. In the absence of baseline information, assume the worst, particularly, when the patient has other symptoms (eg, pain, pallor, paresthesias) to suggest ischemia. Pulses are a palpable physical finding. Doppler signals (sometimes inappropriately called **Doppler pulses**) represent arterial flow that is detectable using an ultrasonic probe. The terms are not interchangeable.

B. Has the patient had arrhythmias? Intermittent atrial fibrillation is notorious for causing arterial emboli.

C. What are the vital signs? Moderate hypotension (typically BP < 70) normally leads to the loss of all extremity pulses. When a patient has preexisting vascular disease affecting only one extremity, mild hypotension may occasionally lead to the loss of pulses in that one extremity.

D. What interventional procedures have been done? Search through progress notes and procedure reports, OR nursing and anesthesia records, and radiology reports. Speak directly to physicians involved in procedures identified, even if a procedure seems unrelated. Unsuccessful portions of procedures may not be adequately documented (eg, unsuccessful arterial cannulation in one extremity followed by successful cannulation in another).

III. Differential Diagnosis

A. Embolism. Emboli originate from many sites. Mural thrombi may accumulate during atrial fibrillation and embolize (particularly if the patient reverts to sinus rhythm). Both valvular debris (either thrombi or vegetations) and atherosclerotic debris (eg, from a proximal aneurysm) may lodge in an artery, obstructing flow to an extremity. Paradoxical embolization occurs when venous clots enter the arterial circulation (eg, through a patent foramen ovale).

B. Thrombosis. Diseased arteries (narrowed or ulcerated from atherosclerotic plaque) may thrombose during low-flow states. A normal artery can thrombose when injured (eg, after an intimal dissection caused by cannulation). Vascular reconstructions thrombose early when there is inadequate inflow (proximal disease), inadequate outflow (distal disease), or technical flaws (eg, kinking or twisting of a graft). Progression of a patient's native disease (eg, worsening distal atherosclerosis) is usually responsible for late thrombosis; hypercoagulable and low-flow states are occasional causes.

C. Vasoconstriction. Vasopressors typically support central BP at the expense of peripheral perfusion. The consequences should be symmetric, reducing all peripheral pulses.

   D. **Inadvertent Arterial Cannulation.** Placing a catheter in an artery that was intended to be placed in a vein may reduce distal arterial flow and pulses. When uncertain about the cannulated vessel (artery vs vein), connect the line in question to a pressure transducer. As a low-tech alternative, allow blood to flow into tubing held vertically. Flow more than 30 cm above the patient strongly suggests arterial cannulation.

   E. **Compartment Syndrome.** Loss of arterial pulses is a very late finding in compartment syndrome. By the time this sign appears, the patient already has neuromuscular damage. Fasciotomy should be performed early, on the basis of ischemic time and mechanism of injury (eg, crush injuries). In borderline cases, intracompartmental pressures can be measured serially.

   F. **Venous Disease.** Massive iliofemoral and saphenous thrombosis can occlude all venous outflow with subsequent loss of pulses. Despite the venous pathophysiology, limb loss is a real threat. Anticoagulation, thrombolytic therapy, and even surgery may be required.

IV. **Database**
   A. **Physical Exam Key Points**
      1. **Pulse exam.** It is crucial to document the patient's pulses at the time of admission, particularly in older patients and patients with known peripheral vascular disease. When evaluating a pulseless patient without a baseline exam, compare one extremity with the other. Also check for the presence of Doppler signals.
      2. **Cardiac exam.** Is the patient's pulse regular? Is there a murmur from valvular disease?
      3. **Anasarca** or focal edema suggest cardiac disease.
      4. **Peripheral vascular findings.** Are the toes (or fingers) pale or blue, cool, with poor capillary filling? Along with pulselessness, these are signs of arterial insufficiency. Distal hair loss is seen with chronic ischemia. Brawny induration and skin ulceration above the ankle suggest venous stasis disease.
   B. **Laboratory Data**
      1. No specific testing is required. When there has been significant tissue ischemia, hyperkalemia and acidosis may be present. When considering a hypercoagulable state (eg, protein C, protein S, AT3 deficiency, lupus anticoagulant, etc), send blood in the proper tubes before starting anticoagulation.
   C. **Radiography and Other Studies**
      1. **EKG.** Identify acute myocardial dysfunction or rhythm disturbances.
      2. **Arteriography.** Diagnose and treat (eg, lytic therapy, balloon dilatation, stenting, etc) arterial lesions. When a revascularized extremity becomes pulseless soon after surgery, arteriography should be done in the operating room at the time of reexploration.

3. **Compartment pressures.** Use proprietary devices or home-made systems (using a needle, tubing, a manometer, an IV bag, and a three way stopcock) to directly measure compartment pressure. The clinical signs of compartment syndrome may be absent in a critically ill patient, and their absence should not preclude making the diagnosis.

V. Plan

A. **Overall plan.** The loss of an extremity pulse represents a limb-threatening emergency. Prompt diagnosis and management are critical for limb salvage. Arteriography is usually necessary, although, in certain circumstances, a careful physical exam may reveal the site and source of the problem. Anticoagulation should be considered early. When appropriate, start heparin while evaluating the patient (before surgery or thrombolytic therapy).

B. **Correct volume depletion.** Dehydration leads to vasoconstriction. Pressors exacerbate this vasoconstriction.

C. **Coordinate services.** Radiography, vascular surgery, anesthesia, and operating room staff may be needed sequentially or simultaneously.

D. **Relief of compartment syndrome.** After several hours of ischemia, assume that the patient has a compartment syndrome. Under such circumstances, fasciotomy will maximize the chance of limb salvage. Limb sacrifice may occasionally be necessary for patient survival. Even when **revascularization** is successful, there may be a reperfusion syndrome. Beware of hyperkalemia, acidosis, and myoglobinuria. Check laboratory values frequently and consider measuring compartment pressures (or empirically performing a fasciotomy). Observation may be hampered by the patient's critical illness.

6. AIRWAY PRESSURE: SUDDEN INCREASE

I. **Problem.** A 52-year-old man on a ventilator 2 d after right lower lobectomy develops a sudden increase in airway pressure.

II. **Immediate Questions**

A. **Is the patient being adequately ventilated?** When in doubt, switch to manual ventilation with a bag-mask device while trouble-shooting. A drop in oxygen saturation will necessitate a rapid intervention.

B. **Is the patient hypotensive?** Rising airway pressure with falling venous return is pathognomonic for tension pneumothorax. Bleeding into the chest, lungs, or airways can also be responsible.

C. **Has the endotracheal tube (ETT) moved?** The tip may be up against the carina, or it may have advanced into the right mainstem bronchus.

    D. Has the ETT been suctioned recently? This will remove mucous plugs and verify that the tube is patent.

    E. Is the patient adequately sedated? A patient experiencing pain or anxiety may bite down on the endotracheal tube or "fight" the ventilator by coughing and straining.

III. Differential Diagnosis

A. Endotracheal Tube Obstruction

1. **External.** The ETT is flexible and can kink or be occluded by a patient biting.
2. **Internal.** Mucus or clots can obstruct the lumen of the tube.

B. Airway Obstruction

1. **Plugging of lumen.** Just as the endotracheal tube can be obstructed by mucus or clots, so can the bronchi. Tissue swelling or sloughing after manipulation or laser treatment may also lead to plugging. In tracheomalacia, the airway's cartilaginous support is damaged, leading to airway collapse during inspiration.
2. **Bronchoconstriction.** Acute bronchospasm can occur in any patient, not just patients with reactive airway disease. Stimulation of the carina by the ETT can cause bronchospasm; other causes include pulmonary embolism, congestive heart failure, drug reactions, and allergic reactions.
3. **Increased intrathoracic pressure.** An enlarging pneumothorax or hemothorax will take up space normally used for lung expansion. In these circumstances, volume-controlled ventilators will attempt to deliver the same volume of air, even as space decreases, by increasing the inflation pressure. A pneumothorax becomes a tension pneumothorax when the pressure increases enough to shift the mediastinum and occlude venous return to the heart. Pneumothorax is a common complication of central line placement and can also result from rib fracture, barotrauma (from mechanical ventilation), or chest tube obstruction. A dramatic increase in intra-abdominal pressure (caused by patient straining, intra-abdominal bleeding, or swelling) may also be transmitted to the intrathoracic space by the upward displacement of the diaphragm. Patients may bite, cough, strain, or fight the ventilator because of pain, anxiety, CNS dysfunction, hypercapnia, or hypoxemia. This commonly occurs when sedation wears off. (See also Ventilator: bucking, high PAP in Problem 88, page 258).

C. Breathing Circuit Obstruction

1. **Expiratory tubing obstruction.**
2. **Misplacement of PEEP valves.**
3. **Mechanical failure of the ventilator.**

IV. **Database**
  A. **Physical Exam Key Points**
    1. **General.** Look for signs of acute distress. Is the patient over-breathing the ventilator? Diaphoresis or cyanosis denote severe limitations in airflow.
    2. **Vital signs.** Falling oxygen saturation, very high or very low heart rates, and/or hypotension suggest imminent arrest.
    3. **Neck and chest.** Listen for wheezing to determine if bronchospasm or pulmonary edema is present.
    4. **Direct laryngoscopy and fiberoptic evaluation.** These exams will identify some causes of obstruction and confirm proper ETT positioning.
  B. **Laboratory Data**
    1. **ABG.** Assess the level of hypoxemia.
  C. **Radiographic and Other Studies**
    1. **Chest radiograph.** Use to rule out pneumothorax, hemothorax, effusion, pulmonary edema, pneumonia, and atelectasis, while confirming proper positioning of the ETT.

V. **Plan**
  A. **Initial Management.** Ensure oxygenation and ventilation. When these are inadequate, verify or re-establish the airway, and switch to manually controlled ventilation (with a bag and mask) until the situation is resolved.
  B. **Specific Treatment Plans**
    1. **Suction the patient.** Passing a suction catheter rules out kinking and clears secretions or clots that may be obstructing the major airways.
    2. **Treat pneumothorax, if present.** Consider the need for needle or tube thoracostomy.
    3. **Treat bronchospasm.** Bronchodilators are the mainstay of therapy. Adjuncts, such as magnesium and lidocaine, should be considered, as well as steroids for refractory cases. Ensure that the patient is adequately sedated. Muscle relaxation (paralysis) may be necessary early in the course of treatment.
    4. **Pass an NG tube.** Decompress the stomach and treat any underlying abdominal processes that may be increasing intra-abdominal pressure.
    5. **Adjust the Ventilator.** New settings may be beneficial when there is mistiming of mechanical breaths with a patient's spontaneous respiratory efforts.

7. ALKALOSIS: METABOLIC

I. **Problem.** A 75-year-old man with history of Type II diabetes mellitus, hypertension, coronary artery disease, ischemic cardiomyopathy, and recent small-bowel obstruction was admitted to the ICU with congestive heart failure after an upper GI bleed, secondary to a duodenal ulcer. He was treated with large doses of intravenous furosemide. A nasogastric tube used to decompress his stomach drained large amounts of bilious fluid. On his third day in the ICU, he became tachycardic (with a heart rate of 120 bpm), with frequent PVCs, with slow shallow respirations (at a rate of 8/min), and was slightly more lethargic on examination. His laboratory values were normal, except for an Na^+ of 148, HCO_3 of 38, Cl^- of 96, and an ABG with a pH of 7.50, a Pco_2 of 47, and a Po_2 of 70.

II. **Immediate Questions:** Consider the common causes for alkalosis.

   A. **What is the patient's volume status?** Loss of extracellular fluid leads to a "contraction alkalosis"

   B. **What is the respiratory rate?** Mechanical hyperventilation (too high a rate or tidal volume) leads to respiratory alkalosis. Spontaneous hyperventilation will be seen as a compensatory response to metabolic acidosis.

   C. **What is being administered to the patient?** Thiazide diuretics, hyperalimentation (containing acetate), Ringer's lactate, and low-chloride IV fluids all cause alkalosis.

   D. **Has the patient been losing "acid"?** Patients vomiting or undergoing continuous NG suction are at risk of developing metabolic alkalosis. Remember though, that the metabolic alkalosis seen in patients undergoing NG suction is not due directly to loss of H^+ ions, but instead to renal losses of H^+ in an attempt to hold onto K^+.

III. **Differential Diagnosis.** Metabolic alkalosis can be divided into two groups: Causes resulting in chloride depletion (hypovolemic) are referred to as **chloride or saline responsive;** causes resulting in chloride expansion (hypervolemic) are referred to as **chloride or saline resistant.**

   A. **Hypovolemic (chloride depleted/responsive)**
      1. **GI loss of hydrogen:** Occurs with vomiting, gastric suction, chloride-rich diarrhea, and rarely with a villous adenoma (usually in the distal sigmoid colon).
      2. **Renal loss of hydrogen:** Can be from diuretics, prolonged hypercapnia, high-dose carbenicillin or penicillin.

   B. **Hypervolemic (chloride resistant):** Causes include renal loss of hydrogen, primary hyperaldosteronism, primary hypercortisolism, adrenocorticotropic hormone excess, exogenous steroid effect, pharmacologic hydrocortisone/mineralocorticoid, licorice, carbenoxolone sodium, renal artery stenosis with right-ventricular hypertension, renin-secreting tumor, hypokalemia, Bartter's syndrome, bicarbonate overdose, pharmacologic overdose of $NaHCO_3$, milk-alkali syndrome, and massive blood transfusion.

IV. Database

A. Physical Exam Key Points

1. **Vital signs.** In addition to causing alkalosis, volume contraction may cause tachycardia or hypotension.
2. **Pulmonary.** With respiratory alkalosis, the patient is usually tachypneic.
3. **Cardiovascular System:** Tachycardia and arrhythmias may occur when the pH > 7.55.
4. **Central Nervous System:** Decreased cerebral blood flow and seizures may occur. Metabolic alkalosis is also associated with paraesthesias of the mouth and face, hyperactive reflexes, tetany, and altered mental status.

B. Laboratory Data

1. **ABG.**
2. **Electrolytes.** Alkalosis leads to hypokalemia and hypocalcemia.
3. **Serum salicylate.** Consider aspirin intoxication.
4. **Urinalysis.** Measuring of urinary chloride (UCl) is helpful in distinguishing the two categories: UCl < 20 mmol/L in chloride depletion and UCl > 20 mmol/L in chloride expansion. In metabolic alkalosis, the UCl is a more accurate reflection of intravascular volume than urine sodium because sodium must be excreted with excess HCO_3. UCl is not reliable in patients on diuretics.

V. Plan

A. General Plan.
Severe metabolic alkalosis is associated with a high mortality rate in critically ill patients. No clinical signs or symptoms are specific. Consideration of the clinical situation, along with measurement of UCl, usually allows appropriate classification.

B.
The causes associated with chloride depletion usually respond to volume replacement (normal saline). Use normal saline, which has more chloride (154 mmol/L) than lactated Ringer's solution (104-to-109 mmol/L), and no acetate.

C.
The causes associated with chloride expansion indicate imbalances in the renal-adrenal axis.

1. Hydrochloric acid is available (a 0.1 N solution) but is rarely necessary.
2. Deliberate hypoventilation is rarely necessary.
3. Acetazolamide (250–375 mg once or twice daily) will increase excretion of HCO_3 but may result in acidemia because of renal loss of potassium.
4. Treat hypokalemia.
5. Discontinue exogenous bicarbonate.
6. A cooperative patient can breathe into a paper bag to transiently increase their F_{ICO_2}.

8. ALKALOSIS: RESPIRATORY

I. **Problem.** A previously healthy 35-year-old woman is admitted to the ICU with acute-onset shortness of breath and right-sided pleuritic chest pain which began 2 d after a long bus ride cross-country. On examination, she is tachycardic, tachypneic, with a low-grade fever and minimal right-calf swelling. Her admitting laboratory values are significant for a pH of 7.50, Pco_2 of 30, Po_2 of 70 (on 100% oxygen with a nonrebreathing mask), serum Na^+ of 140, chloride of 110 and HCO_3 of 24.

II. **Immediate Questions**

A. **What are the patient's vital signs?** Pulmonary embolus should be considered in any hyperventilating patient. When a patient is hypotensive from a pulmonary embolus, they are at high risk of dying. Treatment should be very aggressive in this situation.

B. **Was the patient taking any medications?** Ask about diuretics.

III. **Differential Diagnosis.** Hyperventilation is a component of many diseases. Remember that salicylate ingestion, sepsis, stimulant use and hepatic failure, may have components of primary metabolic acidosis and primary respiratory alkalosis.

A. **Definitions**
  1. **Defect:** Primary hyperventilation.
  2. **Laboratory Manifestations:** Decreased Pco_2 and increased pH.
  3. **Compensation:** There is immediate buffering from proteins and hemoglobin, which release hydrogen, and slow renal compensation, with bicarbonate excretion. Alveolar ventilation is regulated by several factors: chemoreceptors in the medulla (sensitive to H^+) and great vessels (sensitive to oxygen); cortical input (voluntary control); pulmonary chemoreceptors; and stretch receptors. Any of these factors or a combination may trigger hyperventilation.

B. **Hypoxemic drive**
  1. Pulmonary disease with arterial-alveolar gradient.
  2. Cardiac disease with right-to-left shunt.
  3. Cardiac disease with pulmonary edema.
  4. High altitude.

C. **Acute and chronic pulmonary disease**
  1. Emphysema
  2. Other pulmonary diseases
  3. Pulmonary edema

D. **Mechanical overventilation**

E. **Stimulation of the respiratory center**
  1. Neurologic disorders.
  2. Pain.

    3. Psychogenic.
    4. Liver failure with encephalopathy.
    5. Sepsis/ infection.
    6. Salicylates.
    7. Progesterone.
    8. Pregnancy.
    9. Fever.

IV. Database

    A. Physical Exam Key Points. Acute respiratory alkalosis results in numerous clinical manifestations.

      1. Central Nervous System. There may be confusion or dizziness, seizures, paraesthesias, or circumoral numbness.

      2. Cardiovascular System. Tachycardia and arrhythmias occur, especially at a pH > 7.6.

      3. Respiratory System. Hyperventilating patients are usually tachypneic; dyspnea appears when the patient tires.

      4. Muscular System. Alkalosis causes cramps and carpopedal spasm.

    B. Laboratory Data

      1. Metabolic. Expect hypokalemia, hypophosphatemia, and hypocalcemia (check the ionized calcium).

V. Plan. Severe alkalemia is associated with a high mortality and requires aggressive treatment. Therapy is directed at the underlying cause.

    A. Sedation. Mechanically ventilated patients should be sedated to prevent anxiety.

    B. Increase F$_I$CO$_2$. Consider using a rebreathing mask or decreasing the minute ventilation.

    C. Replacement. Use normal saline or, for severe alkalosis, HCl.

    D. Discontinue exogenous bicarbonate administration.

9. ALTERED MENTAL STATUS/HALLUCINATIONS

I. Problem. A 95-year-old woman is transferred to the ICU for acute hypoxemia from severe bacterial pneumonia. During the ensuing 12 h, she develops progressive inattention followed by confusion followed by coma.

II. Immediate Questions

    A. What was the patient's baseline mental status? Is this a "real" change?

    B. What are the vital signs? Mental status changes may be a symptom of hypoperfusion.

    C. What medications was the patient given? Sedatives and narcotics notoriously alter mental status.

D. **Why is the patient in the ICU?** Has the patient had recent head trauma? Is the patient diabetic?

III. **Differential Diagnosis.** Confused thinking and behavior are the hallmarks of altered mental status. In the ICU, irritable and restless behavior will often progress to decreased alertness and motor function, then stupor and coma. Causes are usually multifactorial, with organic, psychological, and environmental factors coalescing to affect the cerebral cortex. Patients fall into two groups:

A. **Those with focal signs usually have the following specific neurologic lesions:**
   1. **Traumatic** (subdural and epidural hematomas)
   2. **Vascular** (intracranial hemorrhage or thrombosis) Thrombosis of the right middle cerebral artery or left posterior cerebellar artery can manifest as confusion.
   3. **Infectious** (meningitis, encephalitis, intracranial abscess)
   4. **Neoplastic** (intracranial space-occupying lesion)
   5. **Congenital** (seizure disorder, cerebral aneurysm)
   6. **Intraventricular** (normal pressure hydrocephalus)

B. **Those with non-focal signs usually have systemic disease, with two exceptions:** (1) Medications are a frequent cause of altered mental status, especially in compensated dementia, and with hepatic or renal dysfunction; and (2) narcotics, benzodiazepines, anticholinergics, cimetidine, corticosteroids, and digitalis are often the culprits.
   1. **Intoxication** (acute or chronic intoxication, withdrawal)
   2. **Vascular** (circulatory collapse, sepsis, and hypertensive encephalopathy)
   3. **Anoxia** (pulmonary or cardiac failure, anesthesia, anemia)
   4. **Degenerative** (exacerbation of underlying dementia)
   5. **Vitamin deficiency** (Wernicke-Korsakoff, niacin, and B12)
   6. **Endocrine-metabolic** (diabetic coma, uremia, hyper-, hypothyroid, hypoglycemia, electrolyte and acid-base disturbance)
   7. **Depression** (pseudodementia and catatonia)

IV. **Database**

A. **History.** Talk to the family and read the chart. Look for a history of substance abuse, prior strokes, or a seizure disorder. Find old neurologic exams to establish a baseline.

B. **Physical Exam Key Points**
   1. **Vital signs.** Immediately evaluate the patient for hypoxia, hypoglycemia, and hypoperfusion. Pay attention to the vital signs and respiratory pattern in particular. For example, an increased blood pressure and low pulse characterize the Cushing Response, a sign of increased intracranial pressure. Cheyne-Stokes breathing (crescendo-decrescendo cycles between apneic periods) sug-

gests metabolic disturbance, congestive heart failure, brain stem lesions, and massive supratentorial lesions.

2. **Neurologic exam.** Is there evidence of head trauma? Does the patient have nuchal rigidity? Focus on asymmetries of motor function in an attempt to focalize findings. Do a thorough eye exam. Cranial nerve deficits may reveal a brainstem lesion.

3. **The mental status exam** reveals the severity of altered consciousness. Decreased attention is a hallmark of delirium and is not usually present with dementia. Have the patient name the months backward, or repeat six digits forward and four backward to assess attention. Test memory and orientation with basic questions about the date, time, and location. Pay attention to the patient's fluency and comprehension of language.

C. **Laboratory Data**
1. **Hemogram.** Rule out infection and anemia.
2. **Electrolytes, BUN, creatinine and glucose.** Are there metabolic causes?
3. **ABG.** Is the patient hypoxic?
4. **Ammonia.** When considering hepatic dysfunction.
5. **Urine.** Toxicology.
6. **Cultures.** As indicated.
7. **INR/PTT.** Assess for coagulopathy.
8. **Other.** Depending on the situation, order a phosphorous level, liver function tests, thyroid function tests, or digitalis level.

D. **Radiographic and Other Studies**
1. **CT or MRI of the head.** The indications include any asymmetric finding on exam, as well as focal processes, falls, and before a lumbar puncture (if increased intracerebral pressure is suspected).
2. **ECG.** When considering hypoperfusion, obtain an ECG to identify myocardial ischemia or arrhythmias.
3. **Chest radiograph.** This should be ordered when hypoxia or abnormal breathing patterns are apparent.
4. **Lumbar puncture.** This should be performed when bacterial meningitis is a possibility (Tube 1: cell count; Tube 2: protein and glucose; Tube 3: Gram stain, culture, and sensitivity; Tube 4: cell count).
5. **EEG.** This is not for emergencies, but is nonetheless underused.

V. **Plan.** Elderly patients are most at risk for altered mental status. Resolution may take days to months. Some never return to baseline. Ensure patient safety first. Confused patients fall, self-extubate, and remove lines and sutures. Try to identify and correct any underlying medical disorder, then focus on symptomatic control.

A. Attempt to control agitation without polypharmacy. Encourage family presence, explain procedures, maximize uninterrupted sleep, dimly light the room, and have eyeglasses and hearing aids readily available.

B. When necessary, **haloperidol** or **olanzapine** are the preferred sedatives for ICU patients, as they have minimal effect on respiration or blood pressure. Contraindications include anticholinergic intoxication, hepatic encephalopathy, withdrawal, or coma. When anticholinergic intoxication is present, stop the offending drug, and give **physostigmine,** but only when arrhythmias or respiratory depression threaten the patient. Hepatic encephalopathy is best treated with short-acting benzodiazepines.

10. ANAPHYLAXIS

Immediate Actions. Identify the allergen and eliminate exposure, assess the airway (consider intubation), administer oxygen, establish large bore IV access (14–16 gauge), give bolus with 500 mL of LR, and administer medications as indicated (diphenhydramine, steroids, epinephrine, or aminophylline).

I. **Problem.** A septic patient is given broad-spectrum antibiotics and rapidly develops flushing, wheezing, and worsening hypotension.

II. **Immediate Questions**

A. **What are the vital signs?** Hypotension and hypoxia require aggressive intervention.

B. **What medications and/or transfusions was the patient given?** Penicillin, cephalosporins, intravenous contrast, aspirin, NSAIDs, and blood transfusions are common causes of anaphylaxis in hospitalized patients. In the outpatient setting, foods and venoms are usually responsible.

III. **Differential Diagnosis.** Anaphylaxis is typically caused by an IgE-mediated release of mast-cell products, including histamine, leukotrienes-C4, D4 and E4, eosinophil-chemotactic-factors, neutrophil-chemotactic-factor, and platelet-activating factor. These mediators and other cytokines lead to bronchospasm, smooth muscle spasm, mucosal edema, inflammation, and increased capillary permeability. Classic IgE-mediated anaphylaxis occurs with antibiotics (eg, penicillin), food, therapeutic agents, and venoms. IV immunoglobulin, blood transfusions, and dialysis membranes cause symptoms of anaphylaxis through the immune complex-complement pathway. Mast cells can also be directly activated by opiates, radiocontrast media, neuromuscular blockers, and dextran. Upper airway obstruction, acute asthma, and pulmonary embolus may mimic anaphylaxis.

IV. Database. Although the signs and symptoms may vary, anaphylaxis typically has a rapid onset and rapid progression. Symptoms may be mild (aura, rhinitis, cough, pruritus, urticaria, rash, conjunctivitis, lacrimation, or flushing), moderate (GI cramps, diarrhea, or vomiting, bronchospasm), or severe (altered consciousness, angioedema, laryngeal edema, pulmonary edema, or cardiovascular collapse).

   A. Physical Exam Key Points
     1. Vital signs. Hypotension and hypoxia are of greatest concern.
     2. Pulmonary. Is there wheezing or stridor? Is ventilation adequate?
     3. Musculocutaneous. Look for cyanosis, a rash, urticaria or pruritus.
     4. Neurologic exam. Be particularly concerned about changes in mental status.

   B. Laboratory Data
     1. ABG. Look for hypoxia and hypercarbia.

   C. Radiographic and Other Studies
     1. Chest radiograph. Rule out CHF, pneumonia, etc.
     2. ECG. Rule out MI.

V. Plan
   A. The most important point to remember when treating a patient for possible anaphylaxis is that benign symptoms can rapidly progress to severe life-threatening symptoms. Establish a secure airway and administer epinephrine as soon as the diagnosis is suspected. The dose is 0.3–0.5 mL of aqueous epinephrine 1:1000 given SQ or IM every 10–15 min × 3. Supplemental oxygen, antihistamines, corticosteroids, and beta-adrenergics should also be initiated promptly.

     Antihistamines (both H1 and H2) should be given in the following dosages:

     Diphenhydramine: 1–2 mg/kg IM, or up to 75 mg IV every 6 h, or by continuous drip at 5 mg/kg every 24 h.
     Ranitidine: 150 mg PO every 8–12 h or 50 mg IV every 6 h, or
     Cimetidine: 300 mg PO every 6–8 h or 200–300 mg IV every 6 h.

     The dosages for corticosteroids are

     Methylprednisolone, 2 mg/kg or 125 mg IV every 6 h, or Hydrocortisone, 5 mg/kg or 300 mg IV, or
     Prednisone, 2 mg/kg or 60 mg PO once a day.

     Beta-adrenergic agonists can be given as
     Albuterol 2.5–5 mg nebulized treatment every 20 min.

   B. Epinephrine and racemic epinephrine can be given as inhalations, particularly for laryngeal edema and bronchospasm. The doses are *epinephrine* 1% solution of 1:100: 1–3 deep inhalations every 3 h, *racemic epinephrine* 2.25% solution of 1:100: 1–3 deep inhalations every 3 h.

C. For hypotension and/or cardiovascular collapse, start with IV fluid, then add pressors (dopamine, epinephrine, or norepinephrine) when needed. The dosages are as follows:
   1. Dopamine: 2–20 µg/kg per min IV drip
   2. Norepinephrine: 0.5–1 µg/min followed by 2–12 µg/min IV drip
   3. Epinephrine: 0.1–0.2 mL 1:1000 in 10mL of NS over 10 min, then 0.25–2.5 mL/min of 1 mL 1:1000 in 500 mL of D_5W.

11. ANEMIA

I. **Problem.** A patient admitted for a varicose vein stripping has a hematocrit of 19% on preoperative laboratory evaluation.

II. **Immediate Questions**

A. **Is the patient hemodynamically stable?** A patient with a chronic anemia is usually somewhat compensated. The evaluation and treatment of those patients can proceed in an orderly fashion. Patients with a low hematocrit secondary to an acute bleed may need urgent volume resuscitation. However, those patients almost always present with clinically apparent bleeding, as opposed to being diagnosed on a routine laboratory test. Tachycardia and determination of postural hypotension are sensitive signs of hypovolemia.

B. **Is the patient's stool positive for occult blood?** On a surgical service, a patient with a new decreased hematocrit should be assumed to have GI bleeding until proven otherwise. Check the indices (MCV, MCH, MCHC) on the CBC, and if they show a microcytic, hypochromic anemia (see Chapter II), chances are even greater that the cause is GI blood loss. Ask about melena (tarry stools) or change in bowel habits. Even if the stool is negative on first check, obtain 2–3 more specimens at different times for a more thorough evaluation.

C. **Does the patient have a history of anemia?** Review the chart or clinic records to find the most recent hematocrit. Ask if the patient has knowledge of an anemia, or if there is a family history of anemia.

D. **Is the low hematocrit result correct?** When the laboratory result is unexpected or when it does not correlate with the clinical appearance of the patient, question the validity of the test. Sources of laboratory error regarding a low hematocrit include (1) the sample was from a different patient; (2) there was a technical problem with the machine; and (3) blood was drawn proximal to an open IV line. Incorrect laboratory results are unusual, but it is worth repeating the test before embarking on an extensive workup. This is true regarding any laboratory result that does not correlate with the clinical situation.

E. **Is there blood available in the blood bank?** When emergency transfusion is considered, call the blood bank to determine whether blood is already set up for the patient. When it has not, obtain the specimens needed to type and cross-match blood. Do not transfuse the patient unless clinically indicated (hemodynamically unstable, etc) or before completing the initial evaluation, confirming the validity of the result, and drawing blood specimens for the laboratory tests discussed below.

III. **Differential Diagnosis.** Anemia is present in many disease states. It can be categorized as inadequate red blood cell production or excessive red blood cell loss or destruction.

A. **Inadequate Red Blood Cell Production**
   1. **Deficient hemoglobin production**
      a. **Iron deficiency:** Usually a result of chronic blood loss or inadequate intake.
      b. **Folate deficiency:** A megaloblastic anemia, common with poor diet (alcoholics, etc).
      c. **Vitamin B$_{12}$:** A megaloblastic anemia can be associated with ileal resection or sprue.
      d. **Thalassemias:** These are inherited deficits in hemoglobin synthesis.
   2. **Inadequate red blood cell production**
      a. **Marrow aplasia:** Caused by drug or chemical exposure.
      b. **Marrow replacement:** Because of neoplasia or fibrosis.
      c. **Chronic disease:** Systemic illnesses can lead to a normochromic, normocytic anemia. Chronic renal failure represents a separate category for this type of anemia owing to the absence of erythropoietin production by the kidneys.

B. **Increased Destruction of Red Blood Cells**
   1. **Intracorpuscular defects**
      a. Hereditary spherocytosis
      b. Enzyme deficiencies
      c. Sickle cell disease
   2. **Extracorpuscular defects**
      a. **Hemolytic anemias:** May be caused by autoimmune reactions that are often drug-induced and may be part of a systemic autoimmune disease.
      b. **Hemolysis:** Caused by prosthetic heart valves.

C. **Acute Blood Loss.** Caused by bleeding from GI tract, GU tract (including menstrual and dysfunctional uterine bleeding in women), retroperitoneal, external bleeding, or operative sites.

IV. **Database**
   A. **Physical Exam Key Points**
      1. **Vital signs.** Orthostatic hypotension and tachycardia may indicate hemodynamically significant anemia.

2. **Skin.** Pallor, pale conjunctiva and nail beds correlate with the degree of anemia reported by the lab.
3. **Abdomen.** Splenomegaly is present in hemolytic anemias, in disorders with intracorpuscular defects leading to RBC destruction, and in myeloid metaplasia. A mass may be present with malignancy.
4. **Rectal exam.** Pay close attention to any mass or the presence of occult blood.
5. **Dressings, drains, and surgical sites.** These should be inspected.

B. **Laboratory Data** (see Section II, page 273 for more details)
1. **Hemogram.** Aside from the hematocrit, look at the WBC and platelet count for evidence of general bone marrow depression or leukemia.
2. **Red blood cell indices.** MCV and MCHC allow a classification of anemia according to RBC size (microcytic, normocytic, or macrocytic) and hemoglobin content (hypochromic or normochromic). Iron deficiency anemia is microcytic and hypochromic, whereas megaloblastic anemia is typically macrocytic.
3. **Peripheral blood smear.** This can also be used to look at the actual size of red blood cells, where the indices may be misleading. For example, if a microcytic and a macrocytic process were occurring together, the MCV may be normal owing to a mixed population of red cells. Examining the shape of the cells (spherocytosis, elliptocytosis, RBC fragments) is sometimes helpful.
4. **Reticulocyte count.** This gives a measure of the production of red cells at the level of the marrow. A low reticulocyte count suggests inadequate production of red cells, whereas an increased count is associated with increased destruction of red cells.
5. **Serum chemistries, BUN, and creatinine.** This may show evidence of renal failure, or elevated indirect bilirubin in hemolytic anemias.
6. **Iron, total iron binding capacity (TIBC).** In iron deficiency, serum iron is decreased and TIBC is increased. In anemia of chronic disease, serum iron is decreased or normal and TIBC is decreased.
7. **Haptoglobin.** Often decreased in hemolytic anemia.
8. **Folate, Vitamin B$_{12}$ levels.** These levels measure deficiencies of specific metabolites.
9. **Coombs' test.** This measures IgM and IgG antibodies in hemolytic anemias.

C. **Radiographic and Other Studies**
1. **Bone marrow biopsy.** When the reticulocyte count is low, this assesses erythrocyte precursors, iron stores, and bone marrow replacement by infiltrative disease processes.

    2. **GI workup.** May include upper GI series, barium enema, upper endoscopy, colonoscopy, angiography, or tagged red blood cell nuclear scans when workup indicates GI source of anemia.

    3. **Ultrasound and CT scans.** May be adjunctive in the evaluation for a tumor.

V. Plan. Notify senior staff as elective operations will often be postponed when an anemia is identified.

    A. Acute Management. When hemodynamically significant anemia is present, start a large bore IV (18 gauge or larger, and draw necessary blood samples for the laboratory and blood bank at the same time) and begin fluid resuscitation when hypovolemia is evident. Check stools for occult blood and when heme-positive, consider passing a nasogastric tube as an initial diagnostic maneuver to check for an upper GI source of bleeding.

    B. Evaluation. Continue with GI workup as described above. When anemia is due to causes other than acute blood loss, gather laboratory data as discussed above, along with a hematology consultation.

    C. Specific Treatments

      1. **Iron deficiency.** Ferrous sulfate or gluconate 325 mg 3 times daily given with a stool softener (eg, docusate sodium), because iron pills cause constipation. Inform patient that the stools will be darkened by the iron.

      2. **Folate deficiency.** 1 mg orally or mixed in IV fluids every day.

      3. **Vitamin B_{12} deficiency.** 1000 mg IM daily for 14 d, then 1000 mg IM monthly.

      4. **Hemolytic anemia.** Often treated with glucocorticoids, such as prednisone, 60–100 mg/d and may require splenectomy.

      5. **Intracorpuscular red blood cell defect.** Splenectomy may be helpful.

      6. **Transfusions.** As needed.

      7. **Operation.** May be needed depending on GI tract evaluation.

      8. **H_2-receptor blockers (eg, cimetidine or ranitidine) and antacids.** Helpful for ulcer disease.

12. ARTERIAL LINE: EXPANDING HEMATOMA, MALFUNCTION

Immediate Actions. When there is an expanding hematoma, apply pressure. When this is unsuccessful, remove the line (and continue to apply pressure).

I. Problem. You are called to the bedside of a 65-year-old man to evaluate an expanding hematoma at the arterial line site. As you approach, you notice a "poor waveform" on the monitor.

II. Immediate Questions

A. Does the patient have a reasonable pulse and blood pressure when measured by noninvasive methods? Remember to evaluate the patient first, when trying to decide whether a "poor waveform" represents a malfunctioning monitor or a true physiologic state. A normal cuff pressure reassures you that the patient is stable.

B. Does the A-line pressure correlate with the blood pressure obtained by cuff? The appropriate difference between invasive and cuff pressures will vary, depending upon cuff and arterial sites. A large discrepancy may suggest that a malfunctioning arterial line is a strong possibility.

C. Is the arterial line still necessary? When it is not, remove it, particularly in the face of a potential complication.

D. Can blood be aspirated from the arterial line? This suggests that the catheter is patent (not kinked or thrombosed) and in the artery.

E. What does the waveform look like? Lack of a waveform suggests a monitoring problem (eg, the transducer is not zeroed, cables are not plugged in, or the catheter is not functional). When a waveform is present, see if it improves with gentle manipulation of the catheter site or with movement of the limb (eg, extension of the wrist). A damped waveform is usually caused by air (or occasionally by clot) in the tubing. Check all parts of the transducing system, as well as the catheter.

F. Is there any vascular compromise of the extremity? Radial artery thrombosis is more common than appreciated after arterial cannulation. When ulnar collateral flow is inadequate, the fingers or hand may become ischemic. Ischemia distal to arterial catheterization may occur at any site and should be treated with immediate catheter removal, plus additional interventions as indicated by the degree and persistence of ischemia.

III. Differential Diagnosis

A. Positioning Problems

B. Profound Hypotension or Arrest. Patients may have no blood pressure. Can a pulse be felt? When patients are unconscious, try a quick chest compression. When they are awake, have them cough. Both maneuvers should show a spike in the pressure tracing (by causing a sudden rise in intrathoracic pressure that is transmitted peripherally). This is a quick and easy way to confirm that the arterial line is transducing in an emergency, and may help to resuscitate a patient.

C. Thrombosed Artery. Arterial thrombosis does occur, although it is much less common than venous thrombosis. Distal spread of thrombus, or thrombosis in the face of compromised collateral blood flow, can threaten the involved extremity. Remove the catheter and obtain a vascular surgical consultation to guide other therapeutic options.

D. Catheter Problems

1. **Out of the artery.** As patients move about with old and loose dressings, the catheter can slip out of the artery. When the catheter is near the arterial puncture site, there may still be a waveform; however, bleeding and hematoma formation are common. Remove the catheter and apply pressure.

2. **Kinked catheter.** This is common when small catheters are used to cannulate peripheral arteries.

3. **Clot in catheter.** Clot may be present at the tip of the catheter or within the lumen. This can be corrected by withdrawing blood, then flushing the line. When the line is flushed without withdrawing blood, the clot may be forced to embolize distally, placing the extremity at risk.

4. **Catheter pressed against vessel wall.** External pressure from tight dressings or angulation of the extremity could potentially occlude the catheter by pressing the tip against the wall of the vessel.

5. **Transducing System Problems.** The electronic system for measuring intravascular pressure consists of four components: the pressure tubing, the transducer, the amplifier, and the display. Problems may be caused by any of these components. For the measuring system to provide accurate information, it must have a reasonable natural frequency and appropriate damping. Detailed explanations are beyond the scope of this chapter, but errors of underdamping or hyperresonance should be minimized and can be accomplished by optimization of the natural frequency of the system, using short, wide, stiff pressure tubing.

6. **Stopcock problems.** Stopcocks may be inadvertently turned off (partially or completely) in the normal course of patient care and movement. Though seemingly simplistic, this is occasionally the source of difficulty.

7. **Zeroing problems.** Has the transducer been zeroed? Some monitors will not provide any waveform or data without zeroing the transducer. In other cases, the waveform may not be seen because it is out of range.

8. **Electronic connection.** The cable connecting the transducer and monitor may be loose.

9. **Transducer malfunction.** Transducers should be rezeroed once a shift as there may be a slight baseline shift. Modern transducers are extremely reliable; however, significant signal drift and out-

right failure can occur, an event for which transducers should be replaced.

10. **Connecting tubing.** Air bubbles, kinks in the pressure tubing, or the use of soft tubing, can cause overdamping, which yields a blunted waveform that underestimates systolic pressure and overestimates diastolic pressure.

IV. Database

A. Physical Exam Key Points

1. **Vital signs**
2. **Blood Pressure.** Obtain serial blood pressures while working on this problem. Again, remember that the arterial line may not be malfunctioning, in which case the patient is in trouble!
3. **Pulse.** Significant brady- or tachycardia may accompany any real drop in blood pressure.
4. **Look for a hematoma at the arterial line site.** When it is present (particularly if expanding), apply direct pressure and remove the catheter.
5. **Distal perfusion.** Check the color and capillary filling to assess peripheral perfusion. Check for sensation whenever possible.
6. **Aspirate blood.**

B. Laboratory Data. Not indicated.

C. Radiographic and Other Studies

1. **ECG.** Look for arrhythmias or ST changes. A normal, regular QRS complex can be falsely reassuring if there is no blood pressure (in pulseless electrical activity [PEA]).
2. **O_2 Saturation.** Good oxygenation is reassuring. Evaluation of the pulse oximeter waveform, if available, helps confirm the presence of reasonable circulation.
3. **Assess the Equipment.** After evaluating the patient and the arterial line site, check the tubing and equipment starting at the patient and working toward the monitor.
4. **Mechanical coupling.** Check the fluid-filled high-pressure tubing that connects the arterial catheter to the pressure transducer. Ensure connections are tight, no kinks are present, and that the tubing is properly filled with fluid. Flush the tubing to remove any tiny air bubbles that may be difficult to see and to ensure patency of the tubing and connections. When the tubing is disconnected from the catheter and gently moved up and down, a waveform should be able to be created, confirming that the equipment is functional. In this case, the catheter is either kinked, clotted, or not in the artery.
5. **Pressure transducer.** Rezero the transducer.
6. **Cable connections.** Occasionally a faulty cable or poor connection will cause problems.
7. **Display.** Check the monitor and the scale on the display.

V. Plan

A. **Treat the patient.** Identify and treat shock as indicated. Apply pressure over any hematoma. Remember to apply pressure over the presumed arterial puncture site, not necessarily over the skin puncture site. Reconsider the need for invasive pressure monitoring.

B. **Ensure that the catheter is in the artery.** Aspirate blood from the catheter or gently flush the catheter after ruling out problems at the insertion site. Consider passing a guide wire to check for catheter and vessel patency. This must be done gently so as not to damage the arterial intima. A new catheter may be exchanged over this guide wire if the original catheter is kinked or damaged. When there is thrombus in the vessel, switch to a new site whenever feasible. When there are no good alternative sites, it may be possible to gently push a wire past the thrombus, then to insert a longer arterial catheter, thereby bypassing the blockage.

C. **Positioning.** Retaping the catheter, repositioning the limb, or using an arm board for support may limit catheter motion and provide more consistent information.

D. **Check the arterial line setup.** Check all connections as described above. Consider trying a whole new arterial line setup if everything seems to be set up properly and a waveform is still not present.

13. ASPIRATION

Immediate Actions. Suction the oropharynx and, if the patient is already intubated, suction the endotracheal tube. When possible, decompress the stomach via an orogastric or nasogastric tube. Stop feeding when applicable. Deliver supplemental oxygen and ensure adequate ventilation.

I. Problem.
A 68-year-old man, postoperative from thoracic aneurysm repair, was discharged to the floor on a regular diet. Now he has become unresponsive and has vomited.

II. Immediate Questions

A. **Is the airway secured?** An intubated patient who vomits is less likely to aspirate than a patient with an unprotected airway, especially if the patient's airway reflexes are compromised. An endotracheal tube also makes it easier to suction the patient and to perform diagnostic and therapeutic bronchoscopy when indicated.

B. **Is the patient tolerating the aspiration?** The quantity and characteristics (bilious, acidic, particulate, etc) of aspirated material and the patient's underlying pulmonary reserve will determine the response to aspiration. Apneic and hypoxic patients should be intubated.

C. **Is the patient being fed?** When he is, stop the feedings to prevent further gastric distention. Gastric acid and particulate matter are particularly caustic; they complicate aspiration and may warrant more aggressive intervention (immediate bronchoscopy and lavage).

D. **Is a gastric tube in place?** When it is not, attempt to place one to decompress the stomach. Remember that placing the tube may transiently lead to gagging or further vomiting.

E. **How is the patient positioned?** Raising the head of the bed minimizes gastroesophageal reflux. Once a patient vomits however, place the patient head-down on the side to encourage drainage out of the mouth, rather than down into the trachea.

III. Differential Diagnosis

A. **Aspiration.** Aspiration refers to the passage of secretions or gastric contents into the trachea and bronchopulmonary tree. Several conditions predispose to aspiration.

   1. **Drugs.** Sedation should be used with caution in any patient with a full stomach. In addition to their sedative effects, narcotics may significantly decrease the cough reflexes and predispose to aspiration.

   2. **CNS Injury.** Neurologic impairment of normal swallowing mechanisms may make it difficult to clear oropharyngeal secretion and predispose to aspiration.

   3. **Hiatal hernia and/or gastroesophageal reflux.** The majority of patients with hiatal hernia do not have reflux and vice-versa. Reflux typically causes heartburn. When there are no symptoms, reflux may be insidious, leading to hoarseness and vocal cord polyps in normal patients and causing silent aspiration (with pneumonia and pulmonary abscesses) in patients with neurologic impairment.

B. **Vomiting without Aspiration.** Aspiration should be considered in any patient who vomits. Nevertheless, monitoring and intervention should be based on the likelihood of aspiration. Healthy alert patients rarely aspirate after vomiting in contrast to patients with airway protective mechanisms.

C. **Pneumonia or Bronchitis.** Sputum cultures may facilitate antibiotic selection. Sputum collected from patients with aspiration, pneumonia, and post-nasal drip from sinusitis may all be similar, however.

IV. Database

A. **Physical Exam Key Points**

   1. **Breath sounds.** Wheezing is a common sequela of aspiration. Clear breath sounds do not rule out aspiration, but suggest a positive prognosis.

   2. **Vital signs.** Patients suspected of aspirating should be monitored with pulse oximetry for at least 2 h. Decreasing oxygen saturation

or an increasing oxygen requirement are the best indicators of developing aspiration pneumonitis.

3. **Quantity of material suctioned.** Patients who aspirate large amounts would seem to be at higher risk of developing aspiration pneumonitis, but for unknown reasons may not be. Likewise, some patients develop a florid pulmonary inflammatory response after aspirating only a small volume of gastric contents.

4. **Characteristics of aspirated material.** The nature of aspirated material may be more important than the volume. The lower the pH, the greater the inflammatory response. Particle size is also important. Poorly masticated regurgitated gastric contents with large chunks can also cause physical airway obstruction. Infected material from sinusitis or dental abscesses can be dangerous as well.

B. Laboratory Data

1. **Pulse oximetry** is the most useful tool to observe these patients. When the SaO_2 remains greater than 90% for 2 h after the event (in the absence of increasing oxygen supplementation), significant aspiration pneumonitis is unlikely.

2. **An ABG** is usually not needed in a patient with good oxygen saturation. It does allow the identification of decreasing oxygen saturation for a patient receiving supplemental oxygen, whereas pulse oximetry may not (since the SaO_2 will remain at 100% for all PaO_2s greater than 100).

C. Radiographic Studies

1. When a chest film is ordered immediately after aspiration, it is typically negative; however, a follow-up film 4–8 h later will commonly show an infiltrate (most often in the right superior basilar segment). The delayed chest radiograph findings are not from the aspirated material but from the inflammatory response caused by the aspirated material. Areas affected will typically appear as fluffy infiltrates.

V. Plan. Intervention should be based on the physiologic consequences of aspiration.

A. Ensure adequate oxygenation and ventilation. Intubation and mechanical ventilation should be instituted early in the course of a significant aspiration. Positive pressure and PEEP will help keep alveoli open. Intubation provides access to the trachea for suctioning and protects the airway from further aspiration.

B. Suctioning. The tracheobronchial tree must be cleared of all particulate matter and any secretions interfering with ventilation. Bronchoscopy may help to identify the extent of airway inflammation, although it is primarily used to remove particulate matter when suction is inadequate. Continued saline lavage is not indicated after the airways are cleared.

C. **Position the patient.** When a patient is noted to be vomiting, place the patient on the side in Trendelenburg position. Vomitus then pools in the oropharynx rather than the hypopharynx (near the cords). Positioning also provides gravity-assisted drainage of the tracheo-bronchial tree and a measure of uphill resistance to further aspiration.

D. **Place NG tube.** Empty the stomach to decrease the likelihood of further vomiting.

E. **Monitor oxygen saturation.** Pulse oximetry should be followed for at least 2 h after the event.

F. **Antibiotics.** The empiric use of antibiotics has not been helpful; however, antibiotics should be considered in neutropenic or immunosuppressed patients, or when there is evidence of a bacterial infection.

G. **Steroids.** Corticosteroids have not been shown to improve outcome after aspiration.

H. **Speech pathology consultation.** Swallowing studies can be done to evaluate airway reflexes. These should be obtained before feeding a patient who is recovering from a stroke or is otherwise at high risk for aspiration.

14. BLEEDING AT THE SITE OF AN INVASIVE LINE/DIC

I. **Problem.** While doing your hospital rounds, you hear that a 38-year-old woman is complaining of bleeding at her IV site.

II. **Immediate Questions**

A. **How much bleeding has occurred?** Blood loss may be visible or occult. Assess vital signs for stability and check for orthostatic blood pressure changes. Significant blood loss will require appropriate resuscitation with crystalloids, colloids, or blood.

B. **Is the bleeding from disconnected IV tubing?** Often IV tubing will loosen and become disconnected from the catheter. Ironically, this can result in substantial blood loss.

C. **Is there bleeding into the local tissues around the IV site that could be immediately problematic?** Hematoma formation around a central line in the neck could lead to airway compromise. Similarly, blood or fluid accumulation in an extremity could result in compartment syndrome.

D. **Is the patient bleeding around the catheter?** This suggests a systemic problem.

E. **Is there evidence of bleeding elsewhere?** Other signs of a systemic bleeding disorder include hematuria, GI bleeding, petechiae, ecchymoses, or bleeding from other line sites or surgical wounds.

F. **Does the patient have other medical conditions that could contribute to bleeding?** Some relationships are obvious (anticoagulated patients or patients with renal or hepatic insufficiency); others are subtle (unusual allergic reactions, autoimmune disorders).

G. **Have there been any recent clinical changes that would result in a bleeding diathesis?** Recent trauma, pregnancy, medication or blood product administration, and sepsis may all lead to systemic bleeding disorders.

III. Differential Diagnosis

A. Non-DIC Causes of Bleeding

1. **Thrombocytopenia.** Spontaneous bleeding occurs when there is an inadequate number of platelets, or when platelet function is impaired. Platelet counts between 50,000 and 20,000 may lead to petechiae or purpura, and counts less than 10,000 may be associated with spontaneous bleeding. Platelet transfusions have a limited longevity. They are indicated to prevent spontaneous bleeding (for counts in the 10,000 range) or for actual bleeding (when the platelet count is less than 100,000). They should be available and may be given before surgery (when the platelet count is < 100,000), although a platelet count of 10,000 may be adequate to perform a splenectomy in a patient with idiopathic thrombocytopenic purpura (ITP) (where platelet function is normal). A platelet count < 100,000 typically prolongs the patient's bleeding time.

2. **Coagulation factor deficiencies.** Hemostasis requires an intact coagulation system. Coagulation factor deficiencies may be associated with many diseases including hemophilia A, von Willebrand's disease, hemophilia B, and Factor XI deficiency.

3. **Mechanical factors.** Trauma to the IV site, too large of a skin nick around a central line, and disconnection of the IV tubing may all lead to bleeding at the local site.

4. **Coexisting disorders**
   a. **Liver disease.** Underlying liver disease may contribute to coagulopathy because of clotting factor deficiencies and thrombocytopenia. It may also predispose to DIC.
   b. **Malabsorption (Vitamin K deficiency/malnutrition).** Has the patient recently had an operation? Patients may be asymptomatic until stressed by surgery or other conditions.
   c. **Medications.** Is the patient receiving subcutaneous heparin, aspirin, or nonsteroidal anti-inflammatory agents? Were they on warfarin before admission? Don't forget that aspirin is present in many compound medications (eg, Percodan) and many over-the-counter medications.

B. Disseminated Intravascular Coagulation (DIC). Inappropriate activation of the coagulation cascade may lead to intravascular coagula-

tion. Ironically, this may be undetectable; however, it consumes coagulation factors and platelets and subsequently activates thrombolysis. This then leads to clinically significant bleeding.

1. **Hemolytic transfusion reaction.** Hemolysis may be caused by the immune-mediated lysis of transfused red cells. Both acute and delayed hemolytic transfusion reactions can activate the coagulation cascade, initiating DIC.

2. **Sepsis.** Bacterial, fungal, or viral septicemia may initiate DIC. Factors released in sepsis may cause platelet activation and aggregation. Hypotension leads to stasis and prevents the normal circulating inhibitors of coagulation from reaching the sites of microthrombi.

3. **Obstetrical.** Placental abruption, amniotic fluid embolism, retained fetal products or placenta, and eclampsia predispose to DIC. Clinically diagnosed amniotic fluid embolism has a mortality rate greater than 50%.

4. **Traumatic injury.** Crush injuries, burns, and head injuries may lead to severe tissue trauma, which is associated with release of tissue thromboplastins, hemolysis and endothelial damage. Each of these may contribute to DIC.

5. **Malignancy.** Various neoplasms, especially leukemia, may be associated with DIC. Although the relationship is not completely understood, tissue factors interacting on the surface of tumor cells may be responsible.

IV. **Database**

A. **Physical Exam Key Points**

1. **Vital Signs.** Fever is seen with sepsis and transfusion reactions. Hemodynamic stability must be assured.

2. **General/Skin.** It is important to check for bleeding at other sites (other IV sites, A-line and chest tube sites, recent surgical wounds). Skin should be examined for petechiae, purpura, and ecchymoses.

B. **Laboratory Studies.** As with most bleeding disorders, a single test cannot be used to diagnose DIC. Instead, the serial results of several tests are examined collectively, including platelets, PT, and PTT.

1. **Platelet count.** The platelet count will be low in both DIC and a myriad of other conditions seen in critically ill patients.

2. **PT and PTT.** These studies are prolonged in any condition where coagulation factors are consumed.

3. **Thrombin time.** This is usually increased with DIC.

4. **Fibrinogen level.** Fibrinogen is reduced through its conversion to fibrin (following the action of thrombin) and its degradation from abnormal increases in plasmin.

5. **Fibrin split/degradation products (FSP/FDP).** FDP and D-dimer are the most useful studies for diagnosing DIC. FDP will be ele-

vated in DIC (and primary fibrinolysis) and normal in other conditions with decreased platelets and a prolonged PT and PTT.

6. **Other coagulation studies.** The workup for a bleeding diathesis depends on whether the primary disorder is bleeding or clotting. The workup may need to be delayed as trauma and surgery affect normal clotting. In addition to a platelet count, PT and PTT, bleeding patients should be tested for platelet function, clotting inhibitors, Von Willebrand's factor, and factor XIII fibrin stabilizing factor. Assays used to work up abnormal clotting include antithrombin III, protein C and S, lupus anticoagulant, lipoprotein A, anticardiolipin, homocysteine, factor V Leiden, prothrombin mutations, and methylene tetrahydrofolate reductase mutations.

7. **Blood smear.** A blood smear may show evidence of schistocytosis or thrombocytopenia.

V. **Plan.** Transfuse and resuscitate the patient as needed. After ensuring that the patient is hemodynamically stable, identify and treat the underlying cause of the bleeding.

A. **Mechanical.** Correct the problem (ie, reconnect the IV tubing or place a suture around the bleeding skin incision site).

B. **Factor deficiencies and thrombocytopenia.** Unless there is concern that allergic reactions to blood components are the cause of the disorder, factor and platelet deficiencies should be corrected. Underlying disorders contributing to these deficiencies should be addressed simultaneously.

C. **DIC.** The treatment of DIC is mainly supportive. Treatment options are often controversial, as DIC is a combination of widespread small-vessel thrombotic deposition and simultaneous systemic bleeding. Underlying conditions causing DIC must be identified and ameliorated as quickly as possible. Get help from experienced practitioners. Blood component therapy (platelets, FFP, cryoprecipitate, etc) may be indicated. Heparin or plasmapheresis may even be of help.

15. BRADYCARDIA

I. **Problem.** A patient admitted with an acute myocardial infarction has a heart rate of 40 bpm. Her blood pressure is 134/86. She has no current chest pain, congestive heart failure, or syncope. Her rhythm strip reveals a Mobitz Type I block (Fig I–3).

II. **Immediate Questions**

A. **What are the patient's vital signs?** For some patients, a slow pulse is inconsequential; for others, it is immediately life threatening. Successful treatment of any arrhythmia depends on recognizing the urgency.

B. **Is the patient symptomatic?** In addition to bradycardia, acute myocardial infarction may cause chest pain, diaphoresis, dyspnea, and

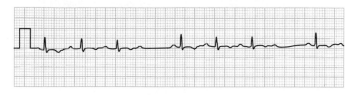

Figure I–3. Second-degree AV block Mobitz type I (Wenckebach) with 4:3 conduction.

nausea. Bradycardia may also cause those symptoms by decreasing cardiac output, which reduces coronary perfusion and exacerbates myocardial ischemia. A symptomatic patient should therefore be treated urgently, even when he/she has a normal blood pressure.

  C. **Was the patient dizzy just before the bradycardia?** These symptoms suggest sinus node dysfunction.

  D. **What medication was the patient given?** Calcium channel blockers, beta-blockers, and digitalis cause bradycardia.

  E. **Does the patient have a pacemaker?** If she does, it may not be working properly.

III. Differential Diagnosis. Common causes of bradycardia include myocardial infarction, myocardial ischemia, digitalis, beta-blockers, calcium-channel antagonists, central venous catheters, and intracranial hypertension.

  A. **Sinus Dysfunction**
    1. **Sick sinus syndrome** aka **"tachy-brady syndrome."** There are intermittent sinus pauses.
    2. **Vasovagal episodes.**
    3. **Increased vagal tone.** Common in athletes and in elderly patients.
    4. **Increased intracranial pressure.** Cushing's reflex.
    5. **Cardiomyopathy.** Ischemic or hypertensive.
    6. **Other causes include** hypothyroidism, hypothermia, and cardiac amyloidosis.

  B. **AV Dysfunction**
    1. **First-degree AV block.** PR > 0.2 s.
    2. **Second-degree AV block Mobitz type I (Wenckebach).** There is progressive prolongation of the PR interval until a beat is eventually dropped.
    3. **Second-degree AV block Mobitz type II.** Regular dropping of ventricular beats (eg, every third or fourth) can progress to complete heart block.
    4. **Third-degree AV block.** Caused by MI, sarcoidosis, amyloidosis, neoplasms, viral myocarditis, Lyme disease, acute rheumatic

fever, and primary degenerative disease of the conduction system.

C. Inferior Wall MI.

D. Drug induced. Digitalis, beta-blockers, and calcium channel antagonists.

IV. Database

A. History. Review medications (particularly those which cause bradycardia). Has the patient had syncope, abdominal pain, or symptoms of congestive heart failure or myocardial ischemia?

B. Physical Exam Key Points
   1. **Vital signs.** The absolute pulse is not as important as the physiologic consequences of bradycardia. Watch for evolving hypotension.
   2. **Cardiopulmonary.** Listen for murmurs, rubs, gallops, and rales.
   3. **Musculocutaneous.** Look for evidence of hypoperfusion (pallor, cool moist skin).
   4. **Neurologic.** In a patient with an altered mental status, bradycardia may indicate increasing intracranial pressure.

C. Laboratory Data
   1. **Electrolytes.**
   2. **Digoxin level.**
   3. **Troponin and CPK/MB.**
   4. **ABG.**
   5. **Thyroid and adrenal hormone levels.**

D. Radiographic and Other Studies
   1. **ECG and rhythm strip.**
   2. **Chest radiograph.**

V. Plan (Fig I–4).

   A. Symptomatic sinus bradycardia, first-degree block and second-degree block may be treated temporarily with atropine.

   B. Sinus bradycardia, first-degree block and Wenckebach block require no treatment unless they cause hypotension or symptoms.

   C. Mobitz block and third-degree block require treatment even when the patient has no signs or symptoms of hypoperfusion.

   D. When patients are unresponsive to atropine but the bradycardia is likely to be self-limited (after medication overdose, myocardial ischemia, or central venous catheter misplacement), temporarily support patients with a dopamine infusion (or glucagon infusion after a beta-blocker overdose) or with temporary transvenous or transthoracic pacing. When the cause is not self-limited, treat patients with early permanent pacer insertion.

   E. Correct digoxin toxicity.

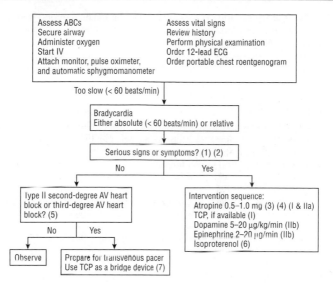

Footnotes
(1) Serious signs or symptoms must be related to the slow rate.
    Clinical manifestations include:
        Symptoms (chest pain, shortness of breath, decreased level of consciousness) and signs (low BP, shock, pulmonary congestions, CHF, acute MI).
(2) Do not delay TCP while awaiting IV access or for atropine to take effect if patient is symptomatic.
(3) Denervated transplanted hearts will not respond to atropine. Go at once to pacing, catecholamine infusion, or both.
(4) Atropine should be given in repeat doses in 3–5 min up to a total of 0.04 mg/kg. Consider shorter dosing intervals in severe clinical conditions. It has been suggested that atropine should be used with caution in atrioventricular (AV) block at the His-Purkinje level (type II AV block and new third-degree block with wide QRS complexes) (class IIb).
(5) Never treat third-degree heart block plus ventricular escape beats with Lidocaine.
(6) Isoproterenol should be used, if at all, with extreme caution. At low doses it is class IIb (possibly helpful); at higher doses it is class III (harmful).
(7) Verify patient tolerance and mechanical capture. Use analgesia and sedation as needed.

Figure I–4. Bradycardia algorithm (patient not in cardiac arrest). (*Reproduced, with permission, from Adult Advanced Cardiac Life Support. JAMA 1992;268:16.*)

F. **Temporary pacing.** This is indicated for transient second-degree AV block (after an MI), drug-induced AV block, and as a bridging measure while waiting for permanent pacemaker insertion.

G. **Permanent pacing.** This is indicated for sinus node dysfunction, second-degree AV block (after an MI), third-degree AV-block, and symptomatic Mobitz type II block.

16. BRAIN DEATH

I. **Problem.** A patient is admitted to the ICU for intubation and mechanical ventilation after a massive embolic stroke. On the second day in the ICU, the patient is unresponsive to pain, pupillary light reflexes, cold caloric responses, and ventilatory drive.

II. **Immediate Questions**

A. **Has the patient suffered permanent neurologic damage?** Gravely ill patients occasionally recover, when they can be supported through their acute illness. Permanent damage is permanent, however, and these patients derive no benefit from aggressive intervention. In such cases, an ICU physician may do the most good by accurately guiding the patient's family as they make treatment decisions.

B. **Can the irreversible cessation of cerebral circulation and respiratory function be documented?**

C. **Can the irreversible cessation of all functions of the entire brain, including the brain stem be documented?**

III. **Differential Diagnosis**

A. The United States federal government codified the **Uniform Determination of Death Act,** which defines death as (1) irreversible cessation of circulatory and respiratory function; or (2) irreversible cessation of all functions of the entire brain, including the brain stem. Criteria for whole brain death vary among states and institutions.

B. Rule out conditions that impair neurologic function, confounding the diagnosis of brain death, such as drug intoxication, hypotension, hypothermia, Guillain-Barré syndrome, subclinical status epilepticus, encephalopathy, severe hypophosphatemia, and brain stem encephalitis.

IV. **Database**

A. **History.** A complete history will elucidate the cause and prognosis of the patient's current condition, and eliminate confounding conditions.

B. **Physical Exam**
   1. **Vital signs.** Check the temperature, pulse, and blood pressure. Are there any spontaneous respirations?

    2. Neurologic exam. Look for any spontaneous movement. Check all cranial nerves. An apnea test will establish the lack of ventilatory drive.

  C. Laboratory data. Usually not indicated.

  D. Other Studies
    1. An EEG may be required to document the lack of electrical activity. Some jurisdictions may require multiple examinations or the opinion of more than one medical doctor.

V. Plan

  A. Care of the Brain-Dead Patient. Brain death has profound effects on circulatory control, hormone production, electrolyte balance, and thermoregulation. These changes must be considered when supporting a brain-dead patient as a potential organ donor. Hypotension should be treated with volume expansion before vasopressors. Patients may not respond to atropine (when medullary compression has eliminated vagal tone), so patients with hemodynamically significant bradycardia may need to be paced. Polyuria often develops as a result of physiologic diuresis after resuscitation, osmotic agents administered to control cerebral edema, hyperglycemia, or diabetes insipidus. Urine output, free water deficit, electrolytes, and glucose should be monitored and corrected. Thermoregulatory control is lost when the hypothalamus stops functioning. Prevent hypothermia by properly insulating the patient.

  B. Discussion with Family. Help the patient's family and loved ones understand brain death. Clarify the applicable legal definition. It may help to explain that physicians are measuring physiologic function and not a patient's "personhood." While evaluating the patient for brain death, also consider the potential for organ donation. When the patient would be an appropriate candidate, notify the applicable organ procurement agency early in the process. In most cases, the physician who tries to "save" the patient should not be the person who discusses organ donation with the family.

17. BURNS

 I. Problem. A 48-year-old woman is brought to the emergency department after being rescued from a house fire.

II. Immediate Questions

  A. Is anything on her body still burning? Stop the fire and wash off any chemicals. Dry chemicals should be brushed off before rinsing.

  B. Is the airway intact?
    1. When the airway is intact, start 100% oxygen via nasal cannula.
    2. Carbon monoxide is a potentially lethal byproduct of combustion. It binds to hemoglobin more tightly than oxygen, so that hemoglo-

bin is no longer available for oxygen transport. Having a patient breathe 100% oxygen will gradually displace bound carbon monoxide.
3. Patients with perioral burns or singed nasal hair are at high risk for airway damage, even if they appear to be breathing comfortably. Early intubation may prevent a later respiratory arrest.
4. Even without facial burns, there can be tracheal edema/spasm from inhaled superheated gases. Question the firemen and/or paramedics and consider early bronchoscopy for patients exposed to smoke.

C. **Are there any other associated injuries?** Perform a full physical exam.

III. **Differential Diagnosis.** Determine the extent and thickness of burned areas and determine the nature of the offending agent.

IV. **Database**
   A. **Physical Exam Key Points**
      1. **Determine the extent of the burn.**
         a. **Differentiate between partial thickness and full thickness burn.**
            i. Viable dermal elements persist in partial thickness (first and second degree) burns, and skin may heal in time without grafting.
            ii. There are no living dermal elements in full thickness (third degree) burns, which will require excision and grafting.
         b. **Determine the total body surface area (TBSA) burned.**
            i. Use the "rule of nines" to determine the surface area (Fig I–5).
            ii. The palm is approximately 1% of the body surface area; this can be used to estimate the size of irregularly shaped burns.
            iii. Relative body proportions are different for children.
         c. **Criteria for transfer to a burn center:**
            i. Second- and third-degree burns on 10% or more of the body for children aged < 10 years or adults aged > 50 years.
            ii. Second- and third-degree burns on 20% of the body for anyone aged between 10 and 50 years.
            iii. Third-degree burns on 5% or more of the body.
            iv. Burns in patients with preexisting medical conditions.
            v. High-voltage electrical and significant chemical burns.
            vi. Burns on hands, feet, eyes, ears, or perineum, leading to a potential for functional or cosmetic disability.
      2. **Examine for associated injuries.** Burns may be obvious; however, beware of other injuries, particularly, when buildings collapse, after car accidents, or after difficult extrications.

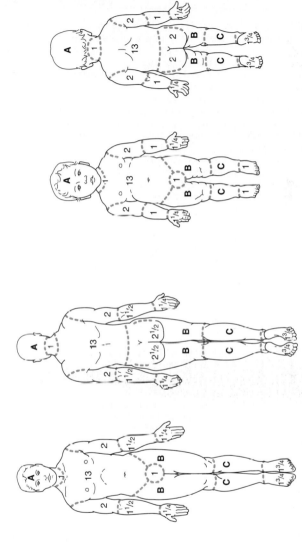

Figure I-5. Tables for estimating the extent of burns in adults and children. In adults, a reasonable system for calculating the percentage of body burned is the "rule of nines": Each arm equals 9%; the head equals 9%; the anterior and posterior trunk each equal 18%; each leg equals 18%; and the perineum equals ¹⁄₂%. (*Reproduced, with permission, from Demling RH, Way LW: Burns & other thermal injuries. In Way LW (editor): Current Surgical Treatment & Diagnosis, 10th ed. Originally published by Appleton & Lange. Copyright © 1994 by The McGraw-Hill Companies, Inc.*)

B. Laboratory Data

1. **Hemogram.** Obtain a baseline study; then, follow trends. The hemoglobin will rise with inadequate fluid resuscitation and will fall when there is bleeding from other injuries.
2. **Electrolytes.** Loss of the skin's barrier function predisposes to electrolyte disturbances. This can be exacerbated by the large volume of fluid needed for resuscitation.
3. **ABG with carboxyhemoglobin determination.** Burns within a closed space may be accompanied by inhalation injury and/or carbon monoxide exposure. All patients should receive supplemental oxygen, and some centers use hyperbaric oxygen for patients with elevated carboxyhemoglobin levels. Keep in mind that significant carboxyhemoglobin levels invalidate the use of pulse oximetry and that smokers may have carboxyhemoglobin levels up to 5% without smoke inhalation.

C. Radiographic and Other Studies

1. **Chest radiograph.** Pneumonitis from thermal or chemical injury may not be visible on the initial films. Nevertheless, an early chest radiograph is important, particularly, when there is concurrent trauma (to rule out a pneumothorax or hemothorax).

V. Plan

A. Obtain adequate IV access and resuscitate the patient.

1. Use large-bore IVs.
   a. Preferably in the arm.
   b. Preferably in unburned skin.
2. Central lines may be placed as needed.

B. Initiate fluid resuscitation (for patients with burns greater than 15% TBSA in children and 20% TBSA in adults).

1. Follow the Parkland formula (or one of the other formulas) for fluid replacement (see Fig I–5) during the first 24 h.
2. Administer half of the estimated fluid during the first 8 h and half during the next 16 h.
3. Closely monitor the urine output (with a Foley catheter) and adjust IV fluids as needed to keep the urine output over 30 cc/h (or at least 1 mL/kg/h for a child < 30 kg).
4. In the second 24 h, as microvascular injury improves and as endothelial cells stabilize, some investigators advocate the use of colloid solutions (0.3 mL/kg per percent burn for 30–50% TBSA or 0.5 mL/kg per percent burn for > 50% TBSA).
5. After 48 h, switch to hypotonic dextrose solutions (D5W or D5¼NS) to replace free water evaporative losses.
6. Expect a total body weight gain of 15–20% during the first 48 h, then a slow return to baseline during the next 7–10 d.

C. **Circumferential and full-thickness burns may require a fasciotomy/escharotomy.**
   1. Tissue edema occurs after all forms of injury. Because burned tissue cannot expand, edema increases tissue pressure leading to ischemia.
   2. Chest wall motion may be sufficiently compromised to prevent effective ventilation.

D. **Treat pain appropriately.** Use intravenous rather than intramuscular or subcutaneous injections, because absorption is erratic after burns.

E. **Metabolic/Nutrition Issues**
   1. The metabolic rate increases with burn size.
   2. This hypermetabolism results in increased oxygen consumption, increased cardiac output, increased minute ventilation, and wasting of lean body mass.
   3. Enteral feeding can be started within the first 24–36 h and is preferred to parenteral nutrition. Enteral feeding releases gut trophic factors and may reduce infectious complications.
   4. Total protein requirements are between 1.5 and 3.0 g/kg. The total calorie to nitrogen ratio should be 100–150:1. Try to meet half of the patient's caloric needs with protein (20% of the total calories) and fat (aim for 30%); the balance should be carbohydrates (about 50%).

F. **Initial Wound Care**
   1. Wash burns gently with a mild disinfectant
   2. Debride small amounts of dead tissue.
   3. Closely monitor the patient's temperature.
   4. Administer tetanus prophylaxis if needed.
   5. Topical antimicrobials can be applied.
      a. Silver sulfadiazine (Silvadene), 1%, penetrates through eschar (although not as well as Mafenide), has a broad spectrum of activity (except for some variants of *Escherichia coli* and *Pseudomonas* spp.), causes no pain, and has no electrolyte consequences. It occasionally causes neutropenia and cannot be used in patients allergic to sulfa.
      b. Mafenide acetate, 11%, diffuses well through eschar and has the broadest antibacterial spectrum (especially against *Pseudomonas* spp.). Unfortunately, application is painful. It also inhibits carbonic anhydrase, which leads to bicarbonate wasting, tachypnea, and metabolic acidosis.
      c. Silver nitrate, 0.5%, is also broad spectrum, but it diffuses poorly through eschar and can cause electrolyte imbalances.

G. **Definitive Wound Care**
   1. Partial-thickness burns will heal in 2 wk unless complicated by infection. Debride nonviable skin but leave blisters/bullae intact.

Clean the area daily and cover it with nonadherent gauze. When the patient is discharged, follow-up in the office every 3–5 d until wounds are healed.

2. When the patient is stable, excise full-thickness burns as soon as possible after resuscitation. The early removal of nonviable tissue improves morbidity and mortality and reduces hospital stay. Excision should be delayed for hemodynamic instability or pulmonary complications. Up to 20% of TBSA can be excised at one setting.

   a. Tangential excision removes successive layers of skin until bleeding is encountered. Deep dermis may be preserved, although blood loss is higher. Topical hemostatic sprays, tourniquets, and the subdermal injection of epinephrine help to limit bleeding.

   b. A full-thickness excision (to investing fascia) can be performed with electrocautery to limit bleeding. This tends to have a poor cosmetic result.

3. A variety of biological dressings are available including

   a. **Cutaneous allograft** can be fresh, cryopreserved, or lyophilized. It becomes vascularized when grafted and promotes granulation tissue, limits infection, decreases fluid loss, and reduces pain. When used as a covering (on nongrafted wounds), it improves healing and allows earlier placement of split-thickness skin grafts. Unfortunately it may carry viruses, certain cancers, and has a limited shelf life.

   b. **Xenografts** (porcine) are in greater supply but are not as effective as allografts, because they are not vascularized by the host. They will encourage granulation and can be replaced with split-thickness skin grafts, once the wound is clean.

   c. **Biobrane** is a collagen-based skin substitute, which is similar to a porcine xenograft. It may be left on partial-thickness burns until there is re-epithelialization.

   d. **Cultured epidermal sheets** are still experimental. They take 3–4 wk to grow, they are fragile, they become infected easily and can scar. They are an option however, when there are not enough donor sites for grafting.

4. **Split-thickness skin grafting** can be applied to wounds with healthy granulation tissue and with surface bacterial counts < 10,000 cfu per gram of tissue. These autografts are typically 0.012 to 0.015 inches thick.

H. **Temperature control.** Burned patients have impaired thermoregulation (as a result of lost skin integrity). This becomes a problem when well-intentioned bystanders or medical personnel apply cold packs to soothe burns. Hypothermia can be minimized by keeping the patient dry and by warming the room.

18. CARDIOPULMONARY ARREST

Immediate Actions
1. Assess responsiveness.
2. When nonresponsive, follow algorithm in Figure I–6 (page 54).

I. **Problem.** One week after a transfemoral amputation, a patient is found unresponsive and pulseless in bed.

II. **Immediate Questions**

   A. **Is the patient responsive?** Basic cardiopulmonary resuscitation (CPR) begins with a vigorous attempt to arouse the patient. Call the patient and shake him or her by the shoulders.

   B. **Is the airway obstructed?** Finger sweep or suction out the patient's mouth. Listen for air movement.

   C. **Are there vital signs?** Check for carotid pulse and blood pressure. After these basic questions are asked and maneuvers performed, begin mouth-to-mouth or, preferably, ventilation with 100% oxygen by bag and mask, and chest compressions. The following questions are then asked as advanced cardiac life support (ACLS) is started.

   D. **What medications is the patient taking?** Cardiac medications are particularly important, especially antiarrhythmics and digoxin. An adverse reaction to a recently administered medication may be determined.

   E. **Are there any recent laboratory values, particularly potassium or hematocrit?** Hyperkalemia (usually 0.7 mEq/L) or severe anemia, usually acute, may cause cardiac arrest.

   F. **What are the patient's major medical problems?** Ask about coronary artery disease, previous myocardial infarction, hypertension, previous pulmonary embolus, and recent surgery.

III. **Differential Diagnosis.** Arrest rhythms include ventricular fibrillation and tachycardia, asystole, bradycardia, and pulseless electrical activity (PEA). Causes of cardiopulmonary arrest may include

   A. **Cardiac**
   1. Myocardial infarction.
   2. Congestive heart failure.
   3. Ventricular arrhythmias.
   4. Cardiac tamponade. Usually posttraumatic.

   B. **Pulmonary**
   1. Pulmonary embolus.
   2. Acute respiratory failure.

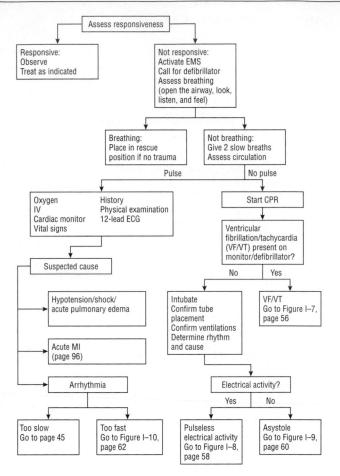

Figure I–6. Universal algorithm for adult emergency cardiac care (ECC). (*Reproduced, with permission, from Adult Advanced Cardiac Life Support. JAMA 1992;268:16.*)

3. Aspiration.
4. Tension pneumothorax.

C. **Hemorrhagic.** Undiagnosed severe bleeding can result in cardiac arrest, such as a ruptured aortic aneurysm.

D. **Metabolic**
1. **Hypokalemia, hyperkalemia.** These may induce arrhythmias.
2. **Acidosis.** Severe acidosis may suppress myocardial function.
3. **Warming from hypothermia.** Arrhythmias may be induced.

IV. Database

A. **Physical Exam Key Points.** As described, check responsiveness and vital signs. Resuscitation should always be initiated before a detailed physical exam is performed.
1. Check ventilation and perform airway opening maneuvers (jaw thrust or chin lift) as needed.
2. Look for tracheal deviation as evidence of a tension pneumothorax.
3. Distended neck veins may indicate pericardial tamponade or pneumothorax.

B. **Laboratory Data.** These should be obtained as soon as possible but should not delay the start of therapy.
1. Arterial blood gas.
2. Serum electrolytes, with special attention to the potassium.
3. CBC. The hematocrit is especially important.

C. **Radiographic and Other Studies**
1. Continuous cardiac monitoring, ensuring correct lead placement.
2. Other studies may be performed after the patient has been resuscitated.

V. Plan.
Therapy for cardiac arrest is based on specific algorithms outlined by the American Heart Association (AHA). Specific AHA algorithms for ventricular fibrillation, ventricular tachycardia, bradycardia asystole, and electromechanical dissociation are shown in Figures I–1 through I–10. Frequently used resuscitation medications are located inside the back cover of this book. Every physician should have these memorized.

In addition, successful resuscitation is based on a team approach, with one leader monitoring the rhythm and ordering therapy according to the appropriate algorithm. Everyone must remain calm and must be assigned to a specific job.

Resuscitation begins with the ABCs: **A**irway (intubate whenever possible), **B**reathing (ventilate), and **C**irculation (chest compression). For adults, the ratio of 5 compressions to 1 breath is used in 2-person CPR.

A. **Ventricular Fibrillation and Pulseless Tachycardia.** See Figure I–7. Torsade de pointes, a rare ventricular arrhythmia, is treated

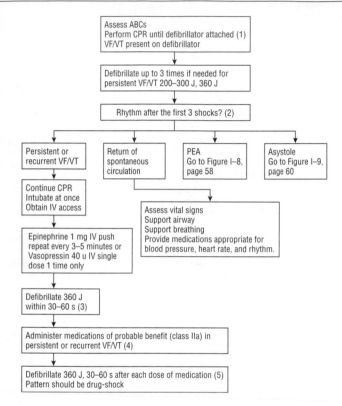

Figure I–7. Algorithm for ventricular fibrillation and pulseless ventricular tachycardia (VF/VT). (*Reproduced, with permission, from Adult Advanced Cardiac Life Support. JAMA 1992;268:16.*)

with a temporary pacemaker, rarely bretylium but never lidocaine. Most often congenital or drug induced, it is characterized by "twisting" or direction changes of the QRS complex around the isoelectric line.

B. Pulseless Electrical Activity (PEA). See Figure I–8. For surgical patients, always consider pulmonary embolism as a cause, especially for those at high risk (obese, previous embolism, certain pelvic and orthopedic cases), and for those with hypovolemia as a cause of PEA. For trauma patients, consider tension pneumothorax and cardiac tamponade. Treat hypovolemia with aggressive fluid resuscita-

Footnotes to Figure I-7
Class I: Definitely helpful.
Class IIa: Acceptable, probably helpful.
Class IIb: Acceptable, possibly helpful.
Class III: Not indicated, may be harmful.

(1) Precordial thump in a class IIb action in witnessed arrest, no pulse, and no difibillator available.
(2) Hypothermic cardiac arrest is treated differently after this point. See section on hypothermia.
(3) Multiple sequenced shocks (200 J, 200-300 J, 360 J) are acceptable here (class I), especially when medications are delayed.
(4) Lidocaine 1.5 mg/kg IV push. Repeat in 3–5 min to total loading dose of 3 mg/kg; then use:
   Amiodarone 300 mg IV push; consider repeating then 150 mg IV push in 3–5 min max. cumulative dose: 2.2 g/24 h.
   Magnesium sulfate 1–2 g IV in torsades de pointes or suspected hypomagnesemic state or severe refractory VF.
   Procainamide 30 mg/min in refractory VF (maximum total 17 mg/kg).
(5) Sodium bicarbonate (1 mEq/kg IV):
   Class IIa
   If known preexisting bicarbonate-responsive acidosis.
   If overdose with tricyclic antidepressants.
   To alkalinize the urine in drug overdoses.
   Class IIb
   If intubated and continued long arrest interval.
   Upon return of spontaneous circulation after long arrest interval.
   Class III
   Hypoxic lactic acids.

tion, tension pneumothorax with tube thoracostomy, and pericardial tamponade with pericardiocentesis.

C. **Asystole.** See algorithm in Figure I-9. The prognosis is poor in cases of asystole. Defibrillate when there is any question about the rhythm being fine ventricular tachycardia.

D. **Bradycardia.** Administer atropine as indicated (see Fig I-4). Pacing may be necessary.

E. **Tachycardia.** See Figure I-10 and Problem 83, page 244. Emergency cardioversion is reviewed in Figure I-11.

F. **Hypotension, Shock, and Acute Pulmonary Edema.** May arise independently or associated with a cardiac event.

19. CENTRAL VENOUS PRESSURE (CVP) CATHETER: CANNOT WITHDRAW BLOOD

I. **Problem.** A nurse comes to you because he is unable to draw a patient's daily laboratory blood tests from the multilumen central venous line.

II. **Immediate Questions**

A. **What is the appearance of the catheter?** Many times the diagnosis can be made by a careful inspection of the site or the catheter itself.

B. **What is the appearance of the CVP tracing/waveform (if available)?** Loss of the usual CVP tracing may indicate dislodgment, clot

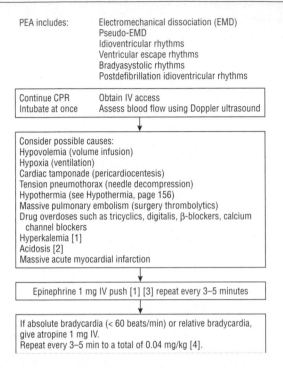

PEA includes: Electromechanical dissociation (EMD)
                         Pseudo-EMD
                         Idioventricular rhythms
                         Ventricular escape rhythms
                         Bradyasystolic rhythms
                         Postdefibrillation idioventricular rhythms

| Continue CPR | Obtain IV access |
| Intubate at once | Assess blood flow using Doppler ultrasound |

Consider possible causes:
Hypovolemia (volume infusion)
Hypoxia (ventilation)
Cardiac tamponade (pericardiocentesis)
Tension pneumothorax (needle decompression)
Hypothermia (see Hypothermia, page 156)
Massive pulmonary embolism (surgery thrombolytics)
Drug overdoses such as tricyclics, digitalis, β-blockers, calcium
   channel blockers
Hyperkalemia [1]
Acidosis [2]
Massive acute myocardial infarction

Epinephrine 1 mg IV push [1] [3] repeat every 3–5 minutes

If absolute bradycardia (< 60 beats/min) or relative bradycardia,
give atropine 1 mg IV.
Repeat every 3–5 min to a total of 0.04 mg/kg [4].

Figure I–8. Algorithm for pulseless electrical activity (PEA) (electromechanical dissociation [EMD]). (*Reproduced, with permission, from Adult Advanced Cardiac Life Support. JAMA 1992;268:16.*)

(of the catheter or the central vein itself), kinking, disconnection, transducer malfunction, or improper catheter location, such as in a noncentral vein. A normal CVP trace should fluctuate appropriately with respiration and cough.

C. **When did the catheter last draw blood easily?** Was blood ever able to be obtained through the catheter? Perhaps the catheter was never properly positioned.

D. **How long ago was the catheter placed?** The older a catheter is, the more likely it will be clotted, infected, kinked, cracked, or fractured. A freshly placed line that is malfunctioning is likely due to misplacement.

E. **What was the intravascular location of the catheter on the last chest film?** When uncertain, another radiograph can be obtained to

Footnotes to Figure I–8
Class I: Definitely helpful.
Class IIa: Acceptable, probably helpful.
Class IIb: Acceptable, possibly helpful.
Class III: Not indicated, may be harmful.

(1) Sodium bicarbonate 1 mEq/kg is class I if patient has known preexisting hyperkalemia.
(2) Sodium bicarbonate 1 mEq/kg:
    Class IIa
    If known preexisting bicarbonate-responsive acidosis.
    If overdose with tricyclic antidepressants.
    To alkalinize the urine in drug overdoses.
    Class IIb
    If intubated and continued long arrest interval.
    Upon return of spontaneous circulation after long arrest interval.
    Class III
    Hypoxic lactic acids.
(3) The recommended dose of epinephrine is 1 mg IV push every 3–5 min. If this approach fails, several
    class IIb dosing regimens can be considered:
    Intermediate: epinephrine 2–5 mg IV push, every 3–5 min.
    Escalating: epinephrine 1 mg–3 mg–5 mg IV push (3 min apart).
    High: epinephrine 0.1 mg/kg IV push, every 3–5 min.
(4) Shorter atropine dosing intervals are possibly helpful in cardiac arrest (class IIb).

check its placement. Does it appear kinked on the film? A well-placed catheter should have its tip well within the vein, but outside of the cardiac chambers, as it can erode through atrial and ventricular walls or cause arrhythmias.

  F. Do the ports flush easily? A catheter that neither flushes nor draws is more likely kinked or clogged. A catheter that easily flushes with no resistance but is difficult to draw from suggests two potential serious difficulties. The application of excessive negative pressure in attempts to aspirate from a lumen may collapse the vein itself or draw the lumen of the catheter against the wall of the vessel. Such may be the case in the hypovolemic patient or one that is sitting with a resulting low or negative venous pressure at the tip of the catheter. Alternatively, the catheter could be in a small venous tributary and not in a central location. Another more troubling possibility is that the catheter is extravascular, the result of erosion or improper initial placement. With a multilumen catheter, be aware that the ability to flush or draw from some, but not all, of the ports, may simply mean some lumens are clogged, or may actually mean that the poorly functioning ports have eroded through or backed out of the vein. These ports may be completely extravascular, and although they do not draw, may flush rather easily into a potential space.

III. Differential Diagnosis

  A. Obstructed Catheter. Small clips intended to prevent back bleeding can occlude a catheter. These may leave a kink that resists flow.

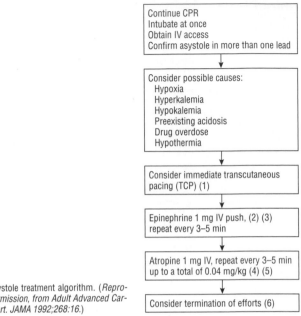

Figure I–9. Asystole treatment algorithm. (*Reproduced, with permission, from Adult Advanced Cardiac Life Support. JAMA 1992;268:16.*)

Clips that hold the catheter and are sutured to the skin may also resist flow, especially if they are positioned slightly askew during initial placement. The latter can be harder to see.

B. Clotted Catheter. The older a catheter is, the more likely it is to be clotted. Slow infusion rates, poorly functioning transducer flush systems, or long intervals between manual flushes may be to blame.

C. Infected Catheter. Indwelling lines are subject to infection and represent a direct route for the entry of bacteria and fungi, possibly resulting in bacteremia or fungemia and systemic septicemia. Suspicious signs of an infected catheter are an erythematous and/or swollen insertion site, elevated WBC, and fever.

D. Misplaced Catheter. Even an initially well-placed catheter may migrate out of place, despite the best suturing and dressing. The markings on the catheter itself can help gauge whether the line has migrated either in or out. Swelling at the site may not only indicate infection but also misplacement. When one of the ports has migrated out of the vein and is immediately subcutaneous, it will be depositing its infusate just below the skin. Depending on the type of infusate

Footnotes to Figure I–9
Class I: Definitely helpful.
Class IIa: Acceptable, probably helpful.
Class IIb: Acceptable, possibly helpful.
Class III: Not indicated, may be harmful.

(1) TCP is a class IIb intervention. Lack of success may be due to delays in pacing. To be effective TCP must be performed early, simultaneously with drugs. Evidence does not support routine use of TCP for asystole.

(2) The recommended dose of epinephrine is 1 mg IV push every 3–5 min. If this approach fails, several class IIb dosing regimens can be considered:
Intermediate: epinephrine 2–5 mg IV push, every 3–5 min.
Escalating: epinephrine 1 mg–3 mg–5 mg IV push (3 min apart).
High: epinephrine 0.1 mg/kg IV push, every 3–5 min.

(3) Sodium bicarbonate 1 mEq/kg is class I if patient has known preexisting hyperkalemia.

(4) Shorter atropine dosing intervals are class IIb in asystolic arrest.

(5) Sodium bicarbonate 1 mEq/kg IV:
Class IIa
If known preexisting bicarbonate-responsive acidosis.
If overdose with tricyclic antidepressants.
To alkalinize the urine in drug overdoses.
Class IIb
If intubated and continued long arrest interval.
Upon return of spontaneous circulation after long arrest interval.
Class III
Hypoxic lactic acids.

(6) If patient remains in asystole or other agonal rhythms after successful intubation and initial medications and no reversible causes are identified, consider termination of resuscitative efforts by a physician. Consider interval since arrest.

(particularly vasoactive drugs and potassium replacements), this may cause skin necrosis and require immediate attention. Central lines may also migrate to other intravascular locations. (Although not commonly needed, a cross-table film may be necessary to rule out migration into the azygous or internal mammary.) Finally, catheters can also erode into extravascular locations, including the pericardial and pleural spaces, and they have been known to fracture and embolize to locations far removed from the original insertion site.

E. **Kinked Catheter.** Internal jugular, subclavian, and femoral lines are all subject to kinking both at the skin and within the vein itself. Subclavian lines in particular have been associated with "pinch off" phenomenon, where the catheter becomes lodged between the clavicle and the first rib, thereby impinging on the lumens and possibly leading to catheter fracture and embolization.

F. **Thrombosis of the Central Vein.** Perhaps it is not merely clotting of the catheter but of the entire central vein itself. Central lines are not only a nidus for infection, but also for clots. When the vein is clotted, showering of clot material to the pulmonary vasculature (ie, pulmonary emboli) may occur, which can dramatically affect a patient's hemodynamic and pulmonary status.

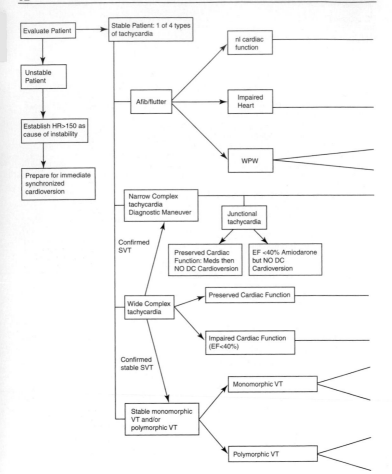

Figure I–10. Tachycardia algorithm. (*Reproduced, with permission, from Adult Advanced Cardiac Life Support. JAMA 1992;268:16.*)

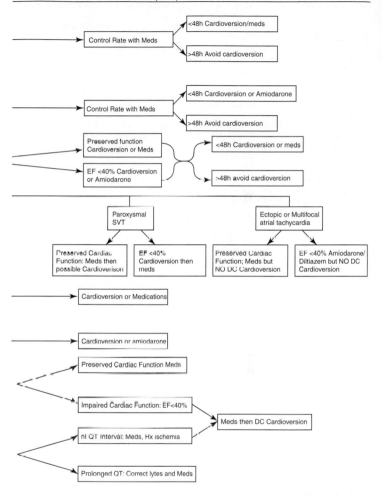

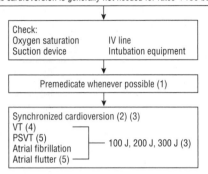

Tachycardia with serious signs and symptoms related to the tachycardia

↓

If ventricular rate is > 150 beats/min, prepare for immediate cardioversion.
May give brief trial of medications based on specific arrhythmias.
Immediate cardioversion is generally not needed for rates < 150 beats/min.

↓

Check:
Oxygen saturation   IV line
Suction device   Intubation equipment

↓

Premedicate whenever possible (1)

↓

Synchronized cardioversion (2) (3)
VT (4)
PSVT (5)   ┐
Atrial fibrillation   ├── 100 J, 200 J, 300 J (3)
Atrial flutter (5)   ┘

Footnotes
(1) Effective regimens have included a sedative (eg, diazepam, midazolam, barbituates, etomidate, ketamine, methohexital) with or without an analgesic agent (eg, fentanyl, morphine, meperidine).
Many experts recommend anesthesia if service is readily available.
(2) Note possible need to resynchronize after each cardioversion.
(3) If delays in synchronization occur and clinical conditions are critical, go to immediate unsynchronized shocks.
(4) Treat polymorphic VT (irregular form and rate) like VF:
200 J, 200–300 J, 260 J.
(5) PSVT and atrial flutter often respond to lower energy levels (start with 50 J).

Figure I–11. Electrical cardioversion algorithm (patient not in cardiac arrest). (*Reproduced, with permission, from Adult Advanced Cardiac Life Support. JAMA 1992;268:16.*)

G. Manufacturer Defect. Before line placement, always flush each of the lumens to rule out manufacturer defect.

IV. Database

A. Physical Exam Key Points

1. Vital signs. Tachycardia and hypotension can indicate infection or hypovolemia. The presence of fever may necessitate that the line be ruled out as a source of infection. Abnormal hemodynamic vital signs and oxygen desaturation can also signal serious problems. In the case of venous thrombosis with resultant showering

of pulmonary emboli, tachycardia, hypotension, low oxygen saturation, and high right ventricular and pulmonary artery pressures
may be seen. Similarly ominous vital signs may accompany pneumothorax and pericardial effusions if they develop tension.

2. **Breath sounds.** Hydrothorax or pneumothorax, the result of
catheter misplacement or migration into the pleural space, may
cause decreased unilateral breath sounds. Tachycardia, hypotension, and low O_2 saturation may also result from such pleural disease. Wheezing can be an early sign of pulmonary embolism.

3. **Heart tones.** Muffled heart tones and elements of Beck's triad
may mean catheter placement or erosion through the myocardium
resulting in tamponade.

4. **HEENT.** Venous congestion of the head and neck may result from
the migration of a subclavian line to the neck, a looped or obstructed catheter, or central venous thrombosis.

5. **Lower extremities.** An ipsilateral congested leg may indicate a
looped or obstructing femoral line, or central venous thrombosis.

B. **Laboratory Data**
   1. **Hemogram.** Elevated WBC may indicate infection.

C. **Radiographic Data and Other Studies**
   1. **Chest radiograph.** Check the position of the catheter on chest
   radiograph. Rule out kinking or malposition. Evidence of pneumothorax and hydrothorax will be apparent. Wedge-shaped in-
   farcts can indicate pulmonary emboli.
   2. **Ultrasound/Doppler studies.** Evidence of thrombosis around a
   central line can often be elucidated with ultrasound.

V. **Plan**

A. **Ensure intravascular position of the catheter.** When it is necessary for infusion of life saving medications, it is important to immediately confirm that the catheter is indeed intravascular in location. The
inability to draw blood samples may be much less important than the
failure to deliver vasoactive substances or potentially life-saving antibiotics to an unstable patient, for example. In rare circumstances,
one could consider the administration of a small amount of a medication whose effects would be discernible, such as isoproterenol,
phenylephrine, or esmolol.

B. **Alter body position.** Adjusting the patient's position may fix the
problem. For example, straightening the leg for a femoral catheter,
turning or tilting the head and neck for a jugular line, or moving the
shoulder on the side of a subclavian site may reduce kinking and improve flow.

C. **Inspect catheter-securing devices.** Ensure that occluding clamps
or clips have been removed and any remaining crimps in the catheter
have also been removed. Ensure that securing clamps are not oc-

cluding flow. These can be temporarily pulled off of the catheter to see whether they were the offending agents. Passage of a sterile wire through these external portions of the catheter can also help alleviate crimps from these devices. Occasionally, additional sutures placed along the catheter for additional security may be tied tight enough to occlude a lumen.

D. **Alter insertion distance.** Pulling a line back slightly or advancing it slightly might result in a more optimal position if the catheter tip was previously against the wall of a vessel. Meticulous sterile technique is required when advancing a catheter.

E. **Alter volume status.** A patient who is hypovolemic may have easily collapsible vessels or a negative venous pressure at the site of the catheter tip. While most central veins will be held open by surrounding tissues, some will not, and more-peripheral veins are subject to this difficulty. Volume replacement, Trendelenburg position, and Valsalva maneuvers may increase venous filling, thus distending the vein.

F. **Flush a clotted catheter.** A gentle flush with saline or heparinized saline may be all that is required. Be sure to use a small (1 cc) syringe. This is rarely dangerous, though the flushed clot can become embolic and may also represent a nidus of infection. Streptokinase or urokinase may be used to "declot" the catheter if available. These are powerful potentially dangerous drugs and should be used only by personnel familiar with their use. Inadvertent administration of too much of these drugs systemically can lead to devastating consequences. On the other hand, salvaging a clotted central line can be very beneficial in situations where replacement of a line carries its own significant risks.

G. **Change the catheter over a guidewire.** Replacing a central line over a guidewire will fix most problems of clotting, clogging, kinking, and leaking or cracked infusion hubs. For improperly positioned lines, it may be possible to effect a change in catheter position with manipulations of a wire. Be watchful for any arrhythmias or changes in vital signs. When an infected catheter is suspected, this may not be sufficient treatment. The site may have to be abandoned, and a new location chosen.

H. **Consider placing a new line.** When all else fails, a new line may need to be placed. It is always important to reconsider whether the need for a central line still exists. Blood samples may be drawn from peripheral veins with standard phlebotomy techniques, and perhaps, there is no longer a need for central access. Central lines represent significant risks, and while incredibly useful in many clinical situations, many patients have suffered complications from these lines when the indications for their use no longer existed. Placement of lines is well covered in other sections of this book.

I. Complications

1. **Embolic complications.** Flushing a line can result in small emboli or an air embolus. The volume of the lumina of most central catheters is quite small, and it is rare for such emboli to have any consequences, let alone serious sequelae. Nevertheless, care should be taken to avoid this problem, if possible. Large-volume cannulas, such as pulmonary artery introducers, without a PA catheter or high-flow trauma lines may result in larger volume clots.

2. **Infectious complications.** The most common late complication is infection. It is estimated that about 5% of all indwelling catheters become infected. The majority of these are due to *Staphylococcus epidermidis, S aureus* (38%, combined), and yeast (24%). Leaving an infected catheter in place can lead to spread of infection. Colonization of the catheter site can spread to the intravascular portion of the line and also the intravascular thrombus that commonly forms around this portion of a catheter. Catheter infections can lead to systemic septicemia and may be life threatening. Any catheter suspected to be infected should be promptly removed.

3. **Catheter damage.** High-pressure flushing and attempts to alleviate obstruction with various maneuvers can damage catheters. Such damage may cause breakage, leading to inadvertent back bleeding or, more commonly, insidious leakage of an infusion, resulting in a patient not receiving desired therapy. Careful inspection of a catheter after any manipulation is always important.

4. **Insertion complications.** Insertion of a new line carries all of the risks present during initial placement, such as arterial puncture (3–9%), pneumothorax (<2%), and more rare complications, such as chylothorax, nerve injury, tracheal puncture, and air embolism. These are discussed elsewhere in this book. All complication rates decrease with increased operator experience.

5. **Late complications.** Other late complications, although very rare, include perforation of the superior vena cava or atrium, leading to tamponade, thrombosis of a central vein with potential thromboembolism, hydrothorax, hydromediastinum, arrhythmias, and catheter fracture with possible catheter embolism.

20. CERVICAL SPINE PRECAUTIONS

I. **Problem.** A 36-year-old man who was involved in a motor vehicle collision has sustained a closed head injury. He has a cervical collar in place. The nurse calls to ask if he can be sat up in a chair.

II. **Immediate Questions**

A. **What kind of collar does the patient have on?** Many trauma patients come to the emergency department in a hard "white" collar.

These collars are for extraction at the scene of an accident and initial transport to the hospital. They should be changed to a softer collar to lessen the risk of skin necrosis. Philadelphia and Miami-J collars are most common.

B. **What radiographs have been performed on the patient?** Because of the urgency of resuscitation, the patient may not have had cervical spine films initially. Until a physical exam is possible, complete evaluation of the cervical spine will not be possible. Radiographic assessment should include ways of evaluating from the odontoid to T1. Under supervision, flexion-extension C-spine films may also be obtained to detect occult instability or determine the stability of a known fracture. CT of the cervical spine has taken an increasing role in further evaluation of known injuries or if adequate visualization is not obtained on plain films.

C. **Does the patient need to be moved?** Spinal precautions should be maintained until a C-spine injury is excluded. When moving the patient is necessary, proper immobilization is achieved with the patient in a neutral position (without rotating or bending the spinal column).

III. **Differential Diagnosis.** All patients presenting in a cervical collar should be suspected of having an injury and treated as such until proven otherwise. Injuries could range from a stable ligamentous injury without sequelae to a high cervical cord injury with resultant quadriplegia and respiratory compromise.

IV. **Database**

A. **Physical Exam Key Points**

1. **Vital Signs.** Neurogenic shock results from impairment of the descending sympathetic pathways in the spinal cord. This type of shock is indicated by the presence of hypotension and bradycardia (failure of tachycardic response to hypovolemia).

2. **Neck.** In the supine position, palpate the spine with the collar removed and note any area of tenderness, step-off, or skin necrosis. Look for injuries that have been obscured by the collar. This initial exam is an opportune time to change from the extraction collar to a more long-term collar.

3. **Neurologic.** A complete neurologic exam should be performed noting any sensory or motor deficit. When there is concomitant head injury, a complete neurologic exam may not be possible. Only the actual exam that is obtained should be documented. Avoid using generic, but nondescriptive terms such as "neurovascularly intact" or "moves all fours."

4. **Pulmonary.** A patent airway is critically important in spinal-cord-injured patients, and early intubation should be accomplished when there is any evidence of respiratory compromise. This can be achieved while maintaining the neck in a neutral position.

5. **Cardiovascular.** Examination should look for evidence of neurogenic shock. Bradycardia and hypotension in conjunction with a neurologic deficit suggest a high cervical spinal cord injury.

B. **Laboratory Data.** No specific laboratory studies are required for cervical spine precautions. A toxicology study may be helpful when there is a question about the patient's ability to relate the presence or absence of neck pain.

C. **Radiographic and Other Studies**
   1. **AP, lateral, open mouth (odontoid) radiographs.** When all 7 cervical vertebrae are not visualized with the lateral radiograph, a swimmer's view is obtained.
   2. **Flexion-extension radiographs.** For a patient with no fractures seen on plain films and who has neck complaints, flexion-extension films may delineate or exclude a ligamentous injury. These films, in general, should be done on awake patients with patient-generated motion. Fluoroscopy is a useful technique.
   3. **CT C-spine.** For patients with known fractures, CT is particularly useful in demonstrating bony detail and the degree of canal compromise. Sagittal reconstructions may be needed in certain fractures. CT has also been used when adequate plain films cannot be obtained.
   4. **MRI.** Provides the most accurate modality in the presence of neurologic deficits. However, it is frequently not feasible to safely obtain an MRI in an unstable patient.

V. **Plan**

A. **Overall Plan.** The overall goal is to prevent spinal cord injury from an unstable fracture or ligamentous disruption. A simultaneous goal is to allow ongoing medical care of the patient.

B. **Specific Plans**
   1. **When in doubt, leave the collar in place.** When the patient has a temporary clouding of sensorium, such as from pharmacologic agents or substances, a repeat physical exam will allow for determination of neck pain. When the patient has a diminished level of consciousness for a prolonged period, the optimal approach is less clear. Coordination between general surgery, orthopedic surgery, neurosurgery, and radiology will be needed to approach these particular patients. Delayed films looking for ligamentous laxity or MRI may be required.
   2. **Consultation** by neurosurgery or orthopedic surgery is indicated in all cases where a spine injury is detected or suspected.
   3. **Establish and maintain proper immobilization** of the patient until the presence of vertebral fractures or spinal cord injuries has been excluded.
   4. **A bed position** of approximately 10 degrees of reverse Trendelenburg (head slightly up) can enhance pulmonary hygiene and

minimize aspiration risks without compromising cervical spine mobility. Patient care and transport should be accomplished with the log-roll technique.

5. **The long spine board** is used predominately for extrication and initial transport efforts. Significant skin breakdown may occur when the patient remains on the board long after the initial evaluation.

21. CHEST PAIN

Immediate Actions. "MONA" treats all chest pain: **M**orphine, **O**xygen, **N**itroglycerin and **A**SA. Additionally, all patients get **stat** cardiac monitoring, ECG and treatment of hyper- or hypotension.

I. **Problem.** A 75-year-old man with a history of severe COPD is admitted to the ICU for severe bacterial community-acquired pneumonia requiring intubation and mechanical ventilation. On his second hospital day, he complains of acute left-sided chest pain at rest, lasting 10 to 15 min with associated tachypnea, diaphoresis, and arterial desaturation. On examination, his blood pressure was 80/40 and his peak airway pressures on the ventilator were 60 cm of H_2O. Auscultation of the chest reveals absent breath sounds on the left side and tracheal deviation to the left.

II. **Immediate Questions**

A. **What are the vital signs?**

B. **What is the appearance of the ECG? Are there any acute changes?**

C. **Did the patient have acute coronary syndrome before transfer to the ICU?** Does the patient have similar pain now?

D. **What kind of operative procedure has the patient undergone?**

E. **What medications were given to the patient?** Did the patient get any sympathomimetics(pitressin for GI bleed)?

F. **What was done to the patient at the time of pain onset? What was he doing?**

G. **What risk factors does the patient have for CAD?** Male, > 35 years; Female, > 45 years, postmenopausal, hypercholesterolemia, hypertension, family history, diabetes, and smoking.

III. **Differential Diagnosis.** The differential diagnosis of patients complaining in the ICU of chest pain is broad, ranging from benign musculoskeletal conditions to pain arising from life-threatening cardiac disease. Patients with chest pain in the ICU should undergo a rapid and focused evaluation. Initially, an effort should be made to exclude life-threatening processes. The "classic symptoms" of myocardial infarction (squeezing chest pressure, pain radiating to the jaw), pericarditis (sharp, catch-like pain), and aortic dissection (excruciating, knifelike or "tearing" pain) should be sought. Atypical chest pain is common in the ICU, and obtaining a specific etiologic diagnosis can be difficult. It is essential to narrow the differential by obtaining a careful history and performing a thorough physical examination.

A. Pulmonary Embolism. Patients with pulmonary embolism may present with the following findings: abrupt onset of dyspnea; chest pain, unrelieved with nitroglycerin; tachycardia; diaphoresis; fever; tachypnea; increased P2; dyspnea at rest; thrombophlebitis of the lower extremity; hypoxemia with a widened alveolar-arterial gradient; sudden onset of pleuritic chest pain; apprehension, cough and hemoptysis (50% of patients); syncope and hypotension (large or multiple emboli); abrupt rise in right atrial, right ventricular, and pulmonary artery pressures (large emboli); and an increase in the difference between the pulmonary artery diastolic and pulmonary artery occlusion pressure.

B. Pneumothorax. Tachypnea, dyspnea at rest, dyspnea with exertion, localized decrease in breath sounds, unilateral decrease in breath sounds, dyspnea of abrupt onset, increased peak airway pressure with normal plateau pressure on mechanical ventilation, sudden hemodynamic instability, arterial desaturation, tracheal deviation, jugular venous distention, and hypotension—all are indicators of a tension pneumothorax that is an immediate life-threatening problem.

C. Aortic Dissection. Patients with aortic dissection may present with the following findings: sudden onset of excruciating chest discomfort, frequently radiating to the back, abdomen, and extremities. Maximal severity usually occurs at onset, with knifelike or "tearing" substernal chest pain. Severe back pain, or chest pain is unrelieved with nitroglycerin. Fever, tachycardia, and elevated diastolic blood pressure may also be present.

1. **Type-A Dissections.** Dissections arising proximal to the left subclavian artery are often seen in young patients with Marfan's syndrome or cystic medial necrosis. Patients with Type-A dissections may present with the following findings: upper-extremity weakness, asymmetric upper-extremity blood pressure, hemiplegia, Horner's syndrome, recurrent laryngeal nerve damage, hemopericardium, and cardiac tamponade. Acute aortic valve insufficiency and dissection of the coronary artery ostium may result in an acute myocardial infarction.

2. **Type-B Dissections.** Dissections arising distal to the left subclavian artery are usually seen in older patients with a history of hypertension and atherosclerotic disease. Patients with Type-B dissections may present with the following findings: paraesthesias, weakness, and pain of the lower extremities; and diminished

or unequal lower-extremity pulses. Manifestations of mesenteric and renal ischemia may also occur.

D. **Acute Pericarditis.** Patients with acute pericarditis may present with the following findings: Chest pain at rest, relieved by leaning forward and worsened by recumbency, inspiration, and cough; chest pain may be band-like with radiation to the arms; pericardial friction rub may be present; chest pain usually lasts longer than 20 min; chest pain not relieved with nitroglycerin; sinus tachycardia may be present, as well as fever, and leukocytosis.

E. **Cardiac Ischemia**
   1. **Angina Pectoris.** Recurrent chest discomfort lasts less than 15 min, is precipitated by stress, and relieved with nitroglycerin or rest. Radiation to the upper extremities, nausea, vomiting, or diaphoresis may be present. Atrial or ventricular arrhythmias may occur. Physical examination is often normal.
   2. **Myocardial Infarction.** Substernal chest pain at rest is similar to but more intense than angina pectoris, and usually lasts longer than 20 min. Chest pain is usually not relieved by nitroglycerin. Certain patients express an overwhelming "sense of doom." Nausea, vomiting, or diaphoresis may be present. Narrow pulse pressure, bradycardia, and atrioventricular blocks may be associated with inferior wall myocardial infarctions. Shock and pulmonary edema may be associated with various large anterior wall myocardial infarctions. Hypotension, clear lungs, and signs of right-heart failure may be associated with right-ventricular infarctions.
   3. **Aortic Stenosis.** Exertional dyspnea, chest pain at rest, heart gallop, harsh systolic murmur radiating to the neck, signs of LVH on examination and ECG, syncope, congestive heart failure—all can be symptoms of aortic stenosis.

F. **Esophageal injury and rupture.** Patients with esophageal injury or rupture usually present with the following histories: atypical chest pain, history of ingestion of toxic agents, such as lye; history of ingestion of pills known to cause mucosal damage; history of traumatic nasogastric tube insertion or other esophageal manipulation; history of retching, vomiting forcefully, heavy lifting, trauma to the chest or straining during defecation; subcutaneous emphysema, left pleural effusion, hydropneumothorax, or mediastinal air on chest radiograph.

G. **Esophageal Spasm.** Squeezing chest pain that may be induced by exercise. Pain is induced by very hot or cold liquids. Dysphagia may be present with liquid and solid food.

IV. **Database.** Chest pain is common in the ICU, and obtaining a specific etiologic diagnosis can be difficult. It is essential to narrow the differential by obtaining a careful history and performing a thorough physical examination.

A. Physical Exam Key Points
1. **Vital signs.**
2. **Pulmonary.** Signs of CHF or pneumonia.
3. **Cardiac.** New onset murmurs, S3 or S4.
4. **Carotid bruits.** Their presence may be an indicator of generalized vascular disease.
5. **Abdomen.** Rule out abdominal disease.

B. Laboratory Data
1. **CK-MB and/or Troponin-T or I.** Cannot use to rule out, only to rule in myocardial injury.
2. **D-Dimer.** Sensitive but poor specificity in PE.
3. **Hemogram, SMA-7 and INR/PTT.**
4. **LFT/Amylase.** When an intra-abdominal cause is considered, pancreatitis and liver disease must be ruled out.
5. **Toxicology.** Cocaine use can cause chest pain.

C. Radiographic and Other Studies
1. **ECG.** STAT repeat 3 times every 20 min.
2. **Chest radiograph.** Look for pneumothorax, pneumonia, CHF, aortic dissection, acute pericarditis, and esophageal rupture.
3. **Ultrasound.** Pericardial or valvular disease, wall motion, transesophageal is useful in aortic dissection, and right ventricular dilation and hypokinesia in PE.
4. **Stress echo.** When indicated.
5. **CT.** In stable aortic dissection.
6. **V̇/Q̇ Scan.**
7. **Angiography.**

V. Plan

A. Specific Management Plans
1. **Pulmonary Embolism.** When there is a high clinical index of suspicion, administer heparin before sending the patient for diagnostic tests. Proceed with diagnostic tests, such as a V̇/Q̇ lung scan, spiral chest CT scan, or pulmonary angiography. Patients too unstable for transport may undergo a lung perfusion scan at the bedside. Consider thrombolytic therapy for patients with massive emboli resulting in acute right ventricular failure. A stat bedside transthoracic echocardiogram may be helpful in certain circumstances.
2. **Pneumothorax.** Obtain a chest radiograph. When a tension pneumothorax is suspected, the pneumothorax should be evacuated before obtaining a chest radiograph. Patients who are critically ill and on mechanical ventilation are at increased risk of pneumothorax. When a ball-valve mechanism develops during positive pressure ventilation, a life-threatening tension pneumothorax may rapidly develop. Loculated pneumothoraces are frequently missed on portable radiographs of critically ill patients. When the diagnosis is clinically suspected, a CT scan of the chest

may be necessary for confirmation. Do not wait for studies such as CT scans in an unstable patient.

3. **Aortic Dissection.** This requires immediate surgical consultation when clinical suspicion is high. Both contrast chest CT scan and transesophageal echocardiography (TEE) are used in the evaluation of aortic dissection. The choice of diagnostic modality depends on the patient (eg, poor renal function may mitigate against obtaining a CT scan with dye) and institutional preferences.

4. **Pericarditis.** Echocardiography visualizes pericardial effusions of various sizes. Electrocardiography may initially show diffuse ST-segment elevation with concurrent PR-depression in the limb and precordial leads. In 24 to 48 h, diffuse T wave inversions followed by ST- and PR-segment normalization may occur. With the development of large pericardial effusions, reduced QRS voltage, oscillatory voltage pattern (electrical alternans), and atrial arrhythmias may be seen. Most patients who are diagnosed with acute pericarditis have an uneventful recovery with bed rest and anti-inflammatory drug therapy. For such patients, aggressive diagnostic strategies, including pericardiocentesis may be warranted. Purulent pericardial fluid, positive Gram's stain/culture or fluid leukocytosis (>2000 WBCs) are suggestive of bacterial pericarditis. Bacterial cultures and serology for antinuclear antibody (ANA), rheumatoid factor, and HIV may be of diagnostic utility for selected patients.

5. **Angina Pectoris.** Electrocardiography may show ST-segment depression, hyperacute T waves, or arrhythmias during ischemia. ECG changes during attacks, stress echocardiography, nuclear medicine scan, exercise stress testing, or cardiac catheterization may be necessary to diagnose cardiac ischemia.

6. **Myocardial Infarction.** Electrocardiography frequently shows ST-segment elevation in at least two contiguous leads with simultaneous Q-wave formation. Nontransmural infarction is not associated with formation of Q waves. Cardiac enzymes should be checked on a regular basis until levels decline. Evaluation and consideration for thrombolytic therapy should be made. Patients with persistent atypical pain and equivocal ECG findings should proceed to coronary angiography. In certain circumstances, echocardiography can be of diagnostic utility in the setting of an acute myocardial infarction (see Problem 31 page 96)

7. **Aortic Stenosis.** Echocardiography or coronary angiography is needed to confirm the diagnosis. Patients with severe aortic stenosis (aortic valve area < 1.0 cm^2) who develop chest pain and hypotension require aggressive management.

8. **Esophageal Spasm.** Various tests, such as esophageal scintography, esophageal manometry, and provocative tests, can be helpful in establishing the diagnosis.

22. CHEST TUBE AIR LEAK

Immediate Action. When there is clinical concern for tension pneumothorax, the involved hemithorax should undergo immediate needle decompression. The presence of a chest tube should not deter the clinician from carrying out this procedure. An angiocatheter (14 gauge or larger) is inserted into the second intercostal space anteriorly. The diagnosis of tension pneumothorax should be clinical and should not wait for or depend on a chest radiograph.

I. **Problem.** A 22-year-old patient develops a chest tube leak after a gunshot wound to the chest.

II. **Immediate Questions**

A. **Is this a new finding or has there been a recent change (small air leak with cough or continuous air leak)?** Small air leaks immediately after surgery or chest tube placement are not unusual. An increase in the amount of air leak warrants further investigation.

B. **Is the patient symptomatic (chest pain, shortness of breath)?** The patient may have a persistent pneumothorax despite placement of a single chest tube and may require a second tube to reexpand the lung. A large air leak with more than one tube in place is suggestive of a bronchial injury.

III. **Differential Diagnosis**

A. **Bronchopleural Fistula.** Trauma or thoracotomy/lung resection may result in a bronchopleural fistula.

B. **System Air Leak.** Occasional detects in the chest tube system can occur. With patient movement for care or studies, the connections may become loose. These should be assessed.

C. **Ruptured Bleb.** Preexisting bleb disease may rupture when the patient is in the hospital.

D. **Large or Persistent Visceral Pleural Injury.** Injury to the visceral pleural may create an air leak too large for one chest tube to handle.

IV. **Database**

A. **Physical Exam Key Points**

1. **Vital signs.** Tachypnea and hypoxia (decreased oxygen saturation) suggest respiratory compromise with possible worsening pneumothorax. Look to see if the patient has had increasing FIO_2 requirements.

2. **Chest/Lungs.** Hyperresonance, decreased breath sounds, or crepitance may indicate persistent pneumothorax. Examine the

chest tube site and ensure a proper airtight seal here. Repositioning of the chest tube is allowed, but advancing chest tubes after
placement is contraindicated. Examine the patient for penetrating
wounds. When the wounds are large enough and not dressed
properly, external air may be drawn into the chest.

3. **Head and neck.** There may be evidence of increasing subcutaneous air with increased facial, neck, and chest swelling.
4. **Examine the chest tube setup.** Clamp the chest tube near the
   chest wall. When the air leak persists, there is a defect in the system. Replacement of the chest tube apparatus will be necessary.
   Examine the junction of the chest tube with the body. Leakage of
   air may also occur around the tube.

B. **Laboratory Data**
   1. **ABG.** Blood gas determination may be helpful if the patient is
      complaining of shortness of breath. ABG may identify gas ex-
      change problems.

C. **Radiography and Other Studies**
   1. **Chest radiograph.** Ensure that the patient is upright when the
      underlying disease state will permit. ICU chest radiographs are
      often obtained with the patient supine. Look closely for pneumo-
      thorax or worsening pneumothorax. This determination may be
      difficult in a patient with massive subcutaneous emphysema.
      Check the position of the chest tube for kinks. Verify that the last
      chest tube hole is actually in the patient's chest. Look for atypical
      locations of pneumothorax, including subpulmonic and medially
      placed pneumothorax.
   2. **Bronchoscopy.** May be indicated when there is a suspected
      bronchopleural fistula.

V. **Plan.** Administer oxygen if needed. Consider repositioning the chest
tube without advancing the tube to correct a kinked tube. Increase suction on chest tube if the apparatus allows. Consider placement of a second chest tube. Resume suction if the patient was recently switched
from suction to water seal. Placement of a second tube may be necessary. When the chest cavity contains adhesions (trapped lung), multiple
tubes may ultimately be required.

23. DEATH

I. **Problem.** You are called to the bedside of a 55-year-old man who was
admitted to the ICU after undergoing repair of a ruptured abdominal aortic aneurysm 3 d ago.

II. **Immediate Questions**
   A. **Does the patient respond to any stimuli?**
   B. **Does the patient have any vital signs?**

    C. Is the patient cold?

    D. Is the patient a potential organ donor? When the patient is brain dead (a "heart-beating cadaver"), then this possibility must be considered.

    E. What is the immediate cause of the patient death? What medications were given to the patient recently?

III. Differential Diagnosis. The physician must recognize that death rarely results from failed medical therapy and is often not to be forestalled. Sophisticated medical devices surround and sometimes remain in the ICU patient after death. In this challenging setting the physician must change the focus from fighting disease to comforting family and loved ones. Numerous conditions are conducive to coma and cardiopulmonary arrest.

        a. Ascertain that ACLS was performed for 20 min before pronouncing the patient dead.

        b. Rule out hypothermia.

IV. Database

    A. Physical Exam Key Points

        1. Vital signs. Check for heart sounds, temperature, breath sounds, and blood pressure.

        2. Other. Check gag reflex, pupils, and response to severe pain.

    B. Laboratory Data (none indicated).

    C. Radiographic and Other Studies.

        1. In some institutions, ECG or EEG in special situations.

V. Plan

    A. The patient's primary doctor and a representative from the hospital's decedent affairs should be called promptly. The primary physician may want to call the patient's family and loved ones personally. However, many times a primary physician will ask a house officer to speak with family and loved ones if he/she is present.

    B. It is critically important to determine whether or not this is a "coroner's case." The laws regarding this determination vary among states. Be aware of the laws in your state, and be sure to call the coroner when indicated. Reasons for a death to be a coroner's case in some states include intra-operative deaths, death within 24 h of admission, or death under unknown circumstances.

    C. When giving bad news, it is best to do it in person. The physician must have an empathetic, professional attitude. The discussion should be clear, using words such as "death" and "dead." Avoid euphemisms. The house officer should be prepared to answer basic questions regarding the death and should allow adequate time for answers and expressions of grief. Emotional responses to death vary greatly; expect a wide range of responses. An offer to call a clergy member or make a difficult phone call to a loved one is also appreciated.

D. Offer the family and loved ones time alone with the deceased. Cover the body to the shoulders and remove all medical devices, unless an autopsy will be performed, or the body will be released to the coroner.

E. A death note should include admission date and diagnosis, complications, reason for, and time of death.

F. Autopsy can often provide a more definitive cause of death and provide closure for loved ones. It is appropriate to offer an autopsy after the news of a death has been given, and the family has had some time to grieve. A family's understanding of the cause of death is very important in the grieving process. The family should be told whether this is a "coroner's case."

G. The physician must play a supportive, reassuring role when counseling a patient's loved ones. A patient's death may have meaning outside of the obvious loss. It is important to be sensitive to cultural differences regarding the perception of death. Death is not simply the failure of medical care.

H. Use judgment when touching family and loved ones when they are grieving. Approximately 50% of family members welcome touching, while the other half does not.

I. A family's reaction to death depends on whether it was expected, how fast it came, and how well everyone was prepared. Acceptance of death comes with the recognition that it is part of life.

24. DECREASED CARDIAC OUTPUT

I. Problem. You are called to evaluate a postoperative patient with a cardiac output (CO) of 2.5 L/min.

II. Immediate Questions

A. Are there accompanying clinical signs of shock? What is the mental status of the patient and has it changed? How long does it take for capillary refill, and what is the urine output? Is the patient diaphoretic?

B. What are the other vital signs? Is the patient hemodynamically stable? Is he breathing and what is the oxygen saturation? Is he febrile? What is the blood pressure? Low blood pressure may necessitate immediate treatment if it is not high enough to ensure adequate perfusion of the brain and coronary arteries.

C. How was the cardiac output measured? How accurate and reproducible is the technique? Is the measurement artifactual or real?

D. What has the cardiac output been? Does this represent a change? Has the change been gradual or of sudden onset? It is always important to examine trends when evaluating "numbers" in patient care. Dramatic changes can signal an acute crisis in contrast to incremental changes that may imply a different set of differential diagnoses.

E. What other clinical changes have occurred? CO is influenced by heart rate, preload, afterload, myocardial compliance and contractility. Decreases in cardiac output may result from any clinical changes that affect these variables. These variables are separate, yet interdependent, and are controlled by the autonomic nervous system as well as humoral mechanisms. Many physiologic and mechanical factors may influence any of these variables.

F. What is the cardiac rhythm? Tachycardia, bradycardia, atrial and ventricular arrhythmias, and heart block can reduce CO by decreasing filling time or causing asynchrony between the atria and ventricles, resulting in ineffective inotropy.

G. What is the central venous pressure (CVP) or pulmonary capillary wedge pressure (PCWP)? Have there been changes in preload measured in other ways, such as by echocardiography? Preload is a major factor affecting cardiac output.

H. Has there been a change in contractility? New onset of myocardial dysfunction will decrease CO. The most obvious cause would be new myocardial ischemia.

I. Is the blood pressure too high? Blood pressure is a major variable affecting ventricular afterload and, hence, the effectiveness of ventricular function and output.

J. What other therapeutic modalities have recently changed or been initiated? Changes in mechanical ventilation may affect cardiac output by decreasing venous return.

K. Is there any evidence of a tension pneumothorax or pericardial tamponade? These conditions can have dramatic effects on CO and will require an urgent intervention.

III. Differential Diagnosis. CO is influenced by heart rate, preload, afterload, myocardial compliance and contractility. These variables are often interdependent and all should be considered when approaching a differential diagnosis. One must always consider that an error in measurement has occurred.

A. Heart Rate and Rhythm

1. **Bradycardia.** Heart rate × stroke volume = CO. Low heart rate leads directly to decreased CO and often is easily treated (see page 42).

2. **Tachycardia.** Rapid heart rate leaves less time for ventricular filling. Inadequate filling leads to lower output. This may be particularly important in the presence of valvular disease (see page 244).

3. **Heart block.** Lack of coordination of the contractions of the atria and ventricles may lead to poor filling of the ventricle and, hence, reduced output.

B. **Preload.** Preload is an important variable affecting filling of the ventricle. It determines the degree of stretch of the sarcomeres and, hence, is an important variable affecting ventricular contraction and cardiac output. Clinical correlations of measured variables must be made with preload, and this process of correlation is complex and often somewhat inaccurate.

   1. **High preload.** Too much filling of the ventricle will stretch the sarcomeres beyond their optimal length and result in diminished contractility. This will reduce CO and may lead to congestive heart failure. This will be manifested by high CVP and/or high PCWP.

   2. **Low preload.** Inadequate preload fails to optimally fill the ventricle and may lead to low CO. This is particularly relevant when there is a coexisting state of low ventricular compliance. Hypovolemia is the usual cause of inadequate preload but may be brought on insidiously by other factors. With a stiff ventricle, insidious decreases in filling pressures may eventually lead to a precipitous drop in cardiac output and blood pressure. Changes in intrathoracic pressure accompanying the institution of mechanical ventilation or changes in ventilatory parameters may also decrease preload.

C. **Pericardial tamponade or tension pneumothorax.** Similar decreases in preload or effective cardiac filling can be the result of increased pressure in the pericardial or pleural spaces. Cardiac tamponade occurs in 3–6% of patients undergoing open-heart surgery. Equalization of diastolic pressures (CVP, pulmonary artery diastolic pressure, PCWP) with decreasing CO, pulses paradoxus, and muffled heart tones signal this acute event and should prompt immediate action. Tension pneumothorax will also lead to ventilatory difficulties and, similarly, demands urgent intervention.

D. **Contractility and valvular function.** Changes in myocardial contractility have profound effects on cardiac output. Although effectiveness of a contraction is also controlled by preload (and resulting sarcomere length) and afterload, the major variable is the state of the myocardium and the functionality of its valves.

   1. **New onset of poor contractility.** New onset of myocardial ischemia will negatively affect contractility directly. There may also be a secondary change in compliance, so that the ventricle is stiffer, and previous levels of preload are no longer adequate to properly fill the ventricle, resulting in a decreased CO. Other conditions may affect contractility, including the presence of significant electrolyte abnormalities or iatrogenic factors, such as the administration of excessive doses of beta-blockers.

   2. **Preexisting poor contractile state.** Poor contractility as a baseline condition predisposes the patient to a deterioration in CO

when any other variable is not optimized. Such conditions include dilated, idiopathic, or infiltrative cardiomyopathy. Increases or decreases in preload may cause a dramatic drop in CO.

3. **New-onset valvular dysfunction.** Rupture or dysfunction of a papillary muscle will dramatically reduce CO.

4. **Increase in contractility.** Certain disease states, such as hypertrophic obstructive cardiomyopathy, may predispose to a decrease in CO when contractility actually increases. The ventricular outflow tract is obstructed and CO decreases when the ventricle is permitted to empty completely. This occurs when contractility increases, such as with the administration of inotropic drugs or a sympathetic response by the patient. It may also occur when preload or afterload decrease and the ventricle does not totally fill or is permitted to empty too easily.

E. **Increased Afterload.** Increased afterload can negatively affect ventricular performance and CO. Afterload is best approximated in clinical practice by blood pressure and vascular tone. Calculation of systemic vascular resistance is often useful when considering afterload, though it does represent an oversimplification. An increase in afterload may lead to a decrease in CO, as an impaired ventricle is unable to effectively contract and produce an adequate stroke volume. Massive increases in afterload can produce cardiac failure even in a normal ventricle, as is the case with neurogenic pulmonary edema.

F. **Incorrect measurement.** Determination of CO is fraught with technical difficulties. There are numerous factors that may lead to a faulty or inaccurate measurement for all methods of CO determination. Variability of 10-25% is not unusual. An understanding of how CO is determined by whatever technique has been used may be helpful in ruling out the presence of a spurious reading. A repeat measurement is always indicated in the absence of clinical correlation after assurance that the patient is stable.

IV. Database

A. **Physical Exam Key Points**
   1. **Mental Status.** An alert oriented patient suggests adequate central perfusion.
   2. **Vital Signs.** Hypotension and hypertension are important factors of patient stability. They may result from or be the cause of decreased CO. Arrhythmias may be suggested by rate and regularity of the pulse. Changes in weight can reflect fluid balance. Tachypnea may suggest acidosis or hypoxia.
   3. **Neck.** Inspect for jugular venous distention. Congestive heart failure, tamponade, and tension pneumothorax can all cause bulging neck veins.

4. **Cardiac.** Muffled heart tones can suggest tamponade. A new gallop may be present with fluid overload or a change in contractility. Listen for new murmurs, arrhythmias, or rubs.

5. **Pulmonary.** Rales imply fluid overload potentially caused by cardiac failure. Decreased breath sounds may indicate pneumothorax.

6. **Abdomen.** Application of pressure on the right upper quadrant of the abdomen can temporarily augment preload and increase BP and CO when hypovolemia is the cause.

7. **Extremities.** Assess perfusion by color and capillary refill. Assess volume status by inspecting for edema or changes in turgor.

B. **Laboratory Data**

1. **Serum electrolytes.** Chronic cardiac failure induces the renin angiotensin aldosterone system altering sodium and potassium balance. Hyper- or hypokalemia or changes in calcium balance can influence contractility. An increased anion gap can signal acidosis.

2. **Hemoglobin.** Counts may be elevated or decreased with hypovolemia or hypervolemia. Post op hemorrhage can be associated with decreased CO. The coexisting presence of anemia in the face of decreased CO is potentially quite serious due to the resulting large decrease in oxygen delivery.

3. **Arterial blood gases.** Acidosis may be the cause or result of decreased CO. Status of oxygenation can be confirmed.

4. **Cardiac injury panel.** CPK, LDH, and troponin levels may reveal evidence of myocardial injury.

C. **Radiographic and Other Studies**

1. **Chest radiograph.** Look for the presence of pneumothorax, widened mediastinum, Kerley-B lines, or increased pulmonary vascular markings. Also check for proper positioning of a thermodilution catheter.

2. **ECG.** Arrhythmias, ST changes, new Q waves or flipped T waves may indicate myocardial ischemia or damage.

3. **Echocardiogram.** Echocardiography may be the gold standard test to assess decreased CO. It can be useful to evaluate contractility and the presence of wall motion abnormalities. It may help assess preload by analyzing the status of ventricular filling. Tamponade, valvular dysfunction, and hypertrophic cardiomyopathy can be ruled out. It may serve to estimate cardiac output and confirm the decreased measurement. It may also be used to differentiate right from left heart failure.

V. **Plan.** Identify and treat the underlying cause.

A. **Initial Management.** Prioritize with the standard ABCs. If the patient deteriorates to the point of requiring intubation, this should be done without hesitation. Once airway protection is ensured, examine for arrhythmias, conduction abnormalities, or tamponade that would necessitate emergency measures. When the patient is stable from a cardiopulmonary standpoint despite low CO, methodically begin to explore other variables.

B. Confirm Low CO. Repeat CO measurements, ensure proper thermodilution technique, and compare with previous measurements to determine trends. Consider other measurements of CO, such as with Doppler techniques, echocardiographic estimations, or CO_2 rebreathing devices.

C. Treatment of Specific Conditions

1. **Bradycardia or heart block.** Initiate chronotropic (isoproterenol) and/or inotropic drugs to increase heart rate. Consider transcutaneous or transvenous pacing (see page 42).

2. **Tachyarrhythmia.** Treatment of a rapid rate in the presence of decreased CO is difficult when there is any question about decreased ventricular function. Use of a short-acting beta-blocker, such as esmolol, may be considered as a trial. When it has adverse effects on inotropy, it may be easily discontinued and other treatment options considered. Rate control is important in the face of stenotic cardiac valvular lesions (see page 244).

3. **Hypovolemia.** Suspicion of hypovolemia (decreasing CVP, decreasing PCWP, tachycardia, and decreasing urine output) should be aggressively tested with a trial of serial fluid boluses. Filling pressures should be optimized. When hemoglobin is low, red blood cell transfusion should be initiated. A search for the cause of hypovolemia should occur simultaneously. Relative hypovolemia may be simulated by any increase in intrathoracic pressures that, in turn, increase right atrial pressure and decrease venous return. A recent change in pulmonary compliance or mechanical ventilatory parameters often has such an effect. Reconsider any recent ventilator changes, and reassess the pulmonary status of the patient.

4. **Hypervolemia.** Fluid overload leading to heart failure should be aggressively treated with diuresis and other supportive measures. Supplemental oxygen, inotropes, narcotics, and PEEP may be used.

5. **Myocardial ischemia.** New ischemia or infarction will decrease ventricular compliance and contractility. The result will be lower cardiac output, high wall tensions, increased oxygen consumption, and a worsening cycle. Interruption of this process requires aggressive therapy on several fronts. Heart rate control with beta-blockade is important to decrease cardiac work and optimize time for perfusion of the coronary arteries. Another primary therapy is control of preload with nitrates that decrease left ventricular end-diastolic pressure and also enhance myocardial perfusion. Ensure adequate oxygen delivery through administration of supplemental oxygen delivery and optimization of hematocrit. Early consultation with cardiologists should be obtained (see page 96).

6. **Cardiogenic shock.** Decreased CO in the face of adequate preload and reasonable afterload will require the administration of inotropic agents and perhaps the use of other therapeutic modalities. Dobutamine, dopamine, epinephrine, or other medications should be considered. Phosphodiesterase inhibitors, such as amrinone and milrinone, are also often used. Consultation with cardiologists and cardiac surgeons should be initiated for consideration of mechanical support of the circulation. The use of intraaortic balloon counterpulsation devices to facilitate ventricular ejection will increase cardiac output (see page 161). Use of such devices may help alleviate myocardial ischemia and can support a failing heart until surgical intervention for ischemia or acute valvular dysfunction can occur. In heroic situations, use of ventricular assist devices can be considered.

7. **Cardiac tamponade or tension pneumothorax.** These conditions can have dramatic effects by compromising cardiac filling and output. They are suspected in the presence of equalization of diastolic pressures including PCWP, CVP, and pulmonary artery diastolic pressures. Echocardiography is used to evaluate and confirm the diagnosis of cardiac tamponade. A chest radiograph best demonstrates tension pneumothorax. Needle aspiration or tube drainage of either space under tension will have dramatic effects and alleviate the drop in CO.

25. DECREASED CENTRAL VENOUS PRESSURE (CVP)

I. **Problem.** You are called to the bedside of a 63-year-old postoperative patient after the nurse reports a significantly decreased CVP reading.

II. **Immediate Questions**

A. **What are the vital signs?** Have blood pressure and heart rate changed? Is the patient hemodynamically stable?

B. **Are there any obvious signs of bleeding?** Is the reading real? Is the transducer open to air? Has it been zeroed recently?

C. **Has the patient's position changed?** Is the transducer at the appropriate height?

D. **What is the patient's urine output?** Has the urine output decreased over the last 4 h?

E. **Is the central venous catheter properly positioned?** Is there a record of how far the central line was inserted originally? Has the insertion distance significantly changed? Is there a recent x-ray verifying its position?

F. **Can you still draw blood from the line?** Inability to draw blood may indicate that the port is clotted and is not accurately reading CVP.

G. **Is the waveform normal?** A dampened waveform may indicate that the catheter is no longer in the proper position. Ideally, the catheter should be positioned within or adjacent to the right atrium.

III. Differential Diagnosis

A. **Spurious Reading.** The transducer may be at the wrong height and has been moved since the last reading.

B. **Hypovolemia.** CVP correlates with the volume of blood returning to the heart from the systemic circulation.

C. **Hemorrhage.** Check any surgical wounds or indwelling drains for bleeding. Check for gastrointestinal blood loss.

D. **Extravascular Catheter Migration.** The catheter may have migrated out of a central vein into an extravascular space.

E. **Normovolemia Following Appropriate Diuresis.** When vital signs are stable, it is possible that the patient has begun to mobilize fluids. Normovolemia may be present with a low CVP, whereas the patient was overhydrated with a higher CVP when the line was first inserted.

F. **Position Change.** The patient's position may have changed without any change in volume status. The transducer may now be above the right atrium point of reference for pressure readings.

G. **Mechanical Problem.** The catheter may be kinked or mechanically obstructed. The transducer may have failed or be open to air. A stopcock may be turned the wrong way.

IV. Database

A. **Physical Exam Key Points**
   1. **Vital signs.** Look for tachycardia and hypotension, or orthostatic blood pressure changes.
   2. **Neck.** Assess jugular veins for correlation with CVP.
   3. **Physical appearance.** Decreased capillary refill, decreased skin turgor, and a pale appearance suggest hypovolemia and hemorrhage as a cause.
   4. **Inspect, palpate, and percuss surgical site.** Look for bleeding.
   5. **Check any indwelling drains. Inspect insertion site of central line.** Examine the insertion site. Measure the length of catheter inside the patient. Look for anything that may be obstructing the catheter or an open connection.

B. **Laboratory Data**
   1. **Hemoglobin.** Assess bleeding as a cause of decreased CVP.
   2. **Type and Hold.** Anticipate the need for blood transfusion.

C. **Radiographic and Other Studies**
   1. **Chest radiograph.** Evaluate the location of the central venous catheter. Look for hemothorax after thoracic surgery.

V. Plan. Remember that the CVP measurement taken in isolation is rarely helpful. The measurement is helpful when it is used to monitor trends. Do not react to a number, but instead, correlate the result to the clinical situation. Ensure that the patient is hemodynamically stable and sort out the cause of decreased CVP. Recognize that a decreased CVP measurement may not be a cause for action.

  A. Initial Management. After ensuring that the CVP is accurate and is a reflection of decreased intravascular volume, give a fluid bolus. Evaluate changes in hemodynamic variables. Monitor urine output in response to fluid.

  B. Transfusion. Consider transfusing patient if there is ongoing blood loss, and the patient is unstable. Treat ongoing blood loss as necessary. Do nothing if patient is normovolemic.

26. DECREASED INTRACRANIAL PRESSURE (ICP)

  I. Problem. You are called about an ICP reading of 4 mm Hg in an 18-year-old patient with severe frontal cerebral contusions and subarachnoid hemorrhage.

  II. Immediate Questions

   A. What are the vital signs? Bradycardia with hypertension and low respiratory rate constitute the classic Cushing's triad and may indicate impending or recent herniation.

   B. What have the recent ICP readings been? Trends in the value create a more meaningful clinical picture.

   C. Has the change been gradual or sudden? Sudden decrease in ICP may indicate that herniation has occurred.

   D. Is the monitor intact? A dislodged or disrupted catheter may lead to aberrant readings.

  III. Differential Diagnosis

   A. Brain death. Complete herniation and decompression of the brain through the skull either through a craniotomy or the brain stem.

   B. Overzealous medical treatment of increased ICP. Excessive hyperventilation, dehydration, sedatives, or barbiturates may all lead to decreases in the ICP. In many instances, there may be consequences to this overtreatment.

   C. Drainage of CSF. Either unintentional via a catheter malfunction or intentional via a ventriculostomy for increased ICP. Examination of the patient and inspection of the ventriculostomy system should be done.

   D. CSF leak. Undiagnosed drainage postoperative (craniotomy, laminectomy, lumbar puncture, epidural). External leakage may be confused with diaphoresis in critically ill patients. Rarely, spontaneous intracranial hypotension can occur.

IV. Database

A. History. Usually limited, because most patients will be intubated in the ICU but may have complaints of headache, which is aggravated by posture. Other symptoms are nonspecific including dizziness, decreased hearing, photophobia, nausea, and vomiting.

B. Physical Exam Key Points
1. **Vital signs.** Hypertension and bradycardia are found with increasing ICP and herniation. For some patients, herniation and loss of brain function will lead to substantial hemodynamic lability.
2. **Neurologic exam.** Limited findings except acutely changed or decreased LOC. A cranial nerve palsy (typically the third or sixth) may possibly be identified.

C. Laboratory Data. There are no specific laboratory studies to establish the cause of decreased ICP.

D. Radiographic and Other Data
1. Diagnosed by a low CSF pressure on the monitor. Integrity of the monitoring system should be checked.
2. When a lumbar puncture has been done, the pressures will be low.
3. **MRI/CT scan** if obtained can show ventricular shrinkage, vertical displacement of the pons and tonsils with the subsequent development of a subdural effusion.

V. Plan

A. Check patient for signs of life.

B. Place in supine position and rehydrate if necessary.

C. Check connections of the ventriculostomy for CSF leaks or malfunction connections. One may need to replace the hardware.

D. De-intensify medical treatment, if possible.

E. Postoperative complications may require a repair with a blood patch or bone flap to control a CSF leak.

27. DELIRIUM TREMENS

I. Problem. An alcoholic is admitted with alcohol withdrawal seizures 2 d after stopping drinking. Despite an as-needed benzodiazepine order, he gets no sleep and 2 d later is hallucinating, severely agitated, tachycardic, and febrile.

II. Immediate Questions

A. What are the patient's vital signs? Autonomic overactivity is common in DT.

B. What is the patient's mental status?

    C. **Is the patient a known alcoholic?** Has the patient progressed to delirium tremens?

    D. **What medications were given to the patient?**

III. **Differential Diagnosis.** Because delirium tremens occurs late in alcohol withdrawal, it rarely presents a diagnostic challenge. For the patient who has advanced to delirium tremens before hospital presentation and for whom history is unobtainable, it may occasionally be confused with stimulant overdose and more rarely with schizophrenia.

    A. **Withdrawal Syndromes**

    B. **Delirium Tremens (DTs).** A person who abuses alcohol may develop delirium 3–5 d after hospitalization.

    C. **Opioid.** Two days after cessation of drug; restlessness, hypertension, nausea, diarrhea, rhinorrhea, and lacrimation.

    D. **Barbiturates.** Like DT.

    E. **Metabolic Alterations.** Electrolytes, hypoxia, and drug intoxications.

    F. **Infectious.** Sepsis, meningitis, and encephalitis.

    G. **ICU Psychosis**

    H. **Endocrine.** Thyroid, adrenal, hypoglycemia, diabetic ketoacidosis, and hyperosmolar coma.

IV. **Database**

    A. **History.** Look for a 3–5-d cessation of alcohol ingestion and preceding anxiety, confusion hallucinations, insomnia, and seizures.

    B. **Physical Exam Key Points**
        1. **Vital signs.** Autonomic hyperactivity; tremor, diaphoresis, tachycardia, and fever.
        2. **Neurologic exam.** Exclude focal findings. Mental status exam will establish the presence of true delirium.

    C. **Laboratory Data**
        1. **ABG.** Assess hypoxemia.
        2. **Electrolytes.**

    D. **Radiographic and Other Studies**
        1. **CT scan of the head.** Patients with confusion and evidence of head trauma may require head CT, to exclude intracranial hemorrhages that may have resulted from seizures.
        2. **Chest radiograph.** Patients with respiratory distress may require chest radiographs to exclude the presence of aspiration sequelae.

V. **Plan.** Delirium tremens is a medical emergency leading to a mortality rate of 20%.

    A. Benzodiazepines must be administered in doses sufficient to allow sleep. Unlike the alcohol withdrawal which precedes it, delirium tremens often require benzodiazepine administration, resulting in respiratory suppression. Patients will require close monitoring for possible intubation and mechanical ventilation.

B. Nonbenzodiazepine anticonvulsants are not indicated unless patients suffer status epilepticus.

C. Correct compounding factors, such as electrolyte abnormalities, hypoxemia, hypoglycemia, and others.

28. DISLODGED ICP MONITOR

I. Problem. A 24-year-old woman who sustained a closed head injury had an ICP monitor placed. The catheter is no longer in its original position.

II. Immediate Questions

    A. What type of catheter is in place? The majority of ICP monitors are secured to the skull with a "wing nut" type of device through which a fiberoptic catheter is inserted.

    B. Is the entire assembly dislodged or only the catheter? The fiberoptic component may dislodge from the system.

    C. What were the indications for ICP monitoring? The clinical situation may have stabilized or changed such that the device is no longer required.

III. Differential Diagnosis

    A. Catheter Malfunction. When the fiberoptic system gets disrupted, the readings may be unobtainable. Inspection of the system will identify the integrity of the catheter to patient junction.

    B. Catheter Dislodgment. The catheter may be completely dislodged from the securing device. Visual inspection will confirm this situation.

    C. "Wing Nut" Dislodgment. The entire system has become disrupted with effective stripping of the threads at the skull system junction.

IV. Database

    A. Physical Exam Key Points

        1. Visual and physical inspection of the ICP system should be undertaken. Laxity in the fit are indicative of entire system dislodgment. Catheter separation will be evident by the absence of the catheter from the securing device.

        2. Neurologic. Global neurologic status and changes from baseline should be documented. Improvement or long-term stability may indicate that monitoring is no longer needed.

    B. Laboratory Data. No specific laboratory studies are indicated.

    C. **Radiographic and Other Data.** No specific radiographic studies are required.

V. **Plan.** Once the type of dislodgment is identified, the appropriate corrective measures may be undertaken (see page 34 for placement of the device).

    A. **Complete System Dislodgment.** A new system with a new twist drill site is necessary when continued monitoring is indicated.

    B. **Catheter Only Dislodgment.** A new fiberoptic catheter may be placed through the wing nut securing system if the wing nut remains secure.

29. DOUBLE LUMEN INTUBATION

I. **Problem.** A 72-year-old man with known lung cancer is being transferred to your unit because of severe respiratory distress caused by hemoptysis, possibly from his tumor. The transferring team requests lung separation by intubation with a double-lumen endotracheal tube.

II. **Immediate Questions**

    A. **Is intubation with a double lumen tube (DLT) indicated?** Absolute indications for the placement of a DLT include prevention of cross-contamination of the uninvolved lung with blood or pus from the involved lung. By keeping the blood (or infected material) confined to the affected side, the gas-exchanging capacity of the normal lung will be preserved. Other absolute indications include instances where differential ventilation of the two lungs may be needed. For example, a patient with a unilateral bronchopleural fistula will require particular ventilator settings to minimize leak and maximize gas exchange in the affected lung versus the intact lung. And finally, in the case of bronchopulmonary lavage, lung separation will allow easy access to the involved lung, while ventilation can continue uninterrupted in the contralateral lumen.

    B. **What contraindications should be considered?** The major contraindication to placement of a DLT is an endobronchial mass or other obstruction along the path of its placement. Relative contraindications include the patient in whom direct laryngoscopy is assessed to be difficult, or the intubated patient who is already very dependent on mechanical ventilation and cannot tolerate its interruption during the exchange to a DLT. Such manipulation could even lead to a lost airway if the patient cannot be reintubated because of airway swelling, bleeding, or trauma. Also, a small patient with a small larynx or prior history of laryngeal surgery or stenosis may preclude placement of a DLT because of the larger outer diameter compared with conventional endotracheal tubes.

    C. **What equipment (and expertise) is needed?** Most importantly, correctly placing a DLT requires an advanced skill level and expertise.

When your experience with this device is limited, consult an anesthesiologist or experienced intensivist before attempting any such intervention. Invariably, this person will have had the most experience with DLTs and will be of great assistance as there are many caveats and details of placement and lung isolation not discussed in this brief text. After calling for the appropriate help, gather the needed equipment. Be sure to have a bag and mask, oxygen source, and suction available. Also, ensure that the patient is appropriately monitored. The only additional equipment that may be needed is a fiberoptic bronchoscope (FOB) that can pass through both lumens of the DLT. Again, if experience is limited, do not begin any maneuver or medicate the patient before the appropriate help and equipment arrives.

III. **Differential Diagnosis.** Not applicable.

IV. **Database**

A. **Physical Exam Key Points**
   1. **Lungs.** Auscultate for bilateral breath sounds.

B. **Laboratory Data**
   1. **ABG.** Pre- and postintubation.

C. **Radiographic and Other Studies**
   1. **Chest radiograph.**

V. **Plan**

A. **Procedure.** How to select and place the appropriate DLT.
   1. **Selecting the appropriate DLT. Right-sided DLT versus left-sided DLT.** DLTs are available in both right- and left-sided models, named according to which mainstem bronchus is intubated. There is no absolute indication for using one side or the other. Known unilateral obstructing lesions or fresh bronchial suture lines may be a consideration. In general, because of the more proximal origin of the right upper lobe (RUL) bronchus, a left-sided DLT is usually easier to place (Figs I–12 and I–13). Furthermore, the RUL bronchus can vary dramatically in its location and, in some patients, may actually originate from the trachea itself. In this case, use of a right-sided DLT is highly problematic. Because of this proximal location of the RUL, a right-sided DLT has a ventilation slot that fits over the RUL bronchial orifice. Correctly placing and maintaining this position can be difficult. The left-sided DLT does not require such a ventilation slot, as the left upper lobe branch-point is more distal than on the right. Consequently there is a significantly larger margin of safety for left-sided tubes, and, therefore, they are more likely to function properly in the event of a slight position change.
   2. **Selecting the appropriate sized DLT.** Choosing the appropriate size depends roughly on the patient's height (and somewhat on body weight). Women tend to require a 35 Fr or 37 Fr, whereas a

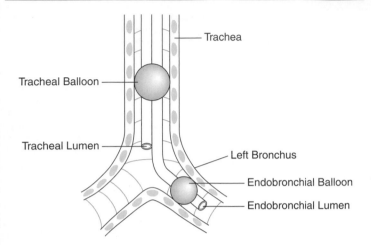

Figure I–12. Correct placement of left-sided double-lumen tube.

39 Fr or 41 Fr is appropriate for most men. Although this can vary, the best sizing method is based on inflation of the bronchial cuff. Once the DLT has been placed, carefully inflate the bronchial cuff. The choice of the correct size is confirmed when only 1–3 cc of air are needed to effect a seal. When more than 3 cc are required to achieve a seal, the tube is too small; a need for less volume suggests the tube may be too large.

3. **Placement.** Hold the DLT with the distal curvature concave to the anterior of the patient, so that the endobronchial portion approaches the vocal cords, just as with a standard single-lumen tube. Visualize the vocal cords with a direct laryngoscope, and place the endobronchial end and its cuff beyond the vocal cords. Once this is done, partially withdraw the stylet from the distal end of the DLT. Advance the DLT while rotating 90 degrees (counterclockwise for left-sided tubes and clockwise for right-sided tubes). This rotation will result in the endobronchial portion angled toward the correct mainstem bronchus.

4. **Verification of placement.** First, verify tracheal intubation by chest rise, auscultation of bilateral breath sounds, capnography, and maintenance of oxygen saturation, just as following conventional intubation. Next, verify correct endobronchial placement by auscultation. For example, with a left-sided tube, clamping the tracheal lumen and ventilating only the bronchial side should result in breath sounds heard only over the left lung field. Clamping the

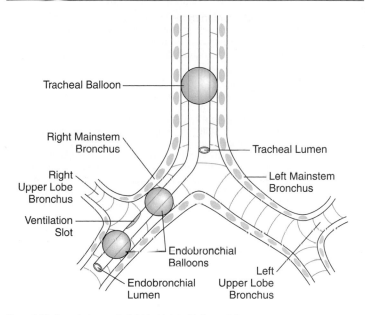

Figure I–13. Correct placement of right-sided double-lumen tube.

bronchial part and ventilating only through the tracheal lumen will leave only right-sided breath sounds. With a right DLT, the results will, of course, be opposite. Direct visual verification and fine adjustments in positioning can be made with the fiberoptic bronchioooope (FOB). Place the FOB into the tracheal lumen of the DLT and advance to the end of the lumen. The carina should be in view along with the intubated bronchus. The bronchial cuff should be barely visible around the circumference of the endobronchial tube. When more than a third of the bronchial cuff is seen, the tube will need to be advanced. Inability to visualize the bronchial cuff suggests that the tube may be in too deep. When needed, fine adjustments in depth can be made under direct visualization with the FOB after deflating both cuffs (tracheal and endobronchial). Next, pass the FOB down the bronchial lumen to make certain that the left upper lobe is not being blocked in the case of a left-sided tube, or that the ventilation slot of the right-sided tube fits nicely over the RUL orifice in the case of a right-sided tube. Beware, however, that direct visualization may not be possible or reliable because of blood or secretions in the airway. Finally, if necessary, check for functional isolation of the lungs, as this is the ultimate goal of lung separation. Again, an experienced practitioner will be of great help. Proper assessment and correction of problems may require a great degree of skill in some settings.

B. Problems and Complications

1. **Malposition.** Although confirmation of correct initial placement of a DLT by auscultation, FOB (if possible), and functional assessment are reassuring, any change in patient position can markedly affect proper placement and, hence, function. For example, flexion of the head can shift the entire DLT caudad, resulting in total mainstem intubation; extension of the head may completely dislodge the endobronchial cuff out of the bronchus. Similar movements may occur with Trendelenburg or reverse-Trendelenburg positioning or lateral positioning. Coughing can also result in tube movement. Reconfirm the position of the DLT after any change in patient position. Always be vigilant for changes in oxygen saturation, airway pressure, auscultation, and capnography, as these are clues to malposition. Always have a low threshold to check the tube's position when there is any question of placement.

2. **Glottic damage.** Care must be taken when placing a DLT so as not to cause damage to the glottis. Despite this, glottic trauma may occur caused by the mere presence of the tube itself, because DLTs have a much larger outer diameter than conventional single-lumen tubes. For example, the outer diameter of the relatively small 35 Fr DLT (O.D. = 11.1 mm) is slightly greater than that of an 8.0 endotracheal tube (O.D. = 10.25 mm).

3. **Tracheal or bronchial rupture.** Most commonly, this occurs along the posterior membranous wall of the trachea during insertion. The likelihood of such damage is lessened if one removes or withdraws the stylet before advancing the DLT (see Placement section) and avoids excessive force. Again, operator experience is vital. Also, excessive bronchial cuff pressure can lead to bronchial wall ischemia, and high volumes could cause rupture. Whenever a DLT is in place, be watchful for pneumothorax, pneumomediastinum, subcutaneous emphysema, or hemodynamic instability. Although a DLT can be a life-saving tool, prolonged use is not desirable. Although no true "time limit" exists, it is considered best to change it to a standard tube as soon as possible to reduce or avoid the aforementioned problems.

DLT Size	Outer Diameter (mm)
35 Fr	11.1
37 Fr	11.8
39 Fr	12.4
41 Fr	13.1

30. DYSPNEA

I. **Problem.** Acute dyspnea develops in a patient immediately after a difficult pulmonary artery catheterization via the right internal jugular vein.

II. **Immediate Questions**

A. **Does the patient have history of asthma or other pulmonary conditions?** Is there any significant cardiac disease?

B. **What are the vital signs?** Does the patient oxygenate well? Is it wheezing or stridor or rales?

C. **Is there associated chest pain?** Pleuritic chest pain?

D. **Did the dyspnea occur abruptly or gradually?** Exertional, hemoptysis, or sputum production?

E. **Is there orthopnea, paroxysmal nocturnal dyspnea, or platypnea?**

F. Have any recent procedures been performed (intubation, central venous catheter, temporary pacemaker or abdominal procedures)?

III. **Differential Diagnosis.** Dyspnea can have numerous possible causes that may involve single or multiple organ systems. It is usually a challenge for physicians to evaluate and diagnose the cause of dyspnea. Dyspnea may be accounted for by a decrease in ventilatory capacity, an increase in ventilatory demand during exercise, or the perception of increased breathing as being uncomfortable.

A. **Limited List of Possible Causes of Dyspnea**
1. **Pulmonary Causes.**
   a. **Airway obstruction.** Laryngospasm, foreign body, tracheal stenosis, tracheomalacia, asthma/COPD exacerbation.
   b. **Pleural/Chest wall.** Pleural effusions, chest wall injury, abdominal distension, pneumothorax, rib fracture, fibrothorax.
   c. **Vascular.** Pulmonary embolus, pulmonary hypertension, vasculitis, veno-occlusive
   d. **Parenchymal.** Pneumonitis, alveolitis, carcinomatosis, metastatic disease, pulmonary fibrosis, ARDS
2. **Nonpulmonary Causes.**
   a. **Cardiac.** Arrhythmia, congestive heart failure, ischemic heart disease, intracardiac shunt, pericardial disease, valvular disease, myxoma.
   b. **Neuromuscular.** CNS disorder, spinal cord injury, systemic muscular disorder, diaphragmatic disorder, myopathy, neuropathy.
   c. **Other.** Anemia, thyroid diseases, GERD, metabolic acidosis, deconditioning, psychogenic.

IV. **Database.** When evaluating a patient with shortness of breath, it would be useful to keep in mind its differential diagnosis, including pulmonary and nonpulmonary (cardiac, neuromuscular and others) causes. A thorough history and physical examination should be performed with close attention to the patient's vital signs, including the oxygen saturation. A chest radiograph, EKG, and ABG should be obtained while the following clinical clues are being processed to further delineate the possible cause(s).

A. **Physical Exam Key Points**
   1. **Vital signs.** Fever, tachypnea, and pulse oxymetry.
   2. **Pulmonary.** Respiratory distress, rales, wheezing, stridor, consolidation, and decreased breath sounds.
   3. **Cardiac.** Evidence of CHF.
   4. **Mental status.**
   5. **Musculocutaneous.** Evidence for potential PE (swelling), pallor, cyanosis, and evidence of CHF.

B. **Laboratory Data**
   1. **Hemogram.**
   2. **ABG.**
   3. **Blood and sputum cultures.**
   4. **Electrolytes.**

C. **Radiographic and Other Studies**
   1. **Chest X-ray.**
   2. **ECG.**
   3. **Other.** PFTs, $\dot{V}/\dot{Q}$-Scan, angiogram, and echocardiogram.

V. **Plan.** Because the list of possible causes of dyspnea is quite extensive, it is important to identify, stabilize, and promptly treat the more life-threatening cause (eg, tension pneumothorax, severe obstructive or stenotic airway, pulmonary edema with cardiogenic shock, or massive pleural effusion). A specific treatment plan for other less emergent causes should be carried out accordingly.

A. **Oxygen.** Maintain Sao_2 at more than 90%.

31. ELECTROCARDIOGRAM (ECG) CHANGES: ACUTE MYOCARDIAL INFARCTION

I. **Problem.** A 55-year-old man with a history of hypertension, hyperlipidemia, and a smoking history of 30 pack-years is admitted with a 1-h history of "crushing" substernal chest pain radiating to his jaw with associated shortness of breath and diaphoresis. His presenting ECG shows sinus bradycardia with a rate of 50 bpm, a 3-mm ST segment elevation in leads II, III, and aVF, and an ST- segment depression in leads V_1–V_3, I, and aVL.

II. **Immediate Questions**

   A. **How many ECGs were done and at what interval?** A single ECG is not the gold standard for the diagnosis of an acute myocardial infarction (AMI). The initial ECG may be nondiagnostic in 20–50% of cases of AMI. It is recommended to do three ECGs every 20 min as soon as the patient complains of chest pain.

B. Does the patient have previously known ECG changes? The ECG diagnosis of AMI may be obscured by many conditions. This is particularly true in the presence of left bundle branch block or left ventricular hypertrophy, which may distort the initial ECG vector and may mimic or mask the changes seen in infarction.

C. Does the patient have a previous history of CAD or risk factors? The decision to admit a patient with chest pain to a coronary care unit should be based on the patient's history and physical exam findings.

D. What is the appearance of the ECG? Observe for the presence of ST segment elevation or depression, Q waves, T-wave inversions, reciprocal changes, presence of confounding factors such as LBBB, LVH, and global changes (not in any one territory). The diagnosis of an AMI is based on at least two of the three following criteria: (1) history of chest pain; (2) characteristic ECG changes; and (3) elevations in cardiac enzymes (Figs I-14, I-15, and I-16).

E. Are there any concomitant cardiac enzyme changes?

III. Differential Diagnosis

A. Acute MI. Early on, a marked increase in R-wave voltage may occur. Hyperacute (prominent) T waves with normal direction occur early (> 5 mm); they are peaked and symmetric. ST segment elevation that is either convex or concave upward may also occur. Q waves > 0.04 s other than in aVR and T-wave inversions or flattening are also a possibility.

B. Predictive Value of Initial ECG in Acute MI (sensitivity/specificity).

New Q wave or ST segment elevation: 40%/>90%
Above ST segment depression: 75%/80%
Above (any) or prior ischemia/infarction changes: 85%/76%
Above (any) or nonspecific ST-T changes: 90%/65%

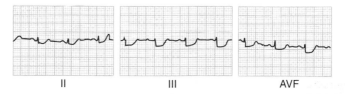

| II | III | AVF |

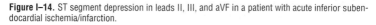

Figure I-14. ST segment depression in leads II, III, and aVF in a patient with acute inferior subendocardial ischemia/infarction.

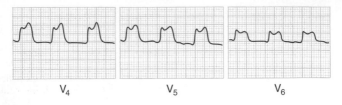

Figure I–15. ST elevation in leads V_4, V_5, and V_6 in a patient with acute anterolateral transmural ischemia/infarction.

C. Pericarditis. ST segment elevation in pericarditis or cardiac contusion usually may be distinguished from acute MI by a "nonstereotyped" ECG pattern failing to correspond to typical distributions for the coronary circulation. Unlike in MI, reciprocal ST segment changes seldom occur in opposing leads. The following are ECG findings in pericarditis:

1. ST elevation is diffuse, involving I, II, and III or two bipolar leads and V_1 to V_6.
2. ST depression is seen in aVR and may also occur in V_1 and II. Typically it is concave upward and < 5 mm in height. Pathologic Q waves are rare.
3. PR segment depression is seen in about 82% of patients.
4. Sequential changes: ST elevation, ST returns to base line, then T wave inversion, then T wave inversion of > 5 mm, then T wave normalizes.
5. Height of ST/T > 0.25 in V_5, V_6, or I.

D. Ventricular aneurysm. The ST segment elevation resulting from a ventricular aneurysm does not evolve on serial EKGs.

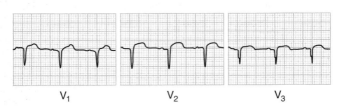

Figure I–16. Q waves in leads V_1, V_2, and V_3 in a patient with an acute anteroseptal transmural myocardial infarction. Note the ST elevation in helping to determine the acute nature of the infarction.

E. Pericardial fluid. Low voltage QRS or electrical alternans.

F. LBBB. Criteria for diagnosis of acute MI in the presence of LBBB.
1. ST elevation ≥ 1 mm in the same direction as QRS: 5 points.
2. ST depression ≥ 1 mm in leads V_1, V_2 and V_3: 3 points.
3. ST elevation ≥ 5 mm opposite with QRS: 2 points. ST elevation ≥ 3 points is 36–78% sensitive and 90–96% specific for acute MI.

G. Benign Early Repolarization
1. Upward concave appearance to ST segment.
2. ST elevations usually ≤ 5 mm. More often in V_3–V_6 than V_1–V_2.
3. Occasional reciprocal ST depressions.
4. Prominent T ≥ 7 mm.
5. Notched J point.
6. Pathologic Qs are rare.

IV. Database

A. Physical Exam Key Points
1. **Vital signs.** Look for signs of cardiac decompensation, adequate oxygenation, ventilation, respiratory distress, and heart rate/rhythm.
2. **Cardiopulmonary.** Notice signs of congestive failure; rales, wheezing, new onset murmurs, S_3 and S_4.
3. **Musculocutaneous.** Cyanosis, pallor and dependent edema.

B. Laboratory Data
1. **Hemogram.** Elevated leukocyte counts, glucose levels, and erythrocyte sedimentation rates in the appropriate clinical setting are suggestive but not diagnostic of acute MI.
2. **CK-MB and Troponin.**
3. **Electrolytes.** Rule out other potentially misleading electrolyte abnormalities.

C. Radiographic and Other Studies
1. **Serial ECGs.** Serial ECGs during the acute phase of suspected AMI are of critical importance. Evolutionary ST segment and T wave changes during an acute transmural MI usually persists for only 1–2 d and are followed after a variable time period by T wave inversions in those ECG leads that showed ST elevation. The ECG can localize the site of infarction or injury with considerable accuracy, based on which leads have abnormal Q waves (>0.03s) or ST-T wave changes. An acute transmural MI has an injury pattern characterized by elevation of the ST segment in different leads, depending on the location of the MI. The earliest change is the development of a hyperacute or peaked T wave that reflects localized hyperkalemia. Thereafter, the ST segment elevates with the following appearance: Initially the J point elevates and the ST

segment retains its concave configuration. Later, the ST segment becomes more pronounced and changes its shape, becoming more convex or rounded upward. The ST segment may eventually become more indistinguishable from the T wave. An initial Q wave develops and the R wave loses amplitude as the ST segment elevates. Later on, ECG changes evolve. The ST segment gradually returns to the isoelectric baseline; the R wave markedly reduces, and the Q wave deepens. In addition, the T wave inverts. These changes can occur within the first few days to weeks after the event.

V. Plan

A. Abnormal Q waves or ST-T wave changes (see Fig I–14)

1. **II, III, aVF: Inferior wall infarction.** Occasionally reciprocal ECG changes are observed in the initial period of the acute infarction, presenting with ST segment depressions in leads V_1 to V_3, I, or aVL. In the setting of an inferior wall infarction, always check for ST segment elevation in right-sided precordial leads (V_4R) to rule out a right ventricular infarction. In addition, tall R waves and/or ST segment depression in V_1 and V_2 and/or ST-T wave changes in extended precordial chest leads (V_7 to V_9) in the setting of an inferior wall infarction may represent a posterior wall infarction. This infarction pattern is most commonly seen in association with inferior wall infarction, as these portions of myocardium share a common blood supply (right coronary artery in 90% of individuals).

2. **V_1–V_6, I, and aVL: Anterolateral infarction** (see Fig I-15). Occasionally reciprocal ECG changes are observed, presenting as ST segment depressions in the inferior leads (I, II, and aVF).

3. **V_1–V_2: Anteroseptal infarction** (see Fig I-16). Occasionally reciprocal ECG changes are observed, with ST segment depressions in the inferior leads (II, III, and aVF) or lateral leads (I, aVL, V_5, and V_6).

4. **V_3–V_4: Anteroapical infarction.** Occasionally reciprocal ECG changes are observed, presenting as ST segment depressions in the inferior leads (II, III, aVF).

5. **V_5, V_6, I, and aVL: Lateral infarction.** Occasionally reciprocal ECG changes are observed, presenting as ST- segment depressions in the inferior leads (II, III, and aVF) and in some cases in leads V_1 and V_2.

B. The patient with ECG changes suggestive of MI should be admitted for continuous ECG monitoring with planned emergent cardioversion, if malignant arrhythmias develop. Unless contraindicated, aspirin and beta-blockers should be given. Depending on the type of MI and local expertise, the patient may benefit from early thrombolytic therapy, emergent angioplasty, or emergent coronary stenting.

32. ENDOTRACHEAL TUBE: AIR LEAK, MALPOSITION, MALFUNCTION

Immediate Actions. Always remember the ABCs of resuscitation. Loss of the airway is an extremely dangerous situation, and arguably the fastest way to accelerate a rapid demise in an already deteriorating situation. Good airway management requires not only skill but also judgment and experience. When you are lacking in any one of these three, call for help early. There are some areas of medicine that an inexperienced practitioner can "muddle through" without catastrophic results; airway management is not one of them.

I. **Problem.** A 27-year-old man after a motorcycle accident with multiple rib fractures, facial trauma, and a closed head injury who is intubated, sedated, and paralyzed has just returned from the CT scanner when the respiratory therapist reports a significant leak around the endotracheal tube.

II. **Immediate Questions**

 A. **Is the patient being effectively ventilated?** A partially dislodged endotracheal tube (ETT) or a ruptured ETT cuff can sometimes allow for suboptimal, yet nevertheless, life-saving ventilation.

 B. **Is the patient breathing?** In this scenario with a paralyzed sedated patient, respiratory effort is less likely. However, if the ETT is obstructed or dislodged, and the patient has some spontaneous ventilatory effort, the situation may be less critical. A spontaneously breathing patient affords some extra margin of safety.

 C. **What is the F_{IO_2}?** Anytime the security of the airway is in question, switch to 100% oxygen, even if the patient is 100% saturated. Should an airway crisis develop, the patient with a higher P_{AO_2} and 100% oxygen in the lungs will have a longer reserve time before becoming hypoxic.

III. **Differential Diagnosis**

 A. **Endotracheal Tube (ETT) Incorrectly Positioned**
  1. **ETT dislodged from trachea.** Unexpected extubation is most likely to occur after a patient has been mobilized or during movement of an inadequately restrained or combative patient. However, even a thoroughly restrained patient can dislodge an endotracheal tube. Unanticipated extubation is a scenario that is likely to require immediate intervention.
  2. **Esophageal Intubation.** Esophageal intubation can result from a failed intubation or an unsuccessful attempt to advance a partially dislodged ETT. This is also a situation that will require immediate intervention.

B. **Endotracheal Tube (ETT) Correctly Positioned but Malfunctioning**
   1. **Cuff not appropriately inflated.** An inadequate volume of air in the cuff can cause a leak around the ETT cuff. Alternatively, there may have been a change in ventilatory conditions, such as a decrease in pulmonary compliance, resulting in higher airway pressures and a new leak around a previously adequately sealing cuff.

C. **Cuff leak.** A cuff leak can result from rupture of the cuff itself, laceration of the pilot tube, or malfunction of the valve at the end of the pilot tube. In most cases, the problem can be temporarily remedied without requiring an ETT change. A partially dislodged ETT with herniation of the cuff across the cords or glottis may appear at first to be ruptured.

IV. **Database**
   A. **Physical Exam Key Points**
      1. **Breath sounds.** Listen to the chest wall in the axillae and lateral chest wall where esophageal sounds are less likely to be transmitted and breath sounds are loudest.
      2. **Vital signs.** Desaturation by pulse oximetry is a late sign of hypoxia. Bradycardia secondary to hypoxia is a very late sign of hypoxia and suggests impending cardiopulmonary arrest.
      3. **Paralysis.** Reintubation and airway management may be facilitated by profound neuromuscular blockade. A peripheral nerve stimulator can be used to determine the level of blockade.
   B. **Laboratory Data**
      1. **ABG.**
   C. **Radiographic and Other Studies**
      1. **Chest radiograph.** A portable or standard chest radiograph or lateral C-spine film can be used to confirm placement of an ETT. However, the results of such studies typically take longer than is required to acutely manage an airway crisis. Save the radiograph for confirmation of ETT placement and tip location after the airway has been secured.
      2. **Other methods to assist in rapid assessment of ETT location.**
         a. **Capnography.** Capnography will detect carbon dioxide in expired gasses and help to confirm tracheal in contrast to esophageal intubation. It will not confirm proper tube location and function, as a herniating tube still occupying the laryngeal inlet will still produce expired CO_2.
         b. **Illuminated intubating stylet.** Passage of an illuminated intubating stylet (Trachlight) down a correctly positioned ETT will result in visualization of a characteristic pattern of transillumination through the upper tracheal rings as the light is passed down the ETT.
         c. **Esophageal detector devices.** Many simple devices have been used to help confirm tracheal versus esophageal intuba-

tion. Rapid aspiration from the top of the ETT using a 60 cc syringe fitted with a 15 mm adapter or the use of a commercially available self-inflating bulb will permit a discrimination to be made in most patients. Air is readily obtained from the trachea but not from the esophagus whose walls will collapse against the end of the tube. This may be unreliable in obese patients or those with severe emphysema but otherwise is quite reliable at picking up esophageal intubation.

    d. Bronchoscopy. When a bronchoscope is available, its passage down the ETT can confirm proper placement (visualization of tracheal rings and the carina). Assessment of distances from the tip of the tube to the carina can be made and may help determine whether a tube is in or out too far. A skilled practitioner can use a bronchoscope to facilitate reintubation if needed.

    e. Direct laryngoscopy. Direct visualization by a skilled practitioner can confirm tube placement and permit immediate reintubation if needed. This may be difficult in a critically ill patient because of swelling from prolonged intubation and pathophysiologic changes accompanying the current illness. Furthermore, adequate sedation and relaxation is usually indicated.

V. Plan. The greatest priority should be given to ensuring good patient oxygenation. Every ICU bed should have immediately available suction, a mask, a self-inflating Ambubag, and an oxygen source. Also, a selection of laryngoscope handles and endotracheal tubes should be nearby and readily available.

    A. Initial Management. This is the time to call for backup if you are uncomfortable managing an airway on your own. Remember that ICU patients rarely have pristine airways; many have been instrumented, bloodied, or anatomically disfigured by edema from prolonged intubation or fluid therapy. Even a skilled practitioner may have difficulty identifying the anatomy during intubation.

    B. Partially Dislodged ETT. When the ETT is partially dislodged, the cuff can be deflated and the ETT gently advanced (20–24 cm at the lip is usually sufficient for most adults). An intubating stylet, such as a gum elastic bougie or an ETT exchanger, passed through the tube first, will maximize the chances of the ETT being redirected into the trachea. Listen for breath sounds, or use portable capnography to confirm tracheal placement of the tube. Alternatively, a fiberoptic bronchoscope could be used in place of the stylet to permit visual confirmation of placement and also be used to redirect a tube back into the trachea. When the tube is not in the trachea or cannot be redirected into the trachea, remove it entirely, and either ventilate the patient by mask or attempt to reintubate the patient when stable.

    C. Esophageal Intubation. Intubation of a non-CO_2-producing end organ (ie, the esophagus) can usually be recognized by the lack of clear bilateral breath sounds and the absence of sustained CO_2 on capnography. It is important to recognize that even skilled practitioners can be fooled using only stethoscopy and that confirmation of correct placement with another method, such as end-tidal CO_2 detection, is vital. Physical exam can be especially misleading in the obese patient and those patients with pulmonary disease. Many anesthesiologists advocate leaving an esophageal ETT in situ to decompress the stomach and to mark the esophagus during subsequent attempts at laryngoscopy. However, when the esophageal ETT hinders mask ventilation, it must be removed promptly.

D. **Cuff Leak.** ETT cuffs are not infallible and are subject to leak for a variety of reasons. The first step in remedying the situation is to determine the source of the leak. The three sources of the leak are the valve, pilot tube, and cuff. The good news is that all can usually be jury-rigged without necessitating an ETT exchange. Cuff pressure is poorly estimated by palpation of the pilot tube balloon; it is more precisely measured with a cuff pressure gauge.

E. **Valve Dysfunction.** Air pressure is maintained in the cuff by a one-way valve located at the proximal end of the pilot tube balloon. Occasionally the valve will stick in the open position and allow air to escape. Placing a 3-way stopcock over the valve, refilling the cuff, and then turning the stopcock so that the off switch points toward the ETT will usually solve this problem. Reassess the cuff pressure in about 10 min.

F. **Pilot Tube Laceration.** The pilot tube is subject to tooth mastication-induced trauma in the patient with intact teeth. Thoroughly sedate and paralyze the patient before inserting your gloved fingers into the patient's mouth to examine the length of the pilot tube for a breech. When a laceration is found, the pilot tube can be carefully cut at the level of the tear. A repair is accomplished by insertion of a blunt 18 gauge needle or 22-gauge IV catheter (with the exposed needle cut off) into the pilot tube. A three-way stopcock is then attached as described previously. Alternatively, a new valve and tube from another ETT can be attached to the cut end. When inspection of the valve and pilot tube do not reveal the source of the problem, the most likely culprit is the cuff. When possible and safe, reintubation may be the best solution. Options include performing laryngoscopy with the ETT in place to be sure that the vocal cords can be visualized. It is important to have a tube one size smaller, in case edema makes reintubation difficult. Other options may include tube exchange, using a commercially available tube exchanger (or NG tube) with a lumen for oxygenation or, perhaps, a gum elastic bougie. A more conservative option for those not comfortable with reintubation for some reason is to frequently reinflate the cuff if the leak is small or consider using a syringe pump to insufflate air continuously into the cuff.

33. FALL FROM BED

I. **Problem.** The day after an open reduction and internal fixation of a humeral fracture, a 60-year-old man fell from bed while trying to go to the bathroom. He has a laceration on his forehead.

II. **Immediate Questions.** Most falls from bed are not associated with serious injury. However, they are extremely upsetting to the patient and the patient's family. Every fall from bed warrants a complete evaluation, documentation of the incident, and thorough search for injury. Pay attention to the "ABCs."

   A. **Is the patient able to speak?** Quickly assess the airway and mental status by having the patient answer the question "What happened?"

   B. **Is the patient back in bed?** To avoid further injury, log-roll patient onto a backboard, use in-line traction or cervical immobilization before placing patient back in bed. Assume a cervical spine injury, and place patient in soft cervical collar.

   C. **Is the patient in pain?** Pain will guide you to the obvious injuries. Perform a thorough physical examination, much like a trauma patient.

III. **Differential Diagnosis.** History obtained from the patient, visitors, and staff may be helpful in determining the underlying reason for the fall. Specific injuries incurred from the fall will not be covered here. Head injury, skeletal fractures, and dislocations lead the list. Review medication list and any recent medications the patient may have received.

   A. **Delirium.** See Problem 27, page 87 for a complete list.

   B. **Dementia.** Preexisting risk factor for falling and should be recognized for prevention. A minimental examination may be helpful.

   C. **Acute Change in Neurologic Status.**
      1. **Delayed recovery from anesthesia.**
      2. **Musculoskeletal weakness in postoperative period.**

IV. **Database**

   A. **Physical Exam Key Points**
      1. **Vital signs.** Fever can cloud the sensorium. Hypotension is seen in septic or cardiogenic shock. Arrhythmias, respiratory rate and pattern should also be evaluated.
      2. **HEENT.** Closely examine scalp and face for signs of head injury. Do a complete cranial nerve exam. Examine teeth.
      3. **Neck.** JVD, C-spine tenderness, nuchal rigidity.
      4. **Chest.** Bilateral breath sounds, wheezing, consolidation, cardiac murmurs, palpate ribs.
      5. **Abdomen.** Tenderness, bowel sounds to screen for abdominal injury.

      6. **Skin.** Bruising, lacerations.
      7. **Extremities.** Tenderness, obvious fractures, check IV lines.

  B. Laboratory Data
      1. **Hemogram.** Anemia, infection.
      2. **Serum electrolytes.** Hypo- and hyperglycemia, kalemia, calcemia, natremia, and magnesemia; uremia, ammonia.
      3. **Cardiac enzymes.** When MI is suspected.
      4. **Toxic drug screen.** When clinically indicated.
      5. **Arterial and venous blood gases.** Acid-base disorders, hypoxia.
      6. **Cultures.** Blood, urine, sputum, if infection suspected.

  C. Radiographic and Other Studies
      1. **ECG.** When MI is suspected or arrhythmia is noted.
      2. **Chest radiograph.** When a respiratory or infectious source is likely and when it is necessary to check for fractures. Rib detail films may be needed to evaluate for fractures.
      3. **Head CT.** For change in mental status.
      4. **Plain radiographs.** Tender extremities and joints to check for fracture or dislocation.
      5. **Lumbar puncture.** When indicated (check for nuchal rigidity).
      6. **EEG.** When indicated (eg, seizure disorder is suspected).
      7. **Pulse oximetry.** Noninvasive means of checking hypoxia.

V. Plan. Overall, an underlying cause for the fall should be sought and treated.

  A. Fractures and Dislocations. These should be splinted and the orthopedic service contacted for definitive care and follow-up. Always check for distal pulses before and after splinting.

  B. Lacerations. These should be cleaned and sutured. Use local wound care for abrasions.

  C. C-spine. When C-spine injury is suspected, immobilize neck and keep patient flat until the spine can be evaluated radiographically.

  D. Prevention of Further Injury. Mild sedation if warranted (perform a brief GCS before sedation). Ensure side rails of bed are up and that the patient is properly oriented to and can reach the nurse call button.

  E. Restraints When Necessary. A bedside commode may be useful both for the weak or elderly patient and also for physical therapy for reconditioning.

  F. Incident Report. Risk management includes completion of the report and documentation of the incident in the chart.

34. FEVER

  I. Problem. The nurse informed you that a 67-year-old patient in the ICU, after a pancreatectomy (Whipple's procedure), has a fever of 39.9 °C.

II. Immediate Questions

A. How high is the "fever?" The Society of Critical Care Medicine practice parameters define fever in the ICU as a temperature > 38.3 °C (>101 °F).

B. How many days postoperatively is the patient?

C. Did the patient have fevers before the operation?

D. Are there any associated complaints? Cough, dysuria, abdominal pain, and so forth.

E. Does the fever have any diurnal pattern?

F. What medications does the patient take? Has he/she stopped taking antibiotics, antipyretics?

III. Differential Diagnosis.

Fever is considered to be a cardinal sign of inflammation or infection. It has been described that certain cytokines, such as interleukin-1, IL-6, tumor necrosis factor-alpha, and interferon-alpha and gamma play a central role in the genesis of fever. Although fever has some harmful and deleterious effects, such as increasing cardiac output, oxygen consumption, carbon dioxide production, and energy expenditure, it also appears to have an adaptive response that helps the host to deal with invading pathogens.

Although **infections** are probably the most common cause of fever in the ICU setting, many noninfectious inflammatory conditions can also cause the release of cytokines, leading to a febrile response. Therefore, the best clinical approach to a febrile ICU patient is to determine whether the fever has an infectious or noninfectious cause. For reasons that are not entirely clear, most noninfectious disorders usually do not lead to a temperature > 38.9 °C (102 °F) except in certain situations, such as a drug fever or after a blood transfusion. Therefore, when the temperature rises above this threshold of 38.9 °C or 102 °F, the cause of the fever should be considered to be an infection.

The most common infections reported in the ICU patients are pneumonia (mainly ventilator-associated pneumonia), sinusitis, blood stream infection, catheter-related infections, and gastrointestinal infections. Although urinary tract infections have been reported to be common in the ICU patients, it is likely that most of these patients have asymptomatic bacteriuria rather than true infections.

Approximately 25% of ventilated patients may have ventilator-associated pneumonia, which can sometimes be a difficult diagnostic dilemma. Semi-invasive and invasive microbiological diagnostic techniques, such as obtaining BAL or protected brush, along with early initiation of appropriated antibiotics have been shown to improve outcome. The initial empiric antibiotic regimen should be broad and cover both gram-positive and gram-negative organisms.

With respect to sinusitis as a cause of fever in the ICU, it occurs more frequently in nasally intubated patients or in patients with long-standing nasogastric tubes. Diagnosis of sinusitis requires a CT scan. The treatment probably involves removing all nasal tubes, drainage of infectious sinusitis by transnasal puncture, and initiation of broad spectrum antibiotics.

About 25% of central venous catheters become colonized with organisms, and approximately 1/3 of these may result in catheter-associated sepsis. *Staphylococcus aureus* and coagulase-negative staphylococci are the most common followed by enterococci, gram-negative bacteria and *Candida* spp. When catheter sepsis is suspected, the catheter should be removed, because replacing it over a guidewire is associated with rapid recolonization of the new catheter. Routine blood cultures and cultures of the catheter tip should be sent prior to the initiation of antibiotics.

A common nosocomial gastrointestinal pathogen is *Clostridium difficile*, which causes pseudomembranous colitis and antibiotic-associated diarrhea. The majority of patients infected with *C difficile* are asymptomatic, because only 30% of infected patients would have diarrhea. When suspected, stools can be sent for fecal leukocytes and for toxins A or B.

Other infections that should also be considered are nosocomial meningitis for patients who have undergone neurosurgical procedure, *Candida* infections in patients who have been in the ICU more than 10 d and have received multiple courses of antibiotics, and intra-abdominal infections in patients who have undergone abdominal surgery.

Besides infections, noninfectious causes of fever should be considered. Even the more common entities can be quite broad: Acute MI, PE, acute pancreatitis, ARDS, posttransfusion fever, adrenal insufficiency, DVT, phlebitis, neoplastic fevers, acalculous cholecystitis, ischemic bowel, cerebral infarction/hemorrhage, subarachnoid hemorrhage, decubitus ulcers, alcohol or drug withdrawal, postoperative fever (48-h postop), and IV contrast reaction.

IV. Database

A. Physical Exam Key Points

1. **Vital signs.**
2. **Musculocutaneous.** Always examine the wound and IV sites. Check for deep venous thrombosis.
3. **HEENT.** Look for URI, otitis, and sialadenitis.
4. **Pulmonary.** Look for pneumonia and atelectasis.
5. **Pelvic, rectal, and buttocks.** Look for abscesses and decubitus ulcers.

B. Laboratory Data

1. **Hemogram.**
2. **Blood cultures.** Most ICU patients who develop a fever should have blood cultures sent.
3. **Urinalysis.** Urine culture is indicated in patients with abnormalities of the renal system or status post urinary tract manipulation.

  4. Stools. Stools should be sent for WBC and *C difficile* toxins for patients with diarrhea.
  5. Wound and sputum cultures.
  6. Thyroid function tests.
  7. Electrolytes.
C. Radiographic and Other Data
  1. Chest radiograph.
  2. CT scan. CT scan of the sinus should be considered for patients with nasal tubes. CT scan of the abdomen is indicated for patients at risk for abdominal sepsis or for patients with abdominal signs.
  3. Venous duplex.
  4. ECG. Postpericardiotomy.
  5. Abdominal ultrasound and HIDA scan.
  6. Gallium scan. In rare cases, using labeled WBC may aide in localizing an occult infectious focus.

V. Plan. Because the differential diagnosis is so broad, specific treatment should be directed toward the presumptive underlying cause(s). These may include empiric antibiotics and central catheter removal for patients with presumptive infections, benzodiazepines for patients with alcohol withdrawal and bromocriptine for patients with malignant neuroleptic syndrome. Central venous catheters > 48 h-old should be removed in patients whose clinical picture is suggestive of infections but where no obvious source has been identified. Empiric antifungal therapy may be initiated for patients with risk factors for candidal infections with persistent fevers, despite the use of empiric antibiotics and where no source of infection has been identified. Because fever may be an adaptive mechanism, cooling measures may be uncomfortable, and routine administration of antipyretics or use of cooling blankets is generally not recommended.

35. FOLEY CATHETER: CANNOT PLACE

I. Problem. A 70-year-old man admitted for a bowel obstruction has had no urine output, and the nurse is unable to place a Foley catheter.

II. Immediate Questions
  A. Is there blood at the urethral meatus? Blood from the meatus is an indication of urethral trauma, including the possibility of creation of a false passage by previous attempts. This question has particular significance when the patient has sustained blunt trauma. In the setting of trauma, the blood at the meatus may represent a urethral tear.
  B. Where was placement of the catheter blocked? When the catheter cannot be introduced into the meatus, a meatal stricture or hypospadias may be present. A smaller catheter may be introduced through a meatal stricture. When this maneuver is unsuccessful, the stricture may need to be dilated or surgically corrected. Hypospadias

needs to be recognized, so that the catheter can be introduced into the meatus at the appropriate location.

   C. **What type of catheter was used?** It is important to note the size and type, because a smaller caliber catheter or a coudé-type catheter may pass easily, where a larger or standard-type catheter could not pass.

   D. **Does the patient have a history of difficulty in voiding or of a weak urinary stream?** These may be symptoms of prostatic enlargement that would explain difficulty in passing the catheter through the prostate. A coudé catheter may also help in this situation.

   E. **Does his medical history include benign prostatic hypertrophy, prostate cancer, urethritis, urethral stricture, or prostate or urethral operation?** Any of these items in the history would suggest the presence of a urethral stricture that would explain the difficulty in placing the catheter.

   F. **When was the last time he voided, what was the volume of the void, and how much fluid has he had?** A small volume with each void may indicate bladder outlet obstruction and subsequent distention. The bladder should be distended when a suprapubic catheter has to be placed.

III. **Differential Diagnosis**

   A. **Hypospadias or Epispadias.** A detailed physical exam should identify these anatomical variants.

   B. **Meatal Stenosis.** When possible, a history of previous catheterization should be obtained. In addition, particular attention should be paid to prior episodes of sexually transmitted diseases.

   C. **Urethral Stricture**
      1. **Prostatic urethra.**
         a. **Benign prostatic hypertrophy (BPH).** A history of urinary tract symptoms, such as frequency, nocturia, and difficulty initiating stream are suggestive of BPH. A rectal exam will usually identify an enlarged prostate.
         b. **Prostatic carcinoma.** Check for nodularity or induration within the prostate on physical exam and for a known history of prostate cancer.
      2. **Membranous urethra.** Stricture may occur in the presence of acute trauma or as a result of remote traumatic injury. Urethral strictures may develop in patients who have undergone pancreatic transplant with bladder drainage.

   D. **Foreign Body**

   E. **Stone**

   F. **Urethral Diverticulum**

IV. Database

A. Physical Exam Key Points

1. **Genitourinary.** Check for hypospadias, epispadias, or meatal stenosis. Ensure that the foreskin retracts, and phimosis is not present. Edema of the penis or scrotum may make it more difficult to grasp the penis during catheter placement.
2. **Rectal exam.** Feel for prostatic enlargement, nodules, and masses.
3. **Abdomen.** Palpate a distended bladder if present.

B. Laboratory Data

1. **Hemogram.** Rule out infection and anemia.
2. **Urinalysis.** Check for UTI and/or blood in the urine.

C. Radiographic and Other Studies

1. Retrograde urethrography may be necessary for diagnostic purposes when urethral laceration is of concern.
2. Cystoscopy with catheter placement may also be diagnostic and therapeutic.

V. Plan

A. Attempt catheter placement with careful attention to technique.

B. When there is difficulty advancing the catheter past the prostatic urethra, a coudé catheter, which has a slightly firmer tip and an upward angle, may help.

C. When a coudé catheter will not pass because of a stricture, filiform bougies and followers may be used to dilate the stricture and allow catheter placement. In many institutions, this procedure may necessitate a consultation with the Urology service.

D. When the filiforms will not pass or there is suspicion of a false urethral passage, further evaluation, including possible cystoscopy, will likely be required.

E. In the presence of significant phimosis, an emergency dorsal slit of the foreskin may be required to allow access for catheterization.

F. When the bladder is distended and a catheter cannot be placed in the usual manner, a suprapubic catheter may be required.

36. FUNGAL INFECTION

I. **Problem.** A patient with chemotherapy-induced neutropenic, septic shock has a new fever and hypotension on day 12 of broad-spectrum antibiotic administration. Urine and skin cultures are positive for *Candida* spp. Blood cultures are negative.

II. Immediate Questions

A. Does the patient have systemic candidiasis?

B. **What (if any) antifungal should he receive?**

III. **Differential Diagnosis**
   A. Because many critical illnesses and/or their treatments result in a compromised immune system, serious, deep-seated fungal infections now develop in many ICU patients. Unfortunately, the stigmata of the systemic inflammatory response that these deep-seated fungal infections provoke are often incorrectly attributed to the patient's underlying medical condition, such as bacterial sepsis, lymphoma, or HIV infection. Whenever immunocompromised patients have an ongoing systemic inflammatory response, the differential diagnosis must distinguish between the underlying disease and a coexisting fungal infection.

IV. **Database**
   A. **History.** Be sure to look for immunocompromising conditions, such as steroid use, broad-spectrum antibiotic use, total parenteral nutrition administration, chronic peripheral venous catheters, neutropenia, heroin addiction, lymphoma, or acquired immunodeficiency syndrome.
   B. **Physical Exam Key Points**
      1. Vital signs, body temperature, a dilated funduscopic exam, and a complete skin and CNS examination.
   C. **Laboratory Data**
      1. **Hemogram.** This should include a leukocyte count.
      2. **Urinalysis.**
      3. **Fungal blood cultures.** Positive peripheral candidal cultures often represent only colonization, but deep-seated infections are rare, unless at least two peripheral sites are positive. Blood cultures positive for *Candida* are specific but not sensitive.
      4. **India ink preparations** and polysaccharide antigen testing of the CSF is necessary when cryptococcal meningitis is suspected.
   D. **Radiographic and Other Studies**
      1. **Chest radiograph** should be obtained.
      2. **Lung biopsy** is necessary to demonstrate invasive pulmonary *Aspergillus.*
      3. **Positive sputum** or BAL cultures cannot diagnose invasive aspergillosis. Zygomycosis is almost always diagnosed by PAS or methenamine silver stains of involved biopsy specimens; blood cultures are almost always negative.

V. **Plan.** Despite its toxicity, amphotericin B is generally the initial therapy for ICU patients with serious fungal infections. Significant exceptions include using fluconazole to treat candidemia in nonneutropenic patients and itraconazole for disseminated histoplasmosis.

37. GASTROINTESTINAL BLEEDING: HEMATOCHEZIA

I. **Problem.** A 79-year-old woman in the ICU with respiratory failure secondary to pneumonia suddenly passes bright red blood per rectum (BRBPR).

II. **Immediate Questions**

A. **What are the vital signs?** When there is any physiologic instability, resuscitate as needed. Preparation for ongoing volume restoration should be made. Tachycardia and hypotension reflect significant volume loss.

B. **How much bleeding has there been and how long has it been going on?** Both clinicians and patients tend to both over- and underestimate the amount of bleeding. Nonetheless, distinction between blood on toilet paper or in the bed versus frank blood should be made.

C. **What is the current blood count?** Although the hematocrit may not accurately reflect the degree of hemorrhage acutely, a low hematocrit is indicative of previous blood loss.

D. **Has there been any transfusion requirement?** Persistent transfusion requirements are indicative of incomplete resuscitation or ongoing hemorrhage.

E. **What is the quality of bleeding** (BRBPR, bloody diarrhea, melena vs occult)? Occult bleeding, or blood that is only detectable on a guaiac test, is generally not reflective of an emergent process. BRBPR may be from an upper source if the bleeding is brisk enough. When hematochezia is from an upper source, there will often be hemodynamic instability. Usually, it represents a lower GI source.

F. **Is there any prior medical history for bleeding episodes?** Known previous upper or lower sources or known liver failure with portal hypertension may suggest the site of bleeding.

G. **Has there been any prior medication use, such as anticoagulants, aspirin, or other non-steroidal anti-inflammatory (NSAID) drugs?** Significant NSAID use may predispose to gastritis or gastric ulceration.

III. **Differential Diagnosis**

A. **Anorectal Disease.** This is a very common cause of bright blood on stools.

1. **Fissure.** This may be visualized as a tear on anoderm. Anoscopy at the bedside is often required to diagnose.

2. **Fissure** is often indicated by blood on stool or on paper.

3. **Hemorrhoids.** These may bleed and/or prolapse. Historical information from the patient or family concerning hemorrhoids may be inaccurate. Hemorrhoids is often used as a generic term for any

anal disease. When cirrhosis is present, the bleeding can be very brisk.

B. Diverticula. This is the most common cause of left colonic bleeding. Despite this fact, the majority of diverticula that bleed are right sided. *Vasa recta* at the neck of the diverticulum rupture, leading to hemorrhage. The volume loss is often significant with hemodynamic instability. Bleeding tends to be episodic. Patients do not always rebleed.

C. Colonic Polyps. Most often, bleeding is minimal and only causes hemepositive stools. When the polyps are larger and more distal, hematochezia may occur.

D. Tumors. These may be indicated by a broad range of bleeding symptoms from hemepositive stool to melena to hematochezia.

E. Angiodysplasia. Multiple lesions are often present. Varying degrees of ectatic vessels can be seen histologically. Actual arteriovenous malformation (AVM) may be present. Multifocality complicates localization efforts.

F. Ischemic Colitis. Once the mucosa sloughs, the colon may bleed.

G. Inflammatory Bowel Disease
   1. Crohn's disease may be indicated by bloody diarrhea.
   2. Ulcerative colitis causes bloody diarrhea from colonic inflammation.

H. Upper GI Source
   1. **Peptic ulcer disease.** Massive bleeding from an ulcer may cause BRBPR with or without hematemesis.
   2. Small bowel tumor.
   3. **Small bowel AVM.** These areas can be difficult to identify. Angiography may be required. Localization during surgery can also be difficult. "On-table" endoscopy can be helpful.
   4. Meckel's diverticula cause lower GI bleeding in children and young adults.

I. Other Sources
   1. Radiation proctitis.
   2. Trauma.
   3. Coagulopathy.
      a. Excessive anticoagulation
      b. Liver failure and portal hypertension via esophageal varices or hemorrhoidal varices

IV. Database

A. Physical Exam Key Points
   1. **Vital signs.** Tachycardia, hypotension, and orthostatic changes are indicative of hypovolemia. The presence of these signs should alert the clinician that aggressive resuscitation is essential.

2. **Skin.** Jaundice and spider angiomas suggest significant hepatic dysfunction. In this clinical setting, variceal hemorrhage may be of concern.
3. **Abdominal exam.** Tumors will occasionally be palpable. Look for incisions indicative of previous surgical interventions. Most conditions leading to hematochezia do not cause peritonitis.
4. **Perianal and rectal exam.** Fissures and hemorrhoids may be identified. Anoscopy will facilitate this diagnostic maneuver. Rectal tumors may be palpable. A sense of the amount of bleeding may sometimes be evident during the exam. Do not discount the possibility that hemorrhoids and a proximal tumor may exist in the same patient.

B. **Laboratory Data**
1. **Hemoglobin and hematocrit.** Values can be used to establish baseline levels. Many of the conditions causing hematochezia will have led to chronic episodic blood loss. The hematocrit may not reflect the actual amount of acute blood loss.
2. **Coagulation studies.** A primary coagulopathy may lead to the development of hematochezia. In addition, ongoing hemorrhage may result in coagulopathy. In either circumstance, replacement with appropriate factors should be part of the ongoing resuscitation.
3. **Blood bank.** The patient should have a sample sent to the blood bank for processing. When hypotension is present, uncross-matched or type-specific blood may be required. Communication of the clinical situation to the blood bank will allow for the patient's needs to be met.
4. **Electrolytes.** Many patients will require angiography as part of a localization strategy. Renal function may be inferred from serum electrolyte measurements.
5. **Ammonia.** When there is preexisting hepatic dysfunction, the protein load from the shed blood may precipitate encephalopathy. Ammonia levels can help in the diagnosis.

C. **Radiographic and Other Studies**
1. **Nuclear scan.** This can identify bleeding as little as 0.1 mL/min. Precision of localization is hampered by both prograde and retrograde intraluminal migration of blood. A nuclear scan may be of use in guidance of the approaches for mesenteric angiography.
2. **Angiography.** This can identify bleeding of as little as 1–2 mL/min. Anatomical specificity is superior to that of nuclear studies. The catheter may even be left in place on the way to the operating room to assist in localization. Therapeutic intervention is also possible with embolization of the source of the bleeding.
3. **Rigid sigmoidoscopy.** This may be done at the bedside. Rectal sources can be visualized. It is useful for patients with acute penetrating trauma.

4. **NG aspiration.** Absence of blood with the presence of bilious fluid excludes an upper gastrointestinal source.
5. **EGD.** When there is clinical suspicion of an upper GI source, EGD should be done. The procedure may be both diagnostic and therapeutic.
6. **Colonoscopy.** When clinically possible, colonoscopy may provide both localization and diagnosis. Occasionally, therapeutic interventions are possible. Incomplete preparation of the bowel, presence of clot, and inability to do a bowel preparation all compromise the utility of the study.

V. Plan

A. **General Plan.** Resuscitation, localization, and control of hemorrhage provide the mainstays of the therapeutic approach to the patient with hematochezia. Instability, anatomical variability, and the episodic nature of the bleeding adds complexity to this approach. Maintenance of hemoglobin levels with transfusion allows some margin of safety for the patient. Significant transfusion requirement in itself may lead to surgical exploration.

B. **Specific Plans**
1. Rule out an upper source with NG tube. When bile is obtained, then the bleeding is almost certain to be past the ligament of Treitz.
2. Melanotic stools are most likely from chronic blood loss; therefore, they should be evaluated by endoscopy.
3. **Hematochezia.**
   a. Bright red blood per rectum in a hemodynamically stable patient should be evaluated by colonoscopy initially.
   b. Resuscitate as needed (packed red blood cells, platelets, coagulation factors, etc).
   c. Bright red blood per rectum in hemodynamically unstable patient should be treated in the following manner.
4. When not in the ICU already, transfer the patient to a critical care setting.
5. Resuscitate as needed. Crystalloid and blood products, such as packed red cells, platelets, and coagulation factors may be required. Notification of the blood bank personnel of the acuity will allow transfusion needs to be met.
6. Rule out an upper GI source of bleeding via NG tube placement.
7. Rule out an anal source via anoscopy and/or rigid sigmoidoscopy.
8. Use a nuclear medicine to isolate the bleeding site (diagnostic only). Surgical planning on the basis of nuclear medicine studies should be based on individual and institutional experiences.
9. When bleeding slows or stops and the patient becomes hemodynamically normal, then prepare for colonoscopy for diagnostic and therapeutic intent. Full bowel cleansing may be possible in this subset of patients.

10. When bleeding continues, and a bleeding source is identified via a nuclear medicine scan, then proceed with angiography with possible vasopressin and/or embolization if the vessel is identified.

11. When the bleeding continues despite embolization, or when embolization is technically unsuccessful, and site is isolated, then proceed with appropriate segmental colonic resection.

12. When the bleeding continues and site is not isolated, then proceed with subtotal colonic resection.

13. When the bleeding stops and no site is identified via nuclear medicine, colonoscopy should be performed. Angiography has a low diagnostic yield if there is not an active hemorrhage.

14. Small bowel enteroscopy or small barium study should be performed if no other disease process is identified.

15. Meckel's scan may also be considered.

38. GASTROINTESTINAL BLEEDING: MELENA

I. **Problem.** A 79-year-old woman in the ICU with respiratory failure secondary to pneumonia is passing dark tarry stools.

II. **Immediate Questions**

A. **What are the patient's vital signs?** As melena reflects blood loss, it is important to ensure that the patient has an optimal volume status. Have the vital signs changed over the last few hours? What is the patient's hemoglobin? Has it fallen? Is her urine output adequate? It may be necessary to consider ordering serial hemoglobin levels or giving intravenous fluid.

B. **Is this the first stool of this quality?** Is this a problem that is in the process of being worked up, or is it a new problem? She most likely will need an upper endoscopy to look for a source of bleeding. Consider a GI service consultation.

C. **Does the patient have a nasogastric tube?** When she does, what does the output look like? Critical patients often suffer from stress gastritis, especially if not on oral feedings. An NG tube should be placed if one is not already present. The return of bright red blood confirms an upper GI bleed. Vascular access should be ensured. The stomach should then be lavaged until clear, serial hemoglobin levels ordered, and an urgent GI consult placed. Check to ensure that the patient is on an H_2-blocker, and consider adding an additional agent.

D. **Is the patient on any anticoagulants, or have there been abnormal coagulation studies for any reason?** Previously stable levels of anticoagulation may become supratherapeutic with the addition of new medications, critical illness, or dietary changes.

   E. **Does she have a history of ulcer disease, esophageal varices, or portal hypertension?** An acute illness may exacerbate a preexisting upper gastrointestinal lesion.

III. **Differential Diagnosis.** Dark, tarry stools are usually due to bleeding from the upper GI tract (proximal to the ligament of Treitz). Rarely, melena may be caused by a jejunal source or right colon source. The dark color is due to the breakdown of blood by enteric bacteria, and may be caused by as little as 50 cc of blood.

   A. **Stress Gastritis.** Predisposing factors include sepsis, major trauma, burn > 35%, ARDS, hypotension, and large transfusion requirements.

   B. **Esophageal Varices.** These are associated with cirrhosis. They are more likely to cause acute hemorrhage. A missed hemorrhagic event, however, may appear as melena.

   C. **Gastric or Duodenal Ulcer.** Fifteen to 20% of these are associated with bleeding. They may be indicated by melena or acute upper GI bleeding.

   D. **Mallory-Weiss Tear.** This may occur after retching or vomiting. It is more likely to cause acute hemorrhage.

   E. **Tumor.** A slowly bleeding right-sided colon tumor can cause bleeding. This bleeding may be either microscopic or of sufficient volume to cause melena.

   F. **Anticoagulation**

IV. **Database**

   A. **Physical Exam Key Points**
      1. **Vital signs.** Check for hypotension and tachycardia. Significant upper gastrointestinal blood loss may cause hypovolemia. Orthostatic determination of vital signs should be done if the patient is not in obvious shock.
      2. **HEENT.** Look for evidence of epistaxis or midface trauma that may have led to swallowed blood.
      3. **Pulmonary.** Look for evidence of aspiration. Also examine for hemoptysis. When the patient is having significant hemoptysis and is swallowing the blood, melena may result.
      4. **Abdomen.** Check the abdomen for increased distention or peritoneal signs.
      5. **Rectum.** Look for the gross characterization of the stool, and assess for microscopic blood with hemoccult test.

   B. **Laboratory Data**
      1. **Hemoglobin.** A baseline level should be obtained, and the trend should be noted. The initial study will not necessarily reflect an acute blood loss.

    2. **Coagulation profile.** A preexisting or acquired coagulopathy may exist.

    3. **Blood bank.** Ensure that a specimen (red-top or clot tube) has been sent to the blood bank.

  C. **Radiographic and Other Studies**

    1. **Radiographs.** Obtain an upright chest radiograph to check for free air when abdominal exam is suspicious. Typically, however, the processes that cause bleeding will be the result of a perforated viscus.

    2. **Nasogastric tube.** When not previously placed, an NG tube can provide initial localizing information.

    3. **EGD.** When an upper GI source is suspected, EGD may be both diagnostic and therapeutic.

V. Plan

  A. **Immediate Plan.** Identify the location of the bleeding and the rate. Peritoneal signs and free air most likely suggest a perforated ulcer and almost always mandate surgical exploration.

  B. **Specific Plans**

    1. **NG tube placement.**

      a. When return is "coffee-grounds," this can be from ongoing gastritis or a source more proximal. Check the nasopharynx for blood. Check to ensure that the patient is receiving an H_2-blocker. If she is, consider adding sucralfate or switching to a PPI.

      b. When the NG tube return is bright red blood, lavage until clear. Obtain an immediate GI consultation for endoscopy. Serial hemoglobin levels should be monitored.

      c. Resuscitate with crystalloid and blood products as needed. Transfusion of multiple units of PRBCs suggests ongoing bleeding and a high likelihood of a surgically correctable lesion.

39. GASTROSTOMY TUBE, DISLODGED

I. Problem. The ICU nurse informs you that a 74-year-old man's feeding gastrostomy has become dislodged.

II. Immediate Questions

  A. **What type of feeding tube is it?** The patient should be examined to determine the type of tube. A percutaneous endoscopic gastrostomy (PEG) will not have an incision on the abdomen, whereas a surgical gastrostomy tube will have one. Check the chart for an operative or procedure note.

  B. **When was the tube placed?** Recently placed tubes that fall out can be more of a problem than those placed remotely. In the acute phase, the stomach may not be adherent to the abdominal wall. This situation is more of a concern with PEG tubes, because the stomach has not been sutured to the abdominal wall.

C. Have there been any changes in the patient's vital signs? Spillage of gastric contents into the peritoneal cavity may cause peritonitis with shock. Aspiration of gastric contents in the setting of a dysfunctional gastrostomy tube may cause respiratory changes.

D. When the patient can communicate, does he have any abdominal symptoms? Abdominal pain may indicate extravasation of spillage of gastric contents.

E. Has the tube been used previously? A previously functional tube that is not working now may be dislodged.

III. **Differential Diagnosis.** Either the tube is dislodged or it is in place. When the tube is completely out of the body, the diagnosis is certain. When the patient has a significantly thick abdominal wall, the tube may be dislodged but not out of the patient.

IV. **Database**

   A. Physical Exam Key Points
   1. **Vital signs.** Tachycardia, tachypnea, and fever can be signs of intraperitoneal spillage of enteral feeds.
   2. **Abdominal exam.** The site of the tube should be inspected, and the technique of placement determined. The presence or absence of the tube should be assessed. When the tube is present, it should be inspected for structural flaws. Aspiration of gastric contents provides supportive evidence that the tube system remains intact. Peritoneal signs on physical examination (eg, rebound tenderness, guarding, etc) may indicate a need for surgical intervention.

   B. Laboratory Data. No specific laboratory study is required. If the initial dislodging event was missed, and the patient is being examined later, a CBC and electrolyte determination may be of help.

   C. Radiographic and Other Studies
   1. **Fluoroscopic evaluation of the tube system.** When the tube has not completely dislodged, a contrast study can confirm a functional system and can also diagnose extravasation. The contrast used must be water soluble. Ideally, the team that placed the tube initially should perform or be present for the study. In the acute postprocedural period, a freshly replaced tube should also be confirmed with a water-soluble contrast study.

V. **Plan**

   A. Overall Plan. To assess need for urgent operation or observation with nasogastric decompression.

B. **Specific Plans**
1. The specific plan depends on the length of time the gastrostomy has been in place and whether it was percutaneously placed or surgically placed. When it is a PEG tube, the stomach is not sutured to the anterior abdominal wall. A nasogastric tube and a tube through the tract should be placed immediately. Operative intervention to correct the gastric wall defect may be required.
2. In a surgical gastrostomy, if the tract is well established, the tube may be replaced with the same size tube. Do not use a larger-bore French tube, as this can cause erosion of the tract and, subsequently, the skin. When the tract is not well formed, the tube should be replaced immediately, and a contrast radiographic study ordered immediately to confirm intragastric placement. Signs of intraperitoneal spillage necessitate an urgent laparotomy to minimize further contamination.

40. HEMATEMESIS

Immediate Actions
1. Assess **A**irway, **B**reathing, and **C**irculation.
2. Obtain vital signs.
3. Intubate, if necessary.
4. Ensure large-bore IV access and begin bolus of 500-mL lactated Ringer's (LR).
5. Obtain blood for transfusion.
6. Place an NG tube.

I. **Problem.** A patient admitted for an elective LeVeen shunt suddenly begins to vomit blood.

II. **Immediate Questions**

A. **What are the blood pressure and orthostatic vital signs?** The initial management focuses on maintaining intravascular volume and perfusion pressure. Blood pressure/orthostatic hypotension is the best on-the-ward estimate of the volume loss.

B. **Are there any bleeding tendencies?** Review available history, physical exam, and laboratory data regarding any correctable coagulation deficit.

C. **Are there any stigmata of alcohol abuse?** Of the major causes of upper GI bleeding, only esophageal varices are associated with any physical signs. Obtain a history and look for physical signs of cirrhosis and portal hypertension, but remember that a diagnosis of cirrhosis does not equate with a diagnosis of variceal bleed.

D. **Did the patient retch or vomit nonbloody material before hematemesis?** A Mallory-Weiss tear is the fourth most common cause of hematemesis in most series, and the patient, nurses, or any observer should be carefully asked about the episode. "Coffee ground" emesis indicates that the blood has been in the stomach long enough to be converted by gastric acid from hemoglobin to methemoglobin.

E. **Does the patient have any history of aortic disease or a prior aortic vascular procedure?** Although low on the list of causes of hematemesis, aortoduodenal fistula should always be included in the initial differential diagnosis of upper GI bleeding. The phenomenon of a sentinel bleed allows some of these patients to be salvaged, but only if the diagnosis is made quickly.

III. **Differential Diagnosis.** Hematemesis is virtually always associated with bleeding proximal to the ligament of Treitz. In the most recent series, ulcer disease, gastritis, esophageal varices, and Mallory-Weiss tears accounted for 90–95% of episodes of hematemesis.

A. **Esophagus**
   1. **Esophageal varices.** These are associated with cirrhosis and portal hypertension.
   2. **Mallory-Weiss tear.** This is usually a mucosal tear at the gastroesophageal junction associated with severe retching with or without vomiting.
   3. **Esophagitis.** Patient has a classic history of heartburn, "water brash" (regurgitation of gastric contents), and worsening of symptoms with recumbency.
   4. **Esophageal tumors.** These are benign, squamous cell carcinomas, or adenocarcinomas.

B. **Stomach**
   1. **Gastritis.** Significant hematemesis usually indicates severe stress gastritis, usually alcohol related.
   2. **Gastric ulcer.** Pain is typically exacerbated by eating but may also be relieved with eating. Up to 42% of these are associated with duodenal ulcer.
   3. **Gastric tumors.**
   4. **Gastric varices.**

C. **Duodenum**
   1. **Duodenal ulcer**
   2. **Aortoduodenal fistula.** This is found almost exclusively in patients who have undergone previous aortic reconstruction.

D. **Hemobilia.** This is usually secondary to trauma, infection, stone disease, or iatrogenic causes.

E. **Systemic Causes**
   1. **Coagulopathy (DIC, leukemia, etc).**

      2. Osler-Weber-Rendu disease. This is associated with multiple telangiectases.

      3. Peutz-Jeghers syndrome. This is associated with multiple hamartomas.

   F. Non-GI Source. Nasopharyngeal bleeding.

IV. Database

A. Physical Exam Key Points

1. **Vital signs.** Orthostatic blood pressure measurements. Determine the pulse and blood pressure with the patient in the supine position for 5 min. Have the patient stand or dangle the legs off the side of the bed. At 1 min, determine BP and pulse. A drop in BP of > 10–20 mm Hg or an increase in pulse of > 10 bpm suggests volume depletion.

2. **Skin.** Cool, moist, pale skin indicates volume loss. Evidence of alcohol abuse is indicated as spider angiomata or palmar erythema. Signs of systemic disease show as multiple bruises, telangiectases, or hamartomas of lips, and oral mucosa.

3. **HEENT.** Look for evidence of epistaxis or other nasopharyngeal source.

4. **Abdomen.** Look for scars from prior ulcer, vascular, or other procedure. Check for pain or evidence of peritoneal signs. Look for signs of portal hypertension, such as splenomegaly, caput medusa, or ascites.

5. **Rectal.** Check for gross blood or melena.

6. **Genitourinary.** Testicular atrophy and gynecomastia are evidence of alcohol abuse.

B. Laboratory Data

1. **Hemogram.** Obtain serial hematocrits, document time drawn, and relation to transfusions.

2. **Platelet count.** Verify there are adequate platelets.

3. **PT/PTT.** Helps identify potentially correctable deficit in the coagulation cascade.

4. **Renal function.** This should be determined as a baseline.

5. **Liver function tests.** These can be used to document liver disease.

6. **Blood bank specimen.** Remember with the initial blood draw to type and crossmatch for up to 6–10 U of blood.

C. Radiographic and Other Studies

1. **Chest radiograph.** This will document aspiration.

2. **Upper endoscopy.** In most hospitals, this is the diagnostic procedure of choice (and sometimes therapeutic).

3. **UGI series.** This may be used when endoscopy is unavailable, and when bleeding has stopped. It interferes with endoscopy and angiography, so it is not usually a first-line study.

     4. Angiogram. This is rarely used unless endoscopy does not identify the source.

V. Plan. Bleeding can be excessive, and as an example, up to 50% of patients with massive UGI bleeding from varices will die. Treat volume loss, establish diagnosis, and implement specific therapies. Continued bleeding in any of these conditions requires the appropriate surgical intervention. However, about 85% of cases of UGI bleeding resolve without operative intervention.

A. Initial Management
    1. Use large-bore IVs (18-gauge or larger) and begin crystalloid.
    2. Type and crossmatch for packed red blood cells (6 units minimum).
    3. Place NG tube. This documents ongoing bleeding and clears the stomach for endoscopy. An Ewald tube may be needed to evacuate large volumes of clot.
    4. Monitor volume replacement
       a. Always chart serial hematocrits, timing, and amount of transfusions, because this measures the rate of bleeding, which is the major criterion to decide whether surgery is needed in many instances.
       b. Foley catheter
       c. Central line if needed, especially, for patients with cardiac or respiratory disease.
    5. Correct coagulopathy with platelets or FFP.
    6. Insert NG tube, and irrigate with saline until clear. The temperature of the irrigant is not as important as clearing the material from the stomach.
    7. Consider intubation to protect the airway from aspiration.

B. Specific Treatment. After acute bleed is stabilized.
    1. Ulcer
       a. Give antacids via NG tube every 1–2 h.
       b. H$_2$-receptor blockers (cimetidine, ranitidine). These may prevent rebleeding, but they probably will not stop ongoing bleeding. They may be used with antibiotics.
    2. Stress gastritis
       a. Antacids.
       b. H$_2$-receptor blockers have no effect in active bleeding.
    3. Esophageal varices
       a. Injection sclerotherapy by endoscopy.
       b. Vasopressin 0.4–0.6 U/min by peripheral IV for 1 h. Repeat every 3 h, if successful.
       c. Balloon tamponade (Sengstaken-Blakemore Tube). Attempt only if experienced, because complications of aspiration, respiratory arrest, and esophageal rupture are possible. Be sure to read the accompanying instruction before attempting placement.

   4. Mallory-Weiss tear
      a. Vasopressin is of unclear effectiveness.
      b. Angiographic embolization.

41. HEMATURIA

I. Problem. A 70-year-old man has hematuria that was noted on his arrival to the ICU after a colon resection.

II. Immediate Questions

A. How long has he had hematuria? Determine whether this is a chronic condition or something that may have been induced by this admission or operation.

B. Is the blood gross or microscopic? Gross hematuria leads to a concern about possible significant blood loss. Gross hematuria may also be associated with blood clots within the bladder. Prevention of occlusion of the catheter in the presence of clots may require a larger-caliber catheter or even an irrigation system (triple-lumen Foley catheter).

C. Does the patient have a Foley catheter or ureteral stents in place? Trauma from placement of these devices may lead to hematuria. Ureteral stents may be placed to aid in intraoperative identification of the ureters in pelvic operations. Stents may also be placed to treat hydronephrosis caused by ureteral obstruction by tumor or stones.

D. What operation was performed? Pelvic surgery, such as low colon resections, risk injury to the bladder and ureters. Injury to the kidneys may occur from retraction. Patients who have had genitourinary tract surgery may routinely have hematuria postoperatively.

E. What is the urine output? No urine output may occur secondary to occlusion of a Foley catheter by blood clots. Urine output is an excellent indicator of kidney perfusion and function.

F. Does the patient have a history of recent prostate or urinary tract surgery? Residual hematuria from transurethral resection of the prostate may persist for several weeks after surgery. History of a previous resection of a urinary tract tumor should cause concern for the possibility of tumor recurrence.

G. Does the patient have dysuria, frequency, or urgency? These symptoms may indicate a urinary tract infection.

H. Does the patient have flank pain? Renal calculi typically cause intermittent flank pain radiating to the groin.

I. What medications is the patient receiving? Check for anticoagulants, which may aggravate bleeding. Also look for cyclophosphamide, which can cause hemorrhagic cystitis.

J. Is this a trauma patient? Particularly with pelvic fractures, suspect injury to the urinary tract.

K. If the patient is a young female, when was her last menstrual bleeding? Urinalysis may be contaminated by bleeding from menses.

III. Differential Diagnosis

A. Iatrogenic. Trauma to the urethra may result from Foley catheter placement. Inflation of the Foley balloon in the urethra or removal of the catheter with the balloon inflated may cause injury. The presence of a catheter may cause bladder irritation. Ureteral stent placement may cause bleeding. Intraoperative injury to the kidneys, ureters, or bladder may occur.

B. Stones. Urinary tract stones may cause microscopic or gross hematuria. They are frequently associated with pain.

C. Tumor. Tumors of the urinary tract or prostate may present as painless hematuria.

D. Infection. Any urinary tract infection may cause hematuria.

E. Trauma. Kidney hematoma or laceration, ureteral, bladder, or urethral injury may result from blunt or penetrating trauma. Pelvic fracture may be associated with urethral injury.

F. Colovesical or Enterovesical Fistula. This usually appears as an infection or pneumaturia and is most commonly associated with diverticulitis.

G. Contamination. This may occur with menstrual bleeding or in a patient with recent trauma. A catheter specimen avoids this problem.

H. Radiation. Radiation cystitis may result from radiation to the pelvis for colorectal or genitourinary malignancies.

I. Anticoagulation. Anticoagulation may unmask otherwise minor bleeding from other causes, such as tumors.

J. Benign Prostatic Hypertrophy

K. Glomerular Hematuria. This may be caused by poststreptococcal glomerulonephritis, systemic lupus erythematosus nephritis, Goodpasture syndrome, Schönlein-Henoch purpura, multiple myeloma, familial hematuria, familial nephritis, minimal change disease, focal glomerulosclerosis IgA nephropathy, membranous glomerulopathy, proliferative glomerulonephritis, hemolytic uremic syndrome, or idiopathic hematuria.

L. Nonglomerular Hematuria. This may be caused by runner's hematuria, drug-induced hematuria, hemophilia, thrombocytopenia, disseminated intravascular coagulopathy, thrombotic thrombocytopenic purpura, hypercalcinuria, hyperuricosuria, medullary sponge kidney, polycystic kidney disease, papillary necrosis, sickle cell disease, analgesic nephropathy, tuberculosis infection, obstructive nephropathy, reflux nephropathy, malignant hypertensive nephropathy, renal artery occlusion, renal vein occlusion, or arteriovenous fistula.

IV. **Database**

A. **Physical Exam Key Points**

1. **Abdominal.** Check for tenderness, masses, distention, wound drainage. If any drains were placed intraoperatively, check nature and volume of output. A urine leak may appear as drainage from drains or wounds.

2. **Rectal exam.** Feel for an enlarged or nodular prostate. When the prostate is "high riding," suspect urethral injury, especially when a pelvic fracture is present.

3. **Urethral meatus.** Gross blood is suspicious for urethral laceration in the setting of a pelvic fracture.

4. **Urine.** When gross blood is present, determine the severity of the hemorrhage. Quantify urine output, because this is an excellent indication of renal function, and lack of any output raises concern of occlusion secondary to blood clots.

B. **Laboratory Data**

1. **Urinalysis.** Look for evidence of a UTI.

2. **Coagulation studies.** Correction of a coagulopathy will potentially resolve the hematuria.

3. **Hemoglobin/Hematocrit.** Determine the severity of hemorrhage and the patient's baseline status.

4. **BUN and creatinine.** Check to reflect renal function.

5. **Urine culture and sensitivity.**

6. **Urine cytology.** For malignancy.

C. **Radiographic and Other Studies**

1. **Abdominal radiograph.** This may show stones in the urinary collecting system.

2. **Intravenous pyelogram.** Provides both anatomic and functional information about the GU tract.

3. **Ultrasound.** Hydronephrosis may be demonstrated on ultrasound exam.

4. **Cystoscopy with retrograde pyelogram.** This enables both the diagnosis and possible treatment of the source of bleeding.

5. **CT scan.** This gives information about presence of masses. Many centers are using noncontrast CT to assess for the presence of ureteral stones.

V. **Plan.** Immediate treatment depends on the severity of hemorrhage. Physical exam, urinalysis, blood count, and coagulation studies will help to determine the urgency of the problem. Hematuria usually does not require emergent intervention.

A. **Immediate Therapy.** Significant hemorrhage may require transfusion with packed cell or other blood products. Coagulopathy may need to be corrected, depending on the cause and severity of bleeding. Clots may be cleared by irrigating the Foley catheter. When clots are a persistent problem, continuous bladder irrigation may be initiated. Continuous irrigation requires the placement of a three-way catheter. The source of the bleeding may then be sought, using the studies above.

B. Treatment of Underlying Problem
 1. **Catheter or stent trauma.** Expectant management.
 2. **Stone.** Hydration and pain control. Stones less than 1 cm usually pass spontaneously. Further evaluation and treatment requires urologic consultation.
 3. **Tumor.** Correction of coagulopathy, if present, may stop bleeding. Urologic consultation is suggested.
 4. **Infection.** Use antibiotic therapy appropriate to setting. Send culture and sensitivity before initiating therapy.
 5. **Trauma.** Hematuria in the trauma patient is usually evaluated by CT scan. An IVP, cystogram, and/or urethrogram may be helpful. Gross blood from the meatus of a trauma patient mandates a urethrogram before placement of a Foley catheter.
 6. **Fistula.** Treatment of an enterovesical or colovesical fistula may require that the patient be NPO, or the fecal stream be diverted surgically.

42. HEMOPTYSIS

I. Problem. A 49-year-old man with a known history of tuberculosis is admitted to the ICU for treatment of a fungal superinfection. The nurse says that there is blood in the material suctioned from the endotracheal tube.

II. Immediate Questions
 A. What is the actual character of the fluid? Small streaks of blood on sputum or secretions have different import than that of frank blood or clots.
 B. What are the vital signs? Fever may reflect an active infection. Hypotension, tachycardia, and orthostatic changes may all indicate intravascular volume depletion. Tachypnea suggests significant pulmonary compromise, possibly from clots within the trachea or the bronchial tree.
 C. What is the baseline status of the secretions? Changes in the volume or the character of the secretions to include blood or clots represent a clinical change. Some conditions have episodic bleeding.
 D. When, and how, was the patient intubated? Traumatic intubation can result in hemoptysis. If a surgical airway is required, there might also be bleeding. Long-term intubation can lead to granuloma formation that can bleed.

E. **Is there a history of tuberculosis or other pulmonary infection?** Bronchitis, TB, fungal infections, and some bacterial pneumonia may all cause bleeding.

F. **Is the bleeding truly hemoptysis?** Epistaxis, oropharyngeal, or upper GI bleeding may all appear as "coughing up blood." The patient's history and a careful physical exam will help clarify the cause.

G. **What is the volume of hemoptysis?** A somewhat arbitrary definition of greater than 500 cc/dL signifies massive hemoptysis and requires immediate diagnosis and treatment. Actual measurement of the blood volume may be difficult.

III. Differential Diagnosis

A. **Infection**

1. **Tuberculosis.** This may appear as a range of hemoptysis from blood-streaked sputum to frank bleeding. Erosion of the pleura into a bronchial or pulmonary vessel may lead to life-threatening hemoptysis. Aneurysms of the pulmonary artery, known as **Rasmussen aneurysms,** are seen in a small percentage of patients with cavitary TB. These aneurysms may rupture, leading to massive hemoptysis.

2. **Fungal.** Either primary infection or superinfection of a cavitary mycobacteria lesion may occur. This additional stimulus is often the factor that leads to hemoptysis. *Aspergillus* species are particularly prone to hemorrhagic events. Mycobacteria infections are not always TB.

3. **Bacterial.** In general, bacterial infections do not generate hemoptysis to any significant degree. There may be blood-tinged sputum with some infections. In cultures, *Serratia* has a pinkish color that may be mistaken for hemoptysis.

4. **Bronchitis.** Most often seen with tobacco use. Tracheobronchitis may occur with patients who have been intubated for significant periods. The degree of hemoptysis is usually minor.

B. **Tumor.** Primary lung cancer will, in general, only result in bloody sputum. When the tumor has progressed clinically, there may be situations where erosion of major pulmonary vessels by the tumor may occur. When this happens, the hemoptysis will be massive.

C. **Trauma.** Trauma, either from the prehospital environment, or from iatrogenesis may cause hemoptysis. Both penetrating and blunt trauma may cause hemoptysis. Penetrating trauma will usually cause a hemothorax (see Problem 43, page 132), but hemoptysis may occur. Procedures in the ICU may lead to hemoptysis if pulmonary laceration occurs. Pulmonary artery catheters may rarely cause significant hemoptysis when there is rupture of a pulmonary artery with decompression into an airway.

D. **Tracheoinnominate Fistula.** This occurs usually after tracheostomy. Often a preceding bleed (often called a "herald bleed") will have occurred. When it is not corrected surgically, the condition is often fatal.

E. **Foreign Body.** An aspirated foreign body may lead to irritation of the airway and subsequent bleeding. When the foreign body is sharp and lacerates the wall of the bronchial tree, bleeding may be significant.

F. **Nonpulmonary Causes.** In patients who are not intubated, blood may come from nonpulmonary sources. Common causes include esophageal varices, peptic ulcers, midface trauma, and oropharyngeal lesions. When the airway is secured with a definitive airway, this confusion is less likely, although not impossible.

G. **Medical Bleeding.** In circumstances of generalized coagulopathy, hemoptysis may result. In most instances, the pulmonary system will not be the only source of bleeding. Identification and correction of the underlying source are essential.

H. **Pulmonary Embolism.** When pulmonary embolism results in a pulmonary infarction, hemoptysis may result. Orthopedic surgery and trauma patients are at particular risk for thromboembolism. Consideration should be given to anticoagulation and, in appropriate circumstances, thrombolytic therapy.

IV. **Database**

A. **History.** Risk factors should be documented, including smoking history, tuberculosis exposure (including night sweats), immune status, trauma, prior procedures, and previous chest radiograph findings.

B. **Physical Exam Key Points**
   1. **Vital Signs.** Tachypnea should be identified, and trends in respiratory rate noted. Tachycardia, hypotension, and orthostatic changes may reflect the severity of the bleeding. Fever may indicate infection.
   2. **Face.** Evidence of trauma should be identified. Trauma from procedures such as NG tube or ET tube placement may lead to significant bleeding that may be confused with hemoptysis. Missing teeth should be sought as a potentially aspirated foreign body.
   3. **Pulmonary.** Decreased breath sounds suggest hemothorax or pleural effusion. Egophony is found with consolidation of pneumonia. Rubs can be found with effusions.
   4. **Cardiac.** Arrhythmias may result from, or lead to pulmonary embolism. Changes from baseline exam are of particular importance. New murmurs should also be evaluated.
   5. **Abdomen.** Evidence of cirrhosis should be sought. When cirrhosis is present, portal venous hypertension may lead to bleeding esophageal or gastric varices. Peptic ulcer disease may present with epigastric tenderness. Both these conditions may be confused with hemoptysis.

6. **Extremities.** Significant ileofemoral DVT may manifest with extremity edema.

C. Laboratory Data

1. **Hemogram.** An increase in the WBC level suggests infection. Diminished hemoglobin levels reflect blood loss. With acute hemorrhage, the hemoglobin level may not be low. Platelets may be low from a consumptive coagulopathy or be a primary cause of coagulopathic bleeding.

2. **Coagulation Profile.** Coagulopathy may be either causative or secondary. When values are elevated, correction with appropriate therapy is indicated.

3. **Sputum.** Studies for culture, Gram's stain and AFB studies should be obtained. In bacterial pneumonia, WBCs and a dominant organism will be seen. AFB stains will not universally be positive even with active TB. Sequential sampling is warranted when clinically indicated. TB cultures are also sent, but several weeks are required. Therapy in the ICU will often be based only on AFB stain. Morning gastric aspirates for AFB are a traditional, but occasionally useful, approach in unclear clinical circumstances.

4. **Cytology.** Either sputum samples or bronchoalveolar lavage (BAL) may be used to obtain tissue for cytologic assessment.

D. Radiographic and Other Data

1. **Bronchoscopy.** Allows both diagnosis and pulmonary hygiene. In most instances, morbidity and mortality from hemoptysis results from airway occlusion by clot. Exsanguination does occur, but with less frequency. Therapeutic maneuvers include placement of a bronchial-occluding balloon.

2. **Chest radiograph.** Contusion, hemopneumothorax, infiltrates, and cavitary lesions may all be seen. Identification of these findings allows therapy to be tailored to possible causes.

3. **Angiography.** Both pulmonary and bronchial angiography may be indicated. Pulmonary embolism may be identified, and when appropriate, lytic therapy instituted. When anticoagulation or thrombolysis are contraindicated, caval filters may be considered. Aneurysms or pseudoaneurysms may be embolized when found.

4. **Chest CT Scan.** Mass lesions and possible TB infections may be identified. When local expertise is available, CT angiography may play a role in the diagnosis of PE.

5. **TB Skin Test.** Both TB and controls should be administered. Acutely ill patients in the ICU may have impaired cellular immunity, and, as such, may be anergic. Anergy should not deter the diagnosis of TB when appropriate findings are present otherwise.

6. **Pulse Oximetry.** With acute hemoptysis, bleeding into the airway may rapidly lead to gas exchange compromise. ABG determination will be insensitive to the acuity of the change.

V. Plan

A. Immediate Plan. Massive hemoptysis requires a concerted team approach. Blood bank, critical care, surgical, radiology, and pulmonary services must all be contacted. Appropriate intravenous access is crucial. When not already done, intubation is indicated, both to protect the airway and to exclude a nonpulmonary source. Control of bleeding with appropriate resuscitation frame the management. Patients with significant unilateral bleeding may benefit from double-lumen tube placement and the use of two ventilators.

B. Specific Plans

1. **Infection.** Appropriate antimicrobial therapy should be initiated. In many locations, TB has developed resistance. Treatment should be tailored on the basis of known pathogens and their sensitivity profiles.

2. **Trauma.** Pulmonary contusion will often exacerbate before clearing. Supportive measures should be instituted, including mechanical ventilation. High clinical suspicion should exist for pulmonary contusions with multiple rib fractures or a flail chest. Hemothorax is managed with chest tube placement. Proximal airway injuries may have both significant bleeding and significant air leak.

3. **Tracheoinnominate fistula.** Bleeding from a patient with a tracheostomy requires immediate assessment with preparation for probable exploration in the operating room. Most instances of bleeding will be preceded by a "minor" episode of bleeding. Surgical exploration with ligation of the vessel and repair of the trachea provide the best options for salvage. Direct digital pressure of the vessel against the sternum or hyperinflation of the cuff may temporize until the patient reaches the OR. No episode of bleeding should be attributed to "suction trauma" or granuloma until direct physical exam is done.

4. **Foreign Body.** Rigid bronchoscopy will allow retrieval of most foreign bodies.

5. **Interventional Radiology.** Thrombolytic therapy, when possible by clinical circumstances, will treat pulmonary embolism. When aneurysmal changes are found, embolization may control hemorrhage and avoid surgical intervention.

6. **Resection.** In circumstances of persistent or uncontrolled bleeding, resections of tumors, injured lung segments, or areas of infection (TB or *Aspergillus*) may be life saving.

43. HEMOTHORAX

I. Problem. A 65-year-old man with a large pancreatic pseudocyst has some mild shortness of breath, and the nurse says that the breath sounds are decreased on the left.

II. Immediate Questions

A. **Is he in respiratory distress?** Respiratory distress generates an emergent situation. The patient must be immediately assessed and treated. In the absence of respiratory distress, the workup may proceed in a more deliberate manner.

B. **What medications is the patient taking?** Aspirin may cause platelet dysfunction. Coumadin effects may vary because of dietary changes or a new medication. Chronicity of therapy does not exclude an overanticoagulated state.

C. **Is the patient anticoagulated for any reason?** In the presence of a hemorrhagic complication, the need for anticoagulation may have to be reevaluated. When the anticoagulation is for venous thromboembolic disease, the patient may require placement of a vena caval filter.

III. Differential Diagnosis

A. **Trauma**
   1. **Penetrating trauma.** Gunshot wounds or stab wounds to the chest, back, flank, or upper abdomen may all result in hemothorax. In thoracoabdominal injury, the bleeding source may be either in the abdomen or the chest.
   2. **Blunt trauma.** Blunt trauma may also cause hemothorax, typically, from rib fractures. Either pulmonary laceration or intercostal vessel injury may be the source of bleeding.
   3. **Iatrogenic.** Complications of procedures may cause a hemothorax. Central line attempts, chest tube placement, and liver biopsies are known causes of hemothorax.
   4. **Operative.** Patients who have undergone thoracic procedures, such as lung biopsy, lobectomy, pneumonectomy, or mediastinoscopy, may all have postoperative bleeding.

B. **Pulmonary Causes**
   1. **Bullous emphysema.**
   2. **Tuberculosis.**
   3. **Pneumonitis.**
   4. **AVM.**
   5. **Cancer.**

C. **Pleural Causes**
   1. **Torn adhesion.**
   2. **Neoplasm.**

D. **Coagulopathies.** Both acquired and congenital

E. **Abdominal causes**
   1. **Pancreatic pseudocyst.**
   2. **Splenic artery aneurysm.**
   3. **Hemoperitoneum.**

IV. Database

   A. **Physical Exam Key Points**

      1. **Vital signs.** Tachypnea, tachycardia, and hypotension indicate significant volume loss and can be a clue to extent of the hemothorax.

      2. **Tracheal deviation** away from the side of the lesion can occur with large hemothoraces.

      3. **Decreased breath sounds.** This finding may be present with either a pneumothorax or a hemothorax. Presence of breath sounds does not exclude a hemothorax.

      4. **Dullness to percussion.** With significant hemothorax, the percussion exam will demonstrate dullness. Looking for this finding can help distinguish hemothorax from pneumothorax.

   B. **Laboratory Data**

      1. **Hemogram.** This provides baseline information. When the bleeding has been over a long period, the hemoglobin level may be low. If thoracentesis fluid is collected, the hemoglobin of the fluid can be compared with the systemic value. Platelet number can also be evaluated.

      2. **Coagulation profile.** When a coagulopathy exists, appropriate corrective therapy should be started.

   C. **Radiographic and Other Studies**

      1. **Chest radiograph.** Obtain a lateral and AP if the patient is stable. Obtain only an AP if he is not. In the supine position, a hemothorax may layer posteriorly. Radiographically, this situation will result in a diffuse haziness in the involved hemithorax. When a chest tube has been previously placed, it should be assessed for position. When the last hole is not within the pleural space, the tube should be replaced at a new site. Look for evidence of previous thoracic procedures.

V. Plan

   A. **Overall Plan.** To evacuate the fluid and determine the cause when unknown. Complete evacuation of the chest cavity is the therapeutic goal.

   B. **Specific Plans**

      1. When the effusion appears small on chest radiograph, a thoracentesis can be performed. In a patient with acute penetrating trauma, the evacuation should be done with a chest tube.

      2. When less than 500 cc is obtained, thoracentesis may be sufficient. (When there is associated pneumothorax for some reason, a tube thoracostomy should be placed without thoracentesis.)

      3. When more than 500 cc is obtained, a tube thoracostomy should be placed.

      4. When an amount greater than 1500 cc is obtained, or output is greater than 200 cc/h for 3 h, a thoracotomy should be performed.

When the hemothorax is in the acute postoperative period after a thoracic surgery procedure, the patient may require a return to the operating room for inspection of suture lines and of the thoracotomy incision.

44. HYPERGLYCEMIA

I. **Problem.** A 98-year-old woman is found unconscious at home by neighbors. Her serum glucose on admission to the ICU is 857 mg/dL and she has diffuse ST-T wave changes on her ECG.

II. **Immediate Questions**

A. **Is there a history of diabetes?** Was the patient given her insulin.

B. **What triggered the hyperglycemia?** A catastrophe, such as sepsis and trauma, can trigger severe hyperglycemia.

C. **Has hypovolemia led to inadequate glucosuria?**

III. **Differential Diagnosis**

A. **Renal impairment.** Most hyperglycemic episodes in the ICU result from inadequate glucosuria in patients with glucose intolerance. Because the renal tubule's threshold for glucose reabsorption is usually no higher than 200 mg/dL, serum glucose can only exceed this value when renal ultrafiltration is inadequate (usually because of massive volume depletion) to allow appropriate glucosuria. Not infrequently, however, intrinsic renal disease, postrenal obstruction, and other prerenal conditions, such as cardiogenic shock, may interfere with glucosuria.

B. **Underlying medical catastrophe.** Even with intact glucosuria, however, ICU patients may suffer hyperglycemia when offending events, such as stroke, myocardial infarction, bowel ischemia, or sepsis mediate massive release of counterregulatory hormones (cortisol, epinephrine, glucogen, or growth hormone). Exogenous administration of massive amounts of counterregulatory hormone, such as pulse steroid administration, may also cause hyperglycemia.

IV. **Database**

A. **History.** Look for the causes listed above, especially diabetes.

B. **Physical Examination Key Points**
1. **Vital signs.** Check for fever, tachycardia, hypotension, and Kussmaul respirations.

C. **Laboratory Data**
1. **Electrolytes.** Check for ketoacidosis, and determine levels of potassium, phosphorus and serial glucose.
2. **ABG.** Check to confirm acidosis (DKA).
3. **Lactic acid.** This test is useful for patients with DKA and patients with sepsis.

4. **Urinalysis.** Determine the presence of glucosuria and urinary ketone bodies.
5. **Cultures.** Obtain a full set of cultures (blood, urine, sputum, etc).

V. Plan

A. When the patient suffers a medical catastrophe causing the hyperglycemia, direct emergent therapy against the catastrophe. When total body volume depletion causes the hyperglycemia, rapid volume infusion with normal saline will correct the hyperglycemia once renal function recovers. Often, this mandates administration of more than 10 L of normal saline both to correct the original massive volume depletion and to compensate for the increasing osmotic diuresis resulting from the ensuing glucosuria. Almost all of these patients will have total body potassium depletion and will require potassium monitoring and replacement. They may also benefit from phosphate administration.

B. Patients with postrenal obstruction, intrinsic renal disease, nonhypovolemic prerenal dysfunction, catastrophic release of counterregulatory hormones, or exogenous administration of steroids should have these conditions corrected. When uncorrectable, the hyperglycemia can be controlled with insulin administration. Although serum potassium levels will often decrease with insulin administration, most of these patients suffer no total body potassium depletion and will require little or no potassium administration.

C. Patients suffering concomitant ketoacidosis will require insulin to correct the ketoacidosis; this will also correct the hyperglycemia. When the hyperglycemia resolves before the ketoacidosis clears, glucose infusion will allow ongoing insulin administration.

45. HYPERKALEMIA

I. Problem. A 75-year-old woman with chronic renal insufficiency secondary to diabetic nephropathy was admitted to the ICU in a hyperosmolar nonketotic state and septic shock secondary to *Escherichia coli* urosepsis. Her initial laboratory data revealed an anion gap and non-anion gap metabolic acidosis and a serum potassium level of 7.4 mEq/L. Her initial ECG showed peaked T waves and PR prolongation (Fig I–17).

II. Immediate Questions

A. What are the vital signs? Check for cardiac effects of hyperkalemia.

B. What is the appearance of the ECG? Look for peaked T waves, flat P waves, prolonged PR interval, and widened QRS complexes. Look for the presence of arrhythmias.

C. What is the renal function of this patient? Check urine output.

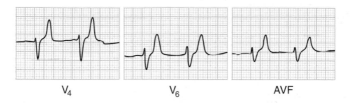

V_4 V_6 AVF

Figure I–17. Diffuse tall T waves in leads V_4, V_6, and aVF with widened QRS and junctional rhythm (loss of P waves), representing hyperkalemia.

D. **Has the patient received exogenous potassium?** Was she recently given an IV solution or administered an intravenous medication (especially some antibiotics)?

E. **Is the laboratory result accurate?** Alterations in serum potassium are best explained by changes in intake, cellular shift, and renal excretion.

III. Differential Diagnosis

A. **Excess intake.** Because the kidney can substantially increase potassium excretion, excess dietary potassium almost never causes hyperkalemia. However, in patients with mild renal impairment, excess potassium intake may be an important cause of hyperkalemia. Potassium supplements, salt substitutes, potassium penicillin, stored blood transfusions, oral tobacco products can all cause this condition.

B. **Transcellular shifts.** These can be caused by beta-blockers, digitalis, aldosterone deficiency, insulin deficiency, hypertonicity, succinylcholine, hyperchloremic metabolic acidosis, cell lysis, rhabdomyolysis, hemolysis, or tumor lysis.

1. **Hyperchloremic acidosis** (but not organic acidoses, such as ketoacidosis or lactic acidosis) is associated with hyperkalemia because of cellular shifts. In these cases, the serum potassium increases by an average of 0.5 mEq/L for each 0.1 increase in pH.

2. **Aldosterone deficiency** increases serum potassium by causing potassium to move out of the cells and by decreasing renal excretion.

3. **Insulin deficiency** and hypertonicity (eg, hyperglycemia) independently cause a cellular-to-serum shift of potassium, which explains the hyperkalemia (and prompt resolution with therapy) so often seen in patients with DKA.

4. **Life-threatening hyperkalemia** can be seen with rhabdomyolysis, tumor lysis syndrome, massive hemolysis, and occasionally with succinylcholine, particularly, with simultaneous renal insufficiency.

C. **Decreased renal excretion.** This can be caused by decreased glomerular filtration rate (GFR < 5 mL/min), decreased tubular secretion, aldosterone deficiency, hypoaldosteronism, hyporeninemia, ACE inhibitors, heparin, tubulointerstitial nephritis, analgesic nephropathy, chronic pyelonephritis, sickle cell disease, renal allograft, obstructive uropathy, drugs, triamterene, amiloride, spironolactone, cyclosporine, trimethoprim, pentamidine, or NSAIDs.

1. **Renal insufficiency** can produce hyperkalemia when the GFR decreases to < 10 mL/min, or urine output decreases to < 1 L/d. Exceptions are interstitial nephritis and hyporeninemic hypoaldosteronism, which more frequently cause hyperkalemia because of a defect in tubular potassium secretion.

2. **Adrenal insufficiency** is a known cause of hyperkalemia from impaired renal potassium excretion but is not commonly seen in the ICU.

3. **Drugs.** The drugs that are generally believed to cause hyperkalemia by inhibiting tubular potassium secretion are potassium sparing diuretics (spironolactone, triamterene, and amiloride), pentamidine, heparin, trimethoprim-sulfamethoxazole, NSAIDs, and ACE inhibitors.

D. **Pseudohyperkalemia.** This can be caused by hemolysis of the specimen, a prolonged period of tourniquet application before blood drawing, or thrombocytosis/leukocytosis (potassium is released as the clot forms).

1. **Pseudohyperkalemia** is the release of potassium when blood clots in a test tube. Patients with severe leukocytosis (> 100,000) or thrombocytosis(> 400,000) are particularly prone to this phenomenon.

2. When this condition is suspected, the serum potassium should be measured in an unclotted blood sample.

IV. **Database**

A. **Physical Exam Key Points**

1. **Cardiovascular system.** The most serious consequence of hyperkalemia is slowing of the electrical conduction of the heart. The ECG can begin to change when the serum potassium reaches 6.0 mEq/L, and it is always abnormal when the serum potassium reaches 8.0 mEq/L. ECG changes include peaked T waves in the precordial leads followed by decreased R wave amplitude, widened PR interval, widened QRS complex, and finally loss of the P wave and the development of the sine wave. The final event is ventricular asystole.

2. **Neuromuscular system.** Paraesthesias and weakness may progress to flaccid paralysis.

B. **Laboratory Data**

1. **Electrolytes, BUN, and creatinine.** Check levels to diagnose hyperkalemia and renal failure.

2. **Hemogram.** Check for fictitious hyperkalemia, thrombocytosis, and leukocytosis.
3. **ABG.** Anion gap acidosis.
4. **Cortisol level or ACTH stimulation test.**
5. **Digoxin level.**
6. **Myoglobin level.** Check especially in trauma patients (crush).

C. **Radiographic and Other Studies**
1. **ECG.** Differentiate between "real" and pseudohyperkalemia.
2. **Ultrasound.** Use sonography to rule out renal obstruction.

V. **Plan.** Although hypokalemia is often well tolerated, hyperkalemia (serum K^+ > 5.5 mEq/L) can rapidly become a serious life-threatening condition.

A. The aggressiveness with which hyperkalemia is treated should parallel the severity of the clinical manifestations of the disorder, largely determined by the ECG manifestations. With serum potassium less than 6 mEq/L, little therapy is required, other than discontinuing the occult sources of dietary potassium listed previously.

B. When the potassium level increases to more than 6 mEq/L and/or peaked T waves appear, volume expansion (as tolerated), loop diuretics, and oral Kayexalate are appropriate.

C. When the potassium level increases to more than 7 mEq/L and/or prolonged PR interval and widened QRS complex appear, more urgent therapy is needed. Driving potassium intracellularly with glucose and insulin (25–50 g dextrose with 10–20 U regular insulin) or albuterol (5–20 mg [1.0–4.0 mL] inhaled) is indicated. Albuterol usually works within 30 min, will decrease serum potassium levels to 0.6–1.0 mEq/L and lasts for 2 h or more. Sodium bicarbonate (2 ampules [100 mEq]) causes an exchange of hydrogen for potassium across the cell membranes, decreasing the serum potassium level within minutes.

D. When the potassium level increases to more than 7.5–8.0 mEq/L and/or hyperkalemia-induced heart block, the sine wave, or ventricular arrest appear, therapy with calcium (10–20 mEq IV over 5 min) should be initiated.

E. Other maneuvers to decrease serum potassium level or to remove potassium from the body must also be promptly initiated. Hemodialysis is the most effective method of decreasing the serum potassium level in patients with renal failure.

46. HYPERNATREMIA

I. **Problem.** An elderly patient found comatose at home with a massive stroke is admitted to the ICU with a serum sodium level of 159 mEq/L, a BP of 85/40 and diffuse ST and T wave changes on his ECG.

II. **Immediate Questions**

A. **Has the hypernatremia caused CNS hemorrhage or edema?**

   B. **Has the patient suffered mental status changes or seizures be-**
      cause of severe hypernatremia?
   C. **Does hyponatremia or hypovolemia pose the bigger threat to**
      the patient?
   D. **What medications is the patient taking?**

III. **Differential Diagnosis.** With the rare exception of overadministration of
    hypertonic solutions (such as overzealous sodium bicarbonate adminis-
    tration during cardiopulmonary resuscitation), hypernatremia results
    from loss of hypotonic body fluids without adequate free water replace-
    ment.

   A. **Inadequate fluid resuscitation.** Check especially in comatose and
      postoperative patients.
   B. **Free water loss.** Most bodily fluids are hypotonic with respect to
      sodium, thus excessive losses will lead to hypernatremia.
      1. **Nonrenal losses:** These are caused by NG suction, diarrhea, fis-
         tulas, insensible pulmonary losses (intubated patients), and in-
         sensible cutaneous losses (in fever up to 0.5 L per 24 h per
         degree centigrade above 38 °C).
      2. **Renal losses:** These are caused by diuretics, nephropathy, dia-
         betes insipidus and mellitus, ATN (polyuric phase), and drugs (Di-
         lantin, mannitol, phenytoin, and lithium).
      3. **Steroid hormones.** These cause hypernatremia by excessive
         administration of steroids, increased/ectopic ACTH production,
         Cushing's syndrome, and primary aldosteronism.

IV. **Database**
   A. **History.** The history should focus on potential fluid-losing conditions,
      how rapidly the hypernatremia developed, and mental status
      changes and seizures.
   B. **Physical Examination Key Points**
      1. **Vital signs.** Orthostatics and tachycardia will indicate hypovolemia.
      2. **Skin.** Inspect for turgor, mucous membranes, and cushingoid fea-
         tures.
      3. **Neurologic.** Include mental status.
   C. **Laboratory Data**
      1. **Electrolytes.** Assessment of BUN/creatinine levels will help de-
         termine dehydration. Other electrolyte abnormalities occur fre-
         quently.
      2. **Hemogram.** Hct will increase in dehydration.
      3. **Urine sodium.** When level is < 20 mEq/L, it suggests extrarenal
         volume losses.
      4. **Serum/Urine osmolality.** This is increased with volume
         losses/hypertonic urine suggesting extrarenal losses and isotonic
         or hypotonic urine suggesting renal losses.

V. Plan

A. When hypovolemic sequelae (such as myocardial ischemia or renal failure) predominate, the hypovolemia should be rapidly corrected with a normal saline IV infusion.

B. When hypernatremic sequelae, such as mental status changes or seizures predominate, free water administration to correct the hypernatremia should take precedence. To avoid the theoretical risk of cerebral edema resulting from rapid rehydration, only half the free water deficit should be replaced on the first day. Because hypernatremic patients usually also have total body sodium depletion, formulas assuming constant total body sodium will underestimate the free water deficit.

The formula to determine free water needed is as follows:

$$\text{Water deficit} = (0.6 \times \text{current weight in kg}) - \text{TBW},$$

where TBW = 0.6 × preadmission body weight in kg.

C. Treat underlying cause of hypernatremia: Check for nonrenal losses, diabetes mellitus, diabetes insipidus, and so forth.

47. HYPERTENSION

I. Problem. After AAA repair, a 65-year-old man is brought to the ICU with a BP of 190/110.

II. Immediate Questions

A. Is this a hypertensive crisis? Hypertensive crisis is defined as a hypertensive emergency or hypertensive urgency. Acute or ongoing vital target organ damage in a patient with severe hypertension is considered a hypertensive emergency. It requires a prompt reduction in blood pressure within minutes or hours. Complications include death, stroke, nephropathy, myocardial ischemia/infarction, nephropathy, retinopathy, or peripheral vascular disease.

B. Is there end organ damage? The absence of target organ damage in the presence of a severe elevation of blood pressure is a hypertensive urgency and requires reduction in blood pressure within 24–48 h. There is a continuum between the clinical syndrome of hypertensive urgency and emergency; hence, their distinction may not always be clear and precise.

C. What medication is the patient taking? Sympathomimetics, steroids, and contraceptives can be associated with acute hypertension.

D. Is there a history of hypertension? Mild elevation may be seen after surgery with large fluid infusions.

E. Does the patient have a chest pain or focal neural findings? Hypertension can induce ischemic syndromes and intracerebral bleeds.

III. Differential Diagnosis

The most common cause of hypertensive encephalopathy is abrupt elevation of BP in the chronically hypertensive patient. Other conditions predisposing a patient to elevated blood pressure can cause the same clinical situation.

A. Postoperative Causes

1. **Pain.**
2. **Hypoxia.**
3. **Vasospasm.**
4. **Carotid sinus reflex abnormalities** (eg, status post carotid endarterectomy)
5. **Fluid overload.**

B. Other Causes

1. **Chronic renal parenchymal disease.**
2. **Acute glomerulonephritis.**
3. **Renovascular hypertension.**
4. **Withdrawal from hypertensive agents (eg, clonidine).**
5. **Encephalitis, meningitis.**
6. **Pheochromocytoma.**
7. **Sympathomimetic agents (eg, cocaine, amphetamines, phencyclidine [PCP], lysergic acid diethylamide [LSD]).**
8. **Eclampsia and preeclampsia.**
9. **Head trauma and acute cerebral vascular events (eg, strokes, hemorrhage, embolus, edema).**
10. **Collagen vascular disease.**
11. **Autonomic hyperactivity.**
12. **Vasculitis.**
13. **Ingestion** of tyramine-containing foods or tricyclic antidepressants in combination with monamine oxidase (MAO) inhibitors.

IV. Database

A. History.

A thorough review of the medical history is essential. The absence of a prior history of hypertension should prompt emphasis on a review of systems, medication list, and medication compliance. Actively seek recreational drug-induced causes. Neurologic complaints are vague and may include headache, confusion, visual disturbances, seizures, nausea, and vomiting. With cardiac ischemia, angina, palpitations, arrhythmias, and dyspnea may be present. Renal involvement may produce hematuria and acute renal failure.

B. Physical Exam Key Points

1. **Neurologic Exam.** A thorough and complete neurologic and funduscopic exam should be used in assessing the extent of cerebral involvement. On funduscopic exam, look for papilledema, hemorrhage, exudates, and cotton-wool spots. Transient and migratory neurologic nonfocal deficits, ranging from nystagmus to weak-

ness, and an altered mental status, ranging from confusion to coma, may be present.

2. **Cardiopulmonary exam.** Signs of heart failure include the presence of an S_3 gallop, distended neck veins, peripheral edema, murmurs, abdominal pulsations, and diminished pulses. Acute renal failure can cause pulmonary and peripheral edema with rales, and wheezes on auscultation.

C. **Laboratory Data**
   1. **Hemogram.** Obtain a CBC and check for the presence of microangiopathic hemolytic anemia.
   2. **Urinalysis, BUN, and creatinine:** With hypertensive nephropathy, an elevated creatinine with hematuria and casts may be present. Urine toxicology screen is important in excluding drug-induced hypertensive encephalopathy.
   3. **Cardiac Enzymes.** Exclude myocardial ischemia by monitoring cardiac enzymes.

D. **Radiographic and Other Studies**
   1. **Head CT.** Scan to evaluate for presence of stroke, hemorrhage, or intracranial masses.
   2. **Chest radiograph.** Obtain to evaluate for possible complications of hypertensive encephalopathy, including aspiration caused by altered mentation. A chest radiograph can also evaluate for other disorders (eg, acute pulmonary edema and aortic dissection).
   3. **ECG.** Perform an ECG to evaluate for the presence of cardiac ischemia.

V. Plan

A. When initiating therapy, the admitting blood pressure should be used as a baseline to avoid overtreatment with resulting relative hypotension and inadequate perfusion. An excessive decrease can compromise blood flow, inducing cerebral ischemia. Decreasing the mean arterial pressure by 25% usually is a safe maneuver; the resulting blood pressure should still be within the autoregulatory cerebral blood flow range.

B. Even in a chronically hypertensive patient with altered baseline cerebral blood flow autoregulation, a 25% decrease in mean arterial pressure would likely fall into the autoregulatory range.

C. The goals of therapy usually are to lower mean arterial pressure by 25% and diastolic blood pressure to 100–110 mm Hg.

D. Intensive care unit monitoring with arterial blood pressure monitoring is required for adequate titration of pharmacologic agents. Routine neurologic reassessment is also necessary to monitor signs of deterioration because of inadequate treatment, progression of neurologic insult, overzealous reduction in blood pressure, or other alternate causes.

E. Quickly and effectively treat severe hypertension to deter the progression to coma and death. When invasive monitoring is not immediately available, initiate alternate therapy with agents that do not require close monitoring until a monitored situation becomes available.

F. Medications

1. **Nitroprusside sodium (Nitropress).** This agent decreases systemic vascular resistance via direct dilatation of arterioles and veins. Although it may increase ICP, it is still considered first-line therapy for its rapid onset and short duration of action (see page 494).

   a. **Adult Dose.** Administer 0.5–1 μg/kg/min IV infusion, and titrate to desired BP.

   b. **Contraindications.** Documented hypersensitivity; idiopathic hypertrophic subaortic stenosis, and atrial fibrillation or flutter.

   c. **Precautions.** Potential for cyanide toxicity occurs with prolonged infusion (> 72 h) and high infusion rate (> 3 μg/kg/min); suspect with hyperreflexia, worsening mental status, and toxicity in presence of metabolic acidosis; treatment for cyanide toxicity includes amyl nitrate, thiosulfate, and hydroxocobalamin; dialysis may be necessary for thiocyanate toxicity; hypoxia by inhibition of hypoxia-induced vasoconstriction in the pulmonary vasculature, causing perfusion to nonventilated areas of the lung.

2. **Labetalol (Normodyne).** Competitive and selective alpha 1-blocker and nonselective beta-blocker with predominantly beta effects at low doses. Onset of action is 5 min with half-life of 5.5 h. Provides a steady consistent drop in BP without compromising cerebral blood flow. Used when invasive blood pressure monitoring is not available for initiation of nitroprusside (see page 481).

   a. **Adult Dose.** 20 mg IV bolus, then 20–80 mg IV bolus every 10 min; not to exceed 300 mg. Alternatively, 2 mg/min IV infusion, titrate to desired BP; not to exceed 300 mg.

   b. **Contraindications.** Documented hypersensitivity; cardiogenic shock, pulmonary edema, bradycardia, atrioventricular block, uncompensated congestive heart failure, reactive airway disease, and severe bradycardia.

   c. **Interactions.** Labetalol decreases effect of diuretics and increases toxicity of methotrexate, lithium, and salicylates; may diminish reflex tachycardia, resulting from nitroglycerin use, without interfering with hypotensive effects; cimetidine may increase labetalol blood levels; glutethimide may decrease labetalol effects by inducing microsomal enzymes.

   d. **Precautions.** Caution in impaired hepatic function; discontinue therapy when there are signs of liver dysfunction; in elderly patients, a lower response rate and higher incidence of toxicity may be observed.

3. **Nitroglycerin (Nitro-Bid).** Provides arteriolar dilation and venodilation. Used in emergencies involving myocardial ischemia caused by the dilatation of coronary arteries (see page 494).
   a. **Adult Dose.** Administer 5–300 μg/min IV infusion, titrate to desired BP.
   b. **Contraindications.** Documented hypersensitivity; severe anemia, shock, postural hypotension, head trauma, closed angle glaucoma, or cerebral hemorrhage.
   c. **Interactions.** Aspirin may increase nitrate serum concentrations; marked symptomatic orthostatic hypotension may occur with coadministration of calcium channel blockers (dose adjustment of either agent may be necessary).
   d. **Precautions.** Caution in coronary artery disease and low systolic blood pressure.
4. **Trimethaphan camsylate (Arfonad).** A ganglionic blocking agent primarily used in aortic dissection. Reduces heart rate and left ventricular ejection rate, thus lowering shearing force (see page 515).
   a. **Adult Dose.** Administer 0.5–10 mg/min IV infusion, and titrate to desired BP.
   b. **Contraindications.** Documented hypersensitivity; anemia; cerebral vascular disease; coronary artery disease; glaucoma; hypovolemia; MI; respiratory insufficiency; shock.
   c. **Interactions.** Coadministration with anesthetic agents may cause hypotension; trimethaphan may potentiate neuromuscular blocking action of nondepolarizing agents and succinylcholine. Precautions: decreased cardiac output and peripheral vascular resistance may occur, causing orthostatic hypotension; ganglionic blockade causes dry mouth, visual changes, urinary retention, and ileus.
5. **Phentolamine (Regitine).** Alpha-1 and alpha-2 adrenergic blocking agent that blocks circulating epinephrine and norepinephrine action, reducing hypertension that results from catecholamine effects on the alpha receptors.
   a. **Adult Dose.** 5–10 mg IV bolus 0.2–5 mg/min IV infusion.
   b. **Contraindications.** Documented hypersensitivity; coronary or cerebral arteriosclerosis and renal impairment.
   c. **Interactions.** Concurrent administration of epinephrine or ephedrine may decrease phentolamine effects; ethanol increases phentolamine toxicity.
   d. **Precautions.** Caution in tachycardia, peptic ulcer, and gastritis; cerebrovascular occlusions and myocardial infarctions can occur following phentolamine administration.
6. **Nicardipine (Cardene).** Calcium channel blocker, potent, rapid onset of action, ease of titration, and lack of toxic metabolites. Effective but limited reported experience in hypertensive encephalopathy (see page 493).
   a. **Adult Dose.** Loading: 5–15 mg/h IV, maintenance: 3–5 mg/h IV.

   b. **Contraindications.** Documented hypersensitivity; severe hypotension, cardiogenic shock, atrial fibrillation, CHF interactions: H_2 blockers may increase bioavailability of nicardipine; coadministration with propranolol or metoprolol may increase cardiac depressant effects on AV conduction.
   c. **Precautions.** Adjust dose in hepatic and renal impairment; may increase frequency and duration of angina attacks.
7. **Hydralazine (Hydrea).** Direct arteriolar dilator, limited role because of reflex tachycardia causing increased cardiac oxygen demand (see page 475).
   a. **Adult Dose.** 5–20 mg IV bolus, 0.5–1 mg/min IV infusion.
   b. **Contraindications.** Documented hypersensitivity; mitral valve rheumatic heart disease interactions: MAO inhibitors and beta blockers may increase hydralazine toxicity; pharmacologic effects of hydralazine may be decreased by indomethacin.
   c. **Precautions.** Has been implicated in myocardial infarction; use with caution in suspected coronary artery disease. Transition to oral antihypertensives should be initiated after end-organ damage has been controlled. In hypertensive urgency, oral antihypertensives can be administered concurrent to any parenteral therapy.

48. HYPOGLYCEMIA

I. **Problem.** A patient with severe pancreatitis becomes diaphoretic and tachycardic, but his mental status is normal. His serum glucose is 28 mg/dL.

II. **Immediate Questions**
   A. **Does the hypoglycemia cause significant sequelae, such as altered mental status, seizures, or coma?**
   B. **What medications were given to the patient?** A diabetic patient may be overmedicated with insulin or oral hypoglycemics.
   C. **What is the "no-hypoglycemia" diagnosis?** Retroperitoneal sarcoma, insulinoma, paraneoplastic syndrome, pancreatic transplant, and liver transplant or resection.

III. **Differential Diagnosis**
   A. **Exogenous causes:** Insulin administration, oral hypoglycemics, pentamidine, beta-blockers, and MAO inhibitors are all associated with hypoglycemia.
   B. **Endogenous causes:** Hepatic failure, adrenal crisis and renal failure. Patients with preexisting hypoglycemic conditions, such as reactive hypoglycemia, insulinomas, islet cell hyperplasia, or growth hormone deficiency can also suffer from these in the ICU. Additionally, retroperitoneal sarcomas, paraneoplastic syndrome, factitious

hypoglycemia (when WBC > 40,000, they can metabolize the glucose in the specimen tube; these patients will be asymptomatic), sepsis, and severe malnutrition.

IV. Database

A. Physical Exam Key Points

1. **Signs of counterregulatory hormone release.** Anxiety, tremor, diaphoresis, and tachycardia.
2. **Neurologic exam.** Headache, altered mental status, focal neurologic deficits, seizures, and coma suggest hypoglycemia.

B. Laboratory Data

1. **Serum glucose.** A serum glucose < 40 mg/dL is compatible with hypoglycemia.
2. **Serum insulin and C-peptide.** Detects endogenous insulin (insulinomas versus surreptitious insulin administration).

C. Radiographic and Other Studies.

May be used in the diagnosis of tumors. Arteriography is more useful in the diagnosis of insulinoma.

V. Plan

A. When the patient has symptoms or signs of counterregulatory hormone release or hypoglycemia, and the serum glucose is < 40 mg/dL, a bolus IV administration initially of 50 g of glucose should correct the hypoglycemia.

B. When the underlying cause cannot be corrected, serum glucose must be monitored, and ongoing glucose should be administered. The amount of glucose necessary to prevent recurrent hypoglycemia may suggest the underlying cause. Low rates of glucose administration (such as 5% dextrose at 150 cc/h) suggest failure of gluconeogenesis, such as occurs from hepatic failure or adrenal crisis. High rate of glucose administration (such as 10% dextrose at 200 cc/h) suggest increased insulin activity, such as occurs from insulin overdoses or insulinomas. If the patient has no venous access, intramuscular glucagon will raise the serum glucose acutely when the patient has sufficient hepatic glycogen.

C. **Liver resections.** Patients should be maintained on 10% dextrose, and glucose level should be checked frequently.

D. **Adjust medications**

49. HYPOKALEMIA

I. **Problem.** A 55-year-old man with a history of severe ulcerative colitis is admitted to the ICU with a 4-d history of severe abdominal pain and bloody diarrhea. Initial laboratory data revealed a hyperchloremic non-anion gap metabolic acidosis and a potassium level of 2.6 mEq/L.

II. Immediate Questions

A. **Is the patient symptomatic?** Is there abdominal tenderness, vomiting, nausea, weakness, and ECG changes (arrhythmias, PACs, PVCs, flattening of T waves, U waves, and S-T segment changes)?

B. **What medications was the patient given?** Loop diuretics, amphotericin B, and digitalis. Hypokalemia will potentiate digitalis toxicity.

C. **What is the potassium level?** Hypokalemia (serum potassium < 3.5 mEq/L) may result from decreased intake, increased losses (vomiting, NG suctioning, and diarrhea are the most common causes), or redistribution of potassium.

III. Differential Diagnosis

A. **Gastrointestinal Losses:** These can be caused by diarrhea, cathartics, fistula, villous adenoma, vomiting, or NG suctioning. Significant GI losses of potassium are usually colonic (diarrhea, cathartic abuse) and accompanied by hyperchloremic acidosis. Although gastric juice contains little potassium (10 mEq/L), vomiting or gastric suction often cause hypokalemia because of concurrent volume contraction, secondary hyperaldosteronism, and renal potassium wasting.

B. **Intracellular Potassium Shift.** This can be caused by alkalosis, insulin administration, refeeding, albuterol, or periodic paralysis.

C. **Renal Losses.** These can be caused by diuretics, antibiotics (carbenicillin, ticarcillin, and amphotericin B), postobstructive diuresis, ATN (diuretic phase), hyperaldosteronism, Cushing's syndrome, adrenal carcinoma, contraction alkalosis, renal artery stenosis, corticosteroid therapy, licorice, nonabsorbable anions, platinum compounds, ketones, increased urine flow, Bartter's syndrome, or magnesium depletion. Renal artery stenosis (secondary hyperaldosteronism) also causes hypokalemia because of urinary potassium loss. Renal wastage is also seen when nonabsorbable anions (ie, carbenicillin) are filtered in to the urine, increasing distal potassium secretion. Any process increasing tubular flow will enhance tubular potassium secretion. Renal tubular acidosis (RTA type I and type II) and Bartter's syndrome are rare causes of renal hypokalemia. In the ICU, hypomagnesemia can also be a cause.

IV. Database. Potassium is an intracellular cation; therefore, a serum level of 3.0 mEq/L represents a total body deficit of 150–200 mEq in the adult patient.

A. **Physical Exam Key Points**
1. **Cardiac.** Look for the P wave of an irregular rhythm.
2. **Neurologic exam.** Paralysis, paraesthesias, and blunting of reflexes.

   3. **Gastrointestinal.** Look for signs of obstruction, ileus, distention, and vomiting (may indicate digitalis toxicity or may be the cause of hypokalemia).
B. **Laboratory Data**
   1. **Electrolytes.** Other electrolyte perturbations may coexist (hypocalcemia or hypomagnesemia).
   2. **ABG.** Acid-base disturbances often accompany hypokalemia.
   3. **Urine electrolytes.** Check levels of sodium, potassium, and osmolality to determine renal wasting (useful only for patients not given diuretics).
   4. **Digoxin level.**
C. **Radiographic and Other Studies**
   1. **ECG and rhythm strip.**

V. **Plan.** Severe hypokalemia (ECG changes or serum level < 3 mEq/L) should be treated more expeditiously.
   A. **Parenteral Replacement**
      1. **Indications.** Digoxin toxicity, arrhythmias, potassium level < 3 mEq/L, those who cannot take potassium replacement orally (ideally via central line).
      2. Maximum replacement via peripheral veins should not exceed 40 mEq/L because of the damaging effect of potassium on the veins (in emergency, 60 mEq/L). Up to 20 mEq/h can be replaced via a central line over an hour (in 100 mL of D5W or NS). Check potassium every 2 h and monitor continuously for arrhythmias.
   B. **Oral replacement.** When potassium is > 3 mEq/L, give 40–120 mEq/d in divided doses. This is the ideal route, because hyperkalemia can almost never occur when the patient has normal renal function.
   C. **Refractory cases.** Correct hypocalcemia and/or hypomagnesemia.

50. HYPONATREMIA

I. **Problem.** An ICU patient admitted with cardiogenic pulmonary edema undergoes vigorous diuresis. On hospital day 2, her serum sodium level decreases from 134 mEq/L to 112 mEq/L, and she suffers a 5-min grand mal seizure.

II. **Immediate Questions**
   A. **Does the patient have mental status changes or seizures not readily explainable by processes other than the hyponatremia?**
   B. **What is causing the hyponatremia?**

III. **Differential Diagnosis**
   A. True hyponatremia usually results from antidiuretic hormone (ADH) causing excess free water retention. Appropriate ADH activity results from hypertonicity or severe hypovolemia. Inappropriate ADH activity

may result in hypervolemic patients whose volume receptors misperceive volume status as being low. The syndrome of inappropriate antidiuretic hormone release (SIADH) occurs when patients release ADH in response to neither hypertonicity nor real nor misperceived hypovolemia.

B. **Common causes of hyponatremia in ICU patients include**
   1. **Hyperosmotic:** Hyperglycemia and mannitol administration.
   2. **Hypovolemia:** Over diuresis, diarrhea, vomiting/gastric suctioning, mineralocorticoid deficiency.
   3. **Hypervolemia misperceived as hypovolemia:** Congestive heart failure, nephrotic syndrome, liver failure, SIADH, pain, narcotic, psychosis, myxedema, glucocorticoid deficiency, and total body potassium deficiency.

IV. **Database.** The history should elicit recent mental status changes and seizures to assess the severity of the hyponatremia. It should also elicit likely causes such as those listed previously.

   A. **Physical Exam Key Points.** The physical exam should assess the mental status and volume status.

   B. **Laboratory Data.** Determine the serum sodium level and tonicity. High BUN, creatinine, BUN/creatinine ratio, and uric acid may all reflect true or misperceived hypovolemia. Urine and serum osmolality, liver function tests, thyroid function tests, cortisol level, and ACTH stimulation tests should also be done.

   C. **Radiographic and Other Studies**
      1. **Chest radiograph.** Looking for failure.
      2. **Head CT.** When indicated.
      3. **Water load Test.** Restrict fluids until serum sodium level is normal; then challenge with 20 mL/kg of water orally; then collect urine for the next 5 h. When < 75% of the water given is excreted or when urine osmolarity fails to decrease < 200, a diagnosis of SIADH may be made.

V. **Plan**

   A. Patients suffering hyponatremic seizures or mental status changes require emergent, rapid correction of their serum sodium to 118 mEq/L or until resolution of their hyponatremic stigmata. Hypertonic saline should not be used. Hypervolemic or SIADH patients may require concomitant diuretic administration.

   B. Acutely ill patients who have corrected their sodium level to 118 mEq/L and nonacute patients should be treated according to the cause of their hyponatremia, and serum sodium should probably be corrected no faster than 0.5 mEq/L/h to avoid an unquantified risk of central pontine myelinolysis. Intravenous normal saline infusion should correct hypovolemic patients. Therapy for hypervolemic patients should address their underlying conditions; treating the hyponatremia per se is usually counterproductive. Therapy for SIADH patients should address the underlying disorder. Free water restriction will treat the hyponatremia nonspecifically; saline infusion may worsen the hyponatremia.

51. HYPOTENSION

Immediate Actions. Hypotension requires immediate assessment and treatment. Ensure intact airway, breathing, and secure large-bore IV access (ABCs). A systolic blood pressure of less than 90 mm Hg is considered hypotension in an adult and suggests compromise of oxygen delivery to vital tissues. Immediate interventions consist of rapid administration of IV fluid and, possibly, the placement of the patient in the Trendelenburg position. In hypovolemic states, positioning may not be therapeutic. A thorough search for active bleeding should be undertaken. This bleeding may be either internal or external. Apply direct pressure to obvious bleeding.

I. **Problem.** A 64-year-old woman who had an elective AAA repair earlier in the day has a BP of 85/65.

II. **Immediate Questions**

   A. **What are the other vital signs?** Sinus tachycardia (although often a late finding) suggests intravascular volume depletion. Large intraabdominal procedures result in "third spacing" of fluids; patients usually need 24–48 h of extra IV fluid to keep the intravascular space replete. An arrhythmia, such as atrial fibrillation or SVT, does not allow the ventricles to fill or empty appropriately.

   B. **How was the blood pressure measured?** Is the pressure from a cuff or from an arterial line? Excessive edema may generate inaccurate pressures as may also an improperly sized cuff. Arterial lines are subject to both dampening of the waveform and a whip artifact that under- and overestimate the actual pressure. When arterial line measurements are used, confirmation with cuff pressure measurements can eliminate the question of artifact.

   C. **What has the urine output been?** Urine output is a marker of perfusion. Roughly 25% of the cardiac output flows to the kidneys. In the presence of normal renal function, urine output provides an accurate reflection of the intravascular volume status. Adults should have 0.5 cc/kg/h. Pediatric kidneys do not have the same capacity to concentrate urine. As such, for pediatric patients, acceptable urine output should be at least 1.0 cc/kg/h.

D. **What surgery was done and when?** Different procedures have different propensities for postoperative volume difficulties. Other procedures are not prone to have "hidden" or silent bleeding or volume loss.

E. **Was an intra-abdominal operation performed?** Significant shifts of intravascular volume may occur. Fluid may enter the bowel lumen, the bowel wall, or the peritoneal cavity. In addition, bleeding may occur postoperatively into the peritoneal cavity.

F. **Was there a large intraoperative blood loss?** Incomplete resuscitation intraoperatively can cause hypotension. Large volume blood loss may also lead to a coagulopathy that extends the degree of bleeding.

G. **Has the patient had recent laboratory determinations?** Anemia, when present, may need correction. An elevation in the white count can suggest a possible infection that may result in sepsis and a low systemic vascular resistance. Elevation in BUN and creatinine levels may make urine output a less reliable marker of volume status.

H. **Does the patient have a cardiac history?** Pump failure may result from either significant myocardial ischemia or infarction. Pacemaker dysfunction may also lead to pump failure. For patients with cardiac diseases, hypotension may generate a secondary insult to the heart, creating an additional source of hypotension.

I. **Are there invasive monitors in place?** A Swan-Ganz catheter allows better determination of pump function by providing a means of calculating cardiac output. CVP and wedge pressures reflect intravascular volume status.

J. **Was there recent administration of anti-hypertensive drugs?** Regimens that have been stable for the patient in the past may overmedicate in the acute phase of an illness or injury.

III. **Differential Diagnosis**

A. **Hypovolemia.** This is by far the most common cause of hypotension immediately postoperatively. Many nonoperative conditions may also generate hypovolemia. Direct initial attention to the patient's ICU flow sheet. When the patient has been to the operating room, the flow sheet may be incomplete. The anesthesia record should be consulted.

B. Incomplete resuscitation from any cause may precipitate hypotension. Unless there are very strong clinical contraindications to intravenous fluids, volume therapy should be initiated. When episodes requiring resuscitation are repeated, ongoing blood loss should be suspected and corrected. DIC may evolve as the patient's illness progresses.

C. Nonhemorrhagic sources of volume loss may also be present. Insensible loss may be significant with persistent fevers. NG suction may generate voluminous fluid losses. Diarrhea may be difficult to measure, but it can generate hypovolemia. Burns and open surgical wounds can be significant sources of hypovolemia (see page 47).

D. Cardiogenic Shock

1. **Primary cardiac dysfunction.** Perioperative or primary myocardial infarction may lead to hypotension. A 12-lead ECG is useful to check for S-T changes or to compare with a preoperative tracing. Comparison with old ECG studies is crucial to avoid missing evidence of ischemia and infarction. Pseudonormalization can obscure S-T segment changes when the preexisting ECG is not normal. Hypothermia from any cause may exacerbate the patient's cardiac function. Large transfusions or non-warmed IV fluid can cause hypothermia, which in turn, can affect cardiac contractility.

2. **Secondary cardiac dysfunction.** Many other clinical conditions result in inadequate cardiac output. Cardiac tamponade, tension pneumothorax, and high levels of PEEP can all impair venous return, and subsequently, cardiac output.

E. Neurogenic Shock.
Trauma patients with cervical spinal cord injuries lose sympathetic regulation, resulting in hypotension. Characteristically, they are hypotensive without a concomitant tachycardia.

F. Septic Shock.
Bacterial toxins cause a decrease in systemic vascular resistance. There is often an associated lactic acidosis. All infections do not generate septic shock, so the mere presence of bacteria on culture reports does not equate to sepsis.

G. Anaphylactic Shock.
This condition can be caused by IV contrast, high dose narcotics, or dextrans. The airway needs to be protected and epinephrine given (1:1000 0.3–0.5 mL SQ). Diphenhydramine may be used as an adjunct.

H. Adrenal Crisis.
The actual incidence of this condition is relatively uncommon. However, concomitant hypoglycemia, hyponatremia, and hyperkalemia suggest the diagnosis. These patients are refractory to volume resuscitation and pressors. Diagnosis is by rapid ACTH stimulation test. When unable to logistically obtain the test, empiric therapy may be instituted. Unstable patients are treated with stress-dose steroids and IV fluid with glucose.

IV. Database

A. Physical Exam Key Points

1. **Vital signs.** Elevation in temperature may be indicative of infection and subsequent sepsis. Relative bradycardia with hypotension suggests spinal cord injury with loss of sympathetic tone. Antihypertensive overdose, most evident with beta blockers may also result in this condition. In athletes and children, hypotension may occur late in hypovolemia. Arrhythmias should be identified.

2. **Global exam.** Look for clinical signs of external bleeding or other fluid loss. Direct attention at any wounds or drains. Blood loss into dressings or linens may be difficult to measure.

3. **Skin.** Patients in hypovolemic shock have cool and clammy skin. Ecchymosis may reflect internal hemorrhage. Traumatic wounds may be evident.

4. **Neck.** Look for jugular venous distention (JVD). This condition reflects an elevated central venous pressure (CVP). The degree of JVD may be used to clinically assess the CVP by direct measurement. Pericardial tamponade, tension pneumothorax, and pump failure may all lead to abnormal amounts of JVD. When the patient is also hypovolemic, tamponade and tension pneumothorax may not lead to JVD.

5. **Cardiovascular.** Listen for muffled heart sounds. Look at the ECG tracing. Identify the presence and the trend of tachycardia. New murmurs can indicate myocardial dysfunction and subsequent pump failure.

6. **Pulmonary.** Changes in the quality of breath sounds can indicate pneumothorax or pleural effusion. Consolidation suggestive of pneumonia may be identified.

7. **Abdomen.** Tenderness, guarding, and hypoactive bowel sounds reflect an acute abdominal process. Peritonitis with subsequent fluid sequestration may be evident. Intraabdominal hemorrhage may also be present. Abdominal distention from intraabdominal bleeding is usually not identified until massive blood loss has occurred.

8. **Extremities.** Increasing edema suggests continued loss of volume into the extravascular spaces. Traumatic wounds may be present and not identified on the initial assessment.

9. **Neurologic.** Decreased mentation suggests poor oxygen delivery to the brain. Cervical cord transection will present with lower extremity flaccidity and loss of rectal tone. Hypotension and bradycardia suggest spinal cord injury.

B. **Laboratory Data**

1. **Hemogram.** Check to make sure the patient has an adequate hemoglobin. Both chronic and acute blood loss will lead to a low hemoglobin level. In the circumstance of acute hemorrhage, the hemoglobin level may not reflect the degree of blood loss. Clinical judgment will direct therapy.

2. **Electrolytes.** Volume shifts that result from the resuscitation or the event leading to the hypotension require that electrolyte levels be monitored. In addition, hypotension may lead to acute tubular necrosis. Frequent electrolyte assessment will allow appropriate intervention (see also Problem 45, Hyperkalemia, and Problem 63, Oliguria/Anuria).

3. **Check coagulation studies.** Coagulopathy will prolong the bleeding and hamper efforts to correct intravascular volume de-

pletion. "Medical coagulopathy" also makes surgical interventions more hazardous. Fresh frozen plasma, platelets, and cryoprecipitate may all be required.

4. **Arterial blood gas.** This determination is essential in determining acid base status. Acidosis reflects inadequate perfusion until proven otherwise. Respiratory alkalosis is seen with early sepsis, followed by metabolic acidosis.

5. **Cardiac enzymes.** Creatinine phosphokinase (CPK) with isoenzymes and troponin assess the presence of myocardial damage. Serial determinations are needed for complete diagnosis.

C. **Radiographic and Other Data**
   1. **Chest radiograph.** This allows for determination of hemothorax, pneumothorax, and occasionally, tamponade. The presence of enlarged cardiac silhouette suggests tamponade or failure, but its absence does not exclude these diagnoses.
   2. **Pulmonary artery catheter.** PA catheter (Swan-Ganz catheter) placement is not, in itself, therapeutic. The data must be interpreted and placed in clinical context. A general summary of information from PA catheters is displayed in Table I–1. Reassessment during volume replacement may provide the greatest utility of the monitoring device.

V. **Plan**

A. **Immediate Plan.** Resuscitation and control of hemorrhage provide the cornerstone of management of hypotension. Definitive diagnosis should not be required before the onset of therapy. Communication between critical care teams, surgery, blood bank, and the operating room are essential.

B. **Specific Plans**
   1. **Hypovolemic shock.** Resuscitate with crystalloid and blood products as necessary. Initial therapy is fluid, not the administration of pressors. Adequate intravascular volume should be insured before *any* pharmacologic therapy is initiated. Apply

TABLE I–1. PULMONARY ARTERY CATHETER TRENDS WITH DIFFERENT CAUSES OF HYPOTENSION.

Cause	CVP/Wedge[a]	CO[b] (4–8)	SVR[c] (800–1400)
Hypovolemic	Down	Down	Up
Cardiogenic	Up	Down	Up
Neurogenic	Normal	Normal	Down
Septic	Normal/up	Up	Down

[a]CVP = central venous pressure; [b]CO = cardiac output; [c]SVR = systemic vascular resistance.

pressure to external bleeding sources, when present. Pressure dressings or occlusion devices are markedly inferior to direct digital pressure. Place a Foley catheter to monitor urine output. When a central line is in place, transduce CVP. When there is a poor response to fluids, consider another cause or ongoing blood loss. When the clinical picture is unclear, or there is suspicion of cardiac dysfunction, consider PA catheter placement.

2. **Cardiogenic shock.** Place PA catheter and support with appropriate pharmacologic agents. Dobutamine, dopamine, epinephrine, norepinephrine, or nitrates may all be required. Supplemental oxygen may be necessary. Morphine for pain may blunt endogenous catecholamine release. Pericardiocentesis may be necessary for tamponade. When the patient is in the acute postoperative period from open heart surgery, emergent opening of the sternotomy may be required in the ICU. When there is suspicion of tension pneumothorax, empiric needle decompression followed by chest tube placement is indicated when there is hemodynamic instability.

3. **Neurogenic shock.** Initial therapy includes volume resuscitation. When hypotension persists, pressor therapy is indicated early. Pulmonary arterial catheter placement can be helpful in the management of these patients.

4. **Septic shock.** Treatment of the underlying infectious process is essential to successful management. PA catheter placement can exclude other causes of hypotension. Treat with fluids to maintain CVP/wedge. Therapy with pressors may be required, but their use should be guided by the clinical situation. The overall goal is to maximize organ perfusion. Culture appropriate body fluids when source is unknown. Aggressive search for any undrained infection should be undertaken. "Mundane" sources may develop during hospitalization, such as appendicitis, diverticulitis, perirectal abscesses, or suppurative thrombophlebitis. A thorough reassessment is indicated when no focal source can be identified.

52. HYPOTHERMIA

I. **Problem.** An elderly man with alcohol intoxication is found unconscious in an alley. Upon admission, his rectal temperature is 30.2 °C, and he is shivering.

II. **Immediate Questions**

   A. **What are the vital signs?** Does the patient have a cardiac arrhythmia?

   B. **What is the core temperature?** Core temperature will guide therapy, passive or active rewarming, cardioversion, or drug therapy.

III. Differential Diagnosis

A. Definitions. Hypothermia, defined by a core temperature < 35 °C. can result from exposure to severe cold, such as a cold water immersion. When it develops in an ICU patient, it typically results from thermoregulatory impairment, such as alcohol intoxication, barbiturate overdose, hypothyroidism, hypoadrenalism, hypopituitarism, massive central nervous system insult, erythroderma, burns, exfoliative dermatitis, and sepsis.

IV. Database

A. History. Look for preceding cold exposure, drug use, and the preexisting medical conditions listed previously that impair thermoregulation.

B. Physical Exam Key Points

1. **Vital signs.** Continuously monitor the core temperature (noninvasive thermometers should be placed at least 5 cm from the anal verge), blood pressure and volume status; take notice of shivering.

2. **Neurologic exam.** Perform a complete neurologic exam, including mental status when patient is not comatose.

C. Laboratory Data

1. **Hemogram.** Rule out complicating conditions, such as sepsis (especially for older patients), and determine the oxygen-carrying capacity of the blood and hemoconcentration.

2. **Electrolytes, BUN, creatinine, and glucose.** Volume status and hypoglycemia.

3. **Urinalysis.** Rule out myoglobinuria (caused by shivering).

4. **ABG.**

D. Radiographic and Other Studies

1. **Continuous core temperature monitoring.** This will guide therapy.

2. **ECG and continuous cardiac monitoring.**

V. Plan. Specific therapy should address an underlying medical condition that impairs thermoregulation. As long as patients remain hypothermic, they risk refractory ventricular fibrillation, which rough handling may provoke.

A. Core temperature exceeds 30 °C and the patient is shivering. Passive rewarming by covering the patient with blankets will safely treat the hypothermia.

B. Patients who are not shivering. Such patients require active rewarming.

1. **External active rewarming.** Heat applied to the body surface avoids invasive devices; however, it may result in rewarming

shock, as cutaneous vascular beds vasodilate, and it may precipitate paradoxical core cooling and acidosis. These may all result in refractory ventricular fibrillation.

Use for patients with core temperatures exceeding 28 °C; core temperatures less than 28 °C mandate internal active rewarming. Most drugs are ineffective in hypothermic patients; however, oxygen and dextrose should be given, and bretylium may be given as prophylaxis against ventricular fibrillation. Even in the absence of vital signs or central nervous system activity, patients should not be declared dead until they have been rewarmed.

2. Internal active rewarming. Heated lavage of the bladder, stomach, or peritoneum, or heated extracorporeal circulation require invasive devices but lessen the chance of rewarming, shock, paradoxical core cooling, and acidosis.

53. INCREASED INTRACRANIAL PRESSURE

I. **Problem.** The intracranial pressure (ICP) in a 26-year-old man who sustained a closed head injury secondary to assault 2 d ago is now 25 mm Hg.

II. **Immediate Questions**

A. **What are the Vital Signs?** Increased ICP related to increased respiratory rate, temperature, and blood pressure can be treated. Overall management is directed to correction of a dysfunctional hyperdynamic state. Cerebral perfusion, however, must be maintained.

B. **Has there been a neurologic change?** When the patient is not intubated and is having symptoms of increased ICP, intubation may be necessary. Sedation and paralytics are useful in intubated patients. Metabolic demands are attenuated and ICP "spiking" is minimized.

III. **Differential Diagnosis**

A. **Physiologic**

1. **Increased $Paco_2$.** Hypercarbia may cause cerebral vasodilatation. Intentional hypocarbia, in most cases, will be done under the direction of a neurosurgeon.

2. **Decreased Serum Sodium.** Sodium plays an important role in serum osmolarity and, subsequently, may worsen cerebral edema. Hyponatremia may exacerbate underlying cerebral injury.

3. **Hyperthermia.** This globally increases the metabolic rate and may increase cerebral metabolic demand.

4. **Agitation.** This generally causes increased activity, and the increased respiratory drive (bucking the ventilator) may lead to increased intracranial pressure (ICP).

5. **Seizure Activity.** Dysfunctional brain activity increases metabolic demand and may subsequently lead to increased cerebral activity. Intracranial pressure may increase.

B. Anatomical

1. **Hydrocephalus.** Subarachnoid blood can alter cerebral spinal fluid absorption and lead to hydrocephalus.

2. **Hematoma.**

   a. **Extra-axial**

   b. **Epidural.** Small hematomas may be observed, but surgical intervention is often required.

   c. **Subdural.** In the presence of increasing ICP, evacuation may be urgently required.

   d. **Intraparenchymal.** The need for surgical intervention is less uniform than in other conditions. The decision to drain surgically is based on the overall clinical course and the appearance of the CT scan.

C. Edema. This may be a result of the original injury or be secondary to the perfusion abnormalities generated by the functional activity of the intracranial process.

IV. Database

A. History. Early symptoms of increased ICP include headache, nausea, vomiting, and blurred vision.

B. Physical Exam Key Points

1. **Vital Signs.** Increased temperature results in an increased need for oxygen to the brain, resulting in increased blood flow to the brain. Increased respiratory rate may signify that a patient is agitated and fighting the ventilator. This condition results in increased intrathoracic pressure and decreased venous return from the head. An increase in BP will increase the ICP.

2. **HEENT.** Papilledema suggests increased ICP. Pupillary dilation, unilateral or bilateral, is suggestive of herniation. Head position should be checked to maximize venous return. Cervical spine immobilization devices may exacerbate this condition, especially when improperly fitted. Pharmacologic dilation of the pupil to facilitate the exam should not be done in the acute period.

3. **Neurologic Exam.** Most patients are sedated, but check for spontaneous movements, pain response, and any sign of neurologic deterioration.

C. Laboratory Data

1. **Arterial blood gases.** Increased $Paco_2$ can be treated by increasing the minute volume of the ventilated patient. Increasing minute volume demands may indicate a patient with deteriorating clinical status.

2. **Serum Chemistry.** Rule out any hypo-osmolar cause. Brain injury may result in SIADH or diabetes insipidus. These conditions may result in a secondary brain injury.

3. **Disseminated vascular coagulation (DIC) panel.** Injured brain tissue releases tissue thromboplastin and may cause or sustain

coagulopathy. Worsening or abnormal coagulation studies may indicate new or continued intracranial hemorrhage.

D. Radiographic and Other Studies

  1. Head CT scan. This should be obtained in all patients with a change in clinical exam associated with an increase in ICP. Check for increasing hematoma, edema, or hydrocephalus. When present, they require immediate attention.

V. Plan. The cause of increased ICP should be determined, but initial treatment should be to decrease the ICP. Any increase in ICP more than 20 mm Hg that cannot be corrected or be explained requires a CT scan for evaluation. This is also true for patients with unexplained neurologic deterioration.

  A. Immediate Action. Acute change in the patient's ICP requires urgent intervention to maximize patient outcome. Neurosurgical input and that of critical care teams should be immediately sought to provide optimal management of the patient. Many maneuvers to enhance cerebral perfusion have systemic sequelae. Implementation will ideally be part of a multidisciplinary approach.

  B. Ventilation. Increase minute volume to normalize the $Paco_2$. Hyperventilation beyond normal $Paco_2$ is controversial but may be used in the short term. With depressed mental status, the patient may require intubation. With acute deterioration of mental status, the patient may need intubation for airway control. Once the patient is intubated, sedation and paralytics are useful to decrease agitation and patient-ventilator mismatch. The BP may improve with these interventions. A sedative plan should be chosen that allows for adequate ventilation and neurologic assessments.

  C. Hematoma. Correct coagulopathy. Patients are often hypofibrinogenic and need cryoprecipitate. When the patient's condition is deteriorating, surgical drainage may be necessary.

  D. Diuretics. Mannitol 20% solution (0.25–1 mg/kg every 4–6 h) over 5–15 min will help control cerebral edema. When a large amount of mannitol is being used, Lasix can be added to give greater overall effect. Give 20–60 mg IV 30 min after mannitol. Lasix has been shown to decrease the production of CSF.

  E. Barbiturates. Phenobarbital coma can be induced and works through an unknown mechanism to decrease ICP. Phenobarbital, however, has been shown to decrease blood pressure, which can be harmful to the brain-injured patient.

  F. Rule out Seizures as a Possible Cause. Brain-injured patients are predisposed to seizures. A postictal state may be difficult to distinguish from an unresponsive state.

54. INTRA-AORTIC BALLOON PUMP: HYPOTENSION

I. **Problem.** A 62-year-old man is in the ICU with an intra-aortic balloon pump after cardiac surgery. He has a sudden drop in BP to 65/35 mm Hg.

II. **Immediate Questions**

A. **What are the patient's vital signs?** Inquire about the recent trend and any acute changes in vital signs. Tachycardia, tachypnea, and hypotension require immediate intervention.

B. **What surgical procedure did the patient have?** Determine the nature of the patient's underlying cardiac disease and what procedure was performed. Was the procedure a primary or a reoperative procedure?

C. **Is the patient preoperative or postoperative?** Often balloon pumps may be placed to sustain the patient until cardiac revascularization can be undertaken. The underlying condition may be deteriorating. Postoperative placement may be required when myocardial function is marginal.

D. **What is the patient's cardiac rhythm?** Rhythm disturbances are common after cardiac surgery and may result in impairment of cardiac output. Tachyarrhythmias may prevent effective counterpulsation of the intraaortic balloon pump leading to hypotension.

E. **What are the balloon pump settings?** Determine whether the balloon pump is timed according to the electrical activity of the heart or to the arterial pressure waveform. Also know the pump ratio, and whether any changes have been made recently.

F. **What other cardioactive agents is the patient receiving?** Vasopressor and inotropic drugs are often necessary after cardiac surgery. Also determine whether afterload-reducing agents are being administered, as they may affect blood pressure.

III. **Differential Diagnosis**

A. **Cardiogenic Shock**

1. **Infarction.** Cardiac failure may result from an ischemic insult to the heart. This condition should always be considered in any postoperative patient requiring an intra-aortic balloon pump.

2. **Arrhythmia.** Cardiac rhythm abnormalities may occur in the postoperative patient, but are particularly common after heart surgery. Atrial arrhythmias, in particular, are common after cardiac surgery.

3. **Valvular disruption.** Cardiac valve disease may result from endocarditis or infarction of the papillary muscle. Acute valvular disruption should be considered in cases of acute cardiac decompensation.

4. **Tamponade.** Mediastinal bleeding is a potential problem after cardiac surgery. Observe chest tube output, and verify tube patency. Sudden cessation of significant mediastinal bleeding may signify the development of cardiac tamponade. When a pulmonary artery catheter is in place, equilibration of intracardiac pressures may be observed. Cardiac tamponade may also result after transmural myocardial infarction and ventricular rupture.

5. **Tension pneumothorax.** Patients requiring positive pressure ventilation are at risk of barotrauma and pneumothorax. Elevated ventilator peak airway pressures are usually present. Most patients with aortic balloon pumps also have central venous catheters in place. Often these procedures are performed intraoperatively. Review of radiographs will identify a pneumothorax, if present.

6. **Pulmonary embolus.** Respiratory and cardiac failure may result from pulmonary embolus, particularly for patients at risk of deep venous thrombosis. Prophylaxis for venous thrombosis should be used for patients having surgery and must be given preoperatively to be effective.

B. **Hypovolemic Shock.** Postoperative bleeding is the most common cause of hypovolemia in the surgical patient. Careful attention to volume resuscitation is essential, and invasive hemodynamic monitoring may be appropriate. Intravascular volume depletion is indicated by a decrease in pulmonary artery wedge and central venous pressures. A compensatory tachycardia may be present. Patients with underlying cardiac disease or on beta blockers may not develop tachycardia.

C. **Intra-aortic Balloon Pump Malfunction**

1. **Balloon migration.** Ideally, the balloon is positioned in the descending aorta just distal to the left subclavian artery. Inappropriate positioning or migration of the balloon may lead to ineffective counterpulsation. Radiopaque markers identify the location of the balloon on chest radiograph.

2. **Balloon rupture.** The balloon may rupture, an event that is usually detected by the appearance of blood in the balloon tubing. This may lead to escape of gas from the balloon into the arterial system.

3. **Balloon volume loss.** A leak in the balloon or tubing may lead to inability of the balloon to inflate fully. This is usually detected by the monitor alarms on the pump. Incomplete counterpulsation will both impair forward flow and reduce the amount of afterload reduction on the heart itself.

4. **Asynchrony of counterpulsation.** Inflation and deflation of the balloon are timed to the patient's cardiac cycle. This cycle may be driven by either using the patient's ECG signal or the arterial waveform. When the ECG signal is used, synchronization may be impaired from tachyarrhythmias, artificial pacemaker function, and

low-voltage ECG signals. When the cycle is triggered by pacer spikes, the spike must be clean and not obscured by noise in the system.

5. **Vascular complication.** Rarely, aortic dissection or rupture may result from intra-aortic balloon placement.

IV. Database

A. Physical Exam Key Points

1. **Vital Signs.** Verify functioning of arterial lines and blood pressure cuffs. Dampening of the arterial waveform may indicate a problem in the tubing or transducer. A temperature spike would suggest possible sepsis from an underlying infection. Arrhythmias should be sought.

2. **Neck.** Assess for jugular venous distention. Significant distention would suggest heart failure, cardiac tamponade, or tension pneumothorax.

3. **Cardiac.** Heart sounds may be faint with auscultation when tamponade is present. New murmurs, rubs, or an irregular rhythm can be detected on examination. With complete valvular disruption, murmurs may not be present.

4. **Lungs.** Breath sounds will be diminished when tension pneumothorax or hemothorax is present. Rales would be detected in patients with congestive heart failure. When a chest tube is present, it should be assessed for function.

5. **Extremities.** Assess for peripheral pulses and capillary refill. Absent or weakened pulses confirms significant hypotension. Pulse examination may detect the presence of an arrhythmia. Pulses distal to the insertion site should also be documented.

6. **Neurologic.** Altered mental status may result from inadequate cerebral perfusion.

B. Laboratory Data

1. **Hemogram.** A blood count may show a low hemoglobin level when hemorrhage is the problem. However, a normal level may be obtained initially during a rapid bleed when fluid equilibration has not occurred. WBC may be increased when sepsis is present.

2. **Electrolytes.** Electrolyte abnormalities may result in cardiac arrhythmias. Potassium and magnesium levels should be monitored and corrected as needed.

3. **Arterial blood gas.** Cardiac function may be impaired when acidosis is present. Blood gas analysis can also reveal abnormalities in oxygenation and ventilation.

4. **Cardiac enzymes.** These can be useful for detecting damage to myocardium; however, time is required for enzymes to become elevated. Serial determinations are often required to make the diagnosis.

5. **Mixed venous oxygen saturation.** Mixed venous oxygen saturation may be measured on a continuous basis with an oximetric pulmonary arterial catheter. Changes in the value may give an early indication of impending tamponade.

C. **Radiographic and Other Studies**

1. **Twelve-lead electrocardiogram.** This can be useful for detecting cardiac rate and rhythm abnormalities. Ischemia and pericarditis may be suggested by ST-segment changes. Lead placement may be altered by the presence of the sternotomy and its dressing.

2. **Chest radiograph.** Tamponade may be seen as an enlarged cardiac silhouette, although the absence of a change does not exclude tamponade. Pneumothorax will be seen when present. Additional information relating to pulmonary disease, such as pulmonary edema, infiltrate, and effusion are visible. The radiopaque markers that indicate the position of the balloon should be identified and should confirm proper positioning.

3. **Pulmonary catheter measurements.** Heart pump function can be determined by measuring the cardiac index. Volume status can be estimated using central venous pressure and pulmonary artery occlusion pressure measurements.

4. **Echocardiogram.** This can detect when cardiac tamponade is present. An echocardiogram will also demonstrate both valvular function and myocardial wall motion and function.

5. **V̇/Q̇ scan and pulmonary angiogram.** These can be useful for diagnosing pulmonary embolus when clinically suspicious. V̇/Q̇ scan may both underdiagnose and overdiagnose pulmonary embolism.

V. **Plan**

A. **Overall Plan.** The primary goal is to support adequate blood pressure to ensure tissue perfusion. Generally, a minimum mean arterial pressure of 55 mm Hg is required to maintain cerebral perfusion.

B. **General Measures**

1. Ensure adequate oxygenation, and supplement with ventilatory support when necessary. Establish venous access if not already done.

2. Tension pneumothorax or tamponade requires immediate treatment. When tension pneumothorax is present, rapid needle decompression of the affected side followed by tube thoracostomy is indicated.

3. Cardiac tamponade requires evacuation of pericardial fluid either by pericardiocentesis or mediastinal reexploration when the patient has had recent heart surgery.

4. Provide fluid resuscitation when hypovolemia is present. Initially, crystalloid should be given intravenously; however, blood or another colloid may be required.

   5. Cardiac rate and rhythm abnormalities must be corrected rapidly. Defibrillate when ventricular fibrillation or tachycardia is present. Atrial fibrillation should be treated with cardioversion.
C. Pump Manipulation
   1. When the balloon pump is set to follow the ECG signal, try switching to the arterial waveform. This may fix problems from an ECG artifact or low-voltage signals.
   2. Note any alarms from the balloon pump. When there is a leak in the balloon or tubing, the balloon should be removed and replaced by a new one.
   3. Note the beat ratio of the balloon pump. When the ratio is low, increasing it may improve augmentation (for example from 1:8 to 1:4 or 1:2).
D. Pharmacologic inotropic support may be appropriate when cardiac output is low, and hypovolemia has been corrected. Dopamine, dobutamine, epinephrine, and milrinone IV drips are most commonly used. Pressor support with ephedrine, Neo-Synephrine, or norepinephrine may be used to support blood pressure from low systemic resistance. A pulmonary artery catheter and arterial line should be used to guide therapy and titrate medications appropriately. Clinical judgment is required to tailor the pharmacologic support to the patient's physiology.
E. Congestive heart failure, as characterized by elevated central venous and wedge pressures and rales on lung examination should be treated with diuretics and afterload reduction.

55. INTUBATION: BRONCHOSPASM

I. Problem. After successfully intubating a patient in the ICU, you auscultate the chest to check for bilateral breath sounds, and you notice expiratory wheezes.

II. Immediate Questions
   A. Is the patient ventilating? Wheezing immediately after intubation usually results from tracheal irritation. Airway reactivity can manifest itself as wheezing with a mild obstructive respiratory pattern all the way to severe bronchospasm with no ventilation and hemodynamic instability. Therefore, it is important to recognize and treat even mild bronchospasm early, before it progresses to a more serious problem.
   B. Does the patient have a history of reactive airways? A past medical history of asthma, chronic obstructive pulmonary disease (COPD), and smoking predisposes patients to bronchospasm after intubation. When the previous medical history is known before intubation, certain prophylactic measures can be taken that will be discussed later.

C. **What are the vital signs?** After any intubation, it is vital to monitor BP, heart rate, oxygen saturation, and the presence of end-tidal CO_2.

III. Differential Diagnosis

A. **Tracheobronchial Irritation.** Most cases of postintubation bronchospasm are due to the endotracheal tube irritating the trachea or carina. Laryngoscopy can also elicit bronchospasm. All patients are at risk; however, the inadequately anesthetized patient and the patient with a history of reactive airway disease are at the highest risk.

B. **Cardiac.** Wheezing is not always pulmonary in origin. Volume overload with pulmonary edema and congestive heart failure can cause wheezing. Pulmonary embolism is also a consideration.

C. **Aspiration.** Aspiration of gastric contents during intubation can also induce bronchospasm and should always be included in the differential diagnosis.

D. **Foreign Body.** The presence of a foreign body in the tracheobronchial tree can also be responsible for bronchospasm.

E. **Mechanical Obstruction.** Obstruction of the endotracheal tube can produce wheezing and, therefore, should be considered and ruled out. Kinking, mucus, blood clot, cuff overinflation, endobronchial intubation, and the bevel of the tube lodged against the carina or trachea are all situations that can obstruct an endotracheal tube.

IV. Database

A. **Physical Exam Key Points**

1. **Vital Signs.** Oxygen saturation via pulse oximetry should be closely monitored. A declining saturation is indicative of poor pulmonary gas exchange. Blood pressure and heart rate are also important signs to monitor, and hemodynamic instability is indicative of a deteriorating situation. Tachycardia is often present initially, and bradycardia follows when oxygenation continues to decline.

2. **Pulmonary.** The presence of expiratory wheezes and a prolonged expiratory phase during auscultation are hallmarks of bronchospasm. Inspiratory wheezes may also be present. The inability to auscultate breath sounds in the presence of a properly placed endotracheal tube may indicate severe bronchospasm with no ventilation, and this situation requires immediate intervention. When rales are noted, the wheezing may be due to pulmonary edema.

3. **Cardiac.** The presence of an S_3 gallop may indicate volume overload and a problem of cardiac origin.

B. **Laboratory Data**

1. **ABG.** Draw an arterial blood gas when time permits. Oxygen and carbon dioxide partial pressures (PO_2 and PCO_2) can determine the effectiveness of ventilation and oxygenation.

C. Radiographic and Other Studies

1. **Chest radiograph.** Often, no time is available for a chest radiograph; however, the chest radiograph can help rule out main stem bronchial intubation and, possibly, the presence of a foreign body.

2. **CO_2 waveform analysis.** The presence of a gradual up-sloping end-tidal CO_2 waveform, which never reaches a plateau, is diagnostic of an expiratory airway obstruction. The normal end-tidal CO_2 waveform has a steep upslope during the beginning of expiration, which then reaches a plateau, followed by a steep downslope as expiration begins. The waveform may also be useful in monitoring the improvement of the obstruction.

3. **Ventilation pressures.** Because bronchospasm is an obstructive process, the peak ventilatory pressure will increase dramatically with little to no change in the plateau pressure. Other common causes of increased peak pressure with no change in the plateau pressure are a kinked breathing circuit (inspiratory limb), mucus plugging/secretions, and an overinflated ETT balloon that is obstructing a mainstem bronchus.

4. **Flow-Volume loops.** Ventilators are now available that will produce a flow-volume loop with each breath (Fig I–18). These "loops" or spirograms are a graphical representation of flow against time. The area produced within the "loop" is vital capacity. Bronchospasm can produce a loop with decreased expiratory flows all the way to decreased inspiratory and expiratory flows as with severe bronchospasm.

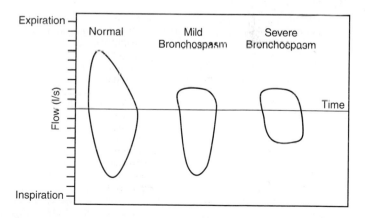

Figure I–18. Flow-volume loops produced by a ventilator demonstrate normal flow in inspiration and expiration. Note the decrease in expiratory flow (mild bronchospasm) or decrease in both expiratory *and* inspiratory flow (severe bronchospasm).

V. Plan

A. Prophylactic Treatment. Ideally, patients with preintubation wheezing or with a history of reactive airway disease should be treated appropriately before intubation, when time allows. This prophylactic treatment should include an anticholinergic (eg, glycopyrrolate) that inhibits reflex bronchospasm and has the added benefit of decreasing irritating airway secretions. An inhaled beta-agonist is also a mainstay of preintubation treatment, ideally via a nebulizer but, at the least, via a multidose inhaler. IV steroids should also be considered in the patient with severe reactive airway disease.

B. Intubation. To prevent bronchospasm, a deeply anesthetized state should be achieved before the airway is instrumented. IV induction agents should be given in the recommended doses—the choice is not as important as the achievement of a deep anesthetic state. Remember that administration of sodium pentothal may cause some histamine release and predispose the patient to bronchospasm. Propofol may actually produce some bronchodilation; it blunts airway reflexes more intensely than sodium pentothal and, therefore, is the agent of choice, assuming no other complicating factors. Etomidate is another reasonable choice, especially for a hemodynamically unstable patient. Ketamine is also an excellent choice and produces bronchodilation via catecholamine release. Treatment with IV lidocaine (1.5 mg/kg) before intubation also helps to blunt airway reflexes. The histamine-releasing paralytic agents (eg, atracurium, curare, and mivacurium) should also be avoided when possible.

C. Postintubation Treatment

1. Mild bronchospasm. After intubation, if wheezing is noted but air exchange is preserved, treatment should focus on treating the mild bronchospasm and preventing further deterioration. An inhaled beta-agonist (albuterol) can be given via a nebulizer through the breathing circuit. Albuterol via an inhaler can also be given but requires a special circuit adapter. Lidocaine can be given intravenously or intratracheally (1.5 mg/kg). An intravenous anticholinergic, such as glycopyrrolate, is also effective and recommended. Steroids should also be considered for their anti-inflammatory effects; they would help reduce the accompanying mucosal edema. It should be noted that the onset of steroids is an hour or longer, and they do not help to improve the immediate situation. The anesthetic should be deepened when possible. This includes another dose of induction agent. When the patient's hemodynamics will tolerate it, ketamine or propofol would be the drugs of choice. The volatile anesthetics are also potent bronchodilators, but these agents are not practical in the ICU. After the bronchospasm is relieved, maintaining sedation while intubated is important to prevent further episodes.

2. **Severe bronchospasm.** When no breath sounds are noted and the trachea has been successfully intubated, then severe bronchospasm may be present. Wheezing might not be heard, because there is little or no air exchange. Immediate treatment with IV epinephrine (1–10 µg/kg) is warranted. Epinephrine is a potent bronchodilator as are all catecholamines. Epinephrine or terbutaline subcutaneously (0.25 mg) is another route but not the first option. Aminophylline can also be given as a 6 mg/kg bolus followed by 0.5–0.9 mg/kg/h. However, aminophylline should be used cautiously for patients already receiving theophylline and they should receive one fourth to one half the normal dose. Also, aminophylline should be used carefully when ketamine has been used, because the combination can precipitate seizures. As with the scenario above, maintenance of sedation and paralysis is key to preventing further exacerbations.

56. LUMBAR DRAIN MALFUNCTION

I. **Problem.** A 56-year-old patient with a severe closed head injury has a lumbar drain in place that had been functioning well, but now the output has nearly stopped.

II. **Immediate Questions**

A. **How long has the drain been in place and has it changed position?** Dislodgment of the catheter during patient care may shear the catheter or kink it.

B. **How much output had there been and what is the change in output over time?** The trends in drainage may indicate whether a purely mechanical problem exists.

C. **Are there any signs of increasing ICP?** If there are, the patient may require surgical decompression.

III. **Differential Diagnosis**

A. **The drain is occluded or kinked.** Inspection of the system with attention to connections and the positioning of the tubing should identify areas that are kinked. In a posttraumatic patient, potential exists for clot.

B. **The drain is dislodged.** Episodes of agitation or patient movement for procedures may dislodge the drainage catheter.

C. **The drain is not at the proper height.** Manipulation of the patient for diagnostic studies or for patient care may have altered the set height of the regulation system.

IV. **Database**

A. **Physical Exam Key Points**
   1. **Vital signs.** Look for respiratory depression or tachypnea.

      2. Neurologic exam. The patient will probably be intubated and sedated. This may limit the completeness of the examination. To the degree that it is clinically possible, a neurologic exam should be undertaken.

  B. Laboratory Data. No specific laboratory study is required.

  C. Radiographic and Other Studies
      1. A CT scan may be warranted when there is evidence of a changing neurologic status.
      2. Radiographs looking for fragments of the drain should be obtained when there is clinical suspicion that the drain has fragmented.

V. Plan

  A. Overall Plan. Assess the need to remove the drain or to revise or drain CSF by a different route.

  B. Specific Plans
      1. Examine the patient and assess the drain. It may simply be a mechanical problem, which may be resolved by repositioning.
      2. When there is no drainage after repositioning, the drain should be flushed with 1–2 mL of sterile saline to check for occlusion. However, caution must be taken to avoid introducing bacteria into the CSF.
      3. If the drain is still not functioning, it should be removed. A radiograph may be obtained to ascertain that there are no remaining fragments.

57. NASAL INTUBATION

I. Problem. A 32-year-old man after a motor vehicle accident is brought to the operating room for repair of multiple facial fractures, which will include wiring shut his mandible for postoperative stabilization.

II. Immediate Questions

  A. Does the patient require nasal intubation? Certain surgical procedures require nasal intubation, such as a situation where the standard oral endotracheal tube might limit surgical exposure. Also, when oral intubation is complicated by intraoral disease, the nasal route should be considered. For this patient, because the mandible will be wired shut postoperatively, nasal intubation is indicated. Many clinicians believe that nasotracheal tubes are more comfortable, and are more easily secured, and they use these advantages as relative indications for nasal intubation. Data to support these beliefs are equivocal.

  B. Are there any contraindications to nasal intubation? Coagulopathy, basilar skull fracture, intranasal disorders (eg, nasal tumor), and CSF leak are contraindications to nasal intubation. Basilar skull fracture precludes blind nasal intubation. These contraindications must be weighed against the need for nasal intubation. For this patient, if mandibular wiring is absolutely necessary, and a contraindication exists, then a tracheostomy should be considered.

C. Should the intubation be performed after the patient is anesthetized, or should it be performed with the patient awake and before anesthesia is induced? The airway should be evaluated in the usual fashion, and a plan should be devised to secure the airway in the safest manner while also accommodating the needs of the surgeon.

D. How is the nose prepared for intubation? See discussion below.

III. Differential Diagnosis. Not applicable.

IV. Database

   A. Physical Exam Key Points

   1. **Oral Airway.** A detailed oral cavity exam should be conducted. Mouth opening should be noted, although trismus or a mandibular fracture may limit its extent. Neck extension should also be examined, and this may also be limited because of associated cervical spine injuries. All of these aspects of the physical exam influence the ease of direct laryngoscopy regardless of technique.

   2. **Nasal Airway.** A significant nasal fracture or mass may preclude nasal intubation. Epistaxis will also increase the difficulty of nasal intubation, especially when a nasal, fiberoptic technique is employed, because visualization may be impaired.

   3. **Head and Neck.** Raccoon eyes and hemotympanum suggest basilar skull fractures that is a contraindication to blind nasal intubation. The neck should always be examined for tracheal deviation and crepitus. These are signs of tracheal injury and can make laryngoscopy and intubation difficult. A neck hematoma might be an indication of an associated vascular injury of the neck, and this will also increase intubation difficulty.

   B. Laboratory Data

   1. **Coagulation studies should be obtained.** Prolongation of PT or PTT and thrombocytopenia are relative contraindications, because nasal intubation can lead to significant epistaxis.

   C. Radiographic and Other Studies

   1. **Skull radiographs.** Basilar fractures should be ruled out before attempting a blind nasal intubation.

   2. **Cervical spine radiographs.** Cervical spine fractures should be ruled out, when possible, before attempting any elective intubation.

V. Plan

   A. Preparation of Nasal Cavity. The nose should always be prepared with a vasoconstrictor before instrumentation. Phenylephrine nose drops (0.25%) or topical cocaine (4%, maximum 1.5 mg/kg) can be used. When the intubation is to be done with the patient awake, the nose should be anesthetized with topical cocaine (4%, maximum 1.5 mg/kg) or topical lidocaine (2–4%, maximum 1.5 mg/kg). Some clinicians also recommend placing successively larger nasal trumpets through the appropriate nostril. These may help to constrict the mucosa and dilate the nasal passage to make advancement of the endotracheal tube easier.

1. **Awake Nasal Intubation.** When the patient has a potentially difficult airway, then he should not be anesthetized until the airway is secure. Assuming proper nasal preparation, airway anesthesia, and sedation, a fiberoptic, nasal intubation or a blind nasal intubation may be done. A blind nasal intubation is a situation where the endotracheal tube is advanced through the nose and then into the trachea without any direct visualization. Proper placement is confirmed by the presence of end-tidal CO_2 and auscultation.

2. **Nasal intubation after anesthetic induction.** Assuming an otherwise normal airway and proper nasal preparation, nasal intubation may be done after anesthetic induction, especially if performed only for surgical convenience. The intubation may be performed with or without paralysis, depending upon ease of mask ventilation. A blind or fiberoptic technique can then be used. An alternative technique is to advance the endotracheal tube nasally while performing direct laryngoscopy. The endotracheal tube is then advanced through the vocal cords with the aid of Magill forceps.

B. **Complications.** Nasal intubations are not benign procedures. The major complication is epistaxis; however, the chance of this is lessened with proper nasal preparation. Epistaxis can also precipitate laryngospasm (blood on the vocal cords can be very irritating) or result in aspiration. Injury to the turbinates and mucosa can also occur. Bacteremia may also occur after nasal intubation; therefore, appropriate bacterial endocarditis prophylaxis should be administered for the at-risk patient. Long-standing nasal intubation is a predisposing factor to sinusitis that can have an insidious onset for the ICU patient. The concomitant presence of a basilar skull fracture changes this risk profile to one including meningitis.

58. NASOGASTRIC TUBE BLEEDING

I. **Problem.** A 52-year-old man has increasing bleeding from his nasogastric (NG) tube 3 d after a total colectomy.

II. **Immediate Questions**

A. **When was the tube placed?** If placed recently, there may be damage from traumatic insertion. There may be evidence of acute bleeding. If placed several days ago, there may be blood from mucosal irritation.

B. **How much drainage has there been and what are its characteristics?** A small amount of drainage is less urgent than a large amount. A sudden change in the output, however, may indicate occlusion of the tube with clot. Bright red blood is more suggestive of active, ongoing bleeding than is "coffee-grounds" material.

C. **What operations has the patient had?** Fresh proximal suture lines may have bleeding that manifests through the NG tube. Prior gastric surgery may be complicated by recurrent ulceration or marginal ulceration.

D. **Does the patient have a history of ulcer disease?** The patient could have an ulcer that is not being treated with his normal medications because of postoperative ileus. The acute stress of recovery from critical illness may exacerbate preexisting disease processes.

E. **Is the patient on H_2 antagonists? What is the fluid pH?** The pH of the fluid should be greater than 4 if the patient is on ulcer prophylaxis; if not, the patient should be started on ulcer prophylaxis.

F. **What type of tube is present?** Most NG tubes in use in the ICU are of a sump design. The tube should be inspected, and the sumping action confirmed. Dysfunction of this aspect of the NG tube can cause mucosal injury from suction.

III. Differential Diagnosis

A. **Traumatic Insertion.** Nasopharyngeal trauma is not uncommon after NG tube placement. Prevention and attention to detail during insertion minimize this risk. Cooperating with the patients physical makeup makes placement technically easier and better tolerated by the patient

B. **Irritation of Gut Mucosa.** Mucosal bleeding may occur from the simple fact that the tube is in place. Usually, however, the tube is not functional. Routine maintenance with irrigation of both suction and sump ports will decrease the likelihood of mucosal damage.

C. **Irritation of Anastomotic Site.** Mechanical trauma at an anastomosis may cause bloody NG aspirate. This situation is more likely in the acute postoperative period.

D. **Epistaxis.** Whether primary or secondary to tube insertion, epistaxis may result in a significant amount of swallowed blood. This blood may then be found in the patient's NG tube.

E. **Ulcerative Disease.** The ulcers may be preexisting or due to the acute disease process. Ulcers may complicate both burns and head injury. Steroid therapy may exacerbate the process.

F. **Gastritis/Varices/Esophagitis.** Investigate for appropriate past history.

G. **Coagulopathic Patient.** Preexisting or acquired coagulopathy may predispose to bloody drainage from the NG tube.

IV. **Database**

A. **Physical Exam Key Points**

1. **Vital signs.** Hypotension and tachycardia are suggestive of hypovolemia from blood loss. Respiratory symptoms may indicate aspiration of blood around the NG tube.

2. **Abdomen.** Look for signs of peritonitis, distention, or epigastric pain.

3. **HEENT.** Examine for evidence of traumatic insertion, epistaxis, or midface trauma.

B. **Laboratory Data**

1. **Hemogram.** Compare with prior hemoglobin/hematocrit levels to see amount of change, if any.

2. **Coagulation Profile.** Check to see whether the patient has become coagulopathic.

3. **Chemistry.** Look for electrolyte abnormalities that will also need to be addressed. Patients on NG suction should have routine assessment of electrolytes.

4. **Gastric pH.** Check for pH < 4, indicative of inadequate antacid therapy.

C. **Radiographic and Other Studies**

1. **KUB radiograph.** Check for tube position.

2. **Chest radiograph, upright.** Evaluate for signs of esophageal perforation, such as mediastinal widening or mediastinal emphysema. The patient will most likely have free air from his recent laparotomy.

V. **Plan**

A. **Overall Plan.** To find the source of bleeding and determine if aggressive therapy is necessary.

B. **Specific Plans**

1. When upper GI bleeding is apparent, establish vascular access, and begin fluid replacement with isotonic solution. Hypotensive patients may require blood component replacement.

2. **Antacids.** When the patient is not on therapy, begin therapy with IV H_2 antagonists. If the patient is on enteral nutrition, proton pump inhibitors are also an option.

3. Irrigate the NG tube with saline solution. This will help establish whether there is further bleeding, and it will also remove old clots that precipitate further bleeding. There is no need for the saline lavage to be cold. Room-temperature saline is sufficient.

4. When there are "peritoneal signs," the patient will usually require emergent laparotomy. When bleeding persists, an upper en-

doscopy will be required. In the acute postoperative period, this decision should be made by the operative team.

59. NASOGASTRIC TUBE REMOVED EARLY

I. **Problem.** A 42-year-old woman who underwent a vagotomy and antrectomy yesterday has pulled out her nasogastric tube.

II. **Immediate Questions**

A. **When was the tube removed?** If the tube was removed recently, observation may be all that is required. If it fell out 4 h ago and the patient is not having any problems, the tube may not require replacement.

B. **Is the patient complaining of nausea or has she vomited?** If either question is answered in the affirmative, then the tube will most likely need to be replaced.

C. **Has there been any change in the patient's vital signs?** Tachypnea may indicate the patient has aspirated gastric contents.

D. **What is the patient's mental status?** When a patient is confused or disoriented, pain medication may be the culprit, but the possibility of a neurologic event must be ruled out.

E. **What volume had the tube been putting out?** If the tube had been putting out only a small amount, and the patient is not nauseated or vomiting, the tube could possibly be removed after evaluation.

III. **Differential Diagnosis**

A. The tube was removed inadvertently either by the patient or the medical staff.

B. The patient is uncooperative.

C. The patient has had a change in mental status or is disoriented.

IV. **Database**

A. **Physical Exam Key Points**
1. **Vital signs.** Tachypnea or tachycardia may indicate respiratory distress caused by aspiration.
2. **Abdomen.** Distention may be present if the tube had been removed and gone unnoticed for some time.

B. **Laboratory Data.** No laboratory work is necessary unless aspiration pneumonia is suspected. Patients on nasogastric suction should have their electrolytes assessed.

C. **Radiographic and Other Studies.** Verification of tube position in obtunded patients should be done with an appropriate radiograph. In certain circumstances, the placement of the new tube may require fluoroscopic guidance. Chest radiograph findings may lag behind clinical pneumonia.

V. Plan

  A. Overall Plan. To assess the possibility of aspiration pneumonia and to reassess the need of continued gastric drainage.

  B. Specific Plans

  1. When the patient is nauseated or vomiting, the tube must be replaced and properly secured.
  2. When the patient is disoriented, the cause must be elicited. Metabolic disturbances, infection, sleep disturbances may all contribute to disorientation (see also pages 87).
  3. When the patient is uncooperative, she may need to be restrained.
  4. When the patient has aspirated, the resulting pneumonia must be treated appropriately.
  5. In this sample case, the tube will require replacement by the most senior physician available.

60. NAUSEA/VOMITING

  I. Problem. A 46-year-old man with gallstone pancreatitis that had initially cleared clinically now has had several recent episodes of emesis.

II. Immediate Questions

  A. Is there an NG tube in place? A dysfunctional tube may lead to both nausea and vomiting. Tube patency should be established (see page 175).

  B. What are the other symptoms? Global impact of critical illnesses may lead to nausea. Abdominal and retroperitoneal processes, in particular, may cause nausea.

  C. What medications are being given? Many medications used in the ICU have gastrointestinal side effects. When the patient has been hospitalized for an extended period, a review of the medication list with simplification of the regimen may be required. A temporal relation to medication dosing strongly suggests a drug effect.

  D. Is the patient on an enteral diet, and has that diet changed recently? Some patients will not tolerate specific formulas. Sudden or overoptimistic advances in the rate of tube feeding may lead to nausea. Previously stable regimens may change in the face of new illness.

  E. If emesis has occurred, what is the nature of the fluid? Blood, bile, tube feeds, or undigested food will all have diagnostic import.

III. Differential Diagnosis

  A. Improper Function of the NG Tube. Tube assessment and verification of the settings should be done. Both suction and sump ports should be checked for patency.

B. Pharmacologic. Medication may lead to nausea, either by a direct effect, or by stagnation of flow through the gastrointestinal tract.
  1. **Narcotics**
  2. **NSAIDs**
  3. **Chemotherapy agents**

C. Gastric Dysfunction. Impaired gastric emptying will lead to nausea and/or vomiting. Critical illness may exacerbate an underlying disease state.
  1. **Atony.** Diabetes, recent gastric surgery, and significant distention of the stomach may all lead to gastric atony.
  2. **Peptic ulcer disease.** Ulcers in the prepyloric, pyloric, or duodenal bulb may all lead to scarring that will impede gastric emptying.
  3. **Bezoar.** Gastric outlet obstruction may be precipitated by a bezoar lodged in the antrum or pylorus.

D. Postoperative Ileus. When enteral nutrition is started too early, either by the patient or by the clinician, emesis and nausea may result. The routine postoperative ileus is somewhat variable in length.

E. Mechanical Obstruction. Complete and high-grade partial obstruction will lead to nausea and vomiting. The emesis will often be feculent in nature. Many different disorders can cause obstruction.
  1. Tumor.
  2. Adhesions.
  3. Hernia.
  4. Abscess.
  5. Crohn's disease.
  6. Diverticulitis.

F. Infection/Inflammation
  1. **Pancreatitis.** Significant phlegmon in the retroperitoneal space will cause a reactive ileus. Direct impairment of gastric emptying may also occur.
  2. **Cholecystitis.** Either calculous or acalculous cholecystitis may present in the critically ill patient.
  3. **Appendicitis.** Appendicitis, when not diagnosed initially, may lead to diffuse peritonitis. Appendicitis may also develop within the hospital.

G. Genitourinary
  1. **Cystitis.** Infection of the bladder may create nausea or emesis.
  2. **Ureteral obstruction.** Kidney stones classically can lead to pain and nausea.
  3. **Pyelonephritis/renal abscess.** Significant infection in the upper genitourinary (GU) tract may lead to nausea or emesis.

H. Gynecologic
  1. **Routine pregnancy.** Emesis and nausea are common aspects of pregnancy, especially in the first trimester. In extreme circumstances, admission to the hospital is required.
  2. **Pelvic inflammatory disease.**

I. Central Nervous System

1. **Tumors.** Intracranial tumors may cause nausea by direct effect or by swelling.
2. **Elevated ICP.** Vomiting and nausea may occur in circumstances of increased ICP.

J. Vascular. Mesenteric ischemia may lead to both diarrhea and vomiting. History may suggest the diagnosis. Angiography provides optimal diagnostic information.

IV. Database

A. Physical Exam Key Points

1. **Vital signs.** Fever, tachycardia, hypotension can all suggest significant functional disease. Both trends and the actual numbers should be recorded.
2. **Abdomen**
   a. **Bowel Sounds.** Significant disease may be present with persistence of bowel sounds; however, their absence supports either a primary or reactive ileus. Hyperactive, high-pitched bowel sounds with rushes support a diagnosis of obstruction.
   b. **Pain.** Pain patterns and location should be documented. Significant pain without physical exam findings should suggest mesenteric ischemia.
   c. **Tenderness/Peritonitis.** Peritoneal inflammation from infection or chemical irritation will be evident by guarding and rebound tenderness.
   d. **Distention.** Abdominal distention may be difficult to identify in the ICU. Its presence requires additional investigation.
3. **Rectal Exam.** Rectal examination may identify impacted feces, pelvic abscesses, or tumors.
4. **Pelvic.** Pelvic inflammatory disease or ovarian disease will be identified on bimanual or speculum exam. The logistical difficulty of such examinations in the ICU should not deter their performance.
5. **Back.** Costovertebral angle tenderness may be found in instances of ascending urinary tract infections.
6. **Neurologic.** New focality to the exam or a global decrease in the level of consciousness should be sought.

B. Laboratory Data

1. **Hemogram.** Leukocytosis or leukopenia indicate a high likelihood of active infection. Anemia from chronic disease, hemorrhage, or hemodilution of resuscitation may also be found.
2. **Electrolytes.** Electrolyte derangements may lead to, or be secondary to, emesis or ileus. Hypokalemia, in particular, may pre-

vent normal motility. BUN and creatinine may increase with the ongoing fluid shifts.

3. **Amylase/Liver function tests.** Hepatitis, cholecystitis, and pancreatitis may all be reflected with abnormalities in liver function tests and pancreatic enzymes.

4. **ABG.** When metabolic acidosis is of concern, ABG will identify the abnormalities.

C. **Radiographic and Other Studies**

1. **Chest radiograph.** Free intraabdominal air may be seen. Pneumonia and pleural effusions also may be diagnosed. An upright chest radiograph remains the optimal film to identify free air.

2. **KUB radiograph.** Bowel gas patterns should be identified. Dilation, stacking, and air fluid levels are all found with obstruction. Flat and upright films are the primary technique; however, in the ICU, lateral decubitus.

3. **Ultrasound.** This can be useful for diagnosing gallbladder disease, and occasionally, pancreatic disease may be seen on the study. It is an excellent study to diagnose cholecystitis.

4. **CT scan.** This permits evaluation of abscesses, pancreas, kidneys, and obstruction. A CT scan also will identify active diverticular disease.

5. **Angiography.** Biplanar angiography remains the diagnostic test of choice when mesenteric ischemia is of concern.

6. **Contrast studies.** Upper gastrointestinal (UGI) studies, usually with Gastrografin, will allow assessment of the stomach and duodenum. Gastrografin enema identifies obstructing colon lesions. To visualize the small bowel, contrast material will often be required. Its use in the critically ill patient should be guided by the surgical and radiologic services.

V. **Plan**

A. **Overall Plan.** General measures include adequate fluid resuscitation and nutritional support. A vigorous search for causal factors should be undertaken in conjunction with the supportive measures.

B. **Abdomen.** Primary evaluation should include ensuring a functional NG tube. Operative intervention will often be required. Coordination of surgery, anesthesia, nursing, and critical care will optimize outcomes.

C. **Other Sites.** Exclusion of a surgical process in the abdomen is of tantamount importance. When such a determination cannot be made, exploration for diagnosis is often the patient's best chance for survival. Identification of a nonabdominal source with correction, when possible, should be done. Only after these maneuvers have been done should antiemetics be considered.

61. NECK SWELLING

I. Problem. A 67-year-old man has undergone a successful carotid endarterectomy. He is brought to the ICU extubated and stable. Thirty minutes after arrival, he is noted to have an expanding neck mass.

II. Immediate Questions

A. Is the patient oxygenating and ventilating? Neck hematomas and swelling can lead to rapid airway compromise and often require urgent intervention. If the patient is stable, give careful consideration to the optimal treatment.

B. Is the patient hemodynamically stable? Airway compromise can quickly lead to hemodynamic instability. Hypertension can also aggravate bleeding from a recent anastomosis or wound closure.

C. Has there been any recent straining, vomiting, or coughing? These movements can compromise a recent anastomosis or wound closure and should be addressed and treated appropriately.

III. Differential Diagnosis

A. Hematoma. Hematoma after any form of neck surgery is the leading cause of neck swelling and subsequent airway compromise. It may be venous or arterial in nature.

B. Thoracic Duct Injury. This is less common than a hematoma but should be considered, especially after a left neck procedure. Also, this condition is not as acute as a hematoma and is unlikely to cause airway compromise.

C. CSF Leak. This is a rare, subacute-to-chronic complication, but it should be considered for a patient who has undergone cervical spine surgery.

D. Angioedema/Anaphylaxis. These are often a result of a recently administered medication or blood product. Airway edema and swelling occur but do not necessarily result in overt neck swelling. Airway compromise can occur quickly. Urgent treatment and stabilization are required.

IV. Database

A. Physical Exam Key Points

1. **Vital Signs.** Monitoring oxygen saturation is crucial and mandatory in this situation. Tachypnea may represent respiratory distress. Hypertension may compromise a recent vascular suture or anastomosis. Bradycardia and hypotension are late findings of severe respiratory compromise that is quickly advancing to a cardiac arrest.

2. **Neck Exam.** The size and location of the neck mass are important to monitor, especially when it is expanding slowly. Tracheal deviation is also important to note.

      3. Lung Exam. The presence of stridor indicates upper respiratory obstruction. Auscultation of breath sounds indicates there is at least some ventilation beyond the neck mass.

B. Laboratory Data

    1. ABG. Often, no time is available for an arterial blood gas determination; however, when the swelling is slow in forming, an ABG might be useful in determining the degree of respiratory distress. A low level of Pco_2 indicates increased work of breathing. An increasing Pco_2 indicates respiratory fatigue and pending failure. The Po_2 is useful when a pulse oximeter is unavailable or a signal cannot be obtained.

C. Radiographic and Other Studies

    1. A neck ultrasound is useful in following a slowly expanding hematoma or mass. It can help pinpoint the location and origin of the swelling (i.e. if it involves the carotid sheath).

    2. A CT scan can also be of aid in monitoring a slowly expanding neck mass. These studies should not be considered when there is a rapidly expanding neck mass with airway involvement.

V. Plan

A. Initial action. The patient should be examined immediately, and, if airway compromise exists, action to resolve the situation must be taken immediately.

B. Open surgical wound and control bleeding. When the patient has recently undergone a neck procedure, then the surgeon must be called immediately to the bedside. The sutures or staples must be removed immediately. Any bleeding must be tamponaded or controlled with direct digital pressure.

C. Secure airway. Once the wound is opened, if respiratory distress persists, the patient must be intubated emergently. This situation presents a difficult airway, because the normal anatomy will be distorted by the swelling. Medium and long-acting paralytics should be avoided. Additional and, when possible, experienced help should be at the bedside. Secondary intubating techniques should be readily available. A surgeon should also be available for a tracheotomy if intubation proves unsuccessful.

D. Be prepared to resuscitate. Respiratory distress can rapidly deteriorate into cardiac arrest. Therefore, proper equipment and medication for a cardiopulmonary resuscitation should be readily available.

E. Definitive closure in OR. Once the patient is stabilized, definitive surgical repair might be indicated in the OR.

F. Neck swelling without airway compromise. When the patient is stable, and the neck swelling is slow in forming, then the patient can be monitored closely.

G. Notify the surgical team immediately. Closely monitor oxygen saturation and ventilation.

H. Treat hypertension aggressively, especially when the patient has recently undergone a vascular procedure. Definitive treatment follows once the cause is determined.

I. Monitor for further swelling. Any suspicion of expansion should probably be treated by immediately returning the patient to the operating room for intubation and surgical exploration. Airway compromise is insidious in onset and can occur quickly. Experienced practitioners know that timely reexploration is preferable to the high risks of airway compromise, inability to intubate, and need for emergency surgical airway interventions.

62. NEEDLESTICK

I. Problem. A 40-year-old man is admitted to the ICU in fulminant hepatic failure. During the placement of central access, you accidentally stick yourself with a hollow needle.

II. Immediate Questions

A. What pathogens have potentially been transmitted? HIV, hepatitis B (HBV), and hepatitis C (HCV) are the most serious bloodborne pathogens, but approximately 20 microbes have been identified that can be transmitted by needlestick injuries.

B. What factors affect the likelihood of disease transmission?
1. The rate of exposure of the health care worker to carrier patients.
2. The mode of exposure (percutaneous > mucosal > cutaneous).
3. The fluid involved (blood carries the highest risk).
4. The volume of fluid.
5. The concentration of the pathogen in the fluid.
6. The pathogenicity of the organism.
7. The type of needle (hollow bore > solid). Host susceptibility (Has the host been vaccinated, or is the host immunocompromised?). To date, no health care worker has contracted HIV from a solid needle stick.
8. The use of gloves. Gloves decrease the likelihood of transmission (see below).

C. What can I do immediately to minimize the possibility of disease transmission?

III. Differential Diagnosis (Not Applicable)

IV. Database

A. Physical Exam Key Points
1. Examine the site of inadvertent stick.
2. Examine the sticking needle, bore size? etc.

B. **Laboratory Data**
   1. **Serology.**
      a. **Hepatitis B Virus (HBV).** There are approximately 8700 new infections each year secondary to occupational exposures of health care workers. Of these, 400 require hospitalization, and 200 eventually die of either acute or chronic infection. Furthermore, HBV is the most prevalent disease acquired by accidental needlestick. The incidence of HBV is declining because of widespread use of the vaccine and universal precautions. There is a 6–30% percutaneous transmission rate in susceptible health care workers (ie, no vaccine).
      b. **Hepatitis C Virus (HCV).** No vaccine is available. A percutaneous transmission rate of 2.7% has been reported.
      c. **Human Immunodeficiency Virus (HIV).** No vaccine is available. A percutaneous transmission rate of 0.35% has been reported.

V. **Plan.** Health care workers are at risk of acquiring bloodborne infections by percutaneous in addition to cutaneous and mucosal exposures. However, percutaneous exposure carries the greatest risk of transmission. For this reason, the Occupational Safety and Health Administration (OSHA) passed the Bloodborne Pathogens Standard in 1992. This requires hospitals to implement policy and engineering strategies to minimize employee exposure and to develop efficient Exposure Control Plans.

A. **Short-term Plan**
   1. **Clean the wound liberally with alcohol.** Apply antibiotic ointment, then dress the wound.
   2. **Contact the ICU supervisor and the occupational health representative as directed by local hospital policy.** This not only facilitates determination of the health care worker and the source's infectious disposition, but also allows for expeditious prophylaxis, if necessary, and for insurance documentation should disability compensation be appropriate.
   3. **According to state law constraints, determine the source and infectious status of the employee with or without consent.**
   4. **Assess options.** When the source is seropositive, and the health care worker is susceptible, decide whether to initiate pharmacologic prophylaxis against seroconversion (preferably with the aid of an infectious disease consultant).
   5. *Note well:* For HBV, two doses of HBV immunoglobulin are 75% effective in preventing conversion. On the other hand, therapy for HCV using anti-HBV immunoglobulin has not been shown to be effective. HCV immunoglobulin is available at this time only on a purely experimental basis with no data to suggest effectiveness. Zidovudine is still recommended for prophylaxis against HIV. How-

ever, its ultimate efficacy is not known. Furthermore, in a source patient already on antiretroviral therapy, AZT may be inappropriate.

B. **Long-term Plan (Prevention or minimization of future exposures).** The cornerstone of exposure prevention is Universal Precautions, as outlined by the CDC and OSHA.

   1. **Barriers.** Wear appropriate barriers when potential exists for cutaneous or percutaneous exposure to blood and body fluids (gloves, goggles, masks, etc). Wearing gloves, although not absolutely protective against needlesticks, reduces the volume of blood transferred by about 50%. Furthermore, double-gloving may reduce the volume even more.

   2. **Avoid recapping contaminated needles.** This represents the most common cause of accidental needlestick injuries.

   3. **Place used sharps in puncture resistant containers.**

   4. **Use needleless systems whenever possible.** This has not been conclusively proven to lessen the risk of needlestick injury, but, in theory, this should reduce the risk and, potentially, the hospital expenses from diagnosis and treatment of bloodborne pathogens.

63. OLIGURIA/ANURIA

Immediate Actions. If hyperkalemia is encountered, immediate steps to stabilize the conduction across the cardiac membranes should be undertaken. Temporizing maneuvers can redistribute the potassium intracellularly while therapy to remove potassium from the body is instituted.

I. **Problem.** A patient is 2 d postoperative after a lysis of adhesions and a small-bowel resection to remove a small-bowel obstruction. The urine output during the past 4 h has been 100 cc, 50 cc, 9 cc, and 2 cc in that order.

II. **Immediate Questions**

A. **Is the Foley catheter patent?** Check that the catheter has been flushed, and if there is any question, place a new catheter. Many catheters, especially those with a temperature probe, become occluded, and although they flush, they will not necessarily drain. Clots, sediment, or calculi may occlude the catheter.

B. **What is the volume status of the patient?** Hypovolemia is the usual cause of decreased urine output in the postoperative or acute trauma patient. Noninvasive clues to volume status, such as heart rate, blood pressure, and body weight are a good start. Of these, body weight may not be as reliable as a result of third spacing. Central venous pressure and left ventricular filling pressures from a pulmonary artery catheter are invasive means of inferring volume status.

C. **Does the patient have baseline renal insufficiency?** A patient with underlying renal insufficiency will have little reserve for further impairment. This makes managing their volume status all the more difficult and important.

D. **Is the patient on any nephrotoxic drugs or recently received IV contrast?** Aminoglycosides and other antibiotics can cause tubular necrosis. Monitor levels closely and hold medications until appropriate dosing is determined. Recent arteriograms or contrast CTs are often overlooked.

E. **Has the patient suffered episodes of hypotension?** Urine output is viewed as a measure of global perfusion. Hypotension may cause ischemic tubular necrosis. Vasoactive medications may impair renal perfusion.

III. Differential Diagnosis (Table I–2)

A. Prerenal

1. **Hypovolemia.** This is the main cause of oliguria in a postoperative or posttrauma patient.
2. **Hemorrhage.** This can be the result of traumatic or continued postoperative bleeding.
3. **Inadequate fluid resuscitation.** The rate of fluid administration must also consider insensible losses, such as intraoperative (open wound) and postoperative (temperature, wounds, ventilator).
4. **Third space.** A relative intravascular depletion secondary to fluid sequestration. Fluid may sequestrate in the interstitium or the bowel lumen. This redistribution of fluid is common after intra-abdominal or retroperitoneal surgery.
5. **CHF.**

TABLE I–2 DIFFERENTIAL DIAGNOSIS OF OLIGURIA.

Index	Prerenal	Renal (ATN)
Uosm (mOsm/kg)	>500	<350
UNa (mEq/L)	<10–20	>30–40
U/PIC	>20:1	<20:1
FeNa[a] (%)	<1	>2
BUN/Cr	>15–20:1	<10:1
Urine sp gr	>1.015	<1.015
Urine/Serum Osm	>1.8	<1.0–1.2

ATN = acute tubular necrosis.

$$^a FeNa = \frac{UNa \times PRCr}{PRNa \times UCr}$$

6. **Cirrhosis.**
7. **Nephrotic syndrome.**
8. **Renal artery occlusion** (especially in acute renal transplant).
9. **Aortic dissection.** May remove one or both renal artery openings from the flow path of the true lumen.
10. **Emboli.** May occlude the renal artery orifice.

B. **Renal**
1. **Acute tubular necrosis.**
2. **Toxic.** Check medications (aminoglycosides, vancomycin, amphotericin B), IV contrast.
3. **Rhabdomyolysis with myoglobinuria.** This may require a forced saline diuresis.
4. **Ischemic.** Check for hypotension/hypoperfusion.
5. **Interstitial nephritis**
   a. **Medications.** Check for nonsteroidals, beta-lactamase-resistant penicillins.
   b. **Hypercalcemia.** This may cause nephrocalcinosis.
   c. **Postrenal.**
6. **Obstructive uropathy.** Look for ureteral obstruction (remember iatrogenic), urethral obstruction, catheter obstruction.

IV. **Database**
A. **Physical Exam Key Points**
1. **Vital signs.** Check for fever (insensible losses), hypotension/tachycardia (hypovolemia), and body weight. Orthostatic measurements may help elicit hypovolemia.
2. **Skin.** Turgor of the tissue should be evaluated. Evidence of edema and the degree of hydration of the mucous membranes should be documented.
3. **Lungs.** Listen for rales and rhonchi.
4. **CV.** Assessment of central venous pressure may be made clinically by documenting the degree of jugular venous distention. Cardiac gallops, when present, should help to assess volume status.
5. **Abdomen.** Bladder distention indicates a dysfunctional drainage system. Ascites, when present, is suggestive of hepatic dysfunction.

B. **Laboratory Data**
1. **Serum chemistry.** This can help to elucidate prerenal versus renal causes.
   a. Electrolyte disturbances, such as hyperkalemia, can be life threatening, necessitating emergent dialysis.
   b. Hyperkalemia should prompt immediate measures, including evaluation by a 12-lead ECG, looking for conduction disturbances. When conduction abnormalities are seen, calcium

should be given intravenously followed by bicarbonate, insulin, and glucose. Maneuvers to remove the potassium from the body should be instituted immediately.

   2. **Urinalysis/urine electrolytes.** Assessment of specific gravity and urine electrolytes assists in determining prerenal and renal causes ($U_{Na} > 20$ renal, $U_{Na} < 20$ prerenal).

   3. **Hemogram.** Check for hemorrhage or anemia.

   4. **Drug levels.**

C. **Radiographic and Other Studies**

   1. **Chest radiograph.** This documents volume overload. It confirms position of monitoring lines, such as CVP or pulmonary artery catheter. An effusion may represent congestive failure.

   2. **Ultrasound.** This documents bladder and renal size. It may show evidence of hydroureter or hydronephrosis.

   3. **Renal scan.** This is a nuclear medicine study that assesses renal blood flow and excretion. It is most useful after a renal transplant or when an embolus to the renal artery is of concern.

   4. **CVP/Pulmonary artery catheter.** This gives useful information about volume status. It requires proper positioning of the catheter and interpretation. Central venous pressure is extremely unreliable as an indicator of volume status.

V. **Plan**

A. **Overall Plan.** Identify reversible causes of oliguria. As a general rule, in adults, the urine output should be 0.5 cc/kg/h.

B. **Specific Plans**

   1. Careful evaluation of input and output status, trends in electrolytes and hemoglobin should help determine cause.

      a. **Prerenal.** Fluid bolus with NS (or PRBCs as indicated). Monitor volume status with invasive and noninvasive measures. Until the functional status of the kidneys is known, resuscitation fluid should be potassium free. When blood is required, the blood bank can be requested to send blood that is fresh.

      b. Monitor urine output hourly.

      c. **Renal.** Monitor volume status. Adjust electrolytes in fluid and TPN accordingly.

      d. Dopaminergic levels of dopamine are controversial, but 2–3 µg/kg/min is a standard dose. Whether the observed clinical effects are through global increases in cardiac output or through renal artery vasodilation are not clear at present.

      e. Although typically given in bolus form, furosemide may have more benefit when given as a continuous infusion (1–9 mg/h).

      f. **Mannitol.** 12.5–25 g induces an osmotic diuresis.

      g. Stop nephrotoxic medications and also adjust renally excreted medications.

      h. **Postrenal.** Flush or replace urinary catheter as necessary. Ureteral stents or nephrostomy may be indicated, depending on the level of obstruction.

64. OPERATING ROOM TRANSPORT: VENTILATOR ISSUES

I. **Problem.** While in the elevator transporting an intubated and ventilated 42-year-old woman from the ICU to the CT scanner, her Sao_2 begins to decrease.

II. **Immediate Questions**

    A. **What is the oxygen saturation and how quickly is it decreasing?** Is the patient still intubated? Is the endotracheal tube secure? Has the tube moved in the process of transport? Is the balloon cuff inflated?

    B. **Is the patient being ventilated?** Is there chest rise with ventilator breaths?

    C. **Can the patient be ventilated manually with a self-inflating bag?**

    D. **Is the patient making spontaneous respiratory efforts?** Is there movement in the reservoir bag?

    E. **Is the source of oxygen properly connected and turned on?** Is the oxygen tank empty?

    F. **Is the oxygen saturation probe properly placed on the patient?**

III. **Differential Diagnosis**

    A. **Unplanned Extubation.** Check for bronchospasm. With movement, the endotracheal tube can irritate the carina and cause bronchospasm (see other sections).

    B. **Mainstem Intubation.** Has the endotracheal tube migrated into the left or right bronchus?

    C. **Pneumothorax.** Has the oxygen source failed? Check for hemodynamic collapse. Hypoxia could be the result of hypotension and decreased cardiac output.

    D. **Incorrect Ventilator Settings.** Inadequate minute ventilation could result from improper settings on the transport ventilator and lead to atelectasis, hypercarbia, and hypoxia. Similarly, inspired oxygen could be set too low.

    E. **Equipment Failure.** Do not presume that equipment failure is the cause until all patient problems have been ruled out.

    F. **Spurious Reading of Pulse Oximeter Probe**

IV. Database

A. Physical Exam Key Points

1. **Lungs.** Look for a rise in the chest with each breath. Auscultate for bilateral breath sounds. No breath sounds or abnormal breath sounds may indicate unplanned extubation or inadvertent mainstem intubation.

2. **Skin.** Assess peripheral perfusion. Look for cyanosis to confirm decreasing saturation. Assess capillary refill.

3. **Inspect endotracheal tube.** Check insertion distance. Palpate the endotracheal cuff.

4. **Ventilator settings.** Inspect current settings. Check inspiratory pressure and tidal volume or minute ventilation settings.

V. Plan.

Ensure adequacy of oxygenation and ventilation. First check the patient and then check the equipment. Verify proper position of the pulse oximeter, but do not waste valuable time. Call for help or get to help quickly.

A. Ensure adequate supply of oxygen.
Check tank pressure and connections. Switch to 100% oxygen.

B. Begin manual ventilation.
Use self-inflating ambulance bag or other means of manual ventilation. Mask ventilate if necessary.

C. Get off elevator and proceed to a patient care area as quickly as possible.

D. Reposition endotracheal tube if necessary.
Prepare for reintubation if needed.

E. Always travel with the necessary equipment and supplies.

F. Treat associated conditions, such as hemodynamic compromise or pneumothorax.

65. OTORRHEA/RHINORRHEA

I. Problem.
A 29-year-old man, who sustained a LeFort's type-I fracture 2 d ago, after a motorbike accident, has been complaining since yesterday about having continuous clear nasal drainage.

II. Immediate Questions

A. Is this an inflammatory or noninflammatory process?
Rhinorrhea is a symptom that has inflammatory and noninflammatory causes. Critically ill patients often have nasogastric tubes, nasotracheal intubation, and may lay supine for prolonged periods. These problems increase the risk of mechanical damage, impaired drainage, and prolonged infection in the nose and sinuses. Sound logic and investigation can usually determine the cause of rhinorrhea.

III. Differential Diagnosis

   A. Inflammatory causes of rhinorrhea include viral or bacterial infections that can extend into the sinuses. Nasotracheal intubation and nasogastric tubes increase the risk of sinusitis. One study found that approximately 40% of critically ill patients with both nasotracheal intubation and nasogastric tube insertion developed sinusitis within 48 h. Decreased sinus drainage secondary to mechanical obstruction probably increases the rate of infection. Noninfectious reasons for inflammatory rhinitis include allergies and seasonal rhinitis with eosinophilia.

   B. Noninflammatory causes of rhinorrhea include CSF leakage and vasomotor rhinorrhea. CSF leaks can result from trauma or invading tumor. The CSF is clear and watery. When a CSF leak is suspected, a sample of fluid should be examined for low-glucose and beta-2-transferrin levels. Do not delay a neurosurgical consultation. Vasomotor rhinorrhea is a diagnosis of exclusion.

   C. Otorrhea has multiple sources and causes. Fluid may come from the external auditory canal, middle ear, or cranial vault. Causes include infections, malignancies, foreign bodies, and trauma. Careful history and physical examination together with inspection of the fluid will lead to a diagnosis.

IV. Data Base

   A. Physical Exam Key Points

      1. Nasal speculum exam. Use a nasal speculum for anterior rhinoscopy. A red mucosa suggests inflammation. Pallor and edema suggest an allergic reaction.

      2. Drainage. Pay attention to the color and odor of the drainage. Yellow drainage suggests a bacterial cause residing in the external auditory canal or middle ear. White drainage suggests fungal infection or a skin disease. Bloody drainage results from foreign body insertion, head trauma, or chronic infection with granulation tissue. Thick, clear fluid may come from a chronic tympanic membrane perforation. Watery, clear fluid should be treated as CSF until proven otherwise. Check the sample for low glucose and beta-2-transferrin levels. A foul odor does not always suggest anaerobic infection. However, it is strongly associated with bone destruction secondary to infection or malignancy.

      3. Head and Neck Exam. A full head and neck examination, palpation of the outer ear, and otoscopic examination should be performed when otorrhea is present. A tender pinna is pathonomic for otitis externa. Debris in the external canal may limit tympanic membrane examination. Do not irrigate the ear. Assume that the tympanic membrane is perforated. When too much debris precludes adequate examination, consult an otolaryngologist. When possible, assess the tympanic membrane for inflammation, perforation, fluid collection, and cholesteatoma. Cholesteatomas are squamous debris that replace portions of the tympanic membrane. When a cholesteatoma is suspected, consult an otolaryngologist.

4. **Hearing test.** Acutely decreased hearing despite an open external auditory canal mandates audiometry to evaluate inner ear function.

4. History and physical usually determine the cause of otorrhea. Further testing is required only when the cause is still in question.

B. **Laboratory Data**
1. **Hemogram.** Elevated white blood cell count may indicate infectious processes.
2. **Drainage fluid analysis.** Evaluate for cerebrospinal fluid versus inflammatory drainage.

C. **Radiographic and Other Studies**
1. **Head CT.** When scull fractures are suspected or visualization of the sinuses is required.
2. **Evaluate** Waters' views of the sinuses to assess for fluid collections, malignancies, and bony deformities.

V. **Plan**

A. **Always treat the underlying cause.** Oral rather than nasal intubation may prevent sinusitis. Rotate nasogastric tubes between nostrils every 3–4 d. Antihistamines and ipratropium bromide treat simple rhinorrhea.

B. Target antibiotics and antifungals at the presumed pathogen. Special consideration should be paid to diabetic patients. Depending on the clinical picture, medications may range from topical to parenteral. Topical steroids reduce inflammation and are often given with antibiotics and antifungals. A surgeon should be consulted for osteomyelitis, malignancies, and CSF leaks.

C. Culture, Gram's stain, and potassium hydroxide preparations should be performed when antibiotics or antifungals fail to treat a presumed infection. Suspected bone destruction necessitates CT imaging with thin axial and coronal cuts of the temporal and mastoid bones.

66. OXYGEN DESATURATION

I. **Problem.** The nurse calls you to a patient's bedside to assess his low oxygen saturation on pulse oximetry.

II. **Immediate Questions**

A. **What is the level of saturation?** Oxygen desaturation is potentially life threatening. An oxygen saturation of < 90%, corresponding to a Po_2 of < 60 mm Hg, is particularly dangerous because of the shape of the oxy-hemoglobin saturation curve and the precipitous drop in oxygen-carrying capacity of blood that occurs at that point. Severe hypoxia will lead to cardiac dysrhythmias, hypotension, brain injury, and death. Higher saturations in the mid or upper 90s may allow some time for a more thorough evaluation, even though they may represent a drop from previous higher levels.

B. Is the patient breathing? Effective respiratory efforts and air movement are necessary to achieve adequate oxygenation. Hypoventilation and obstruction are common predisposing factors to hypoxia.

C. Is the patient intubated? Intubated patients usually have underlying respiratory compromise and pulmonary disease, and the use of mechanical ventilation also introduces a number of variables to consider as possible causes of hypoxia. However, the intubated patient also simplifies the management somewhat, because intubation and ventilation is often a final common pathway in the interventions necessitated by significant desaturation.

D. Is the patient receiving supplemental oxygen? If not, oxygen administration is an obvious initial step in management. Patients already receiving supplemental oxygen must have the supply of oxygen checked to ensure that disconnected tubing or an empty tank is not to blame. The occurrence of an event of desaturation for someone already on supplemental oxygen is worrisome, as it is likely that an exacerbation of an underlying disorder is to blame.

E. Has the patient recently undergone a surgical procedure? Hypoxia in the postoperative period in not unusual. The cause can be as simple as residual anesthesia, sedation, or analgesia resulting in hypoventilation or atelectasis. Alternatively, it could be the result of a more serious postoperative complication, such as pneumothorax or pulmonary embolism.

III. Differential Diagnosis

A. Pneumothorax. Patients with recent trauma, recent thoracotomy, bronchoscopy, or high retroperitoneal dissection, and mechanically ventilated patients are at increased risk for pneumothorax. Recent insertion or attempts at central venous access is another possible cause.

B. Hypoventilation. Hypoventilation from oversedation, CNS dysfunction, or splinting because of inadequate analgesia can all cause hypoxemia by promoting alveolar collapse. This is usually confirmed by hypercapnia on arterial blood gas analysis.

C. Pulmonary Edema. Pulmonary edema causes hypoxia by interfering with gas exchange. Cardiogenic pulmonary edema results from inadequate cardiac output and can be precipitated by fluid overload, dysrhythmias, and myocardial ischemia. Increased pulmonary capillary permeability can also cause pulmonary edema as a result of sepsis, head injury, aspiration, anaphylaxis, or upper-airway obstruction.

D. **Airway Obstruction.** Upper-airway obstruction from floppy or redundant oral pharyngeal tissue can lead to hypoxemia. Mucus plugging or excessive secretions can obliterate bronchial lumens causing lower-airway obstruction and result in alveolar collapse and hypoxemia. Laryngeal swelling from recent intubation or laryngospasm from occult aspiration are other potential causes of upper-airway obstruction.

E. **Pulmonary Embolism.** Patients with deep venous thrombosis, cancer, multiple trauma, or prolonged bed rest are at increased risk of pulmonary embolism. Postoperative patients are at increased risk because of the additive effects of stasis and hypercoagulable changes resulting from surgery. Large pulmonary emboli can cause both cardiovascular collapse and severe hypoxemia.

F. **Equipment Malfunction or Malposition.** Oximetry probes frequently falsely report low oxygen saturation because of a malfunction or malposition. Patients and staff often dislodge the probe accidentally. The sensors are sensitive to movement and may report false readings if the patient is moving. Fluorescent or red lighting or any high ambient light environment can also cause erroneous readings.

G. **Atelectasis.** Atelectasis is a common cause of hypoxia in the ICU. Hypoventilation from pain, sedation, prolonged bed rest, or inadequate mechanical ventilation can result in alveolar, lobar, or segmental collapse. Resulting right-to-left shunting impairs systemic oxygenation. Postoperative atelectasis can result from increased abdominal pressure and distention as well as changes in pulmonary mechanics that result from surgery on the chest or abdomen.

H. **Air Space Disease.** Pneumonia, aspiration, blood, fluid or any other process that compromises alveolar gas exchange will also increase right-to-left shunting with resultant hypoxia.

I. **Myocardial Infarction or Arrhythmia.** Any compromise in cardiac output may result in inadequate perfusion of the lungs and/or peripheral tissues. This can result in severe hypoxia and hypotension. It should be treated emergently.

J. **Bronchospasm.** Reactive airways may cause hypoventilation, CO_2 retention, and hypoxemia. Changes in compliance and hence the time constants of small airways eventually lead to severe air trapping and a poor distribution of ventilation.

IV. Database

A. Physical Exam Key Points

1. **Assessment.** Assessment of breathing effort, work of breathing, intercostal retractions, effort, and stridor should be noted on initial observation.

2. **Vital signs.** Hypertension, hypotension, dyspnea, tachycardia, bradycardia, are all consistent with hypoxia. Hypoxia causing vital sign abnormalities should be corrected emergently.

3. **Heart.** Irregular rate or rhythm, and/or a new murmur or rub in the presence of hypoxia might suggest a cardiogenic source.

4. **Lungs.** Rales, wheezes, or rhonchi may indicate reactive airways or excessive secretions. Decreased or absent breath sounds may indicate effusion or consolidation. If they are combined with hyperresonance and tracheal deviation away from the affected side, then a tension pneumothorax should be considered. Stridor is more indicative of upper-airway obstruction.

5. **Mental status.** Altered mental status, agitation, and obtundation are all signs of hypoxia.

B. **Laboratory Data**

1. **ABG.** A properly obtained arterial blood gas analysis provides an accurate and reliable measurement of oxygenation status that may confirm the hypoxia suggested by oximetry. It also provides other vital information (pH, CO_2, bicarbonate levels) that helps to further delineate the ventilatory status.

2. **Hemoglobin/Hematocrit.** Anemia further impairs the oxygen-carrying capacity of the blood and makes the presence of hypoxia even more dangerous. Severe anemia can suggest an underlying hypovolemia and decreased cardiac output state that can also further compromise oxygen delivery.

3. **White blood cell count.** An elevated white blood cell count supports an underlying pneumonia/infectious process in the proper clinical picture.

4. **CKMB and/or Troponin-I.** When a cardiogenic source is suspected, serial CKMB and/or troponin-I levels can indicate cardiac ischemia.

C. **Radiographic and Other Studies**

1. **Chest radiograph.** A chest radiograph should be immediately obtained to rule out a pulmonary source. Signs of pulmonary edema, atelectasis, lung consolidation or collapse, pulmonary embolus, and pneumothorax can be quickly diagnosed with an adequate chest radiograph.

2. **V̇/Q̇ scan.** When a pulmonary embolus is strongly suspected, then a ventilation/perfusion scan is a good screening tool. This can only be done when the patient is stable enough to travel out of the intensive care unit. The test is usually time consuming.

3. **CT scan.** Newer "spiral CT" scans can be used to diagnose pulmonary embolus. These are done with IV contrast and fine cuts through the lung fields. The test can be done emergently and is not invasive, unlike the pulmonary angiogram.

4. **Lower-extremity Doppler.** When pulmonary embolus is suspected, then bilateral lower-extremity Doppler exam looking for

DVTs as a possible embolic source is an initial screening tool. This can be done at the bedside. A negative test does not rule out the possibility of a pulmonary embolus.

5. **Pulmonary angiogram.** Pulmonary angiography is the gold standard to diagnose pulmonary embolus. Contrast dye is injected directly into the pulmonary vasculature under fluoroscopy. This test is invasive and time consuming and should only be ordered when your clinical suspicion is high, especially when the patient could be compromised by anticoagulation.

6. **Echocardiogram.** Both dysrhythmias and myocardial ischemia/infarction can lead to inadequate cardiac output and hypoxia. A 12-lead ECG should be obtained to rule out a cardiac source.

V. Plan

A. **Provide or Augment Supplemental Oxygen.** The patient should be placed on supplemental oxygen quickly if it has not already been done. This is easy, inexpensive, and can be done with nasal cannulas, face tent, nonrebreather mask, bag-valve-mask, CPAP, or endotracheal intubation—all while troubleshooting and assessing other areas.

B. **Decompress Pneumothorax.** When a thorough physical examination is consistent with a tension pneumothorax, then emergent decompression by needle thoracostomy placed in the second intercostal space is indicated. This is usually followed by tube thoracostomy. Any symptomatic pneumothorax requires some form of thoracostomy.

C. **Attenuate Obstruction.** Upper-airway obstruction can usually be relieved by applying jaw lift or thrust, placing an oral airway, or insertion of a nasal trumpet. Lower-airway obstruction usually requires endotracheal intubation and deep suctioning or bronchoscopy.

D. **Pulmonary Suctioning and Nebulization.** Common causes of hypoxia in the ICU are atelectasis, reactive airway disease, excessive secretions, and mucus plugging. These can all be relieved with aggressive chest physiotherapy: incentive spirometry or deep breathing, coughing, nebulized beta-agonists, deep suctioning, or fiberoptic bronchoscopy.

E. **Ventilate Patient.** When the patient is hypoventilating, either by decreased ventilatory rate or poor tidal volume, they should be assisted. This can be done initially with a bag-valve-mask or, chronically, with endotracheal intubation and mechanical ventilation.

F. **Infarction or Dysrhythmias.** Symptomatic cardiac dysrhythmias should be treated with the appropriate pharmacologic or electric modality or both. Cardiac ischemia or infarction should be treated aggressively and appropriate consult services contacted.

G. **Correct Fluid Abnormalities.** Hypervolemia often leads to pulmonary edema. Patients are frequently admitted to the ICU postoperatively or after other interventions where they have received large amounts of fluid resuscitation. This usually becomes problematic a few days later when fluids are mobilized. Aggressive diuresis will often help relieve pulmonary edema. Hypovolemia can lead to hypoxia from inadequate circulation or perfusion of tissue. Fluid boluses can help correct inadequate volume.

   H. **Antagonize Sedating Agents.** When the patient is overly sedated and hypoventilating, all sedating drugs should be pharmacologically antagonized gradually with the appropriate agent(s), so as not to produce withdrawal or excessive pain.

   I. **Test Monitors.** Place the oximetry probe on another finger or any other potential site. When this does not correct the problem, place the probe on yourself as a final test. Next obtain a new probe/monitor. Always assume the equipment is working properly until proven otherwise, and take other appropriate actions while testing equipment.

   J. **Correct Anemia.** Transfusions with cross-matched packed red blood cells should be given to correct severe anemia.

67. PACEMAKER MALFUNCTION

   I. **Problem.** A patient is admitted to the ICU for continuous ECG monitoring after a suspected acute MI. Throughout the first 4 h he is AV sequentially paced at 72 bpm. He then suffers ventricular fibrillation, is emergently cardioverted with 360 J and returns in a ventricular escape rhythm of 26 bpm.

   II. **Immediate Questions**

   A. **Is the pacemaker functioning?** Pacemaker malfunction in the ICU may have serious consequences. Causes include failure of pacemaker output, failure to capture, undersensing, and inappropriate pacing rates. ECG interpretation is the key to identifying the type of malfunction. The ICU environment itself can lead to both pseudo and bona fide malfunction. Treatments are intended to temporize until a cardiologist can definitively correct the problem.

   B. **What kind of pacemaker does the patient have?**

   III. **Differential Diagnosis**

   A. **Failure of Output.** Failure of pacemaker output can be sudden and catastrophic. Component failure (rare), total battery depletion, lead fracture, lead disconnection, or oversensing lead to failed output. Battery depletion is avoidable and is preceded by end-of-life indicators, such as a rate change. Lead fracture and disconnection are usually sudden, whereas oversensing happens intermittently. Oversensing of ventricular "noise" in single-lead pacemakers results in pauses, whereas oversensing in dual-chamber pacemakers leads to increased rates.

B. **Failure to Capture.** Lead dislodgment, lead insulation break, exit block, metabolic abnormalities, and battery depletion can all result in no action potential when the pacemaker fires. Lead dislodgment usually happens in the first 3 weeks after implantation. Later, fibrosis at the electrode tip can cause an exit block. Metabolic abnormalities, such as hypo- or hyperkalemia or antiarrhythmic medications may also induce failure to capture.

C. **Undersensing.** Undersensing malfunctions are rarely urgent and usually result in pacemaker output that is competitive with the intrinsic rhythm. Lead dislodgment, poor lead position, lead insulation defect, and low-amplitude intracardiac signal may all result in undersensing.

D. **Inappropriate Pacing Rates.** There are few true malfunctions of the pacing system. One lethal malfunction is "runaway pacemaker." This is an emergency that will quickly lead to hemodynamic instability and collapse. Runaway pacemaker can result from battery failure, random component failure, or radiation-induced component failure.

E. **The ICU Environment and Pacemaker Malfunction**
   1. Both equipment and procedures may cause pacemaker malfunction. The abundance of medical equipment and devices creates a potential for radiofrequency interference affecting pacemaker function in the ICU. When the patient remains in a sustained electrical field, the pacemaker can interpret the interference as cardiac activity. This would alter function episodically but would not damage the pacemaker.
   2. Transthoracic defibrillation can permanently damage the pulse generator. When defibrillation is necessary, position paddles anteroposteriorly and as far from the pacemaker and leads as possible. Afterward, the pacemaker should be serviced.

F. **Continuous ECG Monitoring and Pacemakers.** The continuous ECG monitor is the ICU physician's friend or foe. Occasionally, ECG monitors may pick up radiofrequency interference and interpret this as pacemaker spikes. On the other hand, a computer-assisted monitoring system can diagnose pacemaker malfunctions with 94% accuracy.

IV. **Database**

A. **Physical Exam Key Points.** These are usually irrelevant. Ensure that the ECG leads are appropriately connected. Disconnect any potential radiofrequency-producing devices (eg, cell phones, computers, etc).

B. **Laboratory Data**
   1. **Electrolytes.**

C. **Radiographic and Other Studies**
   1. The ECG is the key to diagnosing pacemaker malfunction. Failure of output appears as bradycardia without pacing spikes, or in the case of oversensing with dual-chamber pacemakers, atrial spikes without following ventricular spikes. Failure-to-capture leads to multiple spikes without subsequent QRS complexes. Undersensing appears as pacing spikes during the refractory period. Therefore, no QRS complex is generated after these premature impulses.
   2. Chest radiograph can show fractured leads and lead displacement. Lead fracture often occurs at the costoclavicular space.

V. **Plan.** Always consider transcutaneous pacing when facing pacemaker failure. When this is inadequate, a temporary transvenous pacemaker may be inserted to stabilize the patient. Treatment should be aimed at temporizing until a cardiologist can arrive.

68. PAIN

I. **Problem.** A 65-year-old patient who is 2 d postoperative after left pneumonectomy is experiencing tachycardia and hypertension and complaining of pain.

II. **Immediate Questions**
   A. **Is this an acute onset of pain that may indicate a life-threatening event?**
   B. **Is the patient able to take in adequate breaths?** Are there significant hemodynamic changes?
   C. **Has the character or location of the pain changed?**
   D. **What has the patient been given for pain up to this point?** Does the patient have an epidural in place that may no longer be working?
   E. **Is the patient allergic to any medications? Is the patient anticoagulated?**
   F. **Are there possible contraindications to sedation in the patient?** Systemic pain medications may sedate a patient and lead to deleterious consequences in the presence of preexisting altered mental status.

III. **Differential Diagnosis**
   A. **Emergent Event.** Acute events must be ruled out before any further workup.
   B. **Head.** Check for acute intracranial hemorrhage, epidural or subdural hematoma.
   C. **Chest.** Check for myocardial infarction, aortic dissection, pulmonary embolism.

D. **Abdomen.** Check for bowel ischemia, perforated viscus, ruptured aortic aneurysm.

E. **Extremities.** Check for compartment syndrome, acute arterial occlusion.

F. **Back.** Check for epidural hematoma or abscess.

G. **Postoperative Pain**
1. **Acute.** The patient who is immediately postoperative may be expected to have a significant level of pain, depending on the type of surgery and its location. Incisional, visceral, and referred pain are common.
2. **Subacute.** Patients may continue to require a pain control regimen for a significant time after the initial procedure.
3. **Nonsurgical pain.** Patients may have pain related to their specific diagnosis, including areas of ongoing chronic inflammation, infection, or ischemia.
4. **Chronic pain.** Patients may have preexisting chronic pain issues that require continuation of a specific pain regimen, such as cancer patients on long-acting opioid medications.

IV. **Database**
A. **Physical Exam Key Points**
1. **General.** Signs of acute distress in a specific region help focus the initial exam.
2. **Vital signs.** Signs of hemodynamic instability, such as rapidly dropping blood pressure and low oxygen saturation, may indicate a life-threatening event and dictate the need for immediate action. An elevated blood pressure or tachycardia, or both are general indicators of pain.
3. **Neurologic.** Altered mental status may signify an intracranial event or deteriorating hemodynamic changes. Paralysis may indicate a neuraxial event, such as an epidural hematoma, abscess, or spinal cord ischemia.
4. **Abdomen.** A complete abdominal exam may help to differentiate between an "acute abdomen" and less acute visceral pain. The location of pain (quadrant) helps focus the area of further evaluation.
5. **Extremity exam.** Absence of peripheral pulses and changes in temperature and color can indicate peripheral ischemia.

B. **Laboratory Data**
1. **Hemogram.** A rapidly decreasing Hct may signify an acute bleed as a possible source of pain.
2. **Coagulation studies.** When neuraxial anesthesia, such as an epidural is indicated, coagulation studies should be obtained. Coagulopathy is a contraindication to placement of an epidural

catheter and will influence the decision to use even single-dose intrathecal therapy.

C. **Radiographic and Other Studies**
   1. **Chest radiograph.** This can show signs of acute pulmonary edema secondary to acute MI or aortic dissection or masses that might cause chest pain.
   2. **Head CT scan or MRI.** These show areas of an intracranial bleed, cerebral edema, or masses.
   3. **Abdominal radiograph or CT scan.** This can show evidence of intra-abdominal hemorrhage, visceral perforation or obstruction, edema secondary to ischemia, or masses that might cause pain.
   4. **Angiogram.** This study of a specific vascular distribution can further elucidate thrombosis and hemorrhage.

V. **Plan**

A. **Initial Management**
   1. **Resuscitate.** Begin basic or advanced cardiac life support protocol if resuscitation is required.
   2. **Medicate.** After ruling out emergent situations, check allergies and contraindications to sedation. The immediate administration of pain medication, such as morphine or fentanyl, may be beneficial.
   3. **Anxiolytics.** If anxiety is a significant component of the patient's perception of pain, an antianxiety medication, such as a benzodiazepine, may be helpful.

B. **Specific Treatment Plans**
   1. **Chronic pain.** If the patient has been treated for chronic pain issues, calling in the pain service team (often anesthesiologists, oncologists, or other pain specialists), if available, can help guide pain management.
   2. **Acute pain.** For the patient with acute pain, several options are available, depending on the specific procedure and illness.

C. **Narcotic Medications**
   1. **PCA.** Patient-controlled analgesia (PCA) is a system that provides an optional basal rate of narcotic infusion plus a method for patient self-administration of additional doses for breakthrough pain. A patient in moderate-to-severe pain, particularly in the immediate postoperative period, often requires a basal rate as a component of the PCA prescription. A patient with only moderate pain may only require the PCA dosing regimen. The PCA pump is programmed for each individual patient, with the total dose of narcotic per hour limited by the programmed "lock-out."
   2. **As-necessary medications (prn).** Standing narcotics plus an as-necessary narcotic for breakthrough pain delivered by caretaker may be the appropriate choice for patients who are unable to manage a PCA system, or for patients at high risk of medication

side effects. Such patients must be monitored closely for signs of respiratory depression and oversedation.

3. **Continuous infusion.** A continuous narcotic delivery system, such as a fentanyl drip, is the common method of pain control in the intubated patient and is often provided along with a benzodiazepine infusion for sedation.

4. **Oral narcotics.** For the patient in mild-to-moderate pain who can take oral medications, hydrocodone is a practical option. Patients with more severe or more chronic pain or both may require a long-acting narcotic, such as extended release oral morphine or codeine, or a fentanyl transdermal patch.

5. **Anti-inflammatory medications.** This category includes non-steroidal anti-inflammatory drugs (NSAIDs). These can be an important adjunct to any pain control regimen. Ketorolac is an NSAID that works well for bone and muscle pain and may be given IV or IM. Oral NSAIDs may be considered if tolerated. Contraindications to NSAID therapy include a history of gastritis, renal impairment, platelet dysfunction, and a high risk of bleeding complications. COX II inhibitors may be used for patients at risk of NSAID-related complications.

6. **Epidural analgesia.** This involves the placement of a catheter in the lumbar or thoracic epidural space. A continuous infusion of local anesthetic or preservative-free opioid or both can provide consistent pain relief. This can be administered to the patient with normal coagulation studies and neurologic status and is placed by an anesthesiologist. Patients that will particularly benefit from epidural analgesia include those that have undergone thoracotomy with chest tube placement, major upper-abdominal surgery, lower-extremity orthopedic procedures, and peripheral vascular procedures with residual pain secondary to ischemia.

7. **Regional nerve blocks.** These may be appropriate for defined areas of pain, such as knee or shoulder surgery, and help to delay need for opioid medication for 8–12 h.

8. **Pleural catheter.** This can be used to infuse local anesthetics into the pleural space for chest wall or pleuritic pain without resulting in any direct effect on mental status.

69. PERSISTENT NEUROMUSCULAR BLOCKADE

Immediate Actions. When the patient has persistent or new-onset muscle paralysis, you must first ensure adequate ventilation and oxygenation. This may require intubation and the provision of mechanical ventilation. Once these are ensured, sedation should also be considered in a timely fashion.

I. **Problem.** You are called to the bedside of a 64-year-old woman who is in a postoperative period following a triple coronary artery bypass graft to evaluate persistent paralysis.

II. **Immediate Questions**

A. **Is the patient stable?** With persistent paralysis or a recurrence of paralysis, an airway and mechanical ventilation must be instituted immediately. It is also important to assess whether the patient is stable from a cardiovascular standpoint. Serious cardiovascular deterioration may be the cause of the apparent paralysis.

B. **What paralytic drugs have been administered?** These drugs are the most likely explanation, so obviously, they can be ruled out if they were never administered. There are a number of conditions that can enhance neuromuscular blockade and result in its persistence into the postoperative period.

C. **Was neuromuscular blockade reversed in the immediate postoperative course?** Lack of reversal or inadequate reversal of muscle blockade is not unusual. Additionally, a reversal agent could have been used that has a shorter duration of action than the paralytic drug itself. A "recurarization" or recurrence of paralysis can occur as the reversal agent wears off, though this is a rare event in modern anesthesia practice.

D. **Does the patient truly have a persistent neuromuscular blockade?** This extrinsic cause of paralysis must be distinguished from an intrinsic process immediately. This can easily be done by using a peripheral nerve stimulator. The diagnosis of new paralysis not explained by pharmacologic blockade mandates an immediate search for a diagnosis.

E. **Is pain or impairment of movement secondary to surgery simulating the paralysis?** Inadequately treated pain may cause splinting and reduced motion, as the patient attempts to alleviate discomfort associated with motion, including those movements associated with respiratory efforts. Musculoskeletal surgery may impair motion of muscles and joints. Intraoperative nerve damage could result in local paralysis.

F. **Is the patient adequately sedated?** Neuromuscular blockade agents do not provide sedation, amnesia, or analgesia. If the patient is stable from a cardiovascular standpoint, amnestic or sedative drugs (eg, benzodiazepines) should be administered to avoid recall. Concomitantly, a narcotic infusion should be considered to allow the patient to tolerate the endotracheal tube. Because the patient may be unable to respond with movement or eye opening, an assessment of the autonomic nervous system may help to evaluate for adequate sedation. Large reactive pupils, tearing, diaphoresis, piloerection, tachycardia, and hypertension are some signs of inadequate sedation. In the case of cardiovascular instability, a cardiostable amnestic agent, such as scopolamine, should be considered.

III. Differential Diagnosis

A. **CNS Disease.** One must consider stroke or intracranial hemorrhage as possible causes of new paralysis. Furthermore, spinal cord disease secondary to trauma, vascular accident, or infection must also be considered. There can be a recrudescence or exacerbation of a preexisting neurologic disorder, such as multiple sclerosis in the postoperative period.

B. **Peripheral Nervous System Disease.** The possibility of peripheral neuropathies from ethyl alcohol, HIV, diabetes, porphyria, or sepsis-induced critical illness polyneuropathy (these usually have both sensory and motor involvement) should be excluded. Myopathies, such as polymyositis, HIV, or alcohol-related myopathies should be evaluated. Guillain-Barré can be a cause of progressive, ascending paralysis (usually postinfectious).

C. **Persistent Neuromuscular Blockade.** A number of causes need to be considered from initial drug administration to reversal and associated aggravating conditions.

D. **Use of a Long-Acting Neuromuscular Blocker.** Long-acting drugs may not have been reversed or may have been inadequately reversed (short-acting reversal agent). What specific paralytic (if any) was used for the patient? It is important to determine whether an intermediate- or long-acting (eg, pancuronium, vecuronium, atracurium) versus a short-acting neuromuscular blocker (eg, rapacuronium, mivacurium) was used during the case. Furthermore, the specific reversal agent that was used (if any) should be determined. The possibility exists that paralysis may recur if a long-acting agent was inappropriately reversed with a short-acting reversal agent. Was succinylcholine used? If so, the possibility of an atypical plasma cholinesterase should be considered. This condition blocks the elimination of succinylcholine and turns it into a long-lasting neuromuscular blocker. Also, large doses of this drug may lead to a phase II block that is difficult to reverse.

E. **Potentiation of Residual Blockade by Other Medications.** Is the patient receiving any other medications that can potentiate the effects of nondepolarizing neuromuscular blockers, either by synergistic actions against neuromuscular transmission or by inhibition of elimination of the paralytic drugs? Aminoglycosides and magnesium are the most common drugs implicated in the scenario of potentiation. Many other drugs have been reported to have varying degrees of effects, including local anesthetics, beta-blockers, calcium-channel blockers, class-I antiarrhythmics, polymyxins, trimethaphan, immunosuppressants, benzodiazepines, and dantrolene. Persistent presence of a volatile anesthetic agent early in the postoperative period will potentiate blockade. If the patient is receiving or has received any of these medications, one may see a prolonged duration of action from muscle relaxants (nondepolarizing). Neuromuscular blockers may also predispose the patient receiving exogenous steroids to steroid myopathy.

F. Potentiation of Residual Blockade by Other Conditions. Certain conditions, such as hypothermia, respiratory acidosis, and metabolic alkalosis can potentiate the effects of neuromuscular blocking drugs. Acute electrolyte abnormalities, such as hypophosphatemia, hypokalemia, and hypermagnesemia can aggravate this situation.

G. Prolongation of Duration of Blocking Drugs Secondary to Underlying Abnormalities. Renal or liver insufficiency, as evidenced by elevated creatinine or liver function tests, can cause an accumulation of neuromuscular blockers and their metabolites.

H. Sedation Simulating Paralysis. Medications may have been given that simulate the presence of paralysis by leading to apnea or a decreased level of consciousness. Have any drugs that suppress ventilatory drive been given postoperatively (eg, narcotics)? Long-acting opioids can have a "stockpiling" effect, leading to ventilatory depression and, ultimately, apnea. Anxiolytics and hypnotic medications may have similarly accumulated or are acting synergistically to impair ventilatory drive.

IV. Database

A. Physical Exam Key Points

1. **Vital signs.** Is the patient stable from a cardiovascular and respiratory standpoint? Assess effectiveness or ventilatory efforts if present. Look for signs of cyanosis.

2. **Muscle strength exam.** Clinical evaluation of muscle function should include a 5-s head lift or hand squeeze. These tests of ability to sustain tetanic contraction will help determine whether residual neuromuscular block is present. The ability to sustain such contractions of peripheral muscles virtually eliminates the possibility of residual pharmacologic blockade. Twitching movements that may resemble seizure activity characterize significant weakness and result from an inability to sustain contraction. Good physical examination for muscle strength in the cooperative patient precludes the need to use a nerve stimulator. Pain may preclude some movement and must be taken into consideration.

3. **Peripheral nerve stimulation.** Deliver a train-of-four electrical stimulus to a peripheral nerve, such as the facial or ulnar nerve. The presence of significant residual nondepolarizing neuromuscular blockade is characterized by a progressive loss of number and quality of twitches. An experienced observer may quantify the degree of blockade, but any diminution in number or quality corre-

sponds with the presence of clinically significant neuromuscular blockade. If the train-of-four stimulus appears intact, a tetanic stimulation should be considered. This is painful in the unsedated patient, but it is a more reliable test for small amounts of residual blockade that are clinically more subtle. If tetanic stimulation is not sustained without fading, residual muscle blockade exists. This result may also occur with blockade from succinylcholine in the case of very large doses or in the presence of an atypical plasma pseudocholinesterase.

4. **Neurologic exam.** Determine whether the deficit is strictly motor or whether a component of sensory compromise is present. Look for localization of weakness or sensory changes and changes in cranial nerve and mental status. These could suggest a neurologic cause.

B. **Laboratory Data.** Basic electrolyte studies should be obtained to rule out abnormalities that could contribute to residual blockade. A review of renal and liver panels should be made to look for organ dysfunction that could be impairing the elimination of drugs.

C. **Radiographic and Other Studies**
1. **Head CT/MRI.** If a central process is suspected, cerebral and/or spinal imaging (CT vs MR) is strongly suggested. The aid of specialized consultants should be sought early.

V. **Plan**

A. **Assess and treat the patient.** As previously discussed, if the patient is unstable (from a cardiovascular or a respiratory standpoint), care should be directed immediately toward reversing this situation. If a patient was previously not paralyzed and was spontaneously ventilating, he or she will obviously require immediate intubation.

B. **Consider the pharmacologic reversal of blockade.** After determining whether a paralytic agent was used, check to see whether any reversal agents were given. If a reversal agent was used, ensure that an adequate quantity of drug was used and that a long-acting reversal agent was used to reverse a long-acting paralytic. Reversal should not be attempted if there is no evidence of muscle function after assessment with a twitch monitor, as this represents a level of blockade that is too deep. Wait for further drug elimination before attempting reversal in such a case. Also check for secondary causes of prolongation of blockade at this time. Consultation with experienced practitioners is probably indicated.

1. **Reversal drugs.** Neostigmine is a good choice for reversal, when indicated, and is used in a dose of 0.07 mg/kg (up to 5 mg) along with 0.014 mg/kg (equal volume to that of neostigmine) of glycopyrrolate to counteract the cholinergic excess peripherally. The onset of action for this set of drugs is usually less than 5 min, and the duration of action is greater than 1 h.

C. **Consult and evaluate.** If either succinylcholine or mivacurium was used at any point, a plasma pseudocholinesterase deficiency should be considered. Evaluation and workup of such a problem is potentially complicated and is beyond the scope of this text. An anesthesiologist familiar with such problems should handle such concerns. Therapeutic options usually involve waiting for drug elimination while the patient is supported as necessary.

D. **Other causes.** If paralysis does not appear to be due to the administration of a neuromuscular blocker, sedation should be lightened. This may have been contributing to the problem and will enable a thorough neurologic examination. As mentioned previously, specialists should be consulted.

70. PLEURAL EFFUSION

Immediate actions. Dyspnea or increasing oxygen requirements mandates urgent patient assessment and treatment. Even in a monitored setting with experienced nursing and respiratory therapy staff, a personal assessment by the responsible physician is required to guide therapy. Telephone orders to increase the fraction of inspired oxygen are only symptomatic stop-gap measures.

I. **Problem.** A 57-year-old woman is currently in the telemetry unit with right-sided chest pain and shortness of breath. Routine chest films show a right pleural effusion.

II. **Immediate Questions**

A. **What are the vital signs?** Tachypnea increases the acuity of the clinical situation. Bradycardia is a marker for significant desaturation and is a harbinger for impending arrest. Fever may be a marker for an infectious origin.

B. **Is the patient short of breath?** Loss of functional respiratory units may lead to dyspnea. If the effusion is significant enough, compression of the contralateral side may occur.

C. **Have any procedures been performed?** Central line attempts, chest tube placement, thoracentesis, or thoracic surgery may all lead to fluid or blood accumulation within the pleural space.

D. **Was the effusion present on previous films?** Patients may have chronic pleural effusions. Comparison to previous films or previous records may indicate the chronicity of the process.

III. **Differential Diagnosis**

A. **Infection.** May be primary or secondary seeding of the pleural space.

1. **Parapneumonia/empyema.** Early empyema may present with serous fluid of increasing volume. If a chest tube is in place, the output may pick up as the empyema begins. Bacterial pneumonia may also present with a surrounding pleural effusion. This condition may evolve into an actual empyema.
2. **Tuberculosis.** Pleural effusion results from seeding of the pleural space with TB organisms. The effusion is generally unilateral and is often associated with pleuritic pain. It will often clear with antituberculosis therapy.
3. **Other infections.** Fungal, viral.
4. **Sarcoidosis.** In a minority of cases of sarcoid, a unilateral effusion may be evident. Laboratory study will identify an exudate. Interstitial changes may be seen on chest radiograph. Skin changes are common, but are not uniformly present.

B. **Congestive Heart Failure.** Effusions may be interlobar. Evidence of pulmonary vascular congestion will generally be evident. If a PA catheter is in place, increased pressures are also expected.

C. **Tumor.** Malignant effusions may result from either direct pleural inflammation from the tumor cells or from the blockage of pleural lymphatics. Simple aspiration is essentially ineffectual in the management of malignant effusions.
1. **Lung.** Lung cancer can cause a pleural effusion by spread directly to the pleura, by lymphatic obstruction, or by generating a postobstructive pneumonia with a subsequent effusion.
2. **Mesothelioma.** Incidence is increased with asbestos exposure. Pleural effusion is a common finding.
3. **Metastatic cancer.** The most common primary tumor associated with pleural effusion is breast cancer.

D. **Trauma.** In the acute setting, fluid in the pleural space after trauma should be considered a hemothorax, not a pleural effusion. In the more chronic state, pleural effusions may occur. The fluid may not have been evident on initial exam.

E. **Pulmonary Embolism.** If a pulmonary infarction has occurred, a pleural effusion may result. In most instances, the effusion is small.

F. **Esophageal Rupture.** Mediastinitis may cause direct irritation of the pleura, or the process may decompress into the pleural space.

G. **Collagen Vascular Diseases**
1. **Rheumatoid arthritis.** Pleural involvement is more common in men with this disease.
2. **Systemic lupus erythematosus.** Pleural effusion is a common manifestation of lupus.
3. **Wegener's granulomatosis.** Pulmonary involvement is present in up to 95% of patients and may include pleural effusion.

H. **Chylothorax.** Trauma or tumors may lead to a leak of chyle into the pleural space. If diagnosis in uncertain, stains for fat may be done on aspirated pleural fluid. If trauma is the cause, spontaneous resolution can sometimes occur.

  I. **Intra-abdominal.** In general, abdominal conditions that result in inflammation or evolution of significant amounts of peritoneal fluid can lead to pleural effusions. The finding may be either unilateral or bilateral. Multiple different causes may be present. Treatment of the underlying condition is the first goal of therapy.

    1. Peritonitis.
    2. Cirrhosis.
    3. Pancreatitis.
    4. Subphrenic abscess.
    5. Nephrotic syndrome.
    6. Drug induced (amiodarone, nitrofurantoin, dantrolene).
    7. Idiopathic.

IV. Database

  A. History

    1. Dyspnea on exertion. Both the chronicity and the trend should be identified.

    2. Pleuritic chest pain. Pain is aggravated by coughing or deep respiratory efforts.

  B. Physical Exam Key Points

    1. Vital signs. Respiratory rate and effort should be documented. Tachypnea reflects significant respiratory decompensation.

    2. Lung exam. Clinical findings that indicate the presence of significant pleural effusion include decreased breath sounds, dullness to percussion, absent tactile and fremitus, and displaced mediastinum.

    3. Cardiac exam. New murmurs, rubs, and gallops may all be present. JVD suggests the presence of congestive heart failure.

    4. Abdominal exam. Peritonitis may be evident. Epigastric tenderness can be suggestive of pancreatitis. Ascites and changes consistent with chronic liver disease are usually evident.

    5. Skin exam. Lupus and Wegener's granulomatosis both have skin lesions associated with active disease.

    6. Joint exam. Rheumatoid arthritis will generate characteristic joint changes.

  C. Laboratory Data

    1. Hemogram. WBC will be increased in most circumstances involving infectious sources. Hemoglobin may be low in cases of hemothorax.

    2. Coagulation studies. In patients with cirrhosis, clotting factor levels may be low. If invasive procedures are planned, one should obtain a baseline set of clotting studies.

    3. Electrolytes. Provide baseline for comparison with pleural fluid levels.

    4. Amylase. This is generally elevated with acute pancreatitis.

D. Radiographic and Other Studies

1. **Thoracentesis.** A sample of thoracentesis fluid should be sent for analysis. Not every clinical situation mandates the obtaining of all possible studies. Interpretation of the protein level, pH, and glucose will allow the physician to diagnose whether a transudate or an exudate is present.

   a. **Gram's stain and culture.** Pleural fluid ordinarily is sterile. The presence of organisms on Gram's stain reflects an active infectious process.

   b. **pH.** Low values, (<7.3), reflect an exudative effusion.

   c. **Glucose.** In transudates, the glucose level will be the same as that of serum. Because of the possibility of wide fluctuations of glucose levels during the acute phase of critical illness, simultaneous measurements should be made.

   d. **Amylase.** A reactive effusion to acute pancreatitis will have a high level of amylase. This finding is also present with some cases of esophageal rupture or tumors.

   e. **LDH.** Levels are low with transudates.

   f. **Cell count and differential.** Both WBC and RBC in pleural fluid are elevated with exudates.

   g. **Total protein.** High protein levels are also indicative of an exudate.

   h. **Cytologic examination.** Malignant effusion can be documented with cytology.

   i. **Smears.** An acid-fast smear may occasionally document TB. Pleural biopsy provides a higher yield.

   j. **Lipid analysis.** Fat stain of the pleural fluid can diagnose chylothorax.

   k. **Rheumatoid factor** and complement levels may be elevated with immune origins.

2. **Chest radiograph.** Upright films.

   a. Blunted costophrenic angle requires at least 300–500 cc to be apparent on an upright chest radiograph.

   b. Look for pooling of fluid within interlobar fissures.

   c. Pleural fluid can be loculated in the chest cavity.

   d. With significant pleural fluid, compressive atelectasis is present and may be seen on film.

   e. Look for subpulmonic effusion fluid between lung and diaphragm resembling elevated hemidiaphragm.

   f. In patients who are supine, pleural effusion may only present as diffuse haziness.

3. **Lateral decubitus** films show layering of free pleural fluid to dependent portions of the chest.

4. **Ultrasound.** This may be done at the bedside. It allows for marking of loculated effusions.

5. **CT.**

      a. CT may show fluid in either the abdomen or the chest. With elevated hemidiaphragm, CT may allow localization to above or below the diaphragm.

      b. CT may show atelectasis.

      c. Tumors, if present, may be visualized.

V. Plan

A. Small effusions with an obvious cause require no treatment other than follow-up examinations and treatment of the underlying condition.

B. Large effusions and effusions requiring diagnosis will need thoracentesis, which may be both diagnostic and therapeutic.

C. Localization by exam, radiograph, or fluoroscopic guidance for optimal insertion will be needed.

D. Obtain a completion film to evaluate whether there is a pneumothorax or a newly discovered pulmonary process.

E. Diagnostic Thoracentesis

  1. Transudate. This is due to altered fluid dynamics. It is either abnormal formation of pleural fluid or caused by an obstruction of fluid absorption.

    a. Not related to pleural surface

    b. Low protein content and low specific gravity

    c. Eighty percent caused by congestive heart failure

    d. Straw colored, clear, and odorless

  2. Exudate. Pulmonary or pleural pathology within the lymphatics causing increased capillary permeability

    a. Higher protein content and specific gravity

    b. 40% caused by malignancy

    c. Cloudy, increased WBCs

  3. Therapeutic thoracentesis.

    a. Removal of the majority of fluid with relief of dyspnea or chest pain.

    b. Should be removed slowly, so that coughing and pain does not occur.

    c. If more than **1000 cc** is removed at one time, severe unilateral pulmonary edema can develop and may be fatal. If the patient is in a regular room, pulse oximetry should be used, and a possible transfer to a monitored setting should be considered. In general, no more than 1000 cc should be removed at one time.

    d. Postprocedure film. A chest radiograph should be obtained to follow the results of the intervention. In general, effusions should be tapped dry. Pneumothorax may also result. Residual fluid represents either incomplete removal of fluid or a bleeding complication.

    e. Chest tube insertion is required for empyema or for any fluid that is too thick to drain with a needle. If there is a history of trauma, chest tube insertion represents the therapeutic option of choice.

    f. Malignant effusions. These are highly likely to reoccur. Chest tube placement is required. Once fluid has been evacuated, then pleurodesis with talc, bleomycin, or other agents should be done. Because many of these agents generate significant pain, preparations for analgesia should be made.

    g. Video-assisted thoracoscopy (VATS).

        i. Pleurodesis may be used to encourage obliteration of the pleural space.

        ii. Pleural or lung biopsy for diagnosis can be performed.

        iii. Pleurectomy for definitive management of empyema.

71. PNEUMOTHORAX

I. Problem. A 34-year-old man, a restrained passenger involved in a motor vehicle collision, is being observed in the ICU. He develops shortness of breath, and his oxygen saturation drops into the mid-80s.

II. Immediate Questions

    A. Does he have any other complaints? Pain can cause an inadequate respiratory effort. Dyspnea and desaturation may reflect global decompensation. Vital signs should be assessed.

    B. Was a chest radiograph obtained in the emergency department before his transfer to the ICU? Initial films should be reviewed to look for missed injuries. If no film was obtained initially, a radiograph should be obtained immediately. The films should be scrutinized for associated injuries, including rib fractures and pulmonary contusion.

    C. What is the patient's baseline status? Patients who have preexisting respiratory disease will not as easily tolerate the relative loss of respiratory units from a pneumothorax.

    D. Is or was he on supplemental oxygen? All trauma patients should initially be on oxygen per nasal cannula at a minimum.

    E. Is he able to speak? Inability to speak could be due to aspiration of a foreign body or a loose tooth. In addition, inability to speak may represent significant respiratory compromise from the pneumothorax or an associated lung injury.

    F. Have any procedures been attempted on the patient? Pneumothorax may occur as a complication of line attempts, bronchoscopy, or tracheostomy. These attempts may not have been documented.

III. Differential Diagnosis

    A. Pneumothorax. In blunt trauma, pneumothorax generally is associated with rib fractures. If no rib fractures are seen, an airway or esophageal injury should be suspected. Spontaneous pneumothorax may occur in some patients.

B. Hemothorax. The symptoms from hemothorax may be very similar to that of pneumothorax. Physical exam and radiograph will distinguish these processes.

C. Shock. Desaturation and dyspnea may be part of a pattern of response to shock.

D. Pneumonia. Significant lobar pneumonia may cause tachypnea and desaturation. Physical examination should distinguish this condition from pneumothorax.

IV. Database

A. Physical Exam Key Points

1. **Vital signs.** Tachypnea or tachycardia may lead to the belief that the patient has a pneumothorax.
2. **Neck.** Examine for subcutaneous emphysema, tracheal deviation, penetrating injuries. Examine for evidence of previous central venous access attempts that may not have been documented.
3. **Chest exam.** Decreased breath sounds on the affected side, subcutaneous emphysema, and hyperresonance to percussion are most likely caused by pneumothorax. Dullness to percussion would be more suggestive of hemothorax. If a chest tube is already in place, examine the tube for function. Has the tube been clamped or become clotted? If an air leak is present, is it large? Both hemothorax and pneumothorax may coexist (see also Problem 43, Hemothorax).
4. **Cardiac exam.** Examine for distended neck veins and pulsus paradoxus.

B. Laboratory Data

1. **Obtain an ABG immediately.** Document level of respiratory function. This will guide further therapy.
2. **Sputum for analysis.** If patient has productive sputum, a sample should be sent for analysis.

C. Radiographic and Other Studies

1. **Chest radiograph.** Evaluate for pneumothorax and hemothorax. Comparison to previous films, if any, should be done. Careful attention to atypical presentation of pneumothorax requires review of apices, bases, and mediastinal structures.

V. Plan

A. Overall Plan. To determine the cause of the pneumothorax and dyspnea.

B. Specific Plans

1. **Examine the patient immediately.** Tension pneumothorax should be treated immediately with needle decompression. Typi-

cally, this procedure is done in the second intercostal space anteriorly. If a needle decompression is done, a tube thoracostomy
(chest tube) is always needed. Inspection of the drainage system
of an existing tube should identify functional problems.

2. **Start supplemental oxygen via nasal cannula or face mask.**
   Patients with significant tachypnea will benefit most from face
   mask systems. Although intubation may be required, if a large
   pneumothorax or tension pneumothorax is present, conversion to
   positive-pressure ventilation may exacerbate the problem.

3. **View the chest radiograph and compare with ED chest radiograph for changes.** If a chest tube had been previously placed,
   examine the tube position. The sentinel hole must be within the
   chest cavity. The tube should be free of kinking. Progression of a
   subtle anterior pneumothorax may allow for its identification on
   subsequent exam. Digital view stations allow manipulation of the
   image to minimize the chance of misinterpretation.

4. **Pneumothorax.** If a pneumothorax is seen on the chest radiograph, the patient will need a tube thoracostomy, because the
   patient is symptomatic. Other times, a patient will require a chest
   tube to be included when they are to undergo general anesthesia
   or positive-pressure ventilation.

5. If a pneumothorax is seen on the ED chest radiograph, and it is
   small, the patient may be monitored with serial physical examinations and chest films. Even in the event of a minimal pneumothorax, if the patient is under positive-pressure ventilation or remote
   from examination, a chest tube is required.

72. POLYURIA

I. **Problem.** A patient is in the ICU after massive head and corporeal injuries from a motorcycle accident. During his first hospital day, he is
placed on mannitol and undergoes multiple contrast imaging studies. On
his second hospital day, his urine output is 250 cc/h.

II. **Immediate Questions**

   A. **Is it water diuresis or solute diuresis?** The answer to this question is
   found by taking a thorough history and doing specific laboratory tests.
   Once the origin is clear, treatment should target the underlying cause.

   B. **What medications was the patient given?** Diuretics can cause
   polyuria.

   C. **How much IV fluid was the patient given?**

III. **Differential Diagnosis.** A number of interventions, diseases, and drugs
commonly encountered in the ICU may result in development or exacerbation of polyuria. Polyuria is arbitrarily defined as a urine output > 3 L in
24 h.

A. Appropriate Diuresis. There are circumstances in the ICU when urine output > 3 L/d is appropriate. Massive fluid resuscitation after trauma can result in physiologic diuresis.

B. Water Diuresis. Diabetes insipidus is characterized by urine osmolarity < 250 mOsm/L. There are neurogenic and nephrogenic causes. Neurogenic diabetes insipidus occurs when the neurohypophysis cannot produce antidiuretic hormone (ADH). Head trauma, brain tumors, or Sheehan's syndrome (postpartum hemorrhage) can all ablate the ability of the neurohypophysis to produce ADH. Nephrogenic diabetes insipidus occurs when the renal collecting tubule is insensitive to ADH. Acute causes include hypokalemia, hypercalcemia, or medications, including lithium, amphotericin B, gentamycin, glyburide, and isophosphamide. Chronic causes include renal failure, amyloidosis, and sickle cell nephropathy.

C. Solute Diuresis. Urine osmolarities > 300 mOsm/L suggest solute diuresis. Causes include administration of osmotically active agents, poor glycemic control, high-protein feeds, or the polyuric phase of renal failure. Solute diuresis can occur after administration of glycerol, mannitol, or radiocontrasts. Serum glucose levels beyond the reabsorbing capacity of the nephron also cause an osmotic diuresis. High protein intake increases serum urea levels, an effect that promotes osmotic diuresis.

IV. Database

A full history is key to identifying possible causes (see previous section, Differential Diagnosis) of polyuria.

A. Physical Exam Key Points
1. **Vital signs.** Look for signs of hypotension and cardiac arrhythmias. A thorough assessment of volume status is critical to caring for ICU patients with polyuria.
2. **Neurologic exam.** Look for signs of CNS injury or electrolyte effects.

B. Laboratory Data
1. **Urinalysis.** Urine output should be closely monitored. Remember that ICU patients may not have the capacity to drink or to have access to water. Check urine osmolarity.
2. **Check serum osmolarity, glucose, electrolytes, and calcium levels.**

C. Radiographic and Other Studies
1. When diabetes insipidus is suspected, a water deprivation test can be performed if the patient is not already dehydrated.
2. Determination of serum antidiuretic hormone levels is helpful in diagnosing diabetes insipidus.
3. **Head CT.** Rule out Sheehan's syndrome.

    4. **Renal nuclear scan.** May be helpful in diagnosis of acute tubular necrosis.

V. Plan. Target treatment at the underlying cause.

    A. Replace intravascular volume because of the importance of maintaining electrolytes at normal levels.

    B. Discontinue or substitute for offending medications.

    C. Correct hyperglycemia and reduce high-protein diet.

73. POSTURING: DECORTICATE/DECEREBRATE

I. Problem. A 24-year-old patient who was admitted after sustaining a closed head injury now is exhibiting flexion of the elbows to any stimulation.

II. Immediate Questions

    A. Is the patient anticoagulated? Supratherapeutic anticoagulation may cause intracranial hemorrhage. Brain injury may also cause a relatively anticoagulated state.

    B. Is there a history of head trauma or tumor? Recent head trauma or fall may result in traumatic hemorrhage. Brain tumors can spontaneously bleed or cause mass effect themselves. Patients may bleed into previously operated sites.

    C. Does the patient have a seizure disorder? Many patients will have spasms or seizures that can be confused with posturing. The patient or the family may be able to relate their seizure history. Observation of the event clinically will help distinguish posturing from seizure activity.

    D. Does the patient have a ventriculostomy or ventricular shunt in place? Malfunction of a shunt may cause increased intracranial pressure.

III. Differential Diagnosis

    A. Intracranial Hemorrhage. This can occur as a result of trauma (findings may be delayed, as in the case of subdural hematoma). Hemorrhagic stroke may be seen in the elderly or hypertensive patient.

    B. Excessive Anticoagulation. Heparinization or excessive anticoagulation with Coumadin may cause an intraparenchymal or intracranial bleed. The effect of Coumadin may change with dietary changes or with the addition of new medications. Improper dosing may also lead to an excessive anticoagulated state.

    C. Structural Mass/Tumor. Typically, symptoms are unilateral, and posturing would be a late finding.

   D. Metabolic. Hepatic, uremic, anoxic, hypoglycemic, or sedative drugs
   may all cause symmetric posturing.

IV. Database

A. Physical Exam Key Points

1. **Vital signs.** Hypertension and bradycardia (Cushing's response)
   are indicative of herniation. Hypotension will adversely impact
   cerebral perfusion pressure and should be corrected.
2. **HEENT.** Loss of papillary reflex and dilated pupils are usually unilateral and late findings.
3. **Neurologic.** A symmetric neurologic examination supports a
   metabolic cause. Decorticate posture resembles arms tight to the
   sides with elbows, wrists, and fingers flexed. The legs are extended and internally rotated. Feet are plantar flexed. Decere-
   brate rigidity demonstrates a clenched jaw with extended neck.
   The arms are adducted and stiffly extended at the elbows with
   forearms pronated and wrists and fingers flexed. The legs are
   stiffly extended at the knees with the feet plantar flexed.

B. Laboratory Data

1. **CBC.** Look for evidence of infection or anemia.
2. **PT/PTT/platelets/fibrinogen.** Look for evidence of coagulopathy.
   Replace with appropriate component therapy.
3. **Serum chemistry.** Rule out metabolic causes, such as hypoglycemia, uremia, and others.

C. Radiographic and Other Studies

1. **CT Head.** This evaluates for bleed, tumor, or stroke. When previous studies are available, a comparison should be made.
2. **Drain/ICP.** Evaluate the drain system to see if it is working properly. Look for occlusion, kinking, or inadvertent clamping of the
   tubing.

V. Plan

A. Immediate Plan.
The goal is to find any correctable cause of the
neurologic change. Early and accurate communication with the neurosurgical service is essential. Maintenance of cerebral perfusion un-
derlies most therapeutic maneuvers.

B. Specific Plans

1. Correction of metabolic disturbance if any. This may require dialysis in the case of uremia.
2. Correction of coagulopathy usually with fresh frozen plasma for
   immediate results.
3. Prompt collaboration with the neurosurgical service if intracranial
   bleed or mass effect is seen on CT. The patient may require immediate surgical intervention. Other specific measures that neurosurgery may direct include

a. **ICP monitoring.** This allows determination of cerebral perfusion pressure and serves as the foundation for therapeutic maneuvers.

b. **Head of bed elevation at least 30 degrees.** This minimizes the likelihood of venous congestion. When a cervical collar is in place, it should be inspected to ensure it is not too tight.

c. **Avoid hypercarbia.** Although hyperventilation as a therapeutic maneuver has been used in the past, maintenance of normocarbia and the prevention of hypercarbia are well accepted.

d. **Hyperosmolar agents (mannitol).** The goal of therapy is euvolemia with hyperosmolarity.

e. **Steroids (for tumors).**

74. PREGNANCY

Immediate Actions. ABCs, oxygen, large-bore IV, and aggressive fluid replacement; transfuse blood as indicated. In late pregnancy, position patient with her left side down to relieve pressure on the vena cava.

I. **Problem.** You are called to the ICU to assess a 34-year-old pregnant women with severe vaginal bleed, possible ruptured membranes, and bleeding from her two IV sites.

II. **Immediate Questions**

A. What are the vital signs?

B. Is this spotting or a "real" bleed?

C. What is the color of the blood (vaginal)? Bright red or dark brown.

D. How far is the woman into her pregnancy?

E. What are the vital signs of the fetus?

F. Did the membranes rupture?

G. Does the patient have any other complicating medical conditions?

H. What medications were given to the patient?

III. **Differential Diagnosis**

A. When managing a pregnant patient in the ICU, a physician must differentiate between the normal physiologic changes of pregnancy and a potential early delivery from pathologic changes. Contractions may either be inconsequential or may lead to an early delivery. Fetal distress must always be a consideration when the mother's status changes. Ruptured membranes are part of normal labor but can lead to serious complication if rupture is premature. Lastly, vaginal bleeding may also herald a serious disorder.

B. **Physiologic Changes in Pregnancy.** A woman's basic physiology changes during pregnancy. Maternal blood volume increases to 40% above baseline by the third trimester. Cardiac output increases from 30%–50% above baseline by 25–32 wk. Both an increased heart rate and stroke volume account for the increase. Minute ventilation reaches from 20%–40% above baseline at term. Increased tidal volume results in arterial pH values of 7.40–7.47, PCO_2 values of 28–32 mm Hg, and plasma bicarbonate values of 18–21 mEq/L. Glomerular filtration rate increases to 50% above baseline by the 16th week of gestation.

C. **Contractions.** Uterine contractions may signify the beginning of normal labor any time after 37 weeks of gestation. "Braxton Hicks" contractions are sporadic uterine contractions that occur in the last 4–8 wk of pregnancy. They are not associated with cervical dilation or effacement. In the last month of pregnancy these "false labor" contractions can occur every 10–20 min. Contractions occurring earlier than 37 wk of gestation may signify an impending preterm birth. A preterm delivery that follows a medical or obstetrical disorder that places the mother or fetus at risk is called **an indicated preterm birth.** The most common causes of indicated preterm births are preeclampsia (43%), fetal distress (27%), intrauterine growth retardation, abruptio placentae, fetal demise, hyperthyroidism, heart disease, obstetric cholestasis, hepatitis, and anemia. All of these pose a definite (although unclear) risk of preterm contractions.

D. **Fetal Distress.** Fetal heart rate patterns reflect fetal conditions. Therefore fetal heart rate monitoring is the universally accepted method of assessing fetal well-being. A heart rate between 110 and 160 bpm is the sign of a well-oxygenated, perfused fetus. Any hypoxia or hypoperfusion in the mother may first manifest as an abnormality of fetal heart-rate patterns. Observation of fetal heart rate may assist in management of the mother.

E. **Sustained fetal bradycardia** (<110 bpm) results from structural cardiac defects, fetal heart block, and possibly maternal lupus. Intermittent and prolonged decelerations in fetal heart rate in an ICU patient are very serious. Maternal hypoxia secondary to amniotic fluid embolism, acute respiratory failure, or eclamptic seizure will cause decelerations. Placental abruption occurs in the situation of decelerations superimposed on maternal hypertension, preeclampsia, or trauma. Cord compression or overaggressive blood pressure control can cause decelerations during delivery. Prolonged fetal bradycardia is an emergency that requires prompt correction or delivery.

F. **Fetal tachycardia** (>160 bpm) is usually less ominous than bradycardia. Common causes include premature delivery, maternal fever, and chorioamnionitis. Hyperthyroidism will also increase fetal resting heart rate.

G. **Ruptured Membranes.** The fetal membrane provides a barrier between the sterile fetus and the bacteria-laden vaginal canal. A large gush of clear fluid followed by a persistent leak signifies rupture of membranes. Premature rupture of membranes is defined as membrane breakage and leak of amniotic fluid before labor contractions. Systemic infection in the mother may weaken fetal membranes. Complications of premature rupture of membranes include maternal and fetal infection, premature labor and delivery, and fetal hypoxia secondary to cord compression. Avoid digital intracervical examination, apply an external electronic fetal monitor, and call the obstetrician.

H. **Vaginal Bleeding.** Vaginal bleeding during the second trimester is associated with preterm birth. The two major causes are placenta previa and abruption. Cervical cancer is an uncommon cause but should always be considered. Hydatidiform mole manifests as vaginal bleeding in the first trimester. Vaginal discharge ranges from scant, dark brown to brisk hemorrhage, requiring transfusion.

I. **Preeclampsia.** This condition may be confused with epilepsy, encephalitis, meningitis, brain tumor, intracranial hemorrhage, and hysteria.

IV. **Database**

A. **History.** Determine the time of the last menstrual period, parity, previous OB/gyn complications, and last intercourse.

B. **Physical Exam Key Points**
   1. **Vital signs.**
   2. **Abdominal exam.** Evaluate for tenderness, uterine irritability, and estimate fundal height.
   3. **Pelvic exam.**
      a. **Early pregnancy.** Determine source of bleeding and os patency; evaluate adnexa and uterus for size, tenderness, or abnormalities.
      b. **Late pregnancy.** Do not perform pelvic exam in third trimester until placenta previa is ruled out or patient is in the operating room (may precipitate fatal hemorrhage); listen for fetal heart tones (Doppler test > 10 wk); monitor continuously.

C. **Laboratory Data**
   1. **Hemogram.**
   2. **Quantitative human chorionic gonadotropin (HCG).**
   3. **Type and cross and check Rh factor.**
   4. **Coagulation profile and DIC screen.**
   5. **BUN and creatinine.**
   6. **Urine/blood toxicology.**
   7. **Proteinuria.** Monitor repeatedly.

D. Radiographic and Other Studies
1. **Ultrasound.** Transvaginal detects yolk sack at 5.5 wk or beta HCG = 1500 IU.
2. **Culdocentesis.** Check for intraperitoneal blood.
3. **Head CT and lumbar puncture.** This can be used when intracranial hemorrhage or meningitis is of concern.
4. **Ferning test.** May be used to test for possible ruptured membranes.

V. Plan

A. Contractions. Contact an obstetrician when an ICU patient reports contractions closer than 20–30 min apart. A nonverbal patient should have continuous electronic fetal monitoring to assess for contractions. Tocolytic therapy should only be instituted under a specialist's guidance. Medications include beta-adrenergic agonists, magnesium sulfate, prostaglandin synthesis inhibitors, and calcium antagonists. Administer RhoGAM when patient is Rh negative; administer oxytocin, to control postabortion bleed. Have an immediate obstetrical consultation. Magnesium Sulfate is the first line of drugs in severe preeclampsia. Valium and phenytoin are considered. Delivery is emergent when preeclampsia is severe.

Use hydralazine or diazoxide for hypertension.

75. PRURITUS

I. Problem. A 45-year-old man admitted for ascending cholangitis has multiple excoriations of his arms caused by pruritus.

II. Immediate Questions

A. What is the duration of symptoms? Acute onset of pruritus in the hospital can usually be attributed to an agent new to the patient, such as medications, laundry (gown/sheets), or anesthetic (epidural).

B. Are there any associated physical findings or other symptoms? Rashes, other lesions and their locations may allude to the cause. Elevated temperature may indicate a systemic reaction or process.

C. Has the patient been started on any new medications or supplemental enteral nutrition? Many analgesics may cause pruritus.

III. Differential Diagnosis

A. Dermatologic
1. **Allergic reactions.** Contact dermatitis (tapes, soaps, detergents, latex).
2. **Infection.** Viral illnesses, shingles, scabies, parasite infections.
3. **Xerosis/dry skin.** Cold weather and low humidity within the hospital may exacerbate dry skin conditions.

B. Systemic

 1. **Allergic reactions.** Medications (IV/oral, local/systemic), blood transfusion (patients often have a mild reaction with an elevated temperature, rash, and itching). Ensure, however, that the patient has not received blood with an incompatible blood type. Epidural anesthetics (especially morphine sulfate) are common causes of pruritus.
 2. **Liver dysfunction.** Cholestasis may cause pruritus.
 3. **Uremia.** A direct relation of BUN levels with pruritus has not been shown.
 4. **Hypothyroid.**
 5. **Hyperparathyroid.**
 6. **Gout.**
 7. **Polycythemia.**
 8. **Myeloproliferative disorders.**
 9. **Parasites.**

C. Psychosomatic

IV. Database

A. Physical Exam Key Points

 1. **Vital signs.** Fever may indicate a systemic process.
 2. **Skin.** Take note of any rash (lesions/skin breakdown) and its characteristics and distribution. Look at both involved and uninvolved areas of skin. Distribution of any rash may provide insight into the origin of the pruritus.
 3. **Respiratory.** Stridor and wheezing may be signs of anaphylaxis.

B. Laboratory Data

 1. **LFTs.** Assess to evaluate liver function.
 2. **BUN and creatinine.** Assess to rule out uremia/renal dysfunction.
 3. **Hemogram.** Eosinophilia is suggestive of drug reaction or parasite infestation.

V. Plan.
Pruritus by itself is typically not an emergent situation, but it may be indicative of an impending or evolving process in need of attention. Attention to the symptom of pruritus may lead to the discovery of ongoing medical processes that need treatment.

A. Anaphylaxis. See Problem 10, page 27.

B. Epidural Anesthetic. Notify anesthetist; this cause is typically resistant to antihistamines; however, it may be eliminated by administration of naloxone at a low dose (1–2 µg/kg/h) without antagonizing the analgesic effect.

C. Uremia. May indicate progressive renal failure with eventual need for dialysis.

D. Dry Skin. Hydrate skin with warm water and moisturizers.

E. Contact Dermatitis. Remove offending agent; apply topical 1% hydrocortisone.

F. Medication Reaction. Discontinue or change medications that may have precipitated the pruritus.

G. Liver. Relieve biliary obstruction if possible.

H. Symptomatic Relief. Administer diphenhydramine 25–50 mg orally or IV every 6 h as necessary; Atarax 25 mg orally every 6 h as necessary; or Solu-medrol 125 mg IV/IM or prednisone 10 mg orally for 5 d.

76. PULMONARY ARTERY (PA) CATHETER: CANNOT WEDGE, MALFUNCTION

I. Problem. The waveforms from a patient's pulmonary artery (PA) catheter are unusual (see page 352 for waveforms).

II. Immediate Questions

A. Is the patient hemodynamically stable? Is there a pressure waveform? Most problems with PA catheters are technical in nature, related to issues with the transducing system or the catheter itself. Differentiate between absence of a pressure waveform and a waveform that is simply dampened.

B. Is the balloon inflated? Perhaps the catheter is wedged.

C. How far in is the catheter, and has it shifted since it was inserted? Was the dressing on the catheter recently changed? Has the patient recently been moved? What was the distance when initially placed?

D. Can the catheter be wedged? If the catheter cannot be wedged at this time, when was the last successful wedge and what has happened to the patient in the interim?

E. Is the patient having hemoptysis? New-onset hemoptysis in a patient with a PA catheter must be assumed to be a pulmonary artery rupture until proven otherwise. When PA rupture is suspected, call for help immediately. The incidence of PA rupture is uncommon (0.06–0.2%), but the mortality rate can range from 45–65% with many patients dying within 30 min of the arterial rupture. Other signs of PA rupture can include cough, dyspnea, shock, or chest pain, or both. In this event, the patient should be placed with the affected side of the chest down and intubated into the unaffected bronchus if possible. Definitive treatment of this lesion is surgical. PA rupture can occur when the catheter is advanced with an underinflated balloon, when the catheter is overwedged, or occasionally, in patients with valvular heart disease. Once again, this is a problem with life or death consequences and requires immediate intervention.

III. Differential Diagnosis

A. **Total Loss of Pressure Waveform, Clot in Catheter.** A blood clot in the catheter could cause a loss of the pressure tracing.

B. **Closed Stopcock.** The stopcock must be open to the pulmonary artery to generate a pressure tracing.

C. **Equipment Failure.** This can occur anywhere in the circuit from the monitor to the transducer to the catheter itself and at all points in between. Ensure that all connections are tight. Has the transducer been properly zeroed?

D. **Dampened Waveform.** Overdamping results in a decrease in the quality of the signal in the system. That is, energy associated with the pressure waveform is not fully transmitted to the transducer, because part of its signal is being absorbed elsewhere.

E. **Air Bubble.** Large air bubbles or several small bubbles may result in a dampened waveform. (Very tiny air bubbles can actually lead to underdamping of a system and overshoot of pressure waveforms.)

F. **Partially Clotted Catheter**

G. **Kinking or knotting of the catheter.** This phenomenon may occur at any time, but occurs, particularly, in patients with dilated cardiac chambers. Repeated catheter manipulation also predisposes to knotting. The possibility of a knot in the catheter should be considered when resistance is encountered when attempting to withdraw the catheter. Excessive tightening of devices intended to secure catheters and keep them from moving in or out are often responsible for partial or complete occlusion of one of the many internal lumens.

H. **Inappropriate Scale on Monitor.** This sounds far-fetched, but a normal PA waveform may appear damped when displayed with a scale intended for systemic arterial pressures.

I. **Wedged Catheter.** Changes in body temperature or positioning may result in a catheter spontaneously wedging. Alternatively, the balloon may not have been deflated since it was last wedged. The presumed damped waveform may simply represent the pulmonary capillary pressures and not those of the pulmonary artery. This represents a risk factor for pulmonary infarct.

J. **Cannot Wedge**

1. **Balloon rupture.** This occurs anywhere from 1%–23% of the time when using PA catheters. Hopefully, the balloon was tested before insertion. Slow inflation of the balloon with 1.5 cc of air will be adequate to obtain a pulmonary capillary wedge pressure (PCWP) when the catheter is in the correct position. Multiple inflations will eventually result in an increased risk of balloon rupture. When the catheter is determined to be in the correct position, balloon rupture should be considered. This is especially true when little or no resistance is encountered on balloon inflation.

2. **Catheter too proximal.** When the catheter is not far enough into the pulmonary artery, balloon inflation will not achieve a PCWP tracing. The catheter may have been inadvertently withdrawn. Changes in body position or ventilation may anatomically alter the previous relationship of the PA catheter to the pulmonary vasculature. In time, the catheter may slowly lose some elasticity, and its original curl may lessen, so that the tip is no longer present in a distal portion of the PA vessel.

IV. **Database**

  A. **Physical Exam Key Points**

    1. **Vital Signs.** As mentioned previously, ensure that the patient is hemodynamically stable.

    2. **Catheter insertion site.** Assess insertion distance of the catheter.

  B. **Laboratory Data** (not indicated).

  C. **Radiographic Studies**

    1. **Chest radiograph.** This may be used to assess the location of the catheter tip and to rule out the presence of kinks or knots. Comparison can be made to old films to determine whether the catheter has moved significantly.

V. **Plan.** The plan of action will revolve around several pieces of data, including the stability of the patient, the presence or absence of a pressure waveform, the quality of the waveform if one is present, the ability to wedge the catheter, and the chest radiograph findings.

  A. **Initial Management.** Assuming the patient is reasonably stable, the first step should be to examine the waveform displayed. As discussed previously, the plan of action should be based on the specific problem with the waveform.

  B. **Aspirate from the catheter to ensure that it is patent. Flush as needed.** If the catheter had a small bubble or clot, flushing should correct the problem. Consider using a syringe rather than the flush system on the transducer pressure bag setup, as it will generate more force to move out a small clot in the PA catheter lumen. These maneuvers should be attempted with both absent and dampened waveforms.

  C. **Replace catheter with occluded lumens. Reconsider the need for PA catheter monitoring.** It is not unusual for a reassessment of the patient's condition to result in a decision to discontinue this mode of invasive monitoring.

  D. **Ensure that the entire transducing system is patent.** Check all connections, ensure that stopcocks are in the appropriate positions.

  E. **Confirm the zero setting of transducer.** Try rezeroing the line if necessary.

F. **Check the scale on the monitor to ensure that it is appropriate.**

G. **Replace defective transducing equipment as needed.** If the patient has a functional arterial line setup, try connecting the PA catheter to the A-line transducer to see whether this changes the readings. Assuming the A-line system is working, one can differentiate a catheter problem from a transducer system malfunction.

H. **Check the chest radiograph to verify proper positioning of the catheter.** Rough averages for insertion distances and their characteristic waveforms are as follows:

1. **CVP tracing: 20 cm.**
2. **Right ventricle pressure tracing: 30–35 cm.**
3. **Pulmonary artery pressure tracing: 40–45 cm.**
4. **Pulmonary capillary wedge pressure tracing: 50–55 cm**
5. **Check the procedure note to see where the catheter originally wedged.** When the data indicate the catheter is not distal enough, try inflating the balloon with 1.55 cc of air slowly and advancing it until a wedge is achieved.

I. **Replace the PA catheter when it appears that the balloon has ruptured.** Alternatively, the balloon inflation port can be taped closed, and the catheter can be left in place. PCWP can usually be estimated from PA diastolic pressure readings.

77. PULSE OXIMETER MALFUNCTION

Immediate Actions. Verify that the patient does indeed have a pulse. The pulse oximeter (pulse "ox") could be functioning properly, and the patient could be in shock or cardiac arrest. This sounds intuitive, but squandering precious moments adjusting the probe in such a situation can make the difference between a successful resuscitation and a poor outcome.

I. **Problem.** A 56-year-old woman is in the ICU after an exploratory laparotomy for a motor vehicle accident. The nurse notes that her oxygen saturation measures 89% on the pulse oximeter.

II. **Immediate Questions**

A. **Does the patient have a pulse?** Verify the presence of adequate pulsatile blood flow.

B. **Is the patient breathing, either spontaneously or mechanically ventilated?** Apnea or hypoventilation will result in oxygen desaturation.

C. **Is the patient receiving supplemental oxygen?** Adequate ventilation must be ensured. Patients on room air, breathing spontaneously, have a significantly smaller margin of reserve than those receiving supplemental oxygen.

D. **What is the pulse rate as measured by pulse oximetry?** Does it correlate with the heart rate determined by ECG? Lack of correlation is suggestive of a hardware problem.

E. **What is the appearance of the pulse oximeter waveform (if available)?** The presence of a regular rhythmic waveform in the face of a decreased oxygen saturation (Sao_2) suggests a patient problem. An irregular or absent waveform is more suggestive of a monitoring problem.

III. Differential Diagnosis

A. Patient Problems

1. **Hypoxia.** Hypoxia should always be ruled out before assuming that there may be a hardware problem. Look for clinical signs of hypoxia. Provide supplemental oxygen (or increase the Fio_2) to see if the Sao_2 improves.

2. **Low cardiac output.** Although they are relatively robust, pulse oximeters may not function in the presence of low cardiac output.

3. **Vasoconstriction.** Peripheral vasoconstriction in a patient with hypothermia or other conditions characterized by excessive sympathetic nervous system activity may have decreased pulsatile flow to an extremity, with resulting poor pulse oximeter readings.

4. **Heart rate.** In rare circumstances, extreme bradycardia (<40 bpm) or tachycardia (>130 bpm) may cause loss of the pulse oximeter signal.

5. **Inadequate regional blood flow from mechanical causes.** A common cause of pulse oximeter failure in an extremity is the cycling of a proximally located, noninvasive blood pressure cuff. The pulse oximeter probe ideally should not be located distal to a BP cuff. Suboptimal positioning may also result in poor local circulation, such as with a patient in the lateral decubitus position with a probe on the dependent arm.

B. Monitoring Problems

1. **Motion Artifact.** Pulse oximeters are subject to varying degrees of motion artifact, depending on the probe type and manufacturer. Obtaining reliable post operative pulse oximetry on a combative, shivering, hypothermic patient can try the patience of even the most devoted ICU clinician. Such situations will hopefully become more manageable with the more widespread availability of newer, artifact-filtering technologies, such as the Massimo or Nellcor 395 series oximeters.

2. **Ambient light artifact.** The pulse oximeter probe uses light of two different wavelengths passed through a part of the patient's body. The quantity of ambient light of each specific wavelength is then subtracted from the measured quantity of light that has successfully transilluminated the tissue. The remaining difference determines the quality of the reading, or signal-to-noise ratio; thus, the less ambient light on the probe, the higher the quality of signal. High ambient light conditions may lead to artifactual readings of 85%, the saturation at which oxyhemoglobin and deoxyhemoglobin have similar absorption of these two frequencies of red light.

3. **Nail paint degradation and contamination of signal.** Nail polishes and press-on nails, especially those red in color, can cause erroneous pulse oximeter readings. Measuring from an alternative site or simply turning the probe sideways on the finger will eliminate this problem.

4. **Injectable dye contamination of signal.** Certain injectable dyes, such as methylene blue, when absorbed into the blood stream in sufficient quantity, can cause artifactually low Sao_2 readings (usually 85%).

5. **Probe nonfunctional.** The probe may be nonfunctioning.

6. **Probe poorly positioned.** The probe may not actually be placed on a body part. The lighted portion of the probe may have slipped off the end of the finger. Alternatively, the probe may be on too tightly and be occluding pulsatile flow in the fingertip.

IV. Database

A. Physical Exam Keypoints

1. **Vital signs.** Check blood pressure. Hypotensive patients may not have measurable peripheral tissue perfusion for pulse oximetry on a finger or toe.

2. **Heart rate.** Profound bradycardia or tachycardia may be outside of the range of the machine.

3. **Temperature.** Cold patients may be peripherally vasoconstricted or shivering, either of which may interfere with pulse oximetry function.

4. **Signs of hypoxia.** Examine the color of the patient's lips, nail beds, and skin to look for cyanosis.

5. **Ventilation.** Assess for adequacy of ventilation. Assess respiratory effort and tidal volume and listen for symmetrical, normal breath sounds.

6. **Probe Location.** Be sure that the body part with the probe is well perfused and relatively motionless.

7. **Monitor waveform.** Examine the pulse oximeter waveform. Correlate the waveform with the ECG. Lack of correlation, or the presence of an irregular waveform in the face of a regular pulse, suggests a continued problem with the oximeter.

B. **Laboratory Data**
   1. **ABG.** Obtain an arterial blood gas. If signs of hypoxia are unclear, send an arterial blood gas and check the P_{O_2}.
C. **Radiographic and Other Data** (not indicated).

V. **Plan**

A. **Give Supplemental O_2.** Consider sending an ABG when true oxygen saturation is in doubt. Always ensure the patient is safe before manipulating or troubleshooting the equipment. Although statistically less likely than probe problems, oxygenation desaturation is potentially life threatening and must be treated immediately. Valuable time wasted trying to rule out an artifact could result in a hypoxic arrest that may otherwise have been preventable.

B. **Reposition Probe.** The fingertip is the traditional starting place for pulse oximeter probes. Most finger probes will also function on a toe that may be less prone to movement. Ear probes may be helpful in the vasoconstricted, shivering, or otherwise active patient. When motion artifact is an issue, reposition the probe to a more or less stationary tissue, when available. For a sedated patient, an ear probe may also be used on the cheek or nares. For pediatric patients, a finger probe may be positioned on the side of a hand or foot. Be creative, but be careful that the probe does not damage the area upon which it is placed.

C. **Cover Probe.** Because probes rely upon light absorption, bright light sources can degrade signal quality. Place a towel, sheet, or opaque foil over the probe to eliminate excessive ambient light.

D. **New Probe.** Try a different probe if the probe in question does not function properly when tested on an available normal caregiver.

E. **Reposition Patient.** Ensure that poor positioning does not compromise flow of adequate regional blood.

F. **Optimize Regional Blood Flow.** When vasoconstriction seems to be the problem, warm the extremity with compresses or other techniques, such as forced air warmers. Consider a digital nerve block or injection of 0.5–1.0 cc of lidocaine 1% (without epinephrine!) into the pulp space to improve blood flow to the finger being used. Either will cause a local sympathectomy and improve regional blood flow for the next 1–2 h.

G. **Addendum.** Oximetry relies on the Lambert-Beer law, and bases calculations of Sa_{O_2} on differences in absorption of red and infrared light by oxygenated and reduced hemoglobin. Oxyhemoglobin absorbs infrared light at 990 nm, and reduced hemoglobin absorbs red light at 660 nm. Arterial pulsations are identified by a process called **plethysmography**, which allows for Sa_{O_2} calculations on the basis of blood that flows in a pulsatile manner and allows for correction of nonpulsatile blood flow (venous blood and tissue). This is why pulse oximetry fails during cardiac arrest or cardiopulmonary bypass. Pulse oximetry is very precise and will generally yield the same value for each true reading.

78. SEDATION: INDICATIONS AND TECHNIQUES

I. **Problem.** You are called to sedate a patient for a procedure.

II. **Immediate Questions**

A. **What is the indication?** Does the patient really need sedation? Can the proposed procedure or situation be safely done without sedation? The patient will often tolerate the procedure after a thorough explanation and assurance. Other times, local or topical anesthesia/analgesia can replace systemic sedation.

B. **Is it emergent or elective?** For elective sedation, all preprocedure preparation and evaluation must be completed. For emergent sedation, the steps that can be omitted safely are up to the physician.

C. **Can informed patient consent be obtained?** Patients (or their legal guardians in the case of minors or incompetent adults) should be informed of and agree to the administration of sedation before the procedure begins. This should include the benefits, risks, limitations, and possible alternatives.

D. **When was the time of the patient's last oral intake and what was its nature?** Because sedatives and analgesics tend to impair airway reflexes in proportion to the degree of sedation, there is an increasing risk of aspiration with procedural sedation. Adequate preprocedure fasting is necessary to maximize the likelihood that the stomach is empty. Adults should have nothing solid to eat for 6–8 h and have nothing but clear liquids for 3–4 h. For children aged < 3 y, diet can be liberalized to permit clear liquids until 2–3 h preprocedure though, again, solid foods should be avoided for several hours. Concomitant medical conditions that would delay gastric emptying, such as acute abdominal processes, postoperative ileus, or diabetic gastroparesis will all increase the risk of a full stomach even in the absence of oral intake.

E. **Has the patient had a previous adverse experience with sedation or analgesia?** Sedation or analgesia should be approached with caution for patients with a history of an adverse experience with sedation or analgesia until the exact cause and reaction can be fully investigated. When the history cannot be obtained or is unclear, then sedation should be postponed or a consultation should be obtained. Previous uneventful sedation or analgesia does not rule out future adverse reactions.

F. **What are the patient's current medications or drug allergies?**
    Many drugs have potential reactions with sedative or analgesic medications. A complete list of the patient's current medications should be reviewed, paying special attention to stimulants, sedatives, or cardiac drugs. As always, any allergies the patient might have should be reviewed.

G. **What underlying medical issues may complicate sedation?** A history of tobacco abuse can suggest underlying pulmonary disease (COPD, reactive airway disease, and emphysema) that could potentially complicate sedation. Past alcohol or substance abuse could make the patient tolerant to some medications or could alter liver function. Other conditions may similarly affect pharmacodynamics and pharmacokinetics of sedative medications but are beyond the scope of this text.

H. **Are there any anatomical issues relevant to the airway?** Because of the possibility of loss of airway protective reflexes during procedural sedation, be prepared for an airway intervention. Is there a history of difficult intubation or are there anatomical features that could make airway management difficult? Is there a history of sleep apnea that would place the patient at increased risk for airway obstruction with sedation?

III. **Differential Diagnosis/Indications.** Procedural sedation may be required for various indications. These include pain, anxiety, and a lack of ability or capacity to cooperate.

A. **Toleration of an Unpleasant Procedure.** Some procedures are only slightly uncomfortable, although they may still require sedation. These situations require sedation with an amnestic or anxiolytic medication but not an analgesic.

B. **Toleration of a Painful Procedure or Medical Condition.** Some needed procedures are extremely painful and require sedation with analgesia. Also some medical conditions themselves are painful, and these patients need continuous analgesia to remain comfortable.

C. **Tolerate Mechanical Ventilation or an Endotracheal Tube.** Most patients will require sedation to tolerate mechanical ventilation or an endotracheal tube. This is best done with an analgesic agent as the foundation of the pharmacologic regimen. Benzodiazepines and other sedatives are added as needed.

D. **Patient is Uncooperative or Unable to Lie Still When Needed.** Some procedures are not painful or unpleasant but require that a patient lie absolutely still for the duration. Sedation with an amnestic or anxiolytic will render most patients motionless.

E. **Patient is Combative and a Danger to Himself or Others.** Patients that are combative and dangerous are best restrained in accordance with hospital protocol, which often involves some form of sedative adjuvant.

IV. Database

A. Physical Exam Key Points

1. **Airway.** A patient's airway should be evaluated before any sedation. Positive-pressure ventilation, with or without endotracheal intubation, may be necessary if respiratory compromise develops during sedation. This may be more difficult in patients with atypical airway anatomy.

2. **Habitus.** Significant obesity (especially involving the neck and facial structures) can lead to potential airway compromise in a sedated patient.

3. **Head and Neck.** A short neck, limited neck extension, neck mass, cervical spine disease, and trauma are usually associated with a difficult airway.

4. **Mouth/Jaw.** Small mouth opening (< 3 cm for an adult), protruding incisors, and a nonvisible uvula are also associated with a difficult airway.

5. **Heart.** Cardiac arrhythmias and valvular heart disease can compromise a patient's ability to tolerate sedation. Symptoms and signs of congestive heart failure are suggestive of poor myocardial contractility that can complicate standard sedative protocols.

6. **Lungs.** Auscultation may reveal evidence of an underlying pulmonary process (effusion, atelectasis, pneumonia, reactive airways) that could compromise adequate gas exchange during sedation.

7. **Access.** All patients undergoing sedation must have adequate intravenous access. This access should be maintained throughout recovery until the patient is no longer at risk of cardiorespiratory depression.

B. Laboratory Data

1. **Arterial Blood Gas.** A recent arterial blood gas gives a baseline of a patient's preprocedure oxygenation and ventilation status and can suggest underlying respiratory disease.

2. **Hemoglobin/Hematocrit.** Anemia can compromise oxygen delivery to tissues. This will limit a patient's ability to tolerate even slight hypoventilation or hypoperfusion during sedation.

3. **Coagulation Status.** Although a patient that is coagulopathic may tolerate sedation, abnormal coagulation may complicate the proposed procedure.

4. **Bun/Creatinine.** Because many sedative or analgesic medications undergo renal elimination, their doses should be properly adjusted or they should be avoided altogether for a patient with renal failure.

C. Radiographic and Other Studies

1. **Chest radiograph.** A recent chest radiograph should be evaluated for any cardiopulmonary disease. Any evidence of a pathologic condition should be investigated further before any elective

sedation. Pleural effusion, atelectasis, consolidation or collapse, hyperinflation, pneumothorax, and cardiomegaly are all potential signs of a patient's inability to tolerate even modest sedation.

2. **Pulmonary Function Tests.** Patients with known or clinically significant pulmonary disease should be evaluated before elective sedation. PFTs provide a diagnostic tool for diagnosing and/or quantifying the severity of obstructive, restrictive, or reactive airway disease and can help predict a patient's ability to tolerate altered ventilation.

3. **Stress test.** Patients with known or suspected underlying cardiac disease should undergo an evaluation by a cardiologist before elective sedation unless the patient has been evaluated recently, and there has been no change in symptoms. This often includes a cardiac stress test, which evaluates function during increased demand similar to that during modest sedation and procedural stimulation.

V. Plan. Assess the need for sedation and safely sedate the patient when indicated.

A. Initial Management. The initial patient evaluation, patient counseling, and preprocedure fast should be completed before elective sedation and finished to a satisfactory extent for emergent sedation.

B. Monitoring Level of Consciousness. The response of patients to commands during procedures performed with sedation serves as a guide to their level of consciousness. Conversation also provides an indication that the patient is breathing. Patients who only have reflex responses are deeply sedated and are approaching general anesthesia.

C. Ventilation. Ventilatory function can be monitored by observation of respiratory activity or by auscultation.

D. Oxygenation. All patients undergoing sedation should have their oxygenation continuously monitored with oximetry.

E. Hemodynamics. Patients with hypertension or coronary artery disease should have continuous ECG monitoring during sedation. Patients without cardiovascular disease can be sedated safely with regular vital sign checks.

F. Recording of Monitoring. A patient's monitored variables (1–4 above) should be recorded at regular intervals during the procedure. Sicker patients and patients under deeper sedation require more frequent recording. Additionally, vital signs should be monitored and documented during (1) presedation; (2) after administration of the sedative or analgesic agent; (3) on completion of the procedure; (4) during recovery; and (5) at the end of recovery.

G. Availability of Staff Person for Assistance. A designated individual, other than the person performing the sedation, should be present to aid in recording and other tasks.

H. Availability of Emergency Equipment and Drugs. Pharmacologic antagonists and appropriately sized equipment for establishing a patent airway and providing positive pressure ventilation (bag/mask and intubation equipment) with supplemental oxygen should be immediately available. A defibrillator should be present or readily available nearby, especially, when the patient has significant cardiovascular disease.

I. Use of Supplemental Oxygen. Equipment to administer supplemental oxygen should be on hand and administered when hypoxemia is anticipated or encountered. Routine use of oxygen is prudent even in healthy patients.

J. Titration of Sedative or Analgesic Medication to Desired Effect. Combinations of sedative and analgesic agents should be administered as appropriate for the procedure and the condition of the patient. Each component should be administered individually to achieve its desired effect (analgesic medication to relieve pain and sedative medication to decrease awareness or anxiety). Small incremental doses of sedative or analgesic medication should be given until the desired effect is achieved. Sufficient time must pass (depending on route of administration) between doses to allow the effect of each dose to be assessed before additional drug administration.

K. Recovery. Patients should be observed and vital signs monitored and recorded until the effects of the sedation have dissipated. It is important to remember that there are synergistic effects from some combinations of medications and that effects may be greater than anticipated. Particularly concerning are the combination of narcotics and benzodiazepines that can lead to a higher incidence of apnea, especially, in the absence of stimulation.

L. Consultation if Needed. Whenever possible, appropriate medical specialists should be contacted before administration of sedation or analgesia to patients with significant underlying conditions or when it appears that sedation to the point of unresponsiveness will be necessary.

M. Sedation Protocol. Sedation protocols exist in all institutions as mandated by JCAHO. These should be readily available and reviewed, incorporating institution-specific guidelines into all sedation procedures.

79. SEIZURES

I. Problem. A 29-year-old woman with chronic renal failure caused by sickle cell disease is admitted to the ICU for acute respiratory failure because of acute lung syndrome. After 2 d of high-dose meperidine administration, she suffers her first-ever grand mal seizure.

II. Immediate Questions

A. Is this a new-onset seizure? Severe systemic illness, multiple medications, and abrupt metabolic changes make ICU patients susceptible to seizures. Under these circumstances, lowered seizure thresholds can manifest in patients with no history of the disorder. It is important to determine whether the seizure is new-onset or the result of an existing disease.

B. Is this seizure status epilepticus? Status epilepticus is a true medical emergency and should be dealt with promptly. Comatose patients should undergo EEG testing to rule out nonconvulsive status epilepticus. Always remember that a normal brain can have a seizure under the right conditions, and a true cause may never be found. Review the patient's past medical history for seizure disorders.

C. Does the patient take anticonvulsant medication? Is the patient receiving all previous medications now? Seizures are often caused by withdrawal from antiepileptic medications. A history of head trauma or drug abuse puts a patient at greater risk of seizure.

D. Does the patient have a history of alcohol, drug abuse, or diabetes? Withdrawal syndromes may be confused with hypoglycemia.

E. Is this a generalized or focal seizure? Focal seizures are more consistent with a CNS cause.

F. Were there any electrolyte abnormalities noted in previous laboratory tests?

III. Differential Diagnosis

A. New-Onset Seizure. Reasons for new-onset seizure in the ICU setting include abrupt sedative-hypnotic and narcotic withdrawal, acute metabolic changes, and drug toxicity. Hyponatremia is the most common acute metabolic change responsible for seizures. This can occur with postoperative fluid loading or sepsis. Other metabolic causes include hypocalcemia, acute uremia, hyper-, and hypoglycemia. Medications most likely to lower the seizure threshold are antibiotics (piperacillin, imipenem, and mezlocillin) and antiarrhythmic agents. Unfortunately, the cause of some seizures may never be known.

B. Status Epilepticus. Status epilepticus is defined as a seizure lasting more than 15–30 min, or as recurring seizures with impaired consciousness throughout the interictal periods. Status epilepticus is a true emergency. Cardiorespiratory dysfunction, metabolic disturbances, and hyperthermia can develop when untreated. Irreversible neurologic injury may occur after 50 min of seizure activity.

C. Unrecognized Seizure Activity. Nonconvulsive status epilepticus occurs in approximately 8% of coma patients. Therefore, coma evaluation should always include an EEG.

IV. Database

A. Physical Exam Key Points

1. **Vital signs.** Ensure adequacy of Airway, Breathing, and Circulation. Check for fever.
2. **Neurologic exam.** Assess for focal signs, which may suggest a cause, and signs of trauma. Inspect and palpate the head for evidence of head trauma, new or old. Examine the tongue for lacerations that may have occurred during the seizure. Assess for broken bones and shoulder dislocations that may occur without obvious trauma during a seizure. Check for postictal state.
3. **Do not try to force something into the patient's mouth, such as a tongue depressor.** This can lead to an injury.
4. **Check for aspiration.**
5. **Is there evidence of incontinence?**

B. Laboratory Data

1. **Electrolytes.** Check especially levels of sodium, magnesium, calcium, and potassium. Check for hypoglycemia, blood urea nitrogen, and creatinine
2. **Urinalysis.** Screen urine for toxins.
3. **Arterial blood gases.** Check to rule out hypoxia.
4. **Blood drug levels.**

C. Radiographic and Other Studies

1. **Lumbar puncture.** A lumbar puncture should be done when CNS infection is suspected, such as in immunocompromised, head trauma, and transplanted patients.
2. **EEG.** An EEG should be performed for all new-onset seizures and, especially, for comatose patients.
3. **MRI or CT.** An MRI or a CT should be performed in all new-onset patients to rule out a structural lesion.

V. Plan

A. General Plan.
First follow the ABCs of CPR and prevent self-inflicted injury during the seizure.

B. Administer Drugs.
Lorazepam or diazepam administration followed by phenytoin loading is the treatment of choice. Second-line medications include midazolam, and propofol. Aim therapeutic efforts at the underlying cause.

C. Treat the Underlying Condition.

D. Prognosis.
In a study of ICU patients with new-onset seizures, 50% had recurrences within 24 h. The mortality rate was 34%. Patients with metabolic abnormalities had the highest mortality risk.

80. STRIDOR

I. **Problem.** A 66-year-old woman is emergently transferred to the ICU for acute onset of stridor.

II. **Immediate Questions**

    A. **Are air entry and oxygenation adequate?**

    B. **Is there an obvious deformity of the neck, such as an expanding hematoma that can be decompressed?**

    C. **Has the patient recently undergone surgery?**

    D. **If so, how long ago and what type of surgery?**

    E. **Has the patient been intubated recently for a non-surgical issue?**

III. **Differential Diagnosis**

    A. **Upper-Airway Obstruction**

        1. **External.** Swelling of the neck or upper airway because of development of a hematoma, abscess, fluid collection, or generalized edema may lead to obstruction because of compression of the airway.

        2. **Internal.**

            a. **Laryngospasm.** This is a prolonged glottic closure reflex initiated by irritants, such as blood, mucus, debris, and foreign bodies.

            b. **Laryngeal edema.** This may be caused by allergy (angioedema) or glottic injury, leading to local tissue swelling at any level of the glottis. Injury may be caused by a traumatic or prolonged intubation.

            c. **Foreign body aspiration.** The presence of a foreign body in the airway can cause obstruction itself or initiate laryngospasm.

            d. **Vocal cord dysfunction.** This could be due to bilateral recurrent laryngeal nerve damage caused by surgical transection or traction or injury by an endotracheal or gastric tube, resulting in unopposed vocal cord adduction. Metabolic derangements, such as hypocalcemic alkalosis after parathyroidectomy, can cause tetany of the laryngeal apparatus.

            e. **Tumor.** An airway tumor can lead to acute or chronic obstruction.

    B. **Lower Airway Obstruction**

        1. **Bronchospasm.** Loud wheezing may be misinterpreted as stridor.

        2. **Pulmonary edema.** Noisy breathing caused by excess fluid may sound like stridor.

    C. **Psychological.** Paroxysmal vocal cord motion (PVCM) is characterized by adduction of the vocal cords during inspiration and abduction during expiration. It is associated with anxiety, emotional disorders, conversion disorders, and emotional instability.

IV. Database

A. Physical Exam Key Points

1. **General.** Signs of acute distress, such as extreme work of breathing and cyanosis, denote the severity of the limitation of airflow. The complete absence of sound denotes absence of nearly all airflow.
2. **Vital signs.** Signs of hemodynamic instability, such as abnormal heart rate and decreasing blood pressure, or low oxygen saturation dictate need for immediate action.
3. **Neck and chest.** Loud stridor over the larynx helps localize disease to the upper airway versus the lower airway.
4. **Direct laryngoscopy and fiberoptic evaluation.** These exams may help identify a foreign body or mass, action of the vocal cords, or the presence of edema.

B. Laboratory Data.
When a metabolic derangement, such as hypocalcemia, is suspected, chemistries and an ABG may be helpful.

C. Radiographic and Other Studies

1. **Chest radiograph.** This may show pulmonary edema, which may itself be the cause of breathing difficulties or the result of an inadequate airway. (Strong inspiratory effort against a closed glottis, as in laryngospasm or an obstructed airway, may result in postobstructive pulmonary edema.) Neck masses and laryngeal deviation may also be seen.
2. **MRI.** This study can clearly define the anatomy of the airway.

V. Plan

A. Initial Management

1. **Ensure adequacy of oxygenation and air entry.** When these are inadequate, an airway must be established via oral or nasal airway placement, bag and mask ventilation, intubation, cricothyrotomy, or tracheostomy.
2. **Call in a specialist early.** An otolaryngologist or anesthesiologist can perform direct laryngoscopy or fiberoptic endoscopy to evaluate the patient and to aid in treatment planning.

B. Specific Treatment Plans

1. **Surgical options.** The development of neck swelling may need to be alleviated surgically. Reopening of the sutures, for example, can immediately decompress an expanding hematoma after carotid or thyroid surgery. Less severe swelling may be alleviated by placing the patient in a head-up position.
2. **Laryngospasm.** Although laryngospasm will not be broken with positive pressure, CPAP should be applied to augment any air movement that may occur if the cords should partially relax. The mainstay of treatment is ensurance of ventilation, possibly with the use of a small dose of muscle relaxant (ie, succinylcholine).

Hypocalcemia should be treated when present. Offending airway irritants, such as secretions or blood, should be removed from the pharynx. Adequate sedation may be required.

3. **Inhaled therapy.** Inhalation of bronchodilators will be effective for treatment of bronchospasm but not laryngospasm. Inhaled racemic epinephrine is a controversial treatment for laryngeal swelling. When this treatment is effective, the patient must be observed closely for rebound of stridor. IV steroids may be useful.

4. **PVCM.** This can be treated with an anxiolytic medication.

5. **Nerve dysfunction.** Vocal cord dysfunction caused by mechanical or neurologic damage may necessitate intubation or tracheostomy, as determined by ENT consultants.

81. SUBCUTANEOUS EMPHYSEMA

Immediate Actions. Tension pneumothorax is an emergency and is described classically with physical findings of hypotension and tracheal deviation away from the affected side. The presence of tension pneumothorax may be associated with subcutaneous emphysema. Diagnosis of tension pneumothorax is clinical, and treatment should be immediate with a needle decompression of the involved hemithorax.

I. **Problem.** A 45-year-old man with acute pancreatitis now has subcutaneous emphysema of the anterior body wall.

II. **Immediate Questions**

A. **Does the patient have a known pneumothorax or chest tube?** Pneumothorax or malfunctioning chest tubes are primary causes of subcutaneous emphysema. Causes of pneumothorax in the ICU include line attempts, chest tube placement, and tracheostomy.

B. **Is the patient intubated or on a ventilator?** Subcutaneous emphysema may be a sign of tracheal rupture or rupture of alveoli secondary to barotrauma. Positive pressure ventilation may contribute to the exacerbation of a pneumothorax and the subsequent subcutaneous emphysema.

III. **Differential Diagnosis**

A. **New Pneumothorax.** Air in the pleural space may track subcutaneously and be an indicator of a pneumothorax. A pneumothorax with associated subcutaneous emphysema usually necessitates a tube thoracostomy. New-onset subcutaneous emphysema in mechanically ventilated patients should immediately arouse suspicion of a pneumothorax.

B. **Malfunctioning Chest Tube.** Subcutaneous emphysema is often seen after initial placement of a new chest tube. When it is found at the site of an old chest tube, it is not normal and often indicates migration, inadvertent clamping, or clogging of the tube (ensure that the sentinel hole in the chest tube is in the chest cavity). Any of these situations may require placement of a new chest tube. Large air leaks may require a second chest tube.

C. **Pneumomediastinum.** Air in the mediastinum may track into the subcutaneous space. The origin of this air may still be from a pneumothorax, but a more proximal source should also be considered.

D. **Gas Gangrene.** Subcutaneous emphysema and crepitance are late findings in gas gangrene or other necrotizing infections. The extent of the infectious process extends beyond the regions with obvious skin changes and may require extensive and sequential debridement for patient survival.

E. **Tracheal Injury.** An injury to the trachea can be caused by iatrogenic trauma from tracheostomy or a rupture from prolonged endotracheal intubation. Volumes of air may be large.

IV. **Database**

A. **Physical Exam Key Points**

1. **Vital signs.** Hypotension and tachypnea are suggestive of pneumothorax. Patients with necrotizing infections may be febrile.

2. **Crepitance.** Palpate for subcutaneous emphysema. There is a typical "Rice Krispies" feel to the subcutaneous tissues.

3. **Chest.** Decreased breath sounds are suggestive of a pneumothorax.

4. **Peripheral exam.** Look for evidence of necrotizing soft tissue infections. Skin changes may be minimal and focal. Many patients with these infections have diabetes.

B. **Laboratory Data**

1. **CBC.** This may be helpful when necrotizing soft tissue infection is suspected.

2. **Electrolytes.** Testing may show evidence of hyperglycemia.

3. **ABG.** Assessment of levels can document the degree of respiratory dysfunction, and can also be a guide for supportive therapy.

C. **Radiographic and Other Studies**

1. **Chest Radiograph.** Evaluates for pneumothorax, position, and efficacy of existing chest tube (if any) and demonstrates distribution of subcutaneous emphysema. Overlying subcutaneous air may obscure the underlying pneumothorax as an artifact.

2. **Bronchoscopy.** If tracheal or bronchial injuries are suspected bronchoscopy may be required.

V. **Plan**

   A. **Tube Thoracostomy.** Placement of an anterior chest tube may be the best option when there is a significant amount of subcutaneous emphysema. Control of the pneumothorax provides control of the source of the subcutaneous air. When no lateralizing source is evident on physical or radiographic exam, bilateral chest tubes may be required.

   B. There is no practical reason for the use of subcutaneous chest tubes or for "venting" incisions. The practice of using these approaches indicates a failure to understand the cause of the subcutaneous air and does not address the primary disease process.

   C. **Bronchoscopy.** This can discover tracheal or bronchial injury. Endoluminal treatments exist, but operative repair may be necessary.

   D. **Ventilator Mode Change.** If high peak airway pressures and pneumothorax secondary to barotrauma are present, consider changing mode of ventilation to lower airway pressures. Attention to both peak airway pressures and shear pressures should minimize the chance of ventilator-induced pneumothorax.

   E. **Control of Soft-Tissue Infection.** Necrotizing fasciitis or other forms of necrotizing soft-tissue infection require aggressive, operative debridement for control. Limited incisions and limited debridement will not provide control of the infectious process.

82. SWOLLEN EXTREMITY

I. **Problem.** The right lower extremity of a 58-year-old woman admitted to the ICU after left hip replacement is severely swollen. The patient has a previous history of ovarian cancer and had 1 mo of radiation therapy.

II. **Immediate Questions**

   A. **Does the patient have congestive heart failure?**

   B. **When was the patient seen last before the extremity swelling?** Chronic versus acute phenomena will direct the diagnosis and therapy.

   C. **Are there any precipitating or aggravating factors?** Such factors can include pregnancy, large uterine fibroids, increased abdominal compartment pressure, and salt-retaining drugs.

   D. **Are there any associated symptoms?** Warmth, erythema, pain, and tenderness are common in cellulitis and thrombophlebitis. Pain with calf swelling are associated with thrombophlebitis, compartment syndrome, arterial thrombosis, or a ruptured Baker's cyst. Dyspnea on exertion or orthopnea suggests CHF. Spider angiomata, palmar erythema, hepatomegaly, or jaundice suggest cirrhosis.

III. Differential Diagnosis

A. Systemic Abnormality

1. **Heart failure.** Patient will usually have a previous history of hypertension or CAD. The swelling is usually bilateral, and the patient will complain concomitantly about having dyspnea, orthopnea, and paroxysmal nocturnal dyspnea. The most common eliciting events in the ICU are myocardial infarction, renal failure, and fluid overload.

2. **Cirrhosis.** The patient will have a history of alcoholism, hepatitis, or recent substance intoxication. It is usually bilateral and associated with ascites, jaundice, and abdominal distention.

3. **Nephrotic syndrome and renal failure.** This is a bilateral phenomenon and is associated with polyuria, eyelid swelling, hypertension, and in acute cases of renal failure, oliguria, or anuria, or both. Check for a recent history of major surgery.

4. **Hypoproteinemia.** This may occur in older patients, patients with AIDS, malnourished patients, and patients who underwent major surgery.

B. Venous Insufficiency.
The patient is commonly female with a history of varicose veins. Occurrence is usually unilateral and is decreased on recumbency.

C. Thrombophlebitis.
Usually sudden onset of swelling with erythema and pain. Most often associated with trauma, intravenous devices, immobilization, childbirth, and drugs (estrogens).

D. Mechanical

1. **Ruptured gastrocnemius.** Sudden onset of pain associated with trauma with ecchymoses at the ankle.

2. **Baker's cyst.** The patient usually has a previous history of moderate-to-severe rheumatoid arthritis.

3. **Constrictive garments.** The patient will usually be an obese female, and she will have no associated pain.

4. **Dependency.** The patient will usually have a recent history of a stroke with impaired mobility, venous insufficiency, and pain that is relieved upon movement.

E. Lymphatic.
This is usually congenital with previous history of single or bilateral swelling of the extremity.

F. Secondary Lymphedema.
The patient is usually female, age > 40 y, with a history of pelvic cancer, radiation, and vascular surgery (male most often) with involvement of the dorsal part of the foot.

G. Lymphedema.
The patient is usually obese with bilateral leg swelling not involving the foot.

H. Salt-retaining drugs.
Patient will have bilateral swelling most often caused by IV antibiotics, estrogen, NSAIDs, lithium, and IV vasodilators.

    I. **Cellulitis**

    J. **Deep Venous Thrombosis**

    K. **Compartment Syndrome**

    L. **Arterial Thrombosis**

    M. **Acquired or Inherited Arterio-Venous Fistula.** Very rare.

IV. **Database**

  A. **Physical Exam Key Points**

    1. **Vital signs.** Look for signs of congestive heart failure. Check for fever in a patient with thrombophlebitis.

    2. **Cardiopulmonary.** Look for signs of failure, rales, distended neck veins, S3 and S4, and congestion.

    3. **Extremities.** Inspect and palpate. Determine the exact area of swelling. Check the knee, anserine bursa, infrapatellar fat pad (none of which causes true edema) or the dorsum of the foot (none in lipedema). Lymphedema begins distally at the foot and with a dorsal hump. Homans' sign is sometimes present (positive in only 15% of patients with DVT). Notice any "chordae" and pain on palpation.

    4. **Skin.** Notice the character of the skin over the swollen area. Thick, taut, and fibrotic skin suggest a chronic process. Erythema and lymphangitic streaks suggest cellulitis. Ecchymoses in the dependent part of the ankle with mid-calf pain suggest gastrocnemius tear. In a patient with rheumatoid arthritis, a painful swelling of one calf and a popliteal cyst on the other side suggest pseudophlebitis or a ruptured Baker's cyst. Check for palmar erythema, jaundice, gynecomastia, periorbital edema, and peau d'orange.

    5. **Complete pulse exam.** Use portable bedside Doppler test equipment.

  B. **Laboratory Data**

    1. **Hemogram.** Check for leukocytosis, cellulitis, and other infections.

    2. **Electrolytes, BUN and creatinine.**

    3. **Liver function tests.**

    4. **Urine albumin and cholesterol.** Check to rule out nephritic syndrome.

    5. **Serum protein electrophoresis.** Check in patients with hypoproteinemia.

  C. **Radiographic and Other Studies**

    1. **Chest radiograph.**

    2. **ECG.**

    3. **Echocardiogram.**

    4. **Venography and venous compression duplex or venous Doppler.** Venography is the gold standard for diagnosing DVT. However, venous duplex or Doppler can also be helpful.

5. **CT scan.** This demonstrates the distribution of the edema. Venous obstruction exhibits increased cross-sectional area of muscle and interstitial compartment. Lymphedema exhibits increased fluid in the interstitial space with a honeycomb pattern. Popliteal cyst shows extension of fluid from the joint space to between the muscle planes.
6. **Direct and indirect lymphangiography.** This can show lymphatic obstruction.
7. **Liver biopsy.** As clinically indicated.
8. **Arthrogram.** Use to rule out Baker's cyst.
9. **Compartment pressures.** Striker compartment pressure needle.
10. **Arteriogram.**

V. **Plan.** The most common cause of unilateral swelling on the lower extremity in the ICU is venous insufficiency. Treatment should be directed at the specific cause (see appropriate chapters).

A. **DVT** (in the ICU)
1. **Low-risk patient:** Major surgery (> 30 min) and age < 40 y; < 1% proximal DVT (PDVT) and < 0.01% fatal PE (FPE).
2. **Moderate-risk patient:** Major surgery as above plus age > 40 y, history of DVT/PE, major trauma or burns, acute MI or stroke; PDVT, 1–10%, FPE, 0.1–1%.
3. **High-risk patient:** Major surgery or major trauma plus history of DVT/PE, cancer surgery, hip or knee surgery, hip or pelvic fracture, and lower limb paralysis; PDVT, 10–39%, FPE, 1–10%.
4. **Prophylaxis.**
   a. **Graded compression stockings.** Never use as the sole preventive measure in the ICU. It is synergistic with chemical prophylaxis (eg, heparin).
   b. **Intermittent pneumatic compression boots (35 mm Hg at the ankle and 20 mm Hg at the thigh).** Used during most surgical procedures.
   c. **Low-dose heparin.** Activation of antithrombin III. Does not interfere with other components of the coagulation cascade in these low dosages, give 5000 IU every 12 h. Initial dose should be given 2 h before surgery and continue for 1 wk after the procedure. It is not the method of choice for high-risk patients.
   d. **Low molecular weight heparin.** Advantages over "regular heparin" are more anticoagulant activity, lower dosages, less frequent dosing, lower risk of bleeding, and lower risk of heparin-induced thrombocytopenia. A disadvantage is the cost (10 × more). Administer Lovenox, 30 mg SQ every 12 h; no laboratory monitoring is required.
   e. **Low-dose warfarin.** Give 10-mg oral loading dose, then a daily 2-mg dose. Adjust INR to be between 2 and 3. This is the preferred method for hip fractures.

    f. **Vena cava filters.** Indications include documented iliofemoral thrombosis, documented PE, free floating thrombus, high-risk condition for fetal PE (severe lung disease), and no iliofemoral thrombosis but a need for long-term prophylaxis and a high risk for both thromboembolism and hemorrhage.

  5. **Treatment.**

    a. **Anticoagulation.** Administer IV heparin to keep PTT 1.5–2.5 times the control. Heparin dosing should be based on body weight. Give an initial bolus of 80 IU/kg, then administer a continuous infusion at a rate of 18 IU/kg/h. Check PTT every 6 h. Coumadin should be started on day 1 of anticoagulation; when INR reaches 2–3, discontinue heparin. Follow closely liver function tests (ALT and AST can reach 15 times the normal), 5–10 d after initiation of therapy does not indicate liver dysfunction per se, and potassium, hyperkalemia is common with heparin therapy (because of heparin-induced aldosterone suppression).

    b. **Thrombolytic therapy.** Effective ONLY if given within the first 7 d of DVT; therefore it is contraindicated in proximal DVT (usually silent, and time of onset cannot be determined). This method does not improve mortality or early morbidity rates.

B. Compartment Syndrome. Consider fasciotomy; obtain immediate vascular surgery consultation.

C. Arterial Thrombosis. Obtain an immediate vascular consult; consider thrombectomy when possible.

83. TACHYCARDIA

I. Problem. A chronic alcoholic patient is admitted to the ICU for severe esophageal variceal hemorrhage. He is incoherent throughout his stay. On the third ICU day, he develops sinus tachycardia at 140 bpm and hypertension to 190/120.

II. Immediate Questions

  A. What are the vital signs? Certain tachycardias need immediate cardioversion (ventricular fibrillation, ventricular tachycardia with hypotension or pulseless ventricular tachycardia).

  B. Does the patient have a baseline cardiac arrhythmia? What was the rhythm before?

  C. Does the patient have underlying heart disease? Previous cardiac surgery, myocardial infarction, chest trauma, or other cardiac structural abnormalities.

  D. What medication is the patient taking? If antiarrhythmics, check appropriate doses and levels. Diuretics predispose to electrolyte abnormalities.

III. Differential Diagnosis. Tachycardia is defined as a heart rate greater than 100 bpm. Tachycardias result from increased pacer activity, ectopic activity, or reentrant rhythms. Tachycardias can be separated into two main categories: narrow complex, originating above the atrioventricular node, and wide complex tachycardias, originating below the atrioventricular node.

A. Narrow-Complex Tachycardias. These may be caused by fever, pain, anxiety, hypotension, thyrotoxicosis, pheochromocytoma, drug-related, sepsis, anemia, pregnancy, AV fistula, Paget's disease, heart failure, pneumothorax, pericardial effusion, hypovolemia, ischemic heart disease, and electrolyte abnormalities.

  1. Sinus tachycardia. This condition often appears in ICU patients. It is narrow complex (QRS complex < 0.12 s) and has a regular rhythm with uniform P waves. Sinus tachycardia is usually an adaptive response to an underlying systemic dysfunction. Hypovolemia, pain, hypoxia, sepsis, and adrenergic agents can all induce sinus tachycardia.

  2. Atrial flutter. This is a transient arrhythmia that is usually in a 2:1 block. The rhythm is regular. Heart rate is usually 150 bpm. A characteristic sawtooth pattern is evident on ECG. Atrial flutter usually converts to normal sinus rhythm or progresses to atrial fibrillation (Fig I–19).

  3. Atrial fibrillation with rapid ventricular response. This is a narrow-complex tachycardia with an irregular rhythm and no discernible P waves. Recent cardiac surgery (2–4 d postoperative), lung resection, and acute myocardial infarction put patients at risk for atrial fibrillation (Fig I–20).

  4. Atrioventricular nodal re-entry. This is a regular, narrow complex, with absent P waves. Heart rates range from 140–220 bpm.

  5. Multifocal atrial tachycardia. This condition is indicated by an irregular rhythm of narrow QRS complexes preceded by multiform P waves. Chronic lung disease, hypokalemia, hypomagnesemia, pulmonary embolism, myocardial infarction, and congestive heart failure increase the risk of multifocal atrial tachycardia (Fig I–21).

  6. Wolff-Parkinson-White syndrome. Short PR intervals and delta waves before the QRS complexes. The regular, narrow-complex tachycardia is the result of an accessory pathway.

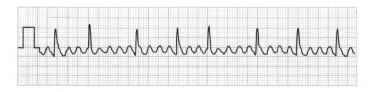

Figure I–19. Atrial flutter with atrioventricular (AV) block (3:1 to 5:1 conduction).

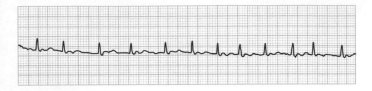

Figure I–20. Atrial fibrillation.

B. **Wide-Complex Tachycardias.** Wide-complex tachycardias can be either ventricular tachycardias or supraventricular tachycardias with atrioventricular delay. Ventricular tachycardias usually have fusion beats and atrioventricular dissociation. Supraventricular tachycardias with delay are usually irregular.

   1. **Torsades de Pointes.** This condition is a wide-complex tachycardia, characterized by QRS complexes of ascending and descending amplitude. A long QT interval puts the heart at risk of torsades. Predisposing medications include quinidine, procainamide, erythromycin, haloperidol, tricyclic antidepressants, and phenothiazines. Electrolyte disturbances that may promote torsades include those involving hypocalcemia, hypomagnesemia, and hypokalemia.

IV. **Database**

   A. **Physical Exam Key Points**

   1. **Vital Signs.** Check pulse rate and regularity, fever, and precipitating factors, such as hypovolemia and pain. Look for serious sequelae, such as systemic hypoperfusion.

   2. **Cardiac.** Check for failure (S_3, S_4), JVD, and murmurs.

   3. **Pulmonary.** Look for evidence of heart failure, rales, or pneumothorax.

   4. **Extremities.** Check for failure, edema, cyanosis, pallor, and temperature.

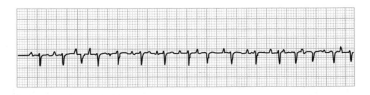

Figure I–21. Multifocal atrial tachycardia.

B. **Laboratory Data**
   1. **Electrolytes.** Check especially levels of potassium, magnesium, and calcium.
   2. **ABG and Sao$_2$.** Evaluate for hypoxia.
   3. **Hemogram.** Evaluate degree of anemia, and sepsis.
   4. **Thyroid function tests.** Check TSH and T$_4$ as necessary.

C. **Radiographic and Other Studies**
   1. **Twelve-lead ECG and rhythm strip, the two most important pieces of information.** Look first for ischemic changes and then work up the differential diagnosis list.
   2. **Chest radiograph.** Look for congestive heart failure and other potential lung disease.

V. **Plan.** First, establish a correct diagnosis, an IV access, and prepare supplemental oxygen.

A. **Atrial Fibrillation and Flutter.** The short-term goal in treating atrial fibrillation and flutter is rate control, not conversion to normal sinus rhythm. Rate control may be accomplished with intravenous digoxin. ICU patients with increased adrenergic tone, however, often require beta blockers or calcium-channel blockers, such as diltiazem, verapamil, esmolol, metoprolol and magnesium. When the patient does not respond to medications and, in addition, is hypotensive with a ventricular rate > 150 bpm and exhibits end-organ dysfunction, then the patient must be cardioverted. Give a sedative (eg, diazepam or midazolam) with or without an analgesic (eg, morphine or fentanyl). Premedicate with procainamide, which transiently enhances AV conduction and is usually used in conjunction with drugs that prolong AV conduction.

B. **Atrioventricular Nodal Reentry.** Carotid massage should be initiated but is often ineffective. Adenosine terminates 90–100% of atrioventricular reentry tachycardias.

C. **Multifocal Atrial Tachycardia.** Treatment includes intravenous magnesium and metoprolol.

D. **Wolff-Parkinson-White syndrome.** Atrioventricular blocking drugs can paradoxically increase the rate via the accessory path (digoxin, calcium-channel and beta-blockers are contraindicated). Therefore, direct cardioversion or procainamide are the treatments of choice.

E. **Ventricular Tachycardia.** Ventricular tachycardia includes 95% of wide-complex tachycardias. When there is evidence of hemodynamic compromise, perform DC cardioversion immediately (when a pulse is present perform synchronized cardioversion, and when it is absent, perform asynchronized). When no hemodynamic compromise exists give lidocaine; if termination is successful, initiate a lidocaine drip (2–4 mg/min). If administration of lidocaine is unsuccessful in terminating the ventricular tachycardia, check the QT interval. If

QT is normal (<0.44 s) give procainamide; however, if the QT is prolonged (>0.44 s), give magnesium.

F. **Torsades de Pointes.** When QT is prolonged, initiate temporary
ventricular pacing (heart rate of 100–120 bpm). When the QT is normal, give traditional antiarrhythmic drugs (eg, lidocaine or procainamide).

84. TACHYPNEA

I. **Problem.** A 57-year-old woman is noted to have a respiratory rate of 35.
She was extubated a few hours ago after returning from the OR following open reduction with internal fixation of a femur fracture suffered after
a fall from a ladder.

II. **Immediate Questions**

A. **Is the patient hypoxic?** Significant hypoxia will result in increased
ventilatory drive.

B. **What other conditions could prove lethal if unrecognized?** A tension pneumothorax can cause tachypnea and dyspnea and may be
quickly fatal if untreated. Similarly, acute respiratory failure can also
be life threatening. Whatever the cause, tachypnea and dyspnea
must be taken seriously, as they often occur late in the course of progression of many conditions.

C. **Does the patient have the accompanying symptom of dyspnea?**
Tachypnea is defined as rapid breathing. Dyspnea is the symptom of
a conscious feeling of "shortness of breath." It usually occurs in situations in which demand for ventilation is out of proportion to the patient's ability to respond. Changes in pulmonary function, such as
bronchospasm, pulmonary edema, or any condition resulting in a decreased pulmonary compliance can lead to tachypnea and dyspnea.

D. **Is the patient ventilating adequately?** Tachypnea with good air
movement can result from metabolic acidosis. Alternatively, tachypnea may result from an inability to achieve an adequate tidal volume,
a condition that is a more ominous situation.

III. **Differential Diagnosis.** Control of ventilation is a complex physiologic
process. Thus, CO_2, and not O_2, plays the dominant role in control of
ventilation. Lesser influences come from the peripheral chemoreceptors
that sense changes in blood pH, PCO_2 and PO_2. There are also pulmonary stretch receptors, irritant receptors, and J receptors that can all
influence ventilation in certain circumstances.

A. **Hypoxia.** There are four types of hypoxia: hypoxic hypoxia (decreased PaO_2), anemic hypoxia, ischemic hypoxia, and histotoxic hypoxia (tissues cannot use oxygen, secondary to effects of toxins).
Regardless of the cause, hypoxia causes increased ventilatory drive
through the stimulation of peripheral chemoreceptors found in the

carotid and aortic bodies. No changes in ventilation occur, however, until arterial P_{AO_2} decreases to < 50 mm Hg.

B. Acidosis. Attempts to compensate for metabolic acidosis may result in tachypnea.

C. Pain. Patients with pain from any body site may hyperventilate. Inadequately treated pain may result in splinting during ventilation that may result in ineffective rapid, shallow breathing.

D. CHF and Pulmonary Edema. Fluid overload, regardless of origin, may push the patient into pulmonary edema. Pulmonary J-receptors are stimulated in this setting and cause dyspnea.

E. Weakness. Residual neuromuscular blockade may cause weakness, or partial airway obstruction in an extubated patient, and may result in ineffective ventilation. Attempts to compensate will result in a higher respiratory rate. As contractions of respiratory and accessory muscles cannot be sustained, the efforts may seem jerky or twitchy.

F. Upper-Airway Obstruction. Upper-airway obstruction may also result from other conditions, such as preexisting airway disease or laryngeal swelling after a recent airway intervention (postextubation). It is characterized by a paradoxical motion of the chest and abdomen (ie, the chest wall expands at the same time as the abdomen moves in and the diaphragm moves up).

G. Reactive Airway. This is a condition that involves input from the medulla, pons, and cerebral cortex. Central chemoreceptors in the brain exert the dominant influence on ventilation CO_2 diffuses across the blood-brain barrier and lowers the pH of CSF. Chemoreceptors sense small changes in CSF pH and adjust respiratory rate. Bronchospasm may stimulate respiratory drive.

H. Pulmonary Embolism. Pulmonary embolism and fat embolism syndromes are characterized by tachypnea and many other signs and symptoms.

I. Other Pulmonary Conditions. The development or aggravation of other pulmonary conditions may cause dyspnea through activation of pulmonary receptors or changes in the work of breathing. These include pneumothorax, pleural effusion, interstitial lung disease, LV failure, exertion or exercise, and pulmonary hypertension.

J. Neurogenic. Head trauma and neurologic abnormalities may result in abnormal central respiratory drive.

K. Fever and Hypermetabolic States

IV. Database

A. Physical Exam Key Points

1. **Vital Signs.** Check blood pressure and pulse rate. Ensure hemodynamical stability. Check respiratory rate. Confirm respiratory

rate. Assess pattern of breathing, and check for abnormal patterns, such as Cheyne-Stokes respirations. Check oxygen saturation. Ensure adequate oxygenation. Do a general assessment. Look for signs of imminent respiratory failure, such as use of accessory muscles, inability to speak, diaphoresis, and so forth. Look for cyanosis or pallor by examining lips, nail beds, and skin.

2. **Chest.** Auscultate for equality of breath sounds over each lung field and for the presence of rales or wheezes. Assess the quality of air movement. Look for chest deformities and retractions with ventilation.

3. **Cardiovascular.** Listen for muffled heart sounds or new gallops or murmurs.

4. **Neurologic.** Assess neurologic status. Assess muscle strength.

5. **Extremities.** Look for signs of DVT. Look for petechiae.

B. **Laboratory Data**
  1. **Arterial blood gas.** An ABG will assess oxygenation in addition to providing information on Pco_2 and pH status.
  2. **End-tidal CO_2.** Capnometry may be helpful, if available, and the patient is intubated.
  3. **Hemoglobin.** Check to rule out anemic hypoxia.

C. **Radiographic and Other Studies**
  1. **Chest radiograph.** Look for pneumothorax, pulmonary edema, pleural effusion, or new infiltrates.
  2. **CT scan.** A chest CT may be helpful for some subtle conditions and, possibly, to rule out pulmonary embolus.
  3. **$\dot{V}/\dot{Q}$ scan.** When a pulmonary embolus is suspected, a $\dot{V}/\dot{Q}$ scan or a pulmonary arteriogram may be indicated. Spiral CT is a newer diagnostic tool for PE but its usefulness varies between institutions.

V. **Plan**

A. **Provide supplemental oxygen as necessary.** Rule out hypoxia.

B. **Alleviate airway obstruction.** Maneuvers can be employed, such as jaw thrust, chin lift, use of oropharyngeal or nasopharyngeal airways, assumption of a sitting position, and CPAP.

C. **Treat pain or anxiety when other serious conditions have been ruled out.**

D. **Impending failure.** Regardless of the cause, when the patient shows signs of impending respiratory failure, consider intubation and mechanical ventilation. Excess work of breathing necessitates assisted ventilation before oxygenation and ventilation fail.

E. **Reverse residual neuromuscular blockade.**

F. **Treat fluid overload.** Diurese appropriately and consider narcotics to decrease preload and alleviate accompanying anxiety.

G. **Correct acidosis and conditions leading to the acidotic state.**

H. **Treat reactive airway disease.** Use inhaled β_2-agonists (albuterol nebulizer treatment). Consider adjuncts, such as anticholinergics, sedatives, relaxants, magnesium, and steroids.

I. Treat underlying pulmonary conditions, such as atelectasis, pulmonary embolism, pleural effusion, or pneumothorax.

85. TRACHEAL DEVIATION

Immediate Action. Two potential life-threatening emergencies require immediate action.

1. **Tension pneumothorax.** When the patient is hemodynamically unstable and has symptoms consistent with a tension pneumothorax (dyspnea, tachypnea, anxiety, pleuritic chest pain, unilateral decreased or absent breath sounds, tracheal deviation), immediate decompression must be performed. This is accomplished by a needle thoracostomy in the second intercostal space in the midclavicular line, followed by tube thoracostomy, usually placed in the anterior midaxillary line in the 4th intercostal space.

2. **Postoperative hematoma.** When the patient is postoperative following head or neck surgery, and a hematoma is suspected to be the cause of the tracheal deviation, the patient must be taken immediately back to the operating room. The airway must be secured and the hematoma opened to release the pressure created by the bleeding.

I. **Problem.** You are summoned by the nursing staff to the ICU to examine a patient after concerns are voiced that his trachea seems to be deviated from the midline.

II. **Immediate Questions**

A. **What are the patient's vital signs?** The question of whether the patient is stable must be determined immediately. Tension pneumothorax may cause hypotension, along with decreased oxygen saturation.

B. **Does the patient currently have any symptoms?** Is the patient resting comfortably or does he appear ill? Chest pain, difficulty breathing, and anxiety may be signs of more serious complications that need immediate action. The presence of stridor is particularly ominous.

C. **Is the patient currently intubated?** If the patient is intubated, have there been any recent changes in the ventilator settings? Intubated patients have a higher incidence of tension pneumothorax. The presenting sign in these patients may be changes in previously stable ventilator settings.

   D. **Has the patient recently had surgery or a traumatic injury?** Any surgical procedure or traumatic injury to the neck can be associated with hematoma and cause tracheal deviation and airway obstruction. This is especially common after carotid artery surgery.
   E. **Has the patient recently had a central line placed?** Pneumothorax is associated with tracheal deviation and may be caused by central line placement, cardiopulmonary resuscitation, previous lung biopsy, or previous neck surgery.
   F. **What is the patient's past medical history?** Was there a preexisting deviation? Thyroid disease or head and neck cancers may be associated with preexisting tracheal deviation.

III. **Differential Diagnosis**
   A. **Acute Changes**
      1. **Tension Pneumothorax. Postoperative Hematoma. Thoracic Aorta Injury.** Thoracic aorta rupture or dissection, usually after a motor vehicle injury, may cause tracheal deviation.
   B. **Chronic Changes**
      1. **Mediastinal Mass.** A preexisting mediastinal mass may cause tracheal deviation. These masses may result in symptoms associated with changes in position or with initiation of positive pressure ventilation.
      2. **Thyroid Disease.** Graves disease may cause a diffuse goiter that will cause tracheal deviation.
   C. **Head or Neck Neoplasm. Esophageal neoplasm. Previous Surgery or Radiation Therapy.** Radiation or previous neck surgery can distort the normal neck anatomy and cause tracheal deviation.

IV. **Database**
   A. **Physical Exam Key Points**
      1. **General.** Assess the generalized appearance of the patient. A calm and relaxed patient is unlikely to be suffering a life-threatening problem.
      2. **Vital Signs.** Low or decreasing oxygen saturation may be consistent with respiratory compromise. Hypotension and tachycardia are symptoms suggesting the need for immediate treatment.
      3. **HEENT.** Check for jugular venous distention (JVD) that is common with tension pneumothorax. Check recent surgical sites and drains for increased bleeding that may indicate formation of a hematoma. Evidence of previous surgical scars may explain a chronic condition associated with tracheal deviation.
      4. **Respiratory.** An initial assessment of the patient's ventilation, including respiratory rate, work of breathing, and use of accessory muscles should be performed. If the patient appears to be having difficulty breathing, the process is more likely to be an acute respir-

atory complication, such as tension pneumothorax, thoracic aorta injury, or postoperative hemorrhage. Decreased or absent breath sounds on one side, possibly with hyperresonance, will occur with pneumothorax. Check also for evidence of stridor, suggesting airway compression.

B. Laboratory Data
1. **ABG.** Hypoxia or hypercarbia may indicate respiratory difficulties.
2. **Hemoglobin.** Check level.

C. Radiographic and Other Studies
1. **Chest radiograph.** The presence of air in the pleural space and the extent of any deviation of the mediastinum and trachea from the effects of tension in one hemithorax can be determined. Evidence of a wide mediastinum suggests the possibility of thoracic aortic disease.
2. **Chest CT.** CT scans provide an excellent view of any tracheal deviation or compression and its cause. This is particularly true for visualization of the trachea below the thoracic inlet, where physical exam is inadequate.
3. **Barium studies.** These should be obtained when the lesion causing tracheal deviation is believed to be an esophageal cancer.
4. **Endoscopy.**
5. **Fiberoptic bronchoscopy or laryngoscopy.** These can be used to assess the degree of airway compression in subtle cases.

V. Plan

A. Initial Management. Of great importance is ensuring that the patient is hemodynamically stable and is adequately ventilating and oxygenating. When assured that the patient is stable, the diagnosis can be made and the need for treatment determined.

B. Specific Therapeutic Interventions
1. **Needle or tube thoracostomy** Tension pneumothorax must be treated immediately when there are signs of hemodynamic or respiratory compromise.
2. **Drainage of postoperative hematoma.** A neck hematoma is a medical emergency and must be treated urgently. The airway must be immediately secured. Airway symptoms are a late sign in the course of this condition. Once lost, the airway may not be easy to control, and intubation may be impossible because of distortion of normal airway anatomy. It is not unusual for a surgical airway to have to be attempted emergently. Neck wounds may be opened at the bedside and be followed up with a return trip to the OR for definitive reexploration and closure.
3. **Tracheostomy.** Symptomatic tracheal deviation in the presence of head and neck neoplasm often requires urgent tracheostomy. Symptoms that usually do not develop until tracheal diameters decrease to 5 mm are rapidly progressive and must be taken seri-

ously. Additional treatment depends on the type of tumor and the degree of spread but may include surgery, radiation, and chemotherapy.

86. TRANSFUSION REACTION

I. **Problem.** During a transfusion of packed red blood cells, a patient's temperature increases to 38.5 °C.

II. **Immediate Questions**

   A. **Vital signs.** Hypotension should be ruled out. Tachypnea is a sign of a significant reaction. Fever is the most common manifestation of a transfusion reaction.

   B. **Does the patient have back or chest pain?** Acute coagulopathy can develop from a major transfusion reaction. Chest pain may develop during hemodynamic stress. Other symptoms may include chills, diaphoresis, hypersensitivity reactions (hives, wheezing, pruritus), or exacerbation of congestive heart failure.

   C. **Has the transfusion been stopped?** If not, do so immediately, and maintain an open IV line with normal saline.

III. **Differential Diagnosis.** Differentiating a fever caused by a transfusion reaction from other causes of postoperative fever is difficult. Assuming no other source, the following transfusion reactions are possible, stated in order of decreasing likelihood and increasing severity.

   A. **White Cell Antigens.** Unlike washed red cells, packed cells contain relatively large numbers of leukocytes. Febrile responses to these cells are usually accompanied by urticaria.

   B. **Minor Protein Reactions.** Allergic reactions to transfused serum proteins can cause fever. Sometimes, anaphylaxis or acute pulmonary edema can occur.

   C. **ABO Incompatibility.** This represents a potentially life-threatening problem, but it occurs rarely. Signs are seen after transfusion of relatively small quantities of blood.

   D. **Contaminated Blood.** Bacterial contamination is rare but should be suspected when high fever and hypotension develop early during a transfusion, because it is often fatal.

IV. **Database**

   A. **Physical Exam Key Points**

      1. **Lungs.** Listen for rales and wheezing.
      2. **Cardiac.** Examine for tachycardia and new flow murmur.
      3. **Abdomen.** Evaluate for pain, especially in the flanks.
      4. **Skin.** Look for rash or hives.

B. **Laboratory Data**

1. **Blood bank specimen.** Two freshly drawn clot tubes (red top tubes) should be returned to the blood bank with the remaining untransfused blood. A repeat crossmatch will be performed. In addition, most blood banks require a heparinized specimen to perform an indirect Coombs' test, looking for previous sensitization.

2. **Urinalysis.** Hematuria after a transfusion reaction represents hemoglobinuria after hemolysis from a major ABO incompatibility.

3. **Hemogram.** Schistocytes may be present in a transfusion reaction; a worsening anemia may develop in the presence of massive red cell destruction.

4. **Serum** for free hemoglobin and haptoglobin. Free hemoglobin will be present with a reaction and haptoglobin will be decreased.

5. **Other laboratory tests.** Coagulation studies and thrombocytopenia may indicate DIC. Monitor renal function by obtaining BUN and creatinine levels along with serum electrolytes. Arterial blood gases rarely are indicated (cardiovascular collapse).

C. **Radiographic and Other Studies.** Not routinely needed, but order when clinically indicated.

V. **Plan**

A. **Immediately Stop Transfusion.** Consultation with the blood bank pathologist usually is indicated to evaluate the reaction and to discuss any further transfusions.

B. **Maintain IV Access.** Monitor urine output and vital signs closely.

C. **Send Blood Bank Appropriate Specimens.** See preceding section, "Laboratory Data." Ensure that the bag is returned to the blood bank immediately.

D. **Mild Reactions.** Usually, the reaction is fever without any evidence of more severe symptoms or hemolysis.

1. Antihistamines (diphenhydramine 25–50 mg IM or IV) and acetaminophen may reverse mild allergic and febrile reactions.

2. Transfusion can usually be restarted.

E. **Severe Reactions.** These usually signify acute hemolysis has occurred. One of the major goals is to prevent renal failure.

1. **Circulatory support.** Maintain adequate blood pressure with volume or pressors. Diuresis with furosemide or mannitol, usually with D_5W, should be started to prevent renal injury in the presence of marked hemolysis. Also, consider alkalinization of the urine with bicarbonate to further protect the kidneys.

2. **Antibiotics.** These will be needed when examination of the remaining untransfused unit reveals evidence of bacterial contamination. The organisms are usually gram-negative bacilli.

F. **Known Reactions.** For patients with known febrile reactions to blood products, the patient can be pretreated with antihistamines (diphenhydramine), or antipyretics, or steroids to avoid the reaction. Blood bank products are discussed in Chapter IV, Fluid and Blood Product Management.

87. VENTRICULAR-PERITONEAL (V-P) SHUNT MALFUNCTION

I. **Problem.** A 27-year-old man with known V-P shunt has an altered level of consciousness with a question of abdominal pain.

II. **Immediate Questions**

   A. **What was the previous level of consciousness and what is the baseline function of the patient?** Patients with V-P shunts may have an altered baseline mental status. It is important to assess the change and not just the current status. Initial neurologic exam in the critical care setting is often limited by the urgency of the admission. Complete neurologic status should be assessed as soon as it is clinically possible.

   B. **Has the shunt been manipulated or accessed recently?** Mechanical obstruction or technical failure of the pump mechanism can occur if manipulation of the shunt occurs.

   C. **Does the patient have meningitis?** Meningitis may cause malfunction of the shunt by either obstructing the catheter with cellular debris or manifesting as a shunt malfunction.

III. **Differential Diagnosis**

   A. **Meningitis.** V-P shunt malfunction may be an early sign of meningitis. This finding may result from obstruction of the catheter from cellular debris.

   B. **V-P Shunt Valve Malfunction.** The one-way valve of the shunt may become nonfunctional, especially if the shunt has been manipulated or "tapped." If the valve becomes inoperable, the shunt is ineffective. Proper function of the shunt valve is essential to the function of the shunt. The check valve status prevents back-flow of peritoneal fluid into the CSF.

   C. **Shunt Tubing Occlusion.** The tubing from the entrance point into the skull to the entrance in the abdomen may become occluded for a variety of reasons, and mechanical obstruction should be ruled out.

   D. **Peritonitis.** Abdominal peritonitis may cause obstruction of the distal end of the shunt causing malfunction. Inflammation may occlude the peritoneal aspect of the shunt. Omentum may also wrap around the abdominal component of the shunt, resulting in occlusion.

IV. Database
  #### A. Physical Exam Key Points
   1. **Vital signs.** Fever may be indicative of meningitis. Hypotension and bradycardia may be indicative of increased ICP and possible herniation.
   2. **Erythema.** Swelling may be signs of local infection of the shunt. Attention should be directed at the region of the reservoir and at the tunneled portion of the catheter.
   3. **Neurologic exam.** Comparison to previous exams may identify changes in neurologic status that may indicate shunt malfunction.
   4. **Abdominal exam.** Peritonitis may be detected as a possible cause of malfunction. Therapy should be directed at the treatment of the primary intra-abdominal component of the patient's condition. Shunt loss from a primary abdominal event is possible but not the rule.
  #### B. Laboratory Data
   1. **Hemogram.** This may show elevated WBC in the case of meningitis or peritonitis.
   2. **CSF.** Check to show indicators of infection (eg, WBCs, bacteria, etc). Fluid may be obtained either from the shunt itself or remotely.
   3. **Electrolytes.** Mental status changes may be secondary to metabolic causes.
  #### C. Radiographic and Other Studies
   1. **Shunt series.** This is a radiographic series used to follow the entire length of the shunt to identify any possible mechanical obstruction. This "shuntogram" provides both anatomic and functional information regarding the patency and capacity of the shunt to drain CSF.
   2. **Head CT.** Used with previous scans to identify any signs of hydrocephalus or meningitis along with positioning of the shunt in the ventricle.
   3. **Abdominal CT.** The scan may show collection of CSF and may indicate the peritoneum is not absorbing the CSF properly and needs repositioning. This CT also may be indicated if the patient exhibits signs of peritonitis. CSF loculation surrounding the shunt may be an early sign of infection of the abdominal component of the V-P shunt system.

V. Plan.
Any decision-making concerning a V-P shunt should be done with the consultation and direction of a neurosurgeon. Elective surgery in the setting of an existing V-P shunt should be modified to direct attention to the presence of the shunt system. A V-P shunt, per se, does not exclude the possibility of laparoscopic interventions. Only older V-P shunts, without appropriate check-valve systems, preclude therapeutic pneumoperi-

toneum. If there is clinical doubt about the integrity of the system, a neurosurgical consultation should be obtained.

A. **Immediate Actions.** V-P shunt malfunctions can cause a variety of symptoms. Malfunction of the shunt should be considered for anyone with mental status changes, neurologic changes, pain and swelling of the apparatus, or signs of peritonitis. Acute change in neurologic status in a patient with an existing ventriculoperitoneal shunt should be considered a shunt failure until proven otherwise.

1. **Exteriorization of the Shunt.** The distal portion of the shunt can be removed from the abdomen and connected to a collection device. This should be done for patients with meningitis, peritonitis, or any other suspected infection. Exteriorization has its greatest utility in the presence of peritonitis. Once the acute infectious phase has cleared, definitive reconstruction may be undertaken.

2. **Tapping of the Shunt.** This may be done for both diagnostic and therapeutic reasons. CSF may be obtained for evaluation and culture, and removal of CSF may resolve the symptoms if caused from increased ICP, secondary to hydrocephalus.

3. **Shunt Replacement.** When mechanical failure of the shunt is the cause, replacement of the shunt should be done under the direction of a neurosurgeon. Either complete reconstruction, or appropriate reconstruction of either aspect of the shunt may be required. A team approach in the setting of required revision may be needed.

88. VENTILATOR: BUCKING, HIGH PEAK AIRWAY PRESSURE (PAP)

I. **Problem.** You are called to the bedside of a 27-year-old man a few hours after craniotomy for evacuation of intracranial hematoma resulting from a high-speed motor vehicle accident. He is "bucking" and the peak airway pressure (PAP) is elevated.

II. **Immediate Questions**

A. **Is the patient properly sedated?** "Bucking" is the term often used to describe a patient coughing on an endotracheal tube (ETT). An ETT can be very irritating to an undersedated patient. Mild-to-moderate sedation will alleviate this problem.

B. **Have the ventilator settings been changed recently?** Ventilator settings that do not provide proper minute ventilation, expiratory time, volume, or pressure can stimulate the patient enough to make him cough despite previously adequate sedation. Inadequate ventilation can lead to spontaneous and mistimed respiratory efforts; the patient may attempt to exhale during the ventilator's inspiratory cycle, leading to elevated PAP.

C. **Has the endotracheal tube been obstructed or moved?** Obstruction, which can cause elevated PAP, may be caused by a number of common occurrences, including a kinked tube, mucus plugging, or the patient biting on the tube. The tube may also be down too far and touching the carina (very sensitive part of tracheobronchial tree) and/or be down a mainstem bronchus. Although an endotracheal tube may have been tolerated previously, the increased stimulation of distal tube movement can result in coughing. Furthermore, tube movement can cause a bout of bronchospasm in a patient who may or may not have been predisposed to reactive airway disease.

D. Could this be a tension pneumothorax? An intubated patient with a developing tension pneumothorax would acutely experience an elevated PAP along with progressive hypoxia and hypotension.

III. Differential Diagnosis. The easiest way to approach this evaluation is to begin with the patient and work toward the ventilator.

A. Inadequate Sedation. A patient with decreasing sedation will eventually cough and buck on the endotracheal tube, as it is very stimulating. Postoperative patients are prone to this as intraoperative sedation and paralysis wear off.

B. Increased Airway Resistance. Patients that are sedated and mechanically ventilated may not adequately clear secretions despite frequent suctioning and oral care. It is not uncommon to have a mucus plug in one of the larger bronchi that will cause elevated PAP, coughing, and inadequate ventilation. Bronchospasm, a foreign body, and airway compression also increase airway resistance and cause elevated PAP.

C. Decreased Pulmonary Compliance. There are many conditions, characterized by reduced pulmonary compliance, that would lead to elevated PAP. Such conditions include pulmonary edema, tension pneumothorax, large pleural effusion, ascites, abdominal packing, or any other abdominal process causing increased abdominal pressure.

D. Seizure. Rarely, seizure activity could result in dramatic increases in abdominal and thoracic muscle tone and lead to increased airway pressure and difficulty with ventilation.

E. ETT Problems. Partial obstruction of an ETT will lead to high airway pressures. This can occur with malposition of the ETT, such as occurs when the tip of the tube slides distally to lie within a mainstem bronchus or if it is up against the wall of the trachea or mainstem bronchus. Kinking, resulting from acute angulation or constriction of the lumen caused by the patient biting down on the tube are obvious mechanical problems.

F. Ventilator Malfunction. The ventilator may be malfunctioning, or it could be set up improperly. The delivery of inappropriate volumes, excessive pressure, or a setting of inadequate exhalation time (stacking) may lead to high airway pressures. Similarly, a lack of ventilator synchronization with a patient's spontaneous breathing can lead to high pressure as a mechanical breath is delivered during exhalation.

IV. **Database**
  A. **Physical Exam Key Points**
      1. **Vital signs.** Check blood pressure and heart rate. BP and HR are fairly nonspecific in this situation, because they will probably be elevated if the patient is stimulated enough to be bucking. However, decreased BP may result from high pleural pressures with impaired venous return (pneumothorax).
      2. **Oxygen saturation.** This will give an indication as to the seriousness of the situation and will determine how quickly it must be diagnosed and corrected. Even if saturation is good, it may not be for long, as a bucking patient is usually not ventilating well.
      3. **Capnometry.** Capnometry is helpful in determining how well a patient is ventilating. Analysis of end-tidal CO_2 concentration correlates with arterial CO_2 tensions. Waveform analysis provides the ability to assess spontaneous respiratory efforts in relation to the mechanical cycles and may provide evidence of mechanical obstruction or reactive disease with prolonged expiratory cycles. Some newer capnometry systems can provide pressure-volume loops that may further elucidate when and how the elevated PAP pressures are arising.
      4. **General assessment.** Determine if the patient is awake enough to respond to any other stimuli, including painful ones.
      5. **HEENT/Neck.** Check where the ETT is taped (should be 20–24 cm at the lips in adults) and feel for a midline trachea.
      6. **Chest.** Listen for bilateral breath sounds and any wheezing or rales.
      7. **Equipment check.**
          a. **Connections.** Check all circuit connections from ET tube to the ventilator.
          b. **Ventilator settings.** Check ventilatory settings, including mode, rate, tidal volumes, I:E ratio, and alarm parameters.
      8. **Plateau pressure.** Check the plateau pressure. A relatively normal plateau pressure in the presence of elevated PAP suggests increased airway resistance or inspiratory flow rate. Elevated plateau pressure indicates a decreased pulmonary compliance.
  B. **Laboratory Data**
      1. In this acute setting, no laboratory data will likely be useful in the actions needed to evaluate, diagnose, and solve the problem quickly.
      2. **ABG.** An arterial blood gas might be useful to confirm oxygenation status and degree of impairment of ventilation, as indicated by elevated carbon dioxide tension.
  C. **Radiographic and Other Studies**
      1. **Chest radiograph.** When time permits, this would be useful, as it could reveal ET tube malposition, pulmonary edema, pleural effusions, or a tension pneumothorax.

      2. Bronchoscopy. If readily available, a bronchoscopic evaluation might be helpful in diagnosing some causes of this problem.

V. Plan

  A. Suctioning. Passage of a suction catheter is helpful in a few ways. When a suction catheter cannot be passed, there is obstruction of the tube, secondary to a kink or occlusion from the patient biting down. A kink can usually be remedied by repositioning, but sometimes the situation requires reintubation with a new ETT. Biting down requires increased sedation and possibly a bite block. Saline lavage accompanied by suctioning can clear secretions and mucus plugging.

  B. Reposition the ETT. Withdrawing the tube back to the correct mid-tracheal position alleviates carinal stimulation and mainstem intubation.

  C. Remove the patient from the ventilator and assist ventilation as needed. A lack of synchronization of the ventilator with spontaneous ventilatory efforts mandates some action. Reconsider the need for mechanical ventilation. Adjust ventilator settings to better mesh with the patient's efforts or use assisted ventilatory modes. Alter patient efforts with sedation.

  D. Sedation. It is essential to ensure that ventilation is possible manually or mechanically before the patient is sedated. When it is not, increased sedation may halt the only ventilation the patient was getting (spontaneous). When ability to ventilate is ensured, quick sedation can be diagnostic and therapeutic. When the patient stops bucking and PAP returns to normal, a sedative infusion may be started or increased as deemed appropriate (opioids, benzodiazepines, hypnotics, etc). When sedation is chosen, ensure that the ventilator is functioning properly. It is wise to have a back-up ventilator ready.

  E. Specific interventions as needed. These are dependent on the cause of the problem. A few are as follows:

    1. Pneumothorax, pleural effusion. Needle decompression (if necessary) and chest tube.

    2. Pulmonary edema. Diurese and treat the underlying causes.

    3. Seizure. A neurology consult may be required if movements seem rhythmic and suggestive of seizure activity.

89. WHEEZING

I. Problem. You are called to evaluate a 38-year-old man reported by the nurse to be wheezing.

II. Immediate Questions

  A. Is the patient oxygenating and ventilating sufficiently?

  B. Is the patient complaining of shortness of breath?

C. Is the airway patent? Is the patient moving air?

D. Can breath sounds be auscultated?

E. Does the patient have underlying COPD or asthma?

F. Has the patient recently received a medication or a blood transfusion?

G. Was the patient recently extubated and is there a history of tracheostomy or other significant instrumentation of the airway? Is the wheezing inspiratory or expiratory?

H. Is there stridor? Is there a known disease that could act like a foreign body and obstruct the airway?

I. Is a nasogastric tube in place? Has the patient aspirated?

J. Has there been any recent chemical, inhalational, or smoke injury to the patient?

III. Differential Diagnosis

A. **Bronchoconstriction.** Not all wheezing is caused by reactive airway disease, though it is the most common cause. Bronchospasm may be an exacerbation of a chronic condition or of new onset.

1. **Chronic bronchospasm.** Preexisting COPD and asthma are common conditions. Smokers may have occult reactive airway disease. Any stimulus may produce an exacerbation of these preexisting conditions or tendencies to wheeze.

2. **Acute bronchospasm.** Many stimuli can cause the new onset of bronchospasm. Common causes include stimulation of the airway by mechanical means, such as by an endotracheal tube or suction catheter, secretions, or blood from pulmonary processes, such as pneumonia or aspiration of oral or gastric fluids. Wheezing, as a component of a systemic reaction, such as anaphylaxis, may accompany a pulmonary embolus or an allergic drug or transfusion reaction.

B. **Upper Airway Obstruction.** The many causes of upper-airway obstruction may produce stridor or sounds like wheezing, as airflow through the upper airway becomes turbulent. This must be discriminated from reactive airway disease, although both causes may coexist.

C. **Chronic preexisting conditions.** Anatomical features, such as a large tongue, redundant pharyngeal tissue, and obesity will predispose to upper-airway obstruction. Sedation or a diminished level of consciousness may compound these underlying tendencies and lead to obstruction. The presence of airway tumors, polyps, mediastinal masses, or oropharyngeal abscesses must also be considered.

D. **Acute conditions.** Glottic or subglottic edema, laryngospasm, or vocal cord dysfunction may cause upper-airway obstruction. Foreign bodies and tubes must be considered.

   E. Heart Failure. Peribronchial accumulation of pulmonary edema fluid will create narrowed airways and may result in wheezing. Contributions are also made by stimulation of various pulmonary receptors.

IV. Database
A. Physical Exam Key Points
   1. **Inspection.** Use of accessory muscles, retractions, or paradoxical motions help to indicate the severity of the situation.
   2. **Vital signs.** Tachycardia and hypotension may be present and require treatment. Fever may suggest an infectious process, such as pneumonia. Measure oxygen saturation.
   3. **Head and neck.** Listen for stridor and inspiratory noises over the larynx as manifestation of upper-airway obstruction.
   4. **Lungs.** Auscultate to check uniformity and symmetry of breath sounds. Harsh, high-pitched sounds suggest airway obstruction. Asymmetric sounds may indicate pneumothorax or pneumonia. Check tidal volumes.

B. Laboratory Data
   1. **ABG.** An arterial blood gas will evaluate oxygenation and the effects on ventilation as revealed by carbon dioxide tension.

C. Radiographic and Other Studies
   1. **Chest radiograph.** Look for hyperexpansion of lung fields and air trapping. Look for air bronchograms or areas of consolidation suggesting pneumonia. Look for signs of pulmonary edema or heart failure (ie, Kerley's B lines, peribronchial cuffing, blunting of costophrenic angles).
   2. **Pulmonary function tests.** Use expiratory flow meter at bedside to assess flow rates.
   3. **Echocardiogram.** Check when your suspicion is high that the wheezing is cardiac in origin.
   4. **Direct or indirect laryngoscopy.** Use to aid in ruling out upper-airway obstruction.

V. Plan
   A. Administer 100% oxygen or at least supplemental oxygen.

   B. Rule out upper-airway obstruction and laryngeal issues.

   C. Treat heart failure if present.

   D. Treat bronchospasm
   1. **Bronchodilators.** The mainstay of treatment is with inhaled beta$_2$ agonists, such as albuterol. A handheld inhaler or nebulizer may be used.
   2. **Anticholinergics.** Consider use of anticholinergics, such as glycopyrrolate to diminish airway secretions.
   3. **Corticosteroids.** Administered by inhaler or systemically, these drugs have a longer time of onset but should be considered for serious bronchospasm.

4. **Consider intubation and mechanical ventilation.** Inability to adequately oxygenate or ventilate or an excessive work of breathing may be indications for these interventions. The patient may need sedation and paralysis, and consideration must be given to the fact that intubation may aggravate bronchospasm by the introduction of an airway foreign body, resulting in stimulation of tracheal mechanoreceptors.

II. Laboratory Tests & Their Interpretation

This section is a selection of the most commonly used lab tests in a critical care unit. If an increased or decreased value is not clinically useful, it is not listed. Because each laboratory has its own set of "normal" reference values, the normals given should be used only as a rough guide. The range for common normal values is given in parentheses and, unless specified, reflects normal adult levels.

ACTH (Adrenocorticotropic Hormone)

(8 AM: 20–140 pg/mL [SI: 20–140 ng/L]; midnight: approximately 50% of 8 AM value).

Increased: Addison's disease (primary adrenal hypofunction), ectopic ACTH production (oat cell and large cell lung carcinoma, pancreatic islet cell tumors, thymic tumors, renal cell carcinoma, bronchial carcinoid), Cushing's disease (pituitary adenoma), congenital adrenal hyperplasia (adrenogenital syndrome).

Decreased: Adrenal adenoma or carcinoma, nodular adrenal hyperplasia, pituitary insufficiency, corticosteroid use.

ACTH Stimulation Test (Cortrosyn Stimulation Test)

Used to help diagnose adrenal insufficiency. Cortrosyn (an ACTH analogue) is given at a dose of 0.25 mg IM or IV in adults or 0.125 mg in children younger than 2 years. Collect blood at 0, 30, and 60 min for cortisol and aldosterone.

Normal response: Three criteria are required: (1) basal cortisol of at least 5 μg/dL, (2) an incremental increase after Cortrosyn injection of at least 7 μg/dL, and (3) a final serum cortisol of at least 16 μg/dL at 30 min or 18 μg/dL at 60 min or a cortisol increase of > 10 μg/dL. Aldosterone increases > 5 ng/dL over baseline.

Addison's Disease (Primary Adrenal Insufficiency): Neither cortisol nor aldosterone increase over baseline.

Secondary Adrenal Insufficiency: Caused by pituitary insufficiency or suppression by exogenous steroids, cortisol does not increase, but aldosterone increases.

Acetone (Ketone Bodies, Acetoacetate)

(normal = negative).

Positive: Diabetic ketoacidosis (DKA), starvation, emesis, stress, alcoholism, infantile organic acidemias, isopropanol ingestion.

Acid Phosphatase (Prostatic Acid Phosphatase, PAP)

(< 3.0 ng/mL by RIA, or < 0.8 IU/L by enzymatic).
   Not a screening test for prostate cancer; most useful as a marker of response to therapy. PSA more sensitive in prostate cancer and largely replacing PAP.

Increased: Carcinoma of the prostate (usually outside of prostate), prostatic surgery or trauma (including prostatic massage), rarely in infiltrative bone disease (Gaucher's disease, myeloid leukemia), prostatitis, or benign prostate hypertrophy.

Albumin

(adult 3.5–5.0 g/dL [SI: 35–50 g/L]; child 3.8–5.4 g/dL [SI: 38–54 g/L]).
   Follows total protein levels but does not detect gamma globulins.

Decreased: Malnutrition, over hydration, nephrotic syndrome, cystic fibrosis, multiple myeloma, Hodgkin's disease, leukemia, protein-losing enteropathies, chronic glomerulonephritis, alcoholic cirrhosis, inflammatory bowel disease, collagen-vascular diseases, hyperthyroidism.

Albumin/Globulin Ratio (A/G RATIO)

(normal > 1).
   A calculated value (total protein minus albumin = globulins. Albumin divided by globulins = A/G ratio). Serum protein electrophoresis is a more informative test.

Decreased: Cirrhosis, liver diseases, nephrotic syndrome, chronic glomerulonephritis, cachexia, burns, chronic infections and inflammatory states, myeloma.

Aldosterone

(Serum: supine 3–10 ng/dL [SI:0.083–0.277 nmol/L] early AM, normal sodium intake [3 g sodium/d]; upright: 5–30 ng/dL [SI:0.138–0.831 nmol/L]; urinary 2–16 μg/d [SI:5.54–44.32 nmol/d]).
   Stop antihypertensives and diuretics 2 wk before test. Upright samples should be drawn after 2 h. Primarily used to screen hypertensive patients for possible Conn's syndrome (adrenal adenoma producing excess aldos-

terone). Urinary studies are of limited utility. Should be done along with a plasma renin.

Increased: Primary hyperaldosteronism (Conn's syndrome), idiopathic hypertrophy bilateral hyperplasia of zona glomerulosa), secondary hyperaldosteronism is more common (CHF, sodium depletion, nephrotic syndrome, cirrhosis with ascites, others), upright posture, very low sodium diet.

Decreased: Adrenal insufficiency (Addison's disease), panhypopituitarism, supine posture.

Alkaline Phosphatase

(adult: 20–70 U/L, child: 20–150 U/L).

A fractionated alkaline phosphatase differentiates the bone or liver origin of the enzyme: heat-stable fraction from liver; heat-labile fraction from bone ("bone burns"). If heat-stable fraction is < 20%, c/w bone origin; if < 25–55%, c/w liver). Largely replaced by the gamma-glutamyl transpeptidase (GGT) and 5'nucleotidase, both increased in liver disease.

Increased: Increased calcium deposition in bone (hyperparathyroidism), Paget's disease, osteoblastic bone tumors (metastatic or osteogenic sarcoma), osteomalacia, rickets, pregnancy, childhood (especially in periods of active growth), healing fracture, liver disease such as biliary obstruction (masses, drug therapy), hyperthyroidism.

Decreased: Malnutrition, excess vitamin D ingestion.

Alpha-Fetoprotein (AFP)

(<16 ng/mL [SI: <16 µL]; third trimester of pregnancy, maximum 550 ng/ml [SI:550 µl])

Increased: Hepatoma (hepatocellular carcinoma), testicular tumor (embryonal carcinoma, malignant teratoma, yolk sac tumor), neural tube defects (in mother's serum [spina bifida, anencephaly, myelomeningocele]), fetal death, multiple gestations, ataxia-telangiectasia, some cases of benign hepatic diseases (alcoholic cirrhosis, hepatitis).

Decreased: Trisomy 21 (Down syndrome) in maternal serum.

ALT (Alanine Aminotransferase, ALAT)

Ammonia

(adult: 10–80 µg/dL [SI:5–50 µmol/L]) (to convert µg/dL to µmol/L, multiply by 0.5872).

Increased: Liver failure, Reye's syndrome, portocaval shunt, medications (5-FU), TPN, inborn errors of metabolism, normal neonates (normalizes within 48 h of birth).

Amylase

(50–150 Somogyi units/dL [SI: 100–300 U/L]).

Increased: Acute pancreatitis, pancreatic duct obstruction (stones, stricture, tumor, sphincter spasm secondary to drugs), pancreatic pseudocyst or abscess, alcohol ingestion, mumps, parotiditis, renal disease, macroamylasemia, cholecystitis, peptic ulcers, intestinal obstruction, mesenteric thrombosis, after surgery.

Decreased: Pancreatic destruction (pancreatitis, cystic fibrosis), liver damage (hepatitis, cirrhosis), normal newborns in the first year of life.

Anion Gap (see Blood Gases, page 270)

Apolipoprotein A & B

(APO-A: male, 80–151 mg/dL; female, 80–170 mg/dL; APO–B: male, 49–123 mg/dL; female, 26–119 mg/dL).
Used to assess risk of CAD. Ratio of Apo-A/Apo-B greater indicator of CAD than LDL/HDL cholesterol.

Autoantibodies

(normal = negative).

Antinuclear Antibody (ANA, FANA): (Normal = negative).
A useful screening test in patients with symptoms suggesting collagen-vascular disease, especially if titer is ≥1:160.

Positive: Systemic lupus erythematosus (SLE), drug-induced lupus-like syndromes (procainamide, hydralazine, isoniazid, etc), scleroderma, mixed connective tissue disease (MCTD), rheumatoid arthritis, polymyositis, juvenile rheumatoid arthritis (5% to 20%). Low titers are also seen in non-collagen-vascular disease.

Anti-DNA (Anti–double-stranded DNA): SLE, chronic active hepatitis, mononucleosis.

Antimitochondrial: Primary biliary cirrhosis, autoimmune diseases such as SLE.

Anti-Smooth Muscle: Low titers are seen in a variety of illnesses; high titers (>1:100) are suggestive of chronic active hepatitis.

Antimicrosomal: Hashimoto's thyroiditis.

ASO (Antistreptolysin O) Titer (Streptozyme)

(<166 Todd units).

Increased: Streptococcal infections (pharyngitis, scarlet fever, rheumatic fever, poststreptococcal glomerulonephritis), rheumatoid arthritis, and other collagen diseases.

AST (Aspartate Aminotransferase, ASAT) (see SGOT)

Base Excess/Deficit

(−2 →+3 mEq/L [SI: −2 →+3 mmol/L] (see Blood gases, page 270).

Increased: Metabolic alkalosis.

Decreased: Metabolic acidosis.

Bicarbonate (or "Total CO_2")

(23–29 mmol/L) (see Carbon Dioxide, page 280).

Bilirubin

(Total, 0.3–1.0 mg/dL [SI: 5.1–17.1 μmol/L]; direct, <0.2 mg/dL [SI: <3.4 μmol/L]; indirect, <0.8 mg/dL [SI: <13.7 μmol/L]) To convert mg/dL to μmol/L, multiply by 17.10.

Increased Total: Hepatic damage (hepatitis, toxins [including many commonly used medications], cirrhosis), biliary obstruction (stone or tumor), hemolysis, congenital liver enzyme anomalies, fasting.

Increased Direct (Conjugated): (NOTE: Determination of the direct bilirubin is usually unnecessary with total bilirubin levels of <1.2 mg/dL [SI:20.5 μmol/L]; this is the form of bilirubin seen in urine). Biliary obstruction/cholestasis (gallstone, tumor, stricture), drug-induced cholestasis, Dubin-Johnson and Rotor's syndromes.

Increased Indirect (Unconjugated): (NOTE: This is calculated as total minus direct bilirubin.) So-called hemolytic jaundice caused by any type of hemolytic anemia (transfusion reaction, sickle cell, etc), Gilbert's disease, physiological jaundice of the newborn, Crigler-Najjar syndrome.

Bilirubin, Neonatal ("Baby Bilirubin")

(Normal levels dependent on prematurity and age in days; "panic levels" usually > 15–20 mg/dL (SI: >257–342 μmol/L in term infants).

Increased: Erythroblastosis fetalis, physiologic jaundice (may be due to breastfeeding), resorption of hematoma or hemorrhage, obstructive jaundice, others.

Bleeding Time

(Duke, Ivy <6 min; Template <10 min).
    Tests only platelet function, not coagulation factors.

Increased: Thrombocytopenia (disseminated intravascular coagulation [DIC], thrombotic thrombocytopenic purpura [TTP], idiopathic thrombocytopenic purpura [ITP]), von Willebrand's disease, defective platelet function including aspirin therapy.

Blood Gases, Capillary

When interpreting a CBG, apply the following rules:

pH: Same as arterial blood gas or slightly lower (N = 7.35–7.40).

Pco$_2$: Same as arterial blood gas or slightly higher (N = 40–45).

Po$_2$: Lower than arterial blood gas (N = 45–60).

O$_2$ Saturation: >70% is acceptable. Saturation is probably more useful than the Po$_2$ itself when interpreting a CBG.

Blood Gases, Arterial & Venous

There is little difference between arterial and venous pH and bicarbonate (except with congestive heart failure and shock); therefore, the venous blood gas may be occasionally used to assess acid-base status, but venous oxygen levels (Po$_2$) are significantly less than arterial levels (Table II–1).

TABLE II–1. NORMAL BLOOD GAS VALUES.

Measurement	Arterial Blood	Mixed Venous[a]	Venous
pH (range)	7.40 (7.36–7.44)	7.36 (7.31–7.41)	7.36 (7.31–7.41)
Po$_2$ (decreases with age)	80–100 mm Hg	35–40 mm Hg	30–50 mm Hg
Pco$_2$	35–45 mm Hg	41–51 mm Hg	40–52 mm Hg
o$_2$ saturation (%) (decreases with age)	>95%	60–80%	60–85%
HCO$_3$	22–26 mEq/L (mmol/L)	22–26 mEq/L (mmol/L)	22–28 mEq/L (mmol/L)
Base deficit (deficit excess)	–2–+3	–2–+3	–2–+3

[a]Obtained from right atrium, usually through a pulmonary artery catheter.

See individual component for differential diagnosis. For acid-base disorders, see the section below and On Call Problems 2 and 3, "Acidosis," and 7 and 8, "Alkalosis."

Metabolic Acidosis: A fall in plasma HCO_3 followed by a compensatory fall in Pco_2. Use the Anion Gap to help establish the diagnosis (Table II–2).

$$Anion\ Gap = Na - (Cl + HCO_3)$$

$$Normal\ Gap = 8 - 12\ mEq/L$$

Differential Diagnosis: (see also On Call Problems 2 and 3, "Acidosis").

Anion gap acidosis ("normochloremic acidosis"): gap >12 mEq/L; caused by a decrease in bicarbonate balanced by an increase in unmeasured acids. Lactic acidosis, ketoacidosis (diabetic, alcoholic, starvation), uremia, intoxication (salicylate, methanol, paraldehyde, ethylene glycol), hyperalimentation.

Non-anion gap acidosis ("hyperchloremic acidosis"): gap between 8–12 mEq/L; caused by a decrease in HCO_3 balanced by an increase in chloride. Renal bicarbonate losses (renal tubular acidosis, spironolactone, carbonic anhydrase inhibitors), GI tract bicarbonate losses (diarrhea, pancreatic fistulas, biliary tract fistulas, ileal loop, ureterosigmoidostomy).

Low Anion Gap: Gap < 8: Not seen with acidosis, but can be seen with bromide ingestion, hyponatremia, and multiple myeloma.

Metabolic Alkalosis: A rise in plasma HCO_3 followed by a compensatory rise in the Pco_2. Spot urine for chloride helps establish the diagnosis (see Table II–2).

Differential Diagnosis: (see also Problems 7 and 8, "Alkalosis").

Urine Chloride < 10 mEq/L ("chloride responsive"): Diuretics, GI tract losses (NG suction, vomiting, diarrhea [villous adenoma, congenital chloride wasting diarrhea in children]), iatrogenic (inadequate chloride intake).

TABLE II–2. SIMPLE ACID-BASE DISTURBANCES.

Acid-Base Disorder	Primary Abnormality	Secondary Abnormality	Expected Degree of Compensatory Response
Metabolic acidosis	$\downarrow\downarrow\downarrow[HCO_3^-]$	$\downarrow\downarrow Pco_2$	$Pco_2 = (1.5 \times [HCO_3^-]) + 8$
Metabolic alkalosis	$\uparrow\uparrow\uparrow[HCO_3^-]$	$\uparrow\uparrow Pco_2$	$\uparrow$ in $Pco_2 = \Delta\ HCO_3^- \times 0.6$
Acute respiratory acidosis	$\uparrow\uparrow\uparrow Pco_2$	$\uparrow[HCO_3^-]$	$\uparrow$ in $HCO_3^- = \Delta\ Pco_2/10$
Chronic respiratory acidosis	$\uparrow\uparrow\uparrow Pco_2$	$\uparrow\uparrow[HCO_3^-]$	$\uparrow$ in $HCO_3^- = 4 \times \Delta\ Pco_2/10$
Acute respiratory alkalosis	$\downarrow\downarrow\downarrow Pco_2$	$\downarrow[HCO_3^-]$	$\downarrow$ in $HCO_3^- = 2 \times \Delta\ Pco_2/10$
Chronic respiratory alkalosis	$\downarrow\downarrow\downarrow Pco_2$	$\downarrow\downarrow[HCO_3^-]$	$\downarrow$ in $HCO_3^- = 5 \times \Delta\ Pco_2/10$

Urine Chloride > 10 mEq/L ("chloride resistant"): Adrenal diseases (Cushing's syndrome, hyperaldosteronism), exogenous steroid use, Bartter's syndrome, licorice ingestion.

Respiratory Acidosis: A primary rise in Pco_2 with a compensatory rise in plasma Hco_3 not higher than 30 mEq/L if acute (see Table II–2).

Differential Diagnosis: (see also Problems 2 and 3, "Acidosis").
Acute: CNS depression (oversedation, narcotics, anesthetic), CNS trauma (CVA, head injury, spinal cord trauma), neuromuscular diseases (myasthenia gravis, Guillain-Barré disease), airway obstruction, laryngospasm, iatrogenic mechanical underventilation, pulmonary lesions (acute pulmonary edema, severe pneumonia), chest trauma (hemothorax, pneumothorax, flail chest).
Chronic: Chronic asthma, emphysema or bronchitis, Pickwickian syndrome.

Respiratory Alkalosis: A primary fall in Pco_2 (see Table II–2).
Differential Diagnosis: (see also Problems 7 and 8, "Alkalosis").
Central nervous system causes: Anxiety, hyperventilation syndrome, pain, head trauma, CVA, encephalitis, CHS tumors, salicylates (early toxicity), fever, early sepsis.
Peripheral stimulation: Pulmonary embolus, CHF, interstitial lung disease, pneumonia, altitude, hypoxemia of any cause.
Miscellaneous: Delirium tremens, cirrhosis, thyrotoxicosis, pregnancy, iatrogenic overventilation.

Blood Urea Nitrogen (BUN)

(Birth–1 year: 4–16 mg/dL [SI: 1.4–5.7 mmol/L]; 1–40 years 5–20 mg/dL [SI: 1.8–7.1 mmol/L]; gradual slight increase with increasing age). To convert mg/dL to mmol/L, multiply by 0.3570.

Increased: Renal failure, prerenal azotemia (decreased renal perfusion secondary to congestive heart failure [CHF], shock, volume depletion), postrenal (obstruction), gastrointestinal (GI) bleeding, stress, drugs (especially aminoglycosides).

Decreased: Starvation, liver failure (hepatitis, drugs), pregnancy, infancy, nephrotic syndrome, overhydration.

BUN/Creatinine Ratio (BUN/Cr)

(mean 10, range 6–20).

Increased: Prerenal azotemia (renal hypoperfusion), GI bleeding, high protein diet, ileal conduit, drugs (steroids, tetracycline).

Decreased: Malnutrition, pregnancy, low protein diet, ketoacidosis, hemodialysis, SIADH, drugs (cimetidine).

CBC Differential Diagnosis (see also Tables II–3 and II–4 for normal ranges).

Basophils: (0–1%).

Increased: Chronic myeloid leukemia, rarely in recovery from infection and from hypothyroidism.

Decreased: Acute rheumatic fever, lobar pneumonia, after steroid therapy, thyrotoxicosis, stress.

Eosinophils: (1–3%).

Increased: Allergy, parasites, skin diseases, malignancy, drugs, asthma, Addison's disease, collagen-vascular diseases (handy mnemonic NAACP: Neoplasm, Allergy, Addison's disease, Collagen vascular diseases, Parasites), pulmonary diseases including Löffler's syndrome and PIE (pulmonary infiltrates with eosinophilia).

Decreased: After steroids, adrenocorticotropic hormone (ACTH), after stress (infection, trauma, burns), Cushing's syndrome.

Hematocrit: (male 40–54%; female 37–47%).

Decreased: Megaloblastic anemia (folate or B_{12} deficiency), iron deficiency anemia, sickle cell anemia, etc), acute or chronic blood loss, hemolysis, dilutional, alcohol, drugs.

Increased: Primary polycythemia (polycythemia vera), secondary polycythemia (reduced fluid intake or excess fluid loss, congenital and acquired heart disease, lung disease, high altitudes, heavy smokers, tumors [renal cell carcinoma, hepatoma], renal cysts).

Hemoglobin: (see Table II–3, page 274 for normal values). See Problem 11, "Anemia."

Increased: Polycythemia vera, secondary polycythemia, high altitude, vigorous exercise.

Decreased: see Hematocrit.

Lymphocytes: (24–44%).

TABLE II-3. NORMAL COMPLETE BLOOD COUNT FOR SELECTED AGE RANGES.

Age	WBC Count (cells/mm)^3 [SI: 10^9/L]	RBC Count 10^6/µL [SI: 10^{12}/L]	Hemoglobin (gm/dL) [SI: g/L]	Hematocrit (%)	MCH (pg) [SI: pg]	MCHC (g/dL) [SI: g/L]^a	MCV (µm)^3 [SI: fl]	RDW
Adult male	4500–11,000 [4.5–11.0]	4.73–5.49 [4.73–5.49]	14.40–16.60 [144–166]	42.9–49.1	27–31	33–37	76–100	11.5–14.5
Adult female	As above	4.15–4.87 [4.15–5.49]	12.2–14.7 [122–147]	37.9–43.9	As above	As above	As above	As above
11–15 y	4500–13,500	4.8	13.4	39	28	34	82	—
6–10 y	5000–14,500	4.7	12.9	37.5	27	34	80	—
4–6 y	5500–15,500	4.6	12.6	37.0	27	34	80	—
2–4 y	6000–17,000	4.5	12.5	35.5	25	32	77	—
4 mo–2 y	6000–17,500	4.6	11.2	35.0	25	33	77	—
1 wk–4 mo	5500–18,000	4.7 ± 0.9	14.0 ± 3.3	42.0 ± 7.0	30	33	90	—
24 h–1 wk	5000–21,000	5.1	18.3 ± 4.0	52.5	36	35	103	—
First day	9400–34,000	5.1 ± 1.0	19.5 ± 5.0	54.0 ± 10.0	38	36	106	—

^{a}To convert from standard reference value to SI units, multiply by 10.

Increased: Virtually any viral infection (AIDS, measles, German measles, mumps, whooping cough, smallpox, chickenpox, influenza, hepatitis, infectious mononucleosis), acute infectious lymphocytosis in children, acute and chronic lymphocytic leukemias.

Decreased: (normal finding in 22% of population), stress, burns, trauma, uremia, some viral infections, AIDS, AIDS-related complex, bone marrow suppression after chemotherapy, steroids.

Lymphocytes, Atypical

>20%: Infectious mononucleosis, cytomegalovirus (CMV) infection, infectious hepatitis, toxoplasmosis.

<20%: Viral infections (mumps, rubeola, varicella), rickettsial infections, TB.

MCH (Mean Cellular [Corpuscular] Hemoglobin): (27–31 pg [SI: 27–31 pg]). The weight of hemoglobin of the average red cell. Calculated by

$$MCH = \frac{Hemoglobin\ (g/L)}{RBC\ (10^6/\mu L}$$

Increased: Macrocytosis (megaloblastic anemias, high reticulocyte counts).

Decreased: Microcytosis (iron deficiency, sideroblastic anemia, thalassemia).

MCHC (Mean Cellular [Corpuscular] Hemoglobin Concentration): (33–37 g/dL [SI:330–370 g/L]). The average concentration of hemoglobin in a given volume of red cells. Calculated by the following formula:

$$MCHC = \frac{Hemoglobin\ (g/dL)}{Hematocrit}$$

Increased: Very severe, prolonged dehydration; spherocytosis.

Decreased: Iron deficiency anemia, overhydration, thalassemia, sideroblastic anemia.

MCV (Mean Cell [Corpuscular] Volume): (76–100 μm^3 [SI: 76–100 fL]). The average volume of red blood cells. Calculated by the following formula:

$$MCV = \frac{Hematocrit \times 1000}{RBC\ (10^6/\mu L}$$

Increased: Megaloblastic anemia (B$_{12}$, folate deficiency), macrocytic (normoblastic) anemia, reticulocytosis, Down's syndrome, chronic liver disease.

Decreased: Iron deficiency, thalassemia, some cases of lead poisoning.

Monocytes: (3–7%).

Increased: Bacterial infection (TB, subacute bacterial endocarditis [SBE], brucellosis, typhoid, recovery from an acute infection), protozoal infections, infectious mononucleosis, leukemia, Hodgkin's disease, ulcerative colitis, regional enteritis.

Platelets: (150–450,000 µL).
   Platelet counts may be normal in number, but abnormal in function as occurs in aspirin therapy. Abnormalities of platelet function are assessed by bleeding time.

Increased: Sudden exercise, after trauma, bone fracture, after asphyxia, after surgery (especially splenectomy), acute hemorrhage, polycythemia vera, primary thrombocythemia, leukemias, after childbirth, carcinoma, myeloproliferative disorders.

Decreased: Disseminated intravascular coagulation (DIC), idiopathic thrombocytopenic purpura (ITP), thrombotic thrombocytopenic purpura, congenital disease, marrow suppressants (chemotherapy, thiazide diuretics, alcohol, estrogens, x-rays), burns, snake and insect bites, leukemias, aplastic anemias, hypersplenism, infectious mononucleosis, viral infections, cirrhosis, massive transfusions, eclampsia and pre-eclampsia, more than 30 different drugs.

PMNs (Polymorphonuclear Neutrophils): (40–76%).

Increased:

- Physiologic (normal): Severe exercise, last months of pregnancy, labor, surgery, newborns, steroid therapy.
- Pathologic: Bacterial infections, noninfective tissue damage (myocardial infarction, pulmonary infarction, crush injury, burn injury), metabolic disorders (eclampsia, diabetic ketoacidosis, uremia, acute gout).

Decreased: Pancytopenia, aplastic anemia, PMN depression (a mild decrease is referred to as neutropenia, severe is called agranulocytosis), marrow damage (radiographs, poisoning with benzene or antitumor drugs), severe overwhelming infections (disseminated TB, septicemia), acute malaria, severe osteomyelitis, infectious mononucleosis, atypical pneumonias, some viral infections, marrow obliteration (osteosclerosis, myelofibrosis, malignant infiltrate), drugs (more than 70, including chloramphenicol, phenylbutazone, chlorpromazine, quinine), B_{12} and folate deficiencies, hypoadrenalism, hypopituitarism, dialysis, familial decrease, idiopathic causes.

RDW (Red Cell Distribution Width): (11.5–14.5).
A measure of the degree of anisocytosis (variation in RBC size) and measured by the automated hematology counters (eg, Coulter Counter).

Increased: Many anemias (concomitant macrocytic and microcytic anemia).

White Blood Cell Count: (see Tables II–3 and II–4, pages 274, 278).

Increased: Infections (especially bacterial), leukemia, leukemoid reactions, tissue necrosis, postsplenectomy, exercise, fever, pain, anesthesia, labor.

Decreased: Sepsis, overwhelming bacterial infections, certain nonbacterial infections (influenza, hepatitis, mononucleosis), aplastic anemia, pernicious anemia, hypersplenism, cachexia, chemotherapeutic agents, ionizing radiation.

C-PEPTIDE

(Fasting, <4.0 ng/mL [SI: <4.0 µg/L]; male >60 years, 1.5–5.0 ng/mL [SI: 1.5–5.0 [m}g/L]; female 1.4–5.5 ng/mL [SI: 1.4–5.5 µg/L]).
Differentiates between exogenous and endogenous insulin production/administration.

Increased: Insulinoma, pancreas transplant, oral hypoglycemic agents (sulfonylureas).

Decreased: Diabetes (decreased endogenous insulin), insulin administration (factitious or therapeutic), hypoglycemia.

Captopril Test

Used in the evaluation of renovascular hypotension, captopril is an angiotensin converting enzyme (ACE) inhibitor that blocks angiotensin II. Captopril is administered (25 mg IV at 8 AM). Aldosterone decreases 2 h later from baseline in normal or essential hypertension, but it is not suppressed in patients with aldosteronism. For renovascular hypertension, the plasma renin activity (PRA) increases > 12 ng/mL/h. An absolute increase of 10 ng/mL/h plus a 400% increase in PRA is noted when the pretest level is < 3 ng/mL/h, and the PRA is more than 150% over baseline when the pretest PRA is > 3 ng/mL/h. The test is now also combined with a nuclear renal scan to identify renal artery stenosis.

CA 15-3

Used to detect breast cancer recurrence in asymptomatic patients and monitor therapy. Levels related to stage of disease.

TABLE II–4. NORMAL PLATELET AND WHITE BLOOD CELL DIFFERENTIAL FOR SELECTED AGES.

Age	Platelet Count (10³ µL) [SI: 10⁹/L]	Lymphocytes Total (% WBC Count)	Neutrophils, Band (% WBC Count)	Neutrophils, Segmented (% WBC Count)	Eosinophils (% WBC Count)	Basophils (% WBC Count)	Monocytes (% WBC Count)
Adult male	238 ± 49	34	3.0	56	2.7	0.5	4.0
Adult female	270 ± 58	As above	As above	As above	As above	As above	As above
11–15 y	282 ± 63	38	3.0	51	2.4	0.5	4.3
6–10y	351 ± 85	39	3.0	50	2.4	0.6	4.2
4–6 y	357 ± 70	42	3.0	39	2.8	0.6	5.0
2–4 y	357 ± 70	59	3.0	30	2.6	0.5	5.0
4 m–2 y	As above	61	3.1	28	2.6	0.4	4.8
1 wk–4 mo	As above	56	4.5	30	2.8	0.5	6.5
24 h–1wk	240–380	24–41	6.8–9.2	39–52	2.4–4.1	0.5	5.8–9.1
First day	As above	24	10.2	58	2.0	0.6	5.8

Increased: Breast cancer, benign breast disease, and liver disease.

Decreased: Response to therapy (25% change considered significant).

CA 19-9 (<37 U/mL [SI: <37 kU/L]).

Increased: Gastrointestinal cancers such as pancreas, stomach, liver, colorectal, hepatobiliary, some cases of lung and prostate, pancreatitis.

CA 125 (<35 U/mL [SI: <35 kU/L])

Not a useful screening test for ovarian cancer when used alone; used in conjunction with ultrasound and physical exam for detection. Rising levels after resection predictive for recurrence.

Increased: Ovarian (serous), cervical adenocarcinoma, endometrial and colon cancer, endometriosis, inflammatory bowel disease, pelvic inflammatory disease, pregnancy, breast lesions and benign abdominal masses (teratomas).

Calcitonin (Thyrocalcitonin)

(<19 pg/mL [SI: <19 ng/L]).

Increased: Medullary carcinoma of the thyroid, C-cell hyperplasia (precursor of medullary carcinoma), small cell carcinoma of the lung, newborns, pregnancy, chronic renal insufficiency, Zollinger-Ellison syndrome, pernicious anemia.

Calcium, Serum

(infants to 1 mo: 7–11.5 mg/dL [SI: 1.75–2.87 mmol/L]; 1 mo to 1 year: 8.6–11.2 mg/dl [SI: 2.15–2.79 mmol/L]; >1 year and adults: 8.2–10.2 mg/dL [SI: 2.05–2.54 mmol/L]; ionized: 4.75–5.2 mg/dL [SI: 1.19–1.30 mmol/L]). To convert mg/dL to mmol/L, multiply by 0.2495).

When interpreting a total calcium value, the total protein and albumin must be known. If these are not within normal limits, a corrected calcium can be roughly calculated by the following formula:

Corrected Total Ca = 0.8 (Normal albumin − measured albumin) + reported Ca

Values for ionized calcium need no special corrections.

Increased: (NOTE: Levels > 12 mg/dL [2.99 mmol/L] may lead to coma and death.) Primary hyperthyroidism, parathyroid hormone (PTH) secreting tumors, vitamin D excess, metastatic bone tumors, osteoporosis, immobilization, milk-alkali syndrome, Paget's disease, idiopathic hypercalcemia of infants, infantile hypophosphatasia, thiazide drugs, chronic renal failure, sarcoidosis, multiple myeloma.

Decreased: (NOTE: Levels < 7 mg/dL [<1.75 mmol/L] may lead to tetany and death.) Hypoparathyroidism (surgical, idiopathic), pseudohypoparathyroidism, insufficient vitamin D, calcium and phosphorus ingestion (pregnancy, osteomalacia, rickets), hypomagnesemia, renal tubular acidosis, hypoalbuminemia (cachexia, nephrotic syndrome, cystic fibrosis), chronic renal failure (phosphate retention), acute pancreatitis, factitious decrease because of low protein and albumin.

Calcium, Urine (24-Hour Urine)

On a calcium-free diet (<150 mg/d [3.7 mmol/d]); average calcium diet (600–800 mg/d) 100–250 mg/24 h [2.5–6.2 mmol/d].

Increased: Hyperparathyroidism, hyperthyroidism, hypervitaminosis D, distal renal tubular acidosis (type I), sarcoidosis, immobilization, osteolytic lesions (bony metastasis, multiple myeloma), Paget's disease, glucocorticoid excess.

Decreased: Thiazide diuretics, hypothyroidism, renal failure, steatorrhea, rickets, osteomalacia.

Carbon Dioxide ("Total CO_2" or Bicarbonate)

(adult 23–29 mmol/L, child 20–28 mmol/L) (see also P_{CO_2} values).

Increased: Compensation for respiratory acidosis, metabolic alkalosis, emphysema, severe vomiting, primary aldosteronism, volume contraction, Bartter's syndrome.

Decreased: Compensation for respiratory alkalosis, metabolic acidosis, starvation, diabetic ketoacidosis, lactic acidosis, alcoholic ketoacidosis, toxins (methanol, ethylene glycol, paraldehyde), severe diarrhea, renal failure, drugs (salicylates, acetazolamide), dehydration, adrenal insufficiency.

Carbon Dioxide, Arterial (P_{CO_2})

(see Table II–1).

Increased: Respiratory acidosis, compensatory increase in metabolic alkalosis.

Decreased: Respiratory alkalosis, compensatory in metabolic alkalosis.

Carboxyhemoglobin (Carbon Monoxide)

(nonsmoker <2%; smoker <9%; toxic > 15%).

Increased: Smokers, smoke inhalation, automobile exhaust inhalation, normal newborns.

Carcinoembryonic Antigen (CEA)

(nonsmoker <3.0 ng/mL [SI: <3.0 µg/L], smoker <5.0 ng/mL [SI: <5.0 µg).
   Not a screening test; useful for monitoring response to treatment and tumor recurrence of adenocarcinomas of the gastrointestinal tract.

Increased: Carcinoma (colon, pancreas, lung, stomach), smokers, nonneoplastic liver disease, Crohn's disease, ulcerative colitis.

Catecholamines, Fractionated, Serum

(Values are variable and depend on the lab and method of assay used. Normal levels below are based on an HPLC technique.)

Catecholamine	Plasma (supine) levels
Norepinephrine	70–750 pg/mL [SI:414–4435 pmol/L]
Epinephrine	0–100 pg/mL [SI:0–546 pmol/L]
Dopamine	<30 pg/mL [SI: 196 pmol/L]

Increased: Pheochromocytoma, neural crest tumors (neuroblastoma), with extra-adrenal pheochromocytoma; norepinephrine may be markedly elevated compared with epinephrine.

Catecholamines, Fractionated (24-h Urine)

(Values are variable and dependent on the assay method used.) Norepinephrine: 15–80 µg/d [SI: 89–473 nmol/d]; epinephrine: 0–20 µg/d [0–118 nmol/d]; dopamine: 65–400 µg/d [SI: 384–2364 nmol/d].
   Used to evaluate neuroendocrine tumors including pheochromocytoma and neuroblastoma. Avoid caffeine, and methyldopa (Aldomet) prior to test.

Increased: Pheochromocytoma, neuroblastoma, epinephrine administration, drugs (methyldopa, tetracyclines are false increases).

Chloride, Serum

(97–107 mEq/L [SI: 97–107 mmol/L]).

Increased: Diarrhea, renal failure, nephrotic syndrome, renal tubular acidosis, mineralocorticoid deficiency, hyperalimentation, medications (acetazolamide, ammonium chloride, hydrochlorothiazide).

Decreased: Vomiting (includes NG suction), diarrhea, diabetes mellitus with ketoacidosis, mineralocorticoid excess, (SIADH), excessive diuretic use, chronic respiratory acidosis, renal disease with sodium loss.

Cholesterol (Total)

(normal, see Table II–5); to convert mg/dL to mmol/L, multiply by 0.02586. Fasting specimen recommended because triglyceride levels may be affected.

Increased: Idiopathic hypercholesterolemia, secondary hyperlipoproteinemias (nephrotic syndrome, biliary cirrhosis, nephrosis, hypothyroidism), pancreatic disease (diabetes), pregnancy, oral contraceptives, steroid administration, hyperlipoproteinemia (types IIb, III, V).

Decreased: Liver disease (hepatitis, malignancy, etc), hyperthyroidism, malnutrition (cancer, starvation), chronic anemias, burns, lipoproteinemias.

High Density Lipoprotein-Cholesterol (HDL, HDL-C)

(fasting: 30–70 mg/dL [SI: 0.8–1.80 mmol/L]; female 30–90 mg/dL [SI: 0.80–2.35 mmol/L]).
   HDL-C has the best correlation with the development of coronary artery disease; decreased HDL-C in males leads to an increased risk. Levels < 45 mg/dl are associated with increased risk of coronary artery disease.

Increased: Estrogen (females), exercise, ethanol.

Decreased: Males, uremia, obesity, diabetes, liver disease, Tangiers's disease.

Low Density Lipoprotein-Cholesterol (LDL, LDL-C)

(50–190 mg/dL [SI: 1.30–4.90 mmol/L]).

TABLE II–5. NORMAL TOTAL CHOLESTEROL
LEVELS BY AGE.

Age (y)	Standard Units (mg/dL)	SI Units (mmol/L)
Infant	<65–175	<1.68–4.52
1–19	<120–220	<3.10–5.68
20–29	<200	<5.20
30–39	<225	<5.85
40–49	<245	<6.35
>50	<265	<6.85

Increased: Excess dietary saturated fats, myocardial infarction (MI), hyper-lipoproteinemia, biliary cirrhosis, endocrine disease (diabetes, hypothyroidism).

Decreased: Malabsorption, severe liver disease, abetalipoproteinemia, nicotinic acid.

Clostridium Difficile Toxin Assay

Fecal (normal = negative).
  Majority of patients with pseudomembranous colitis have positive *C difficile* assay; use endoscopy to confirm plaques. Often positive in antibiotic-associated diarrhea and colitis. Can be seen in some normals and neonates.

Clotting Time, Activated (ACT)

(5–15 minutes).
  Most often used in the OR or dialysis unit to monitor acute anticoagulation status.

Increased: Heparin therapy, plasma-clotting factor deficiency (except Factors VII and XIII). (NOTE: This is not a sensitive test, therefore it is not considered a good screening test.)

Cold Agglutinins

(<1:32).

Increased: Atypical pneumonia (mycoplasmal pneumonia), other viral infections (especially mononucleosis, measles, mumps), cirrhosis, parasitic infections.

Complement C3

(85–155 mg/dL, [SI: 800–1500 ng/L]).

Increased: Rheumatoid arthritis (variable finding), rheumatic fever, various neoplasms (gastrointestinal, prostate, others).

Decreased: Erythematosus, glomerulonephritis (poststreptococcal and membranoproliferative), sepsis, subacute bacterial endocarditis (SBE), chronic active hepatitis.

Complement C4

(20–50 mg/dL [SI: 200–500 ng/L]).

Increased: Rheumatoid arthritis (variable finding), neoplasia (gastrointestinal, lung, others).

Decreased: SLE, chronic active hepatitis, cirrhosis, glomerulonephritis, hereditary angioedema.

Complement CH50 (Total)

(33–61 mg/ml [SI: 330–610 ng/L]).
   Tests for complement deficiency in the classic pathway.

Increased: Acute phase reactants (tissue injury, infections, etc).

Decreased: Hereditary complement deficiencies.

Coombs' Test, Direct (Direct Antiglobulin Test)

(normal = negative).
   Uses patient's erythrocytes; tests for the presence of antibody on the patient's cells.

Positive: Autoimmune hemolytic anemia (leukemia, lymphoma, collagen-vascular diseases), hemolytic transfusion reaction, some drug sensitizations (methyldopa, levodopa, cephalothin), hemolytic disease of the newborn (erythroblastosis fetalis).

Coombs' Test, Indirect (Antibody Screening Test)

(normal = negative).
   Uses serum that contains antibody, usually from the patient.

Positive: Isoimmunization from previous transfusion, incompatible blood because of improper cross-matching.

Cortisol, Serum

(8 AM, 5.0–23.0 µg/dL [SI: 138–365 nmol/L]; 4 PM, 3.0–15.0 µg/dL [SI: 83–414 nmol/L]).
   Most useful when used with ACTH stimulation test (page 265) or dexamethasone suppression test (page 287).

Increased: Adrenal adenoma, adrenal carcinoma, Cushing's disease, non-pituitary adrenocorticotropic hormone (ACTH)-producing tumor, steroid therapy, oral contraceptives.

Decreased: Primary adrenal insufficiency (Addison's disease), congenital adrenal hyperplasia, Waterhouse-Friderichsen syndrome, ACTH deficiency.

Cortisol, Free (24-h Urine)

30–100 µg/d.
Used to evaluate adrenal cortical function, screening test of choice for Cushing's Syndrome.

Increased: Cushing's syndrome (adrenal hyperfunction), stress during collection, oral contraceptives, pregnancy.

Counterimmunoelectrophoresis (CIEP, CEP)

(normal = negative).
An immunologic technique that allows rapid identification of infecting organisms from fluids including serum, urine, cerebrospinal fluid (CSF), and other body fluids. Organisms identified include *Neisseria meningitidis, Streptococcus pneumoniae, Haemophilus influenzae,* and group B *Streptococcus.*

Creatine Phosphokinase (CPK)

(25–145 mU/mL [SI: 25–145 U/L]).

Increased: Muscle damage (acute myocardial infarction, myocarditis, muscular dystrophy, muscle trauma [injection], after surgery), brain infarction, defibrillation, cardiac catheterization and surgery, rhabdomyolysis, polymyositis, hypothyroidism.

CPK Isoenzymes

MB: (normal <6%, heart origin), increased in acute myocardial infarction (begins in 2–12 h, peaks at 12–40 h, returns to normal in 24–72 h), pericarditis with myocarditis, rhabdomyolysis, crush injury, Duchenne's muscular dystrophy, polymyositis, malignancy hyperthermia, and cardiac surgery.
MM: (normal 94–100%, skeletal muscle origin) increased in crush injury, malignant hyperthermia, seizures, IM injections.
BB: (normal 0%, brain origin) brain injury (cerebrovascular accident [CVA], trauma), metastatic neoplasms (prostate), malignant hyperthermia, colonic infarction.

Creatinine, Serum

(adult male: <1.2 mg/dL [SI: 106 µmol/L], adult female: <1.1 mg/dL [SI: 97 µmol/L], child: 0.5–0.8 mg/dL [SI: 44–71 µmol/L]).To convert mg/dL to µmol/L, multiply by 88.40.

Increased: Renal failure (prerenal, renal, or postrenal obstruction), gigantism, acromegaly, ingestion of roasted meat, aminoglycosides and other drugs (cimetidine, some cephalosporins, ascorbic acid, others), false positive with DKA.

Decreased: Pregnancy, decreased muscle mass, severe liver disease.

Creatinine (Urine) & Creatinine Clearance

(adult Male: total creatinine, 1–2 g/d [8.8–17.7 mmol/d]; clearance, 85–125 mL/min per 1.73 m^2; adult female: total creatinine, 0.8–1.8g/d [7.1–15.9 mmol/d]; clearance, 75–115 mL/min per 1.73 m^2 [1.25–1.92 mL/s per 1.73 m^2]); child: total creatinine, (> 3 years) 12–30 mg/kg/d; clearance 70–140 mL/min per 1.73 m^2[1.17–2.33 mL/s per 1.73 m^2].

Decreased: A decreased creatinine clearance results in an increase in serum creatinine usually secondary to renal insufficiency.

Increased: Early diabetes mellitus, pregnancy.

Calculation of Creatinine Clearance: Order a concurrent serum creatinine and a 24-h urine creatinine. A shorter time interval can be used; for example, 12 h, but remember that the formula must be corrected for this change and that a 24-h sample is less prone to collection error.

   Example: (A quick formula is also found on page 518 under "Aminoglycoside Dosing.")

   Calculation of the creatinine clearance from a 24-h urine sample with a volume of 1000 mL, a urine creatinine of 108 mg/100 mL, and a serum creatinine of 1 mg/100 mL (1 mg/dL):

$$\text{Clearance} = \frac{\text{Urine creatinine} \times \text{total urine volume}}{\text{Plasma creatinine} \times \text{time (1440 min if 24 - h collection)}}$$

$$\text{Clearance} = \frac{(108 \text{ mg} / 100\text{mL}) \times (1000 \text{ mL})}{(1 \text{ mg} / 100 \text{ mL}) (1440 \text{ min})} = 75 \text{ mL} / \text{min}$$

Some clinicians advocate a preliminary determination to see if the urine sample is valid by determining first if the sample contains at least 18–25 mg/kg/24 h of creatinine for adult males or 12–20 mg/kg/24 h for adult females. This preliminary test is not a requirement, but can help with the determination if a 24-h sample was collected or if some of the sample was lost.

   If the patient is an adult (150 lb = body surface area of 1.73 m^2), adjustment of the clearance for body size is not routinely done. Adjustment for pediatric patients is a necessity. If the values in the previous example were for a 10-year-old boy who weighed 70 lb (1.1 m^2; see page 534 for the conversion formula), then the clearance would be

$$\frac{75 \text{ mL} / \text{min} \times 1.73 \text{ m}^2}{1.1 \text{ m}^2} = 118 \text{ mL} / \text{min}$$

Dehydroepiandrosterone (DHEA)

(male: 2.0–3.4 ng/mL [SI: 5.2–8.7 µmol/L]; female, premenopausal: 0.8–3.4 ng/mL [SI: 2.1–8.8 µmol/L]; postmenopausal: 0.1–0.6 ng/mL [SI: 0.3–1.6 µmol/L]).

Increased: Anovulation, polycystic ovaries, adrenal hyperplasia, adrenal tumors.

Decreased: Menopause.

Dehydroepiandrosterone Sulfate (DHEA-S)

(male: 1.7–4.2 ng/mL [SI: 6–15 µmol/L]; female: 2.0–5.2 ng/mL [SI: 7–18 µmol/L]).

Increased: Hyperprolactinemia, adrenal hyperplasia, adrenal tumor, polycystic ovaries, lipoid ovarian tumors.

Decreased: Menopause.

Dexamethasone Suppression Test

Used in the differential diagnosis of Cushing's syndrome (elevated cortisol).

Overnight "Rapid" Test: 1 mg of dexamethasone at 11 PM is given PO, and a fasting 8 AM plasma cortisol is obtained. Normally the cortisol level should be < 5.0 µg/dL [138 nmol/L]. If the value is > 5 µg/dL [138 nmol/L], this usually confirms the diagnosis of Cushing's syndrome; however obesity, alcoholism, or depression may occasionally show the same result. In these patients, the best screening test is a 24-h urine for free cortisol.

Low Dose Test: After collection of baseline serum cortisol and 24-h urine free cortisol levels, dexamethasone 0.5 mg PO is administered every 6 h for 8 doses. Serum and urine cortisol are repeated on the second day. Failure to suppress to a serum cortisol of < 5.0 µg/dL [138 nmol/L] and a urine free cortisol of < 30 µg/dL (82 nmol/L) confirms Cushing's syndrome.

High Dose Test: After the low-dose test, dexamethasone, 2 mg PO every 6 h for 8 doses will cause a fall in urinary free cortisol to 50% of the baseline value in patients with bilateral adrenal hyperplasia (Cushing's disease), but not in patients with adrenal tumors or ectopic adrenocorticotropic hormone (ACTH) production.

Erythropoetin (EPO)

5–36 mU/L (5–36 IU/L).

Increased: Pregnancy, secondary polycythemia (high altitude, COPD, etc), tumors (renal cell carcinoma, cerebellar hemangioblastoma, hepatoma, others), PCKD, anemias with bone marrow unresponsiveness (aplastic anemia, iron deficiency, etc).

Decreased: Bilateral nephrectomy, anemia of chronic disease (ie, renal failure, nephrotic syndrome), primary polycythemia (NOTE: The determination of EPO levels before administration of recombinant EPO for renal failure is not usually necessary).

Erythrocyte Sedimentation Rate (ESR)

(see Sedimentation Rate, page 307).

Estradiol, Serum

Serial measurements useful to assess fetal well being, especially in high risk pregnancy.

Phase	Normal Values(Female)
Follicular Phase	25–75 pg/mL
Midcycle Peak	200–600 pg/mL
Luteal Phase	100–1–5 ng/mL
Pregnancy 1st trimester	5–15 ng/mL
2nd trimester	10–40 ng/mL
3rd trimester	5–25 pg/mL
Postmenopause	

Estrogen & Progesterone Receptor Assays

(<3–5 fmol/mg negative, >10 fmol/mg positive, >100 fmol/mg highly positive).

Determined on fresh surgical specimens but also can be determined on fixed specimens. The presence of the receptors is associated with a longer disease-free interval and survival from breast cancer and is more likely to respond to endocrine therapy.

Fecal Fat

(2–6 g/d on a 80–100 g/d fat diet; 72-h collection time).

Increased: Cystic fibrosis, pancreatic insufficiency, Crohn's disease, chronic pancreatitis, sprue, diarrhea states with or without fat malabsorption (NOTE: Barium can interfere).

Ferritin

(male: 15–200 ng/mL [SI: 15–200 µg/L]; female: 12–150 ng/mL [SI: 12–150 µg/L]).

Increased: Hemochromatosis, hemosiderosis, sideroblastic anemia.

Decreased: Iron deficiency (earliest and most sensitive test before red cells show any morphologic change), severe liver disease.

Fibrin D-Dimer (D-DIMER)

(normal = negative).
   Useful in screening for DIC.

Increased: DIC, DVT, acute MI, PE, arterial thrombosis.

Fibrin Degradation Products (FDP), Fibrin Split Products (FSP)

(<10 µg/mL).

Increased: Disseminated intravascular coagulation (DIC) (usually > 40 µg/mL), any thromboembolic condition (deep venous thrombosis, myocardial infarction, pulmonary embolus), hepatic dysfunction, fibrinolytic therapy.

Fibrinogen

(200–400 mg/dL [SI: 2.0–4.0 g/L]).

Increased: Inflammatory reactions, oral contraceptives, pregnancy, cancer (kidney, stomach, breast).

Decreased: Disseminated intravascular coagulation (sepsis, amniotic fluid embolism, abruptio placentae), surgery (prostate, open heart), neoplastic and hematologic conditions, acute severe bleeding, burns, venomous snake bite, congenital.

Folic Acid, Serum Folate

(> 2.0 ng/mL [SI: >5 nmol/L]).

Folic Acid, RBC

(125–600 ng/mL [283–1360 nmol/L]).
   Serum folate can fluctuate with diet. RBC levels are more indicative of tissue stores. B_{12} deficiency can result in the inability of RBC to take up folate in spite of normal serum folate levels.

Increased: Folic acid administration.

Decreased: Malnutrition/malabsorption (folic acid deficiency), massive cellular growth (cancer), medications (trimethoprim, some anticonvulsants, oral contraceptives), vitamin B_{12} deficiency (low RBC levels), pregnancy.

Follicle Stimulating Hormone (FSH)

males: <22 IU/L; females: non-midcycle, <20 IU/L; midcycle surge, <40 IU/L (midcycle peak should be 2 times basal level; postmenopausal, 40–160 IU/L).

Increased: (Hypergonadotropic >40 IU/L), postmenopausal, surgical castration, gonadal failure, gonadotropin-secreting pituitary adenoma.

Decreased: (Hypogonadotropic <5 IU/L prepubertal), hypothalamic and pituitary dysfunction, pregnancy.

FTA-ABS (Fluorescent Treponemal Antibody Absorbed)

(normal = nonreactive).

Positive: Syphilis (test of choice to confirm diagnosis), other treponemal infections.(NOTE: May be negative in early primary syphilis and remain positive in spite of adequate treatment.)

Fungal Serologies

(negative <1:8).
    This is a complement-fixation fungal antibody screen that usually detects antibodies to members of the genera *Histoplasma, Blastomyces, Aspergillus,* and *Coccidioides* spp.

Gastrin, Serum

(fasting: <100 pg/mL [SI: 47.7 pmol/L], postprandial: 95–140 pg/mL [SI: 45.3–66.7 pmol/L]). NOTE: Patient must be off proton pump inhibitors or H_2 blockers.

Increased: Zollinger-Ellison syndrome, pyloric stenosis, pernicious anemia, atrophic gastritis, ulcerative colitis, renal insufficiency, steroid and calcium administration.

GGT (Gamma-Glutamyl Transpeptidase, SGGT)

(male 9–50 U/L; female 8–40 U/L).
    Generally parallels changes in serum alkaline phosphatase and 5′ nucleotidase in liver disease.

Increased: Liver disease (hepatitis, cirrhosis, obstruction, both intrinsic and extrinsic), pancreatitis, primary and metastatic neoplasms, medications (phenytoin, alcohol, barbiturates).

Glucose

(fasting, 70–105 mg/dL [SI: 3.89–5.83 nmol/L]; 2 h postprandial: <120 mg/dL [SI: <6.67 nmol/L]). To convert mg/dL to nmol/L, multiply by 0.05551.

Increased: Diabetes mellitus, Cushing's syndrome, acromegaly, increased epinephrine (injection, pheochromocytoma, stress, burns, etc), acute pancreatitis, adrenocorticotropic hormone (ACTH) administration, spurious increase caused by drawing blood from a site above an IV line containing dextrose, elderly patients, pancreatic glucagonoma, drugs (glucocorticoids, some diuretics).

Decreased: Pancreatic disorders (pancreatitis, islet cell tumors), extrapancreatic tumors (carcinoma of the adrenals, stomach), hepatic disease (hepatitis, cirrhosis, tumors), endocrine disorders (early diabetes, hypothyroidism, hypopituitarism), functional disorders (after gastrectomy), pediatric problems (prematurity, infant of a diabetic mother, ketotic hypoglycemia, enzyme diseases), exogenous insulin, oral hypoglycemic agents, malnutrition, sepsis.

Glucose Tolerance Test, Oral

(NOTE: If fasting blood glucose is > 140 mg/dL, the GTT is unnecessary.) Used to aid in the diagnosis of diabetes mellitus, especially when diagnosis cannot be made on the basis of fasting blood sugar levels. The test is unreliable in severe infection, prolonged fasting, or after insulin. After an overnight fast, a fasting blood glucose is drawn, and the patient is given a 75-g oral glucose load (100 g for gestational diabetes screening, 1.75 mg-kg ideal body weight in children up to 75 g). Plasma glucose is then drawn at 30, 60, 120, and 180 min.
Interpretation:
Adult Onset Diabetes: Any fasting blood sugar >140, or >200 at both 120 min and one other time interval measured.
   Gestational Diabetes: At least two of the following: any fasting blood sugar >105, at 60 min >190, at 120 min >165, or at 180 min >145.

Glycohemoglobin (Hemoglobin A$_{1c}$, Glycosylated Hemoglobin) (4.6–7.1%)

Increased: Diabetes mellitus (uncontrolled; reflects levels over preceding 3–4 mo).

Decreased: Chronic renal failure, hemolytic anemia, pregnancy, chronic blood loss.

Gram's Stain

Used in the identification of gram-negative and gram-positive bacteria.

Technique

1. Smear the specimen (sputum, peritoneal fluid, etc) on a glass slide in a fairly thin coat. If time permits, allow the specimen to air dry. The

smear may also be fixed under very low heat (excessive heat can cause artifacts). When a Bunsen burner is not available, other heat sources include a hot light bulb, or an alcohol swab set on fire. Heat the slide until it is warm, but not hot when touched to the back of the hand.

2. Timing for the stain is not critical, but at least 10 s should be allowed for each set of reagents.

3. Apply the crystal violet (Gram's stain), rinse the slide with tap water, apply iodine solution, and rinse with water.

4. Decolorize the slide carefully with the acetone-alcohol solution until the blue color is barely visible in the runoff. (This is the step where most Gram's stains are ruined.)

5. Counterstain with a few drops of safranin, rinse the slide with water, and blot it dry with lint-free bibulous or filter paper.

6. Use the high dry and oil immersion lenses on the microscope to examine the slide. If the Gram's stain is satisfactory, any polys on the slide should be pink with light blue nuclei. On a Gram's stain of sputum, an excessive number of epithelial cells means the sample was more saliva than sputum.

Gram's Stain Characteristics Of Common Pathogens

Gram-Positive Cocci: *Staphylococcus, Streptococcus, Diplococcus, Micrococcus, Peptococcus* (anaerobic), and *Peptostreptococcus* (anaerobic) species. (If *Staphylococcus* initially is reported as coagulase positive, suspect *S aureus;* if coagulase is negative, suspect *S epidermidis.*)

Gram-Positive Rods: *Clostridium* (anaerobic), *Corynebacterium, Listeria,* and *Bacillus* species.

Gram-Negative Cocci: *Neisseria (Branhamella)* species.

Gram-Negative Coccoid Rods: *Haemophilus, Pasteurella, Brucella,* and *Bordetella* species.

Gram-Negative Straight Rods: *Escherichia, Salmonella, Shigella, Proteus, Enterobacter, Klebsiella, Serratia, Pseudomonas, Providencia, Yersinia, Acinetobacter (Mima, Herellea), Eikenella, Legionella, Bacteroides* (anaerobic), *Fusobacterium* (anaerobic), and *Campylobacter* (comma-shaped) species.

5-HIAA 5-Hydroxyindoleacetic Acid (24-h Urine)

(2–8 mg [SI: 10.4–41.6] μmol/24-h urine collection).

5-HIAA is a serotonin metabolite and is useful to diagnose carcinoid syndrome.

Increased: Carcinoid tumors (usually metastatic), certain foods (avocado, banana, pineapple, tomato), phenothiazine derivatives.

Haptoglobin

(40–180 mg/dL [SI: 0.4–1.8 g/L]).

Increased: Obstructive liver disease, any cause if increased erythrocyte sedimentation rate (ESR) (inflammation, collagen-vascular diseases).

Decreased: Any type of hemolysis (transfusion reaction, etc), liver disease, anemia, oral contraceptives.

Helicobacter Pylori Serology

(normal = negative).
  Most patients with gastritis and ulcer disease (gastric or duodenal) have chronic *H pylori* infection that should be treated. Positive in 35–50% asymptomatic patients (increases with age). Use in dyspepsia controversial.

Hepatitis Testing

Recommended hepatitis panel tests based on clinical settings is shown in Table II–6. Interpretation of testing patterns is shown in Table II–7.

Specific Hepatitis Tests

HBsAg	Hepatitis B surface antigen (formerly Australia antigen, HAA). Indicates either chronic or acute infection with hepatitis B. Used by blood banks to screen donors.
Total Anti-HBc	IgG and IgM antibody to hepatitis B core antigen; confirms either previous exposure to hepatitis B virus (HBV) or ongoing infection. Used by blood banks to screen donors.
Anti-HBc IgM	IgM antibody to hepatitis B core antigen. Early and best indicator of acute infection with hepatitis B.
HBeAg	Hepatitis Be antigen; when present, indicates high degree of infectivity. Order only when evaluating a patient with chronic HBV infection.
Anti-HBe	Antibody to hepatitis Be antigen; presence associated with resolution of active inflammation, but often signifies virus is integrated into host DNA, especially if the host remains HBsAg positive.
Anti-HBs	Antibody to hepatitis B surface antigen; when present, typically indicates immunity associated with clinical recovery from HBV infection or previous immunization with hepatitis B vaccine. Order only to assess effectiveness of vaccine and request titer levels.
Anti-HAV	Total antibody to hepatitis A virus; confirms previous exposure to hepatitis A virus.

TABLE II–6. HEPATITIS PANEL TESTING TO GUIDE IN THE ORDERING OF HEPATITIS PROFILES FOR GIVEN CLINICAL SETTINGS.

Medical Setting	Test	Purpose
Screening tests		
Pregnancy	• HBsAg	All expectant mothers should be screened during 3rd trimester.
High risk patients on admission (homosexuals, dialysis patients)	• HBsAg	To screen for chronic or active infection.
Percutaneous inoculation (donor)	• HBsAg • Anti-HBc IgM • Anti-hepatitis C	To test patients blood (especially dialysis patients and HIV-infected individuals) for infectivity with HBV and HCV if health care worker exposed.
Percutaneous inoculation (victim)	• HBsAg • Anti-HBc • Anti-hepatitis C	To test exposed health care worker for immunity or chronic infection.
Pre-HBV vaccine	• Anti-HBc • Anti-HBs	To determine if an individual is infected or has antibodies to HBV.
Screening blood donors	• HBsAg • Anti-HBc • Anti-hepatitis C	Used by blood banks to screen donors for hepatitis B and C.
Diagnostic tests		
Differential diagnosis of acute jaundice, hepatitis, or fulminant liver failure	• HBsAg • Anti-HBc IgM • Anti-HAV IgM • Anti-hepatitis C	To differentiate between HBV, HAV, and HCV in acutely jaundiced patient with hepatitis or fulminant liver failure.
Chronic hepatitis	• HBsAg +HBeAg +Anti-HBe +Anti hepatitis D (total +Igm)	To diagnose HBV infection + if positive for HBsAg to determine infectivity + if HBsAg patient worsens or is very ill, to diagnose concomitant infection with hepatitis delta virus.
Monitor		
Infant follow-up	• HBsAg • Anti-HBc • Anti-HBs	To monitor the success of vaccination and passive immunization for perinatal transmission of HBV 12–15 mo after birth.
Postvaccination screening	• Anti-HBs	To ensure immunity has been achieved after vaccination (CDC mends titer determination, but usually qualitiative assay adequate).
Sexual contact	• HBsAg • Anti-HBc • Anti-hepatitis C	To monitor sexual partners of patient with chronic HBV or HCV.

Source: Reproduced, with permission, from Gomella LG (editor): Diagnosis: Chemistry, Immunology, and Serology. In: Clinician's Pocket Reference, *9/e, McGraw Hill, 2000.*

TABLE II–7. INTERPRETATION OF VIRAL HEPATITIS SEROLOGIC TESTING PATTERNS.

Anti-HAV (IgM)	HBsAg	Anti-HBc (Igm)	Anti-HBc (Total)	Anti-HCV (Elisa)	Interpretation
+	—	—	—	—	Acute hepatitis A
+	+	—	+	—	Acute hepatitis A in hepatitis B carrier
—	+	—	+	—	Chronic hepatitis B[a]
—	—	+	+	—	Acute hepatitis B
—	+	+	+	—	Acute hepatitis B
—	—	—	+	—	Past hepatitis B infection
—	—	—	—	+	Hepatitis C[b]
—	—	—	—	—	Early hepatitis C or other cause (other virus, toxic, etc)

[a]Patients with chronic hepatitis B (either active hepatitis or carrier state) should have HBeAg and Anti-HBc checked to determine activity of infection and relative infectivity. Anti-HBs is used to determine response to hepatitis B vaccination.
[b]Anti-HCV often takes 3–6 months before being positive. Replaced by more sensitive tests, eg, HCV-RNA PCR.

Anti-HAV IgM	IgM antibody to hepatitis A virus; indicative of recent infection with hepatitis A virus.
Anti-HDV	Total antibody to delta hepatitis; confirms previous exposure. Order only in patients with known acute or chronic HBV infection.
Anti-HDV IgM	IgM antibody to delta hepatitis; indicates recent Infection. Order only in patients with known acute or chronic HBV infection.
Anti-HCV	Antibody against hepatitis C (formerly known as non-A, non-B hepatitis) and is the major cause of post-transfusion hepatitis. Used by blood banks to screen donors. Many false positives.
HCV-RNA PCR	Useful to detect Hepatitis C infection before antibodies rise; associated with viremia.

High Density Lipoprotein Cholesterol (see Cholesterol, page 282)

HLA (Human Leukocyte Antigens; HLA Typing)

This test identifies a group of antigens on the cell surface that are the primary determinants of histocompatibility and are useful in assessing transplantation compatibility. Some are associated with specific diseases, but are not diagnostic of these diseases.

HLA-B27: Ankylosing spondylitis, psoriatic arthritis, Reiter's syndrome, juvenile rheumatoid arthritis.

HLA-DR4/HLA DR2: Chronic Lyme disease arthritis.

HLA-DRw2: Multiple sclerosis.

HLA-B8: Addison's disease, juvenile onset diabetes, Grave's disease, gluten sensitive enteropathy.

Human Immunodeficiency Virus (HIV) Testing

(Normal = negative).
   Used in the diagnosis of acquired immunodeficiency syndrome (AIDS) and to screen blood for use in transfusion. NOTE: CDC guidelines indicate that any HIV-positive person older than 13 years with a CD4+ T-cell level < 200/µL or an HIV-positive person with a series of indicator conditions (such as pulmonary candidiasis, disseminated histoplasmosis, HIV wasting, Kaposi's sarcoma, TB, various lymphomas, *Pneumocystis carinii,* pneumonia, and others) is considered to have AIDS. If HIV-EIA is positive, confirm with Western blot. Next, confirm with HIV RNA viral load and CD4/CD8 ratio to stage disease.

HIV-EIA: Enzyme-linked immunosorbent assay to detect HIV antibody; a positive test should be confirmed by Western blot.

Positive: AIDS, asymptomatic HIV infection, false-positive (recent administration of flu vaccine, dialysis, alcoholic hepatitis, positive RPR, hypergammaglobulinemia, others).

HIV Western Blot

(normal = negative).
   The reference procedure for confirming the presence or absence of HIV antibody, usually after a positive HIV antibody by ELISA determination. Polymerase chain reaction (PCR) may become the confirmatory test for HIV.

Positive: AIDS, asymptomatic HIV infection (if indeterminate, repeat in 1 mo).

HIV RNA ("Viral Load")

Earliest marker of HIV infection, positive within 2 wk of infection. Used to monitor therapy and/or progression.

P24 Antigen Assay: Specific for HIV infection; largely replaced by RNA assay.

HIV CD4 Counts

Widely used predictor of opportunistic infection and HIV progression (likely with counts <200 cells/µL). Used to guide therapeutic intervention (usually < 500 cells/µL).

Human Chorionic Gonadotropin, Serum (HCG, Beta Subunit)

(Normal, <3.0 mIU/mL; 7–10 d post-conception, >3 mIU/mL; 30 d, 100–5000 mIU/mL; 10 wk, 50,000–140,000 mIU/mL; >16 wk, 10,000–50,000 mIU/mL; thereafter, levels slowly decline) [SI units IU/L equivalent to mIU/mL](see also Urinary HCG).

Increased: Pregnancy, testicular tumors, trophoblastic disease (hydatidiform mole, choriocarcinoma levels usually > 100,000 mIU/mL).

Iron

(males: 65–175 µg/dL [SI: 11.64–31.33 µmol/L]; females: 50–170 µg/dL [SI: 8.95–30.43 µmol/L]). To convert µg/dL to µmol/l , multiply by 0.1791.

Increased: Hemochromatosis, hemosiderosis caused by excessive iron intake, excess destruction or decreased production of erythrocytes, liver necrosis.

Decreased: Iron deficiency anemia, nephrosis (loss of iron-binding proteins), normochromic anemia of chronic diseases and infections.

Iron-Binding Capacity (Total) (TIBC)

(250–450 µg/dL [SI: 44.75–80.55 µmol/L]).
    The normal iron/TIBC ratio is 20–50%; <15% is almost diagnostic of iron deficiency anemia. Increased ratio is seen with hemochromatosis.

Increased: Acute and chronic blood loss, iron deficiency anemia, hepatitis, oral contraceptives.

Decreased: Anemia of infection and chronic diseases, cirrhosis, nephrosis, hemochromatosis.

17-Ketogenic Steroids (17-KGS, Corticosteroids) (24-h Urine)

(males: 5–24 mg/d [17–83 µmol/d]; females: 4–15 mg/d [14–52 µmol/d]).
    Overall adrenal function test, largely replaced by serum or urine cortisol levels.

Increased: Adrenal hyperplasia (Cushing's syndrome), adrenogenital syndrome.

Decreased: Panhypopituitarism, Addison's disease, acute steroid withdrawal.

17-Ketosteroids,Total (17-KS) (24-h Urine)

(adult male: 8–20 mg/d [28–69 μmol/L]; adult female: 6–15 mg/dL [21–52 μmol/L] (NOTE: Lower values in prepubertal children).

Measures dehydroepiandrosterone (DHEA), androstenedione (adrenal androgens); largely replaced by assay of individual elements.

Increased: Adrenal cortex abnormalities (hyperplasia [Cushing's disease], adenoma, carcinoma, adrenogenital syndrome), severe stress, adrenocorticotropic hormone (ACTH) or pituitary tumor, testicular interstitial tumor and arrhenoblastoma (both produce testosterone).

Decreased: Panhypopituitarism, Addison's disease, castration in men.

KOH Preparation (Potassium Hydroxide Wet Mount)

KOH preps are used for diagnosis of fungal infections.

Technique

1. Apply the specimen (vaginal secretion, sputum, skin scrapings) to a slide.
2. Add 1–2 drops of 10% KOH solution and mix. Gentle heating may help.
3. Put a coverslip over the specimen and examine the slide for branching hyphae and blastospores that indicate the presence of a fungus. KOH should destroy most elements other than fungus. If there is dense keratin and debris, allow the slide to sit for several hours and then repeat the microscopic examination. Lowering the substage condenser will give better contrast between organisms and the background.

Positive: Filaments, hyphae, spores, budding yeast suggest fungal infection; note that false positives can be seen with cotton or cellulose fibers that may be mistaken for hyphae.

Lactate Dehydrogenase (LDH)

(adults <200 U/L, higher levels in childhood).

Increased: Acute myocardial infarction, pulmonary embolus, cardiac surgery, pernicious anemia, malignant tumors, AIDS-related lymphoma, *Pneumocystis carinii* pneumonia, hemolysis (prosthetic valve, anemias or factitious), renal infarction, muscle injury, megaloblastic anemia, liver disease (hepatitis, obstructive jaundice, medications).

LDH Isoenzymes (LDH 1 to LDH 5): Normally, the ratio LDH 1/LDH 2 is <0.6–0.7. If the ratio becomes >1 (also termed "flipped"), suspect a recent myocardial infarction (change in ratio can also be seen in pernicious or hemolytic anemia). With an acute myocardial infarction, the LDH will begin to rise at 12–48 h, peak at 3–6 d and return to normal at 8–14 d. LDH 5 is >LDH 4 in liver diseases.

Lactic Acid (Lactate)

(4.5–19.8 mg/dL [SI: 0.5–2.2 mmol/L]).

Increased: Lactic acidosis due to hypoxia, hemorrhage, shock, sepsis, cirrhosis, exercise, ethanol, DKA, regional ischemia (extremity, bowel) spurious (prolonged tourniquet).

LE (Lupus Erythematosus) Preparation

(normal = no cells seen).

Positive: Systemic lupus erythematosus (SLE), scleroderma, rheumatoid arthritis, drug-induced lupus (procainamide, others).

Lipase

(0–1.5 U/mL [SI: 10–150 U/L] by turbidimetric method).

Increased: Acute and chronic pancreatitis, pancreatic pseudocyst, pancreatic duct obstruction (stone, stricture, tumor, drug-induced spasm), gastric malignancy, intestinal perforation, fat embolus syndrome, renal failure, diabetes (usually in DKA only), dialysis (usually normal in mumps).

Low Density Lipoprotein-Cholesterol (LDL, LDL-C)

(see Cholesterol, page 282).

Luteinizing Hormone, Serum (LH)

(males: 7–24 IU/L; females: 6–30 IU/L, midcycle peak increase 2–3-fold over baseline).

Increased: (Hypergonadotropic >40 IU/L), postmenopausal, surgical or radiation castration, ovarian or testicular failure, polycystic ovaries.

Decreased: (Hypogonadotropic <40 IU/L prepubertal), hypothalamic, and pituitary dysfunction, Kallmann's syndrome.

Lyme Disease Serology

(normal varies with assay).

Most useful when comparing acute and convalescent serum levels to compare titers. Marked interlaboratory variability is present.

Positive: Infection with *Borrelia burgdorferi* (some cross reactivity with antibodies to Epstein-Barr, syphilis, rickettsia).

Lymphocyte Subsets

Specific monoclonal antibodies are used to identify specific T and B cells. Lymphocyte subsets (also called lymphocyte marker assays, or T- and B-cell assay) are useful in the diagnosis of acquired immune deficiency syndrome, and various leukemias and lymphomas. The designation CD ("clusters of differentiation") has largely replaced the older antibody designations (such as Leu 3a, or OKT3). Results are most reliable when reported as an absolute number of cells/μL rather than a percentage of cells. CD4/CD8 ratio < 1 is seen in patients with AIDS. Absolute CD4 count is used to guide HIV therapy.

Normal Lymphocyte Subsets

- Total lymphocytes 0.66–4.60 thousand/μL
- T-cell 644-2201 μL (60–88%)
- B-cell 82-392 μL (3–20%)
- T-helper/inducer cell (CD4,Leu 3a,OKT4) 493–1191 μL (34–67%)
- Suppressor/cytotoxic T cell (CD8, Leu 2, OKT8) 182–785 μL (10–42%)
- CD4/CD8 ratio > 1

Magnesium

(1.6–2.6 mg/dL [SI: 0.80–1.30 mmol/L]).

Increased: Renal failure, hypothyroidism, magnesium-containing antacids, Addison's disease, diabetic coma, severe dehydration, lithium intoxication.

Decreased: Malabsorption, steatorrhea, alcoholism and cirrhosis, hyperthyroidism, aldosteronism, diuretics, acute pancreatitis, hyperparathyroidism, hyperalimentation, nasogastric suctioning, chronic dialysis, renal tubular acidosis, drugs (cisplatin, amphotericin B, aminoglycosides), hungry bone syndrome, hypophosphatemia, intracellular shifts with respiratory or metabolic acidosis.

Metanephrines (24-h Urine)

<1.3 mg/d [<7.1 μmol/d] for adults, but variable in children.

These are metabolic products of epinephrine and norepinephrine, a primary screening test for pheochromocytoma.

Increased: Pheochromocytoma, neuroblastoma (neural crest tumors), false positive with drugs (phenobarbital, guanethidine, hydrocortisone, others).

MHA-TP (Microhemagglutination, *Treponema pallidum*)

(normal < 1:160).

Confirmatory test for syphilis, similar to FTA-ABS. Once positive, it remains so; therefore, it cannot be used to judge the effect of treatment. False positives with other treponemal infections (pinta, yaws, etc), mononucleosis, and systemic lupus.

Monospot

(normal = negative).

Positive: Mononucleosis, rarely in leukemia, serum sickness, Burkitt's lymphoma, viral hepatitis, rheumatoid arthritis.

Nucleotidase

(2–15 U/L).

Used in the workup of increased alkaline phosphatase and biliary obstruction.

Increased: Obstructive/cholestatic liver disease, liver metastasis, biliary cirrhosis.

Osmolality, Serum

(278–298 mOsm/kg [SI: 278–298 mmol/kg]).

A rough estimation of osmolality is [2(sodium) + BUN/2.8 + glucose/18]. Measured value is usually greater than calculated value. If measured is 15 mOsm/kg > than calculated, consider methanol, ethanol, or ethylene glycol ingestion.

Increased: Hyperglycemia, alcohol ingestion, increased sodium because of water loss (diabetes, hypercalcemia, diuresis), ethylene glycol ingestion, mannitol.

Decreased: Low serum sodium, diuretics, Addison's disease, inappropriate antidiuretic hormone (ADH) (syndrome of inappropriate ADH [SIADH], seen in bronchogenic carcinoma, hypothyroidism), iatrogenic causes (poor fluid balance).

Osmolality, Urine (see Urine, Spot)

Oxygen, Arterial (Po$_2$) (see Table II–1)

See Section VI and Problem 74 "Ventilator Management."

Decreased: Ventilation-perfusion ($\dot{V}/\dot{Q}$) abnormalities, COPD (asthma, emphysema), atelectasis, pneumonia, pulmonary embolus, respiratory distress syndrome, pneumothorax, TB, cystic fibrosis, obstructed airway.

Alveolar hypoventilation: Skeletal abnormalities, neuromuscular disorders, Pickwickian syndrome.

Decreased pulmonary diffusing capacity: Pneumoconiosis, pulmonary edema, pulmonary fibrosis (Bleomycin).

Right to left shunt: Congenital heart disease (Tetralogy of Fallot, transposition, etc).

pH, Arterial

(see Table II–1).

Increased: Metabolic and respiratory alkalosis (see also On Call Problems 2, "Acidosis: Metabolic," and 3, "Acidosis: Respiratory").

Decreased: Metabolic and respiratory acidosis (see also On Call Problems 7, "Alkalosis: Metabolic," and 8, "Alkalosis: Respiratory").

P-24 Antigen (HIV Core Antigen)

(normal = negative).
   Used to diagnose recent acute HIV infection; can be positive as early as 2–4 wk but becomes undetectable during antibody seroconversion (periods of latency). With progression of disease, P-24 usually becomes evident again.

Parathyroid Hormone (PTH)

(normal based on serum calcium provided on the lab report; values vary depending on whether the N-terminal, C-terminal, or mid-molecule is measured. PTH mid molecule, 0.29–0.85 ng/mL [SI: 29–85 pmol/L]; with calcium, 8.4–10.2 mg/dL [SI: 2.1–2.55 mmol/L]).

Increased: Primary hyperparathyroidism, secondary hyperparathyroidism (hypocalcemic states such as chronic renal failure, others), drugs (furosemide, lithium).

Decreased: Hypercalcemia not due to hyperparathyroidism (ie, malignancy), hypoparathyroidism, hyperthyroidism.

Partial Thromboplastin Time (Activated Partial Thromboplastin Time, PTT, APTT)

(27–38 s).

Increased: Heparin and any defect in the intrinsic coagulation system (includes Factors I, II, V, VIII, IX, X, XI, and XII), prolonged use of a tourniquet before drawing a blood sample, hemophilia A and B.

Decreased: DIC.

Phosphorus

(adult: 2.5–4.5 mg/dL [SI: 0.81–1.45 mmol/L], child: 4.0–6.0 mg/dL [SI: 1.29–1.94 mmol/L]). To convert mg/dL to mmol/L, multiply by 0.3229.

Increased: Hypoparathyroidism (surgical, pseudohypoparathyroidism), excess vitamin D, secondary hyperparathyroidism, renal failure, bone disease (healing fractures), Addison's disease, childhood, factitious increase (hemolysis of specimen).

Decreased: Hyperparathyroidism, alcoholism, diabetes, hyperalimentation, acidosis, alkalosis, gout, salicylate poisoning, IV steroid, glucose and/or insulin administration, hyperparathyroidism, hypokalemia, hypomagnesemia, diuretics, vitamin D deficiency, phosphate-binding antacids.

Potassium, Serum

(3.5–5 mEq/L [SI: 3.5–5 mmol/L]).

Increased: Factitious increase (hemolysis of specimen, thrombocytosis), renal failure, Addison's disease, acidosis, dehydration, hemolysis, massive tissue damage, excess intake (oral or IV), potassium-containing medications, drugs (spironolactone, triamterene, pentamidine, NSAIDs).

Decreased: Diuretics, decreased intake, vomiting, nasogastric suctioning, villous adenoma, diarrhea, Zollinger-Ellison syndrome, chronic pyelonephritis, renal tubular acidosis (I and II), metabolic alkalosis (primary aldosteronism, Cushing's syndrome).

Potassium, Urine

(see Urine, Spot, page 315).

Progesterone

Used to confirm ovulation and corpus luteum function.

Phase	Normal Values(Female)
Follicular	<1 ng/mL
Luteal	5–20 ng/mL
Pregnancy 1st trimester	10–30 ng/mL
2nd trimester	50–100 ng/mL
3rd trimester	100–400 ng/mL
Postmenopause	<1 ng/mL

Prolactin

(males 1–20 ng/mL [SI: 1–20 µg/L]; females 1–25 ng/mL [SI: 1–25 µg/L]).

Increased: Pregnancy, nursing after pregnancy, prolactinoma, hypothalamic tumors, sarcoidosis or granulomatous disease of the hypothalamus, hypothyroidism, renal failure, Addison's disease, phenothiazines, haloperidol.

Prostate-Specific Antigen (PSA)

(<4 ng/dL by monoclonal, eg, Hybritech assay).

Most useful as a measure of response to therapy of prostate cancer; approved for screening for prostate cancer. Although any elevation increases suspicion of prostate cancer, levels > 10.0 ng/dL are associated with carcinoma at the 90% confidence level. Age-corrected levels gaining popularity (40–50 y, 2.5 ng/dl; 50–60 y, 3.5 ng/dl; 60–70 y, 4.5 ng/dl; >70 y, 6.5 ng/dl).

Increased: Prostate cancer, acute prostatitis, some cases of benign prostatic hypertrophy (BPH), prostatic infarction, prostate surgery (biopsy, resection), vigorous prostatic massage (routine rectal exam does not elevate levels).

Decreased: Radical prostatectomy, response to therapy of prostatic carcinoma (radiation or hormonal therapy).

PSA Density (PSAD): Ratio of prostate specific antigen (PSA) level to prostate size, as measured by transrectal ultrasound (TRUS). Proposed as a method to differentiate an elevated PSA between 4.0 and 10.0 ng/mL. A PSAD of 0.15 or greater would warrant prostate biopsy.

PSA Velocity: A rate of rise in PSA of 0.75 ng/mL or greater per year on the basis of at least three separate assays 6 mo apart is suspicious for prostate cancer.

PSA Free and Total: Patients with prostate cancer tend to have lower free PSA levels in proportion to total PSA. Measurement of the free/total PSA can improve the specificity of PSA as a screening test. In mildly elevated PSA (4.0–10.0 ng/mL), patients should have a prostate biopsy only if the free PSA percentage is low. Threshold for biopsy is controversial, ranging from less than 15% to less than 25%, with a higher threshold having improved sensitivity and a lower threshold having improved specificity.

Protein, Serum

(6.0–8.0 g/dL).

Increased: Multiple myeloma, Waldenström's macroglobulinemia, benign monoclonal gammopathy, lymphoma, chronic inflammatory disease, sarcoidosis.

Decreased: Malnutrition, inflammatory bowel disease, Hodgkin's disease, leukemias, any cause of decreased albumin.

Protein, Urine

(24-h Urine, < 150 mg/d [< 0.15 g/d]).

Increased: (see Urinalysis Differential Diagnosis, page 314), nephrotic syndrome usually associated with >4 g/d.

Prothrombin Time (PT)

(11.5–13.5 seconds).

(Some labs report the International Normalized Ratio [INR] instead of the Patient/Control ratio to guide anticoagulant [Coumadin] therapy.)

	PT Patient/Control Ratio	INR
Normal	0.9–1.1	0.75–1.30
Therapeutic	1.5–2.5	2.0–4.5

PT evaluates the extrinsic clotting mechanism that includes Factors I, II, V, VII, and X and not altered by heparin.

Increased: Drugs (sodium warfarin [Coumadin]), vitamin K deficiency, fat malabsorption, liver diseases, prolonged use of a tourniquet before drawing a blood sample, disseminated intravascular coagulation (DIC).

RBC Morphology

The following lists some erythrocyte abnormalities and the associated conditions. General terms include poikilocytosis (irregular RBC shape such as sickle and Burr) and anisocytosis (irregular RBC size such as microcytes and macrocytes).

Basophilic Stippling: Lead or heavy metal poisoning, thalassemia, severe anemia.

Howell-Jolly Bodies: After splenectomy, some severe hemolytic anemias, pernicious anemia, leukemia, thalassemia.

Sickling: Sickle cell disease and trait.

Nucleated RBCs: Severe bone marrow stress (hemorrhage, hemolysis, etc), marrow replacement by tumor, extramedullary hematopoiesis.

Target Cells (Leptocytes): Thalassemia, hemoglobinopathies, obstructive jaundice, any hypochromic anemia, after splenectomy.

Spherocytes: Hereditary spherocytosis, immune or microangiopathic hemolysis, severe burns, ABO transfusion reactions.

Helmet Cells (Schistocytes): Microangiopathic hemolysis, hemolytic transfusion reaction, transplant rejection, other severe anemias, TTP.

Burr Cells (Acanthocytes): Severe liver disease, high levels of bile, fatty acids, or toxins.

Polychromasia (Basophilia): The appearance of a bluish-gray red cell on routine Wright's stain suggests reticulocytes.

Renin, Plasma (Plasma Renin Activity [PRA])

(adults: normal sodium diet, upright 1–6 ng/mL/h [SI: 0.77–4.6 nmol/L/h]. Renal vein renin: L & R should be equal).

Useful in the diagnosis of hypertension associated with hypokalemia. Values highly dependent upon salt intake and position. Stop diuretics, estrogens for 2–4 wk before testing.

Increased: Medications (ACE inhibitors, diuretics, oral contraceptives, estrogens) pregnancy, dehydration, renal artery stenosis, adrenal insufficiency, chronic hypokalemia, upright posture, salt-restricted diet, edematous conditions (CHF, nephrotic syndrome), secondary hyperaldosteronism.

Decreased: Primary aldosteronism (renin will not increase with relative volume depletion, upright posture).

Renin, Renal Vein

(normal L & R should be equal).

A ratio of > 1.5 (affected/non-affected) suggestive of renovascular hypertension.

Reticulocyte Count

(normal corrected reticulocyte count is < 1.5 %).

This is reported as a percentage, and you should calculate the corrected reticulocyte count for interpretation of the results (corrected reticulocyte count = reported count × patient's HCT/normal HCT). This corrected count is an excellent indicator of erythropoietic activity. Normal marrow responds to a decrease in erythrocytes (shown by a decreased hematocrit) with an increase in the production of reticulocytes. Lack of increase in a reticulocyte count in an anemic patient suggests a chronic disease, a deficiency disease, marrow replacement, or marrow failure.

Retinol-Binding Protein (RBP)

(adults: 3–6 mg/dL; children: 1.5–3.0 mg/dL).

Decreased: Malnutrition, vitamin A deficiency, intestinal malabsorption of fats, chronic liver disease.

Rheumatoid Factor (RA Latex Test)

(< 15 IU by Microscan kit or <1:40).

Increased: Rheumatoid arthritis, systemic lupus erythematosus (SLE), syphilis, chronic inflammation, subacute bacterial endocarditis (SBE), some lung diseases.

Sedimentation Rate (Erythrocyte Sedimentation Rate, ESR)

Wintrobe Scale: Males: 0–9 mm/h, females: 0–20 mm/h.

ZETA Scale: 40–54%, normal; 55–59%, mildly elevated; 60–64%, moderately elevated; >65%, markedly elevated.

Westergren Scale: Males: <50 years, 15 mm/h; >50 years, 20 mm/h; females: <50 years, 20 mm/h; >50 years, 30 mm/h.
   ESR is a very nonspecific test. ZETA rate is not affected by anemia.

Increased: Any type of infection, inflammation, rheumatic fever, endocarditis, neoplasm, acute myocardial infarction.

Semen Analysis

After 48–72 h of abstinence, semen specimen is collected in a wide mouth polypropylene container with a screw top. The sample is kept as close to body temperature as possible and delivered to the lab within 1 1/2 h. The following are general reference parameters and are typically determined on at least two specimens.

- Volume: 1.5–5.0 mL
- Appearance: white, viscid, opaque
- pH: 7.2–8.0
- Sperm density: >20 × 10^6/mL
- Total sperm count: >40 × 10^6/mL
- Motility: >60%
- Forward Progression: >50%
  or >2+ on a scale 0–4 (0, no movement; 4, excellent forward progression)
- Morphology: (>} 60% normal
- Viability: > 50% (by dye exclusion)
- Fructose, quantitative: > 13 micromol per ejaculate
- Liquification: 10–0 min (measured on a scale 0–4)
- Agglutination: Minimal clumping (increased clumping suggests inflammatory/immunologic process)

SGOT (Serum Glutamic-Oxaloacetic Transaminase) or AST (Serum Aspartate Aminotransaminase)

(8–20 U/L).
Generally parallels changes in SGPT in liver disease.

Increased: Acute myocardial infarction, liver disease, Reye's syndrome, muscle trauma and injection, pancreatitis, intestinal injury or surgery, factitious increase (erythromycin, opiates), burns, cardiac catheterization, brain damage, renal infarction.

Decreased: Beriberi, severe diabetes with ketoacidosis, liver disease.
SGPT (Serum Glutamic-Pyruvic Transaminase) or ALT (Alanine Aminotransaminase)
(8–20 U/L).
(NOTE: SGPT is elevated more than SGOT in viral hepatitis; SGOT is elevated more than SGPT in alcoholic hepatitis.)

Increased: Liver disease, liver cancer and metastasis, liver abscess, liver injury (ischemia, hypoxia), biliary obstruction, pancreatitis, liver congestion (CHF), medications.

Sodium, Serum

(136–145 mmol/L).

Increased: Associated with low total body sodium (glycosuria, mannitol, urea, excess sweating), normal total body sodium (diabetes insipidus [central and nephrogenic], respiratory losses, and sweating), and associated with increased total body sodium (administration of hypertonic sodium bicarbonate, Cushing's syndrome, hyperaldosteronism).

Decreased: Associated with excess total body sodium and water (nephrotic syndrome, congestive heart failure [CHF], cirrhosis, renal failure), associated with excess body water (syndrome of inappropriate antidiuretic hormone [SIADH], hypothyroidism, adrenal insufficiency), associated with decreased total body water and sodium (diuretic use, renal tubular acidosis, use of mannitol or urea, mineralocorticoid deficiency, vomiting, diarrhea, pancreatitis) and pseudohyponatremia (hyperlipidemia, hyperglycemia, and multiple myeloma).

Note: In factitious hyponatremia due to hyperglycemia, for every 100 mmol/L blood glucose above normal, serum sodium decreases 1.6. For example, assume a patient with a blood glucose of 800 mmol/L and a serum sodium of 129 mmol/L. This would factitiously lower serum sodium by about (7 × 1.6) or 11.2 mmol/L. Corrected serum sodium would therefore be 129 + 11 = 140 mmol/L.

Sodium, Urine (see Urine, Spot)

Stool, Occult Blood [Fecal Occult Blood] (Hemoccult Test) (negative)

Repeat three times for maximum yield. A positive test more informative than a negative test.

Positive: Swallowed blood, ingestion of rare red meat, any gastrointestinal (GI) tract ulcerated lesion (ulcer, carcinoma, polyp, diverticulosis, inflammatory bowel disease), hemorrhoids, telangiectasis, drugs that cause GI irritation (eg, NSAIDs), false positives (horseradish, large doses of vitamin C (>500 mg/d) and antacids interfere with test (false negatives).

Stool For White Blood Count (WBC)

(occasional WBC normal).

Increased: (usually polymorphonuclear leukocytes), *Shigella, Salmonella* spp, enteropathogenic *Escherichia coli,* ulcerative colitis, pseudomembranous colitis.

T$_3$ RIA (Triiodothyronine)

(120–195 ng/dL [SI: 1.85–3.00 nmol/L]).

Increased: Hyperthyroidism, T$_3$ thyrotoxicosis, oral estrogen, pregnancy, exogenous T$_4$.

Decreased: Hypothyroidism and euthyroid sick state, any cause of decreased thyroid-binding globulin.

T$_3$ RU (Resin Uptake)

(24–34%).

Increased: Hyperthyroidism, medications (phenytoin [Dilantin], steroids, heparin, aspirin, others), nephrotic syndrome.

Decreased: Hypothyroidism, pregnancy, medications (estrogens, iodine, propylthiouracil, others).

T$_4$ Total (Thyroxine)

(5–12 µg/dL [SI: 65–155 nmol/L]; males: >60 years, 5–10 µg/dL [SI: 65–129 nmol]; females: 5.5–10.5 µg/dL [SI: 71–135 nmol/L]).
Good screening test for hyperthyroidism.

Increased: Hyperthyroidism, exogenous thyroid hormone, estrogens, pregnancy, severe illness, euthyroid sick syndrome.

Decreased: Euthyroid sick syndrome.

Testosterone

(male free: 9–30 ng/dL, total, 300–1200 ng/dL; female, see following list).

Phase	Normal Values (Female)
Follicular	20–80 ng/dL
Midcycle peak	20–80 ng/d
Luteal	20–80 ng/dL
Postmenopause	10–40 ng/dL

Increased: Adrenogenital syndrome, ovarian stromal hyperthecosis, polycystic ovaries, menopause, ovarian tumors, hyperthyroidism, cirrhosis, adrenocortical tumors, trophoblastic disease during pregnancy, medications (oral contraceptives, anticonvulsants).

Decreased: Hypogonadism (primary and secondary testicular failure), LH-RH agonists, orchiectomy, uremia, hepatic failure, hypopituitarism, Klinefelter's syndrome, spironolactone, digoxin.

Thrombin Time

(10–14 s).
Elevation caused by failure of conversion of fibrinogen to fibrin.

Increased: Systemic heparin, disseminated intravascular coagulation (DIC), fibrinogen deficiency, congenitally abnormal fibrinogen molecules, systemic amyloidosis, fibrinolytic therapy.

Thyroxine Binding Globulin (TBG)

(21–52 µg/dL [SI: 270–669 nmol/L]).

Increased: Hypothyroidism, pregnancy, oral contraceptives, estrogens, hepatic disease, acute porphyria.

Decreased: Hyperthyroidism, androgens, anabolic steroids, prednisone, nephrotic syndrome, severe illness, surgical stress, phenytoin, hepatic disease.

Thyroglobulin

(1–20 ng/mL).

Increased: Differentiated thyroid carcinomas (papillary, follicular), Graves' disease, nontoxic goiter.

Decreased: Hypothyroidism, total thyroidectomy, testosterone, steroids, phenytoin.

Thyroid-Stimulating Hormone (TSH)

(0.7–5.3 mU/mL).
Newer sensitive assay is an excellent screening test for hyperthyroidism as well as hypothyroidism. Allows differentiation between a low normal and a decreased TSH.

Increased: Hypothyroidism.

Decreased: Hyperthyroidism. Less than 1% of hypothyroidism is from pituitary or hypothalamic disease resulting in a decreased TSH.

Transferrin

(220–400 mg/dL [SI: 2.20–4.0 g/L]).

Increased: Acute and chronic blood loss, iron deficiency.

Decreased: Anemia of chronic disease, cirrhosis, nephrosis, hemochromatosis.

Triglycerides

(recommended values: males: 40–160 mg/dL [SI: 0.45–1.81 mmol/L]; females: 35–135 mg/dL [SI: 0.40–1.53 mmol/L]). Can vary with age.

Increased: Hyperlipoproteinemias (types I, IIb, III, IV, V), hypothyroidism, liver diseases, alcoholism, pancreatitis, acute myocardial infarction, nephrotic syndrome, familial increase.

Decreased: Malnutrition, congenital abetalipoproteinemia.

Troponin

(Troponin I < 0.35 ng/mL; Troponin T < 0.2 µg/L).
Used to diagnose acute MI; increases rapidly and may stay elevated for 5–7 d. More cardiac specific than CK-MB.

Uric Acid

(males: 3.4–7 mg/dL [SI: 202–416 µmol/L]; females: 2.4–6 mg/dL [SI: 143–357 µmol/L]). To convert mg/dL to µmol/L multiply by 59.58.

Increased: Gout, renal failure, destruction of massive amounts of nucleoproteins (leukemia, anemia, chemotherapy, toxemia of pregnancy), drugs (especially diuretics), lactic acidosis, hypothyroidism, polycystic kidney disease, parathyroid diseases.

Decreased: Uricosuric drugs (salicylates, probenecid, allopurinol), Wilson's disease, Fanconi's syndrome.

Urinalysis

Normal Values

1. Appearance: "yellow, clear," or "straw colored, clear."
2. Specific gravity: neonate: 1.012; Infant: 1.002–1.006; child and adult: 1.001–1.035 (with normal fluid intake 1.016–1.022).
3. pH: newborn/neonate: 5–7; child and adult: 4.6–8.0.
4. Negative for: bilirubin, blood, acetone, glucose, protein, nitrite, leukocyte esterase, reducing substances.
5. Trace: urobilinogen.
6. Sediment:
   Red Blood Count (RBC): male, 0–3/high power field (HPF); female 0–5/HPF.
   White Blood Count (WBC): 0–4/HPF.
   Epithelial cells: Occasional.
   Hyaline casts: Occasional.
   Bacteria: None.
   Crystals: Warm, fresh urine, none. (NOTE: Refrigeration or urine left standing at room temperature may precipitate various crystals.)

Differential Diagnosis for Routine Urinalysis

A. **Appearance**
   1. **Colorless:** Diabetes insipidus, diuretics, excess fluid intake.
   2. **Dark:** Acute intermittent porphyria, malignant melanoma.
   3. **Cloudy:** Urinary tract infection (pyuria), amorphous phosphate salts (normal in alkaline urine), blood, mucus, bilirubin.
   4. **Pink/red:** Blood, hemoglobin, myoglobin, food coloring, beets, ibuprofen.
   5. **Orange/Yellow:** Phenazopyridine (Pyridium), bile pigments.
   6. **Brown/black:** Myoglobin, bile pigments, melanin, cascara, iron, Macrodantin, alkaptonuria.
   7. **Green:** Urinary bile pigments, indigo carmine, methylene blue, Urised.
   8. **Foamy: Proteinuria, bile salts.**
   9. **pH**
   10. **Acid:** High protein (meat) diet, ammonium chloride, mandelic acid and other medications, acidosis, ketoacidosis (starvation, diabetic), chronic obstructive pulmonary disease (COPD).

11. **Basic:** Urinary tract infections (UTI), renal tubular acidosis, diet (high vegetable, milk, immediately after meals), sodium bicarbonate therapy, vomiting, metabolic alkalosis.

B. **Specific Gravity**
Usually corresponds with osmolarity except with osmotic diuresis. Value > 1.023 indicates normal renal concentrating ability.

Increased: Volume depletion; congestive heart failure (CHF); adrenal insufficiency; diabetes mellitus; inappropriate antidiuretic hormone (ADH); increased proteins (nephrosis); if markedly increased (1.040–1.050), suspect artifact or excretion of radiographic contrast media.

Decreased: Diabetes insipidus, pyelonephritis, glomerulonephritis, water-load with normal renal function.

C. **Bilirubin**

Positive: Obstructive jaundice (intra- and extrahepatic), hepatitis.

D. **Blood**

Positive: Stones, trauma, tumors (benign and malignant, anywhere in the urinary tract), urethral strictures, coagulopathy, infection, menses (contamination), polycystic kidneys, interstitial nephritis, hemolytic anemia, transfusion reaction, instrumentation (Foley catheter, etc).

Note: If the dipstick is positive for blood, but no red cells are seen, there may be free hemoglobin from trauma or a transfusion reaction or from lysis of RBCs (RBCs will lyse if the pH is < 5 or > 8), or there is myoglobin present because of a crush injury, burn, or tissue ischemia.

E. **Glucose**

Positive: Diabetes mellitus, pancreatitis, pancreatic carcinoma, pheochromocytoma, Cushing's disease, shock, burns, pain, steroids, hyperthyroidism, renal tubular disease, iatrogenic causes. (NOTE: Glucose oxidase technique in many kits is specific for glucose and will not react with lactose, fructose, or galactose.)

F. **Ketones** Detects primarily acetone and acetoacetic acid and not beta-hydroxybutyric acid.

Positive: Starvation, high fat diet, diabetic ketoacidosis, vomiting, diarrhea, hyperthyroidism, pregnancy, febrile states (especially in children).

G. **Nitrite** Many bacteria will convert nitrates to nitrite. (See also Leukocyte Esterase, below.)

Positive: Infection (A negative test does not rule out infection since some organisms such as *Streptococcus faecalis* and other gram-positive cocci will not produce nitrite, and the urine must also be retained in the bladder for several hours to allow the reaction to take place.)

H. Protein Persistent proteinuria by dipstick should be quantified by 24-h urine studies.

Positive: Pyelonephritis, glomerulonephritis, Kimmelstiel-Wilson syndrome (diabetes), nephrotic syndrome, myeloma, postural causes, pre-eclampsia, inflammation and malignancies of the lower tract, functional causes (fever, stress, heavy exercise), malignant hypertension, congestive heart failure (CHF).

I. Leukocyte Esterase

Positive: Infection (false positive with vaginal contamination).

J. Reducing Substance

Positive: Glucose, fructose, galactose, false positives (vitamin C, salicylates, antibiotics, etc).

K. Urobilinogen

Positive: Cirrhosis, congestive heart failure (CHF) with hepatic congestion, hepatitis, hyperthyroidism, suppression of gut flora with antibiotics.

Urine Sediment

Red Blood Cells (RBCs): Trauma, pyelonephritis, genitourinary TB, cystitis, prostatitis, stones, tumors (malignant and benign), coagulopathy, and any cause of blood on dipstick (see above).

White Blood Cells (WBCs): Infection anywhere in the urinary tract, TB, renal tumors, acute glomerulonephritis, radiation, interstitial nephritis (analgesic abuse).

Epithelial Cells: Acute tubular necrosis, necrotizing papillitis (most epithelial cells are from an otherwise unremarkable urethra).

Parasites: Trichomonas vaginalis, Schistosoma haematobium.

Yeast: Candida albicans (especially in diabetics, immunosuppressed patients, or if a vaginal yeast infection is present).

Spermatozoa: Normal in males immediately after intercourse or nocturnal emission.

Crystals:
Abnormal: Cystine, sulfonamide, leucine, tyrosine, cholesterol.
Normal (in small numbers)

Acid urine: Oxalate (small square crystals with a central cross), uric acid.
Alkaline urine: Calcium carbonate, triple phosphate (resemble coffin lids).
Contaminants: Cotton threads, hair, wood fibers, amorphous substances (all usually unimportant).
Mucus: Large amounts suggest urethral disease (normal from ileal conduit or other forms of urinary diversion).
Glitter Cells: White blood cells (WBCs) lysed in hypotonic solution.
Casts: The presence of casts in a urine localizes some or all of the disease process to the kidney itself.
Hyaline Cast: (acceptable unless they are "numerous"), benign hypertension, nephrotic syndrome, after exercise.
Red Blood Cell (RBC) Cast: Acute glomerulonephritis, lupus nephritis, subacute bacterial endocarditis (SBE), Goodpasture's disease, after a streptococcal infection, vasculitis, malignant hypertension.
White Blood Cell (WBC) Cast: Pyelonephritis.
Epithelial (tubular) Cast: Tubular damage, nephrotoxin, virus.
Granular Cast: Breakdown of cellular casts, lead to waxy casts. "Dirty brown granular casts" typical for acute tubular necrosis.
Waxy Cast: (end-stage of granular cast). Severe chronic renal disease, amyloidosis.
Fatty Cast: Nephrotic syndrome, diabetes mellitus, damaged renal tubular epithelial cells.
Broad Cast: Chronic renal disease.

Urine, Human Chorionic Gonadotropin (HCG)

(negative).
See also Serum HCG.

Positive: Pregnancy (may be positive by day 4, most positive by 14 d after expected menstrual date), testicular carcinoma (choriocarcinoma) hydatidiform mole.

Urine, Indices

Urinary indices are useful in the differential diagnosis of oliguria. They help differentiate prerenal from intrinsic renal causes (see Table II–8).

Urine, Spot (Random) Studies

The so-called spot urine is often ordered to aid in diagnosing various conditions, relying on only a small sample (10–20 mL) of urine.

TABLE II–8. URINARY INDICES.

Index	Prerenal	Renal (ATN)[a]
Urine osmolality (mOsm/kg)	>500	<350
Urinary sodium (mEq/L)	<20	>40
Urine/Serum creatinine	>40	>20
Urine/Serum osmolarity	>1.2	<1.2
Fractional excreted sodium (%)[b]	<1	<1.2
Renal failure index (RFI)(%)[c]	>1	>1

[a] Acute tubular necrosis (intrinsic renal failure)

[b] Fractional excreted sodium (%) $= \dfrac{\text{Urine Sodium / Serum Sodium}}{\text{Urine Creatinine / Serum Creatinine}} \times 100$

[c] Renal Failure Index (%) $= \dfrac{\text{Urine Sodium}}{\text{Urine Creatinine / Serum Creatinine}} \times 100$

Spot Urine for Electrolytes

The usefulness of this assay is limited because of large variations in daily fluid and salt intake, and the results are usually indeterminate if a diuretic has been given.

1. **Sodium** <10 mEq/L [mmol/L]: Volume depletion, hyponatremic states, prerenal azotemia (congestive heart failure [CHF], shock, etc), hepatorenal syndrome.
2. **Sodium** >20 mEq/L [mmol/L]: SIADH, acute tubular necrosis (usually > 40 mEq/L).
3. **Chloride** <10 mEq/L [mmol/L]: Chloride-sensitive metabolic alkalosis (vomiting, excessive diuretic use), volume depletion.
4. **Potassium** <10 mEq/L [mmol/L]: Hypokalemia, potassium depletion, extrarenal loss.

Spot Urine for Protein

(normal <10 mg/dL [0.1 g/L] or <20 mg/dL [0.2 g/L] for a sample taken in the early AM) (See page 314 for the differential diagnosis of protein in the urine.)

Spot Urine for Osmolality/Osmolarity

250–900 mOsm/kg [mmol/kg] (varies with water intake). Patients with normal renal function should concentrate > 800 mOsm/kg [mmol/kg] after a 14-h fluid restriction; <400 mOsm/kg [mmol/kg] is a sign of renal impairment.

Increased: Dehydration, syndrome of inappropriate antidiuretic hormone (SIADH), adrenal insufficiency, glycosuria, high-protein diet, intraoperatively, hypovolemia, medications (cyclophosphamide, vincristine).

Decreased: Excessive fluid intake, diabetes insipidus, acute renal failure, medications (acetohexamide, lithium, others).

Spot Urine for Myoglobin

(qualitative negative).

Positive: Skeletal muscle conditions (crush injury, electrical burns, carbon monoxide poisoning, delirium tremens, surgical procedures, malignant hyperthermia), polymyositis.

Vanillylmandelic Acid (VMA) (24-H Urine)

(<7–9 mg/d [SI: 35–45 µmol/L]).

VMA is the urinary product of both epinephrine and norepinephrine; good screening test for pheochromocytoma; also used to diagnose and follow-up neuroblastoma and ganglioneuroma.

Increased: Pheochromocytoma, other neural crest tumors (ganglioneuroma), factitious (chocolate, coffee, tea, monoamine oxidase [MAO] inhibitors, methyldopa).

VDRL Test (Venereal Disease Research Laboratory) or Rapid Plasma Reagin (RPR)

(normal = nonreactive).

Good for screening syphilis. Almost always positive in secondary syphilis but frequently becomes negative in late syphilis. Also, in some patients with HIV infection, the VDRL can be negative in primary and secondary syphilis.

Positive (Reactive): Syphilis, systemic lupus erythematosus, pregnancy and drug addicts. If reactive, confirm with FTA-ABS (false positives with bacterial or viral illnesses).

Vitamin B₁₂ (Extrinsic Factor, Cyanocobalamin)

(>100–700 pg/mL [SI: 74–516 pmol/L]).

Increased: Excessive intake, myeloproliferative disorders.

Decreased: Inadequate intake (especially strict vegetarians), malabsorption, hyperthyroidism, pregnancy.

WBC (White Blood Cell Count)

(see CBC, page 273).

WBC (White Blood Cell) Morphology

The following gives conditions associated with certain changes in the normal morphology of WBCs.

- Auer Rods: Acute myelogenous leukemias.
- Döhle's Inclusion Bodies: Severe infection, burns, malignancy, pregnancy.
- Hypersegmentation: Megaloblastic anemias.
- Toxic Granulation: Severe illness (sepsis, burn, high temperature).

Zinc

(60–130 µg/dL [SI: 9–20 µmol/L]).

Increased: Atherosclerosis, coronary artery disease.

Decreased: Inadequate dietary intake (parenteral nutrition, alcoholism), malabsorption, increased needs such as pregnancy or wound healing, acrodermatitis enteropathica.

III. Bedside Procedures

Before performing invasive procedures, you should remember the most important procedures of all—the patient's history and physical exam. The astute clinician using simpler, less-invasive studies can often obtain the same results as with a more complicated or more invasive procedure. When less invasive procedures do not aid in diagnosis or management, it is then that these advanced procedures should be used, accepting the associated risks and complications.

The key to any procedure, simple or difficult, is the setup. Anything that is or may be required should be on hand and ready to be used immediately before beginning the procedure.

Universal precautions should be used for any invasive procedure during which the operator can be exposed to potentially infectious body fluids. Not all patients infected with transmissible pathogens can be identified at the time of hospital admission or even later in their course. Because blood and body fluid-transmissible pathogens pose a hazard to personnel caring for these patients (primarily at the time of invasive procedures), certain precautions are now required for routine care of all patients regardless of whether they have been placed on isolation precautions of any type. The CDC defines universal precautions as follows:

1. Hands must be washed before and after all patient contact.
2. Hands must be washed before and after all invasive procedures.
3. Gloves must be worn in every instance in which contact with blood is certain or likely. For example, gloves must be worn for all venipunctures, IV starts, IV manipulation, wound care, etc.
4. Gloves must be worn once and discarded. They may not be worn to perform tasks on two different patients or two different tasks at different sites on the same patient.
5. Gloves must be worn in every instance in which contact with any body fluid is likely, including urine, feces, wound secretions, respiratory tract care, thoracenteses, paracenteses, etc.
6. A gown must be worn when splatter of blood or of body fluids on clothing seems likely.
7. Additional barrier precautions may be necessary for certain invasive procedures in which significant splatter or aerosol generation seems likely. This should not occur during most routine patient care activities. It may occur in certain instances in the operating room, emergency room, the ICUs, and during invasive procedures or cardiopulmonary resuscitation. Masks should always be worn when goggles are worn.

Patients should be counseled before any procedure about its necessity and its potential risks and benefits. Explaining the various steps can often make the patient more cooperative and the procedure easier. Some procedures (eg, bladder catheterization, nasogastric intubation, or venipuncture) do not require a written informed consent beyond normal hospital admission protocols. More invasive procedures (eg, thoracentesis, central venous catheterization or lumbar puncture) require a patient's written consent. Check your institution's practice guidelines for more information.

I. Arterial Line

(See also Section I, Problem 12, page 32).

Indications:
1. Frequent sampling of arterial blood.
2. Hemodynamic monitoring when continuous blood pressure readings are needed (eg, a patient on pressors).

Materials: Prepackaged arterial line set (eg, Arrow) or 20 gauge (or smaller) 1–2-inch IV catheter over needle assembly (Angiocath or other), arterial line setup per ICU routine (transducer, tubing and pressure bag with preheparinized saline), armboard, sterile dressing, povidone-iodine, 3-0 suture and instruments, lidocaine, 25-gauge needle and syringe.

Procedure:
1. Arteries in the order of preference are radial, femoral, and brachial. When using the radial artery, perform the modified Allen test to verify collateral flow in the ulnar artery. Be sure to document the results. Have the patient make a tight fist with the hand slightly flexed. Occlude both the radial and ulnar arteries at the wrist and have the patient open his hand. While maintaining pressure on the radial artery, release the ulnar artery. If the ulnar artery is patent, the hand should flush red within 6 s. If the Allen test is positive (no radial flow), the artery should probably not be used. If the Allen test is difficult to interpret, then use ultrasound to determine arterial flow.
2. When using the femoral artery, remember the mnemonic **NAVEL** to aid in locating the important structures in the groin. Palpate the femoral artery just below the inguinal ligament. From lateral to medial, the structures are **N**erve, **A**rtery, **V**ein, **E**mpty space, **L**ymphatic. The clinician may inject 1% lidocaine subcutaneously for anesthesia. Palpate the artery proximally and distally with two fingers or trap the artery between two fingers placed on either side of the vessel. When you are using the upper extremity, hyperextension of the joint will often bring the radial and brachial arteries closer to the surface.
3. Place the extremity on an armboard with a gauze roll behind the wrist to hyperextend the joint. Prepare the skin with povidone-iodine and drape the extremity with towels. The operator should wear gloves and mask, if possible.

4. Raise a tiny skin wheal at the puncture site with 1% lidocaine using a 25-gauge needle. Carefully palpate the artery and choose the puncture site where it appears most superficial.

5. **Standard technique:** See Figure III–1. While palpating the path of the artery with the left hand, advance the 20-gauge (preferably 2 in long) catheter over needle assembly into the artery at a 30-degree angle to the skin. Once a "flash" of blood is seen in the hub, advance the entire unit 1–2 mm, so that the needle and catheter are in the artery. If blood flow in the hub stops, carefully pull the entire unit back until flow is reestablished. Once the catheter is in the artery, hold the needle steady and advance the catheter over the needle into the artery. The catheter should slide smoothly into the artery. Withdraw the needle completely and check for arterial blood flow from the catheter. Briefly occlude the artery with manual pressure while the pressure tubing is being connected.

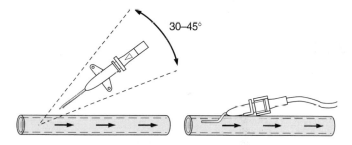

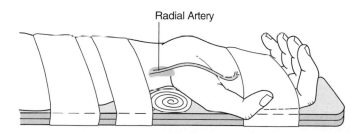

Figure III–1. Technique of radial artery catheterization. (*Reproduced, with permission, from Gomella TL (editor): Arterial Access. In:* Neonatology, *4th ed. Originally published by Appleton & Lange. Copyright © 1999 by The McGraw-Hill Companies, Inc.*)

Note: The pressure tubing system must be preflushed to clear all air bubbles before connection.

6. **Prepackaged technique:** Kits are available with a needle and guidewire that allow the Seldinger technique to be used. The entry needle is placed at a 30-degree angle to the skin site and is inserted until there is a flash of blood that rises in the catheter. The guidewire (orange handle in some kits) is inserted in the vessel and the catheter is advanced. The wire is removed and connected to the pressure tubing.

7. Alternative procedure ("through and through" technique): The approach to the artery is the same as in step no. 5, however, the artery is purposely punctured through both the anterior and the posterior walls. This method is probably most useful in children and infants. Once a flash of blood is seen in the hub, the entire unit is advanced together until blood no longer fills the hub. (This can be done in a single motion.) The entire unit is then withdrawn s-l-o-w-l-y until blood starts to fill the hub. The catheter is then advanced while the needle is withdrawn. The tubing is then connected as in step no. 5.

8. Suture in place with 3-0 silk and apply a secure and sterile dressing. Flush systems as necessary to ensure patency and also flush transducers to allow continuous blood pressure monitoring.

Complications: Infection, hemorrhage, thrombosis of the artery, emboli, pseudoaneurysm formation.

II. Bronchoscopy

Indications: Depending on the indication, either rigid or flexible fiberoptic bronchoscopy may be indicated.

1. Pulmonary toilet. For severe atelectasis, pneumonia, or aspiration. (rigid or flexible)
2. Foreign body retrieval (rigid)
3. Hemoptysis (rigid)
4. Assess injury (rigid or flexible)
5. Aid in a difficult intubation (flexible)

Equipment: Bronchoscope, either flexible or rigid, light source, sterile saline, suction, supplemental oxygen, monitors (pulse oximeter), (Fogarty catheters, epinephrine, gauze packing, for interventions as needed), sedatives, paralytics, topical lidocaine spray with epinephrine.

Procedure:

1. Often the ICU patient requiring bronchoscopy is already on a ventilator.
2. Ensure that the patient is adequately sedated, and if necessary, paralyzed for the procedure. Monitors (pulse oximeter, blood pressure)

should be on and properly functioning. The ventilator should be in a continuous mandatory mode and set to 100% oxygen.

3. A special connector is attached that will keep the tubing circuit closed and allow the flexible bronchoscope to be introduced without a break in the system and a loss of oxygen. Spray the posterior pharynx with topical lidocaine with epinephrine.

4. The flexible scope can then be passed through either the endotracheal or tracheostomy tube, ensuring that the tube is either securely in place or being held by an assistant. As a general rule, the endotracheal tube or the tracheostomy tube should be 1 mm more than the bronchoscope.

5. Pass the carina and examine both main bronchi and distal bronchioles.

6. For pulmonary toilet, irrigate with sterile saline, and suction secretions.

In an awake nonintubated patient, the preparation is the same. Sedation without paralysis is important as well as application of topical anesthetic to the posterior naso- and hypopharynx. Supplemental oxygen should be available. The patient's head should be extended. (Often a shoulder roll is helpful.) The flexible scope may be passed via the nose or mouth. When using the rigid scope, often, although not always, general anesthesia may be required. An oxygen source is connected to the rigid scope, and it is placed orally through the airway, allowing visualization of the trachea and mainstem bronchi. Interventions may then be performed through the rigid scope, as indicated.

Complications:

1. Trauma (to the oral cavity and tracheobronchial tree, with the use of the rigid scope)
2. Arrhythmias
3. Aspiration
4. Hypoxemia

The rigid bronchoscope is a special instrument rarely used outside of the operating room and, thus, it is not generally applicable to the critical care unit. The main advantage of this instrument is that a ventilator can be connected directly to it and the patient can be ventilated through the scope. This instrument requires special expertise to be used correctly.

III. Central Venous Catheterization

(See also Section I, Problem 19, page 58 and Peripherally Inserted Central Catheters, page 349).

Indications:

1. Administration of fluids and medications, especially when there is no peripheral access.

2. Administration of hyperalimentation solutions.
3. Measurement of central venous pressure (CVP).
4. Adjunct to placement of a pulmonary artery catheter or transvenous pacemaker.
5. Acute dialysis or plasmapheresis (Shiley catheter).
6. Trauma/shock resuscitation.

Materials: Minor procedure tray and instrument tray, gloves, hat, mask, gown (especially for hyperalimentation lines), central venous catheter of choice (Intracath, Cordis or Swan-Ganz introducer, subclavian line, triple lumen catheters, Shiley for dialysis), IV fluid, and tubing.

Procedures: There are several different sites for inserting a "deep line," including the subclavian, internal jugular, supraclavicular, external jugular, antecubital, and femoral. The first two are most commonly used. The subclavian sites are better tolerated by conscious patients and are easier to maintain. Shiley catheters for dialysis are typically placed in the subclavian or femoral veins. Coagulation studies should be available for review.

A. Subclavian Technique (Fig III–2):

1. Use sterile technique (povidone-iodine preparation, gloves, mask, and a sterile field).
2. Place the patient flat or head down in the Trendelenburg position with the head in the center or turned to the opposite side (the "ideal" position is somewhat controversial, and is left up to the individual's preference). The left subclavian vein provides a gentle curve into the superior vena cava, and therefore, it is often the vein of choice for long lines. However, remember that the thoracic duct is on the left side, and the dome of the pleura rises higher on the left. It may be helpful (this is also a controversial point) to place a towel roll along the patient's spine.
3. Use a 25-gauge needle to make a small skin wheal with 1% lidocaine (mixed 1:1 with sodium bicarbonate 1 mEq/L helps remove the sting) 2 cm below the midclavicle. At this point, a larger needle (eg, 22 gauge) can be used to anesthetize the deeper tissues and locate the vein.
4. Attach a large-bore, deep-line needle (a 14-gauge needle with a 16-gauge catheter at least 8–12 inches long) to a 10–20-mL syringe and introduce it into the site of the skin wheal.
5. Advance the needle under the clavicle aiming for a location halfway between the suprasternal notch and the base of the thyroid cartilage. The vein will be encountered under the clavicle, just medial to the lateral border of the clavicular head of the sternocleidomastoid muscle. In most patients this is roughly two fingerbreadths lateral to the sternal notch. Gentle pressure on the needle at the skin entrance site will assist in lowering the needle under the clavicle.

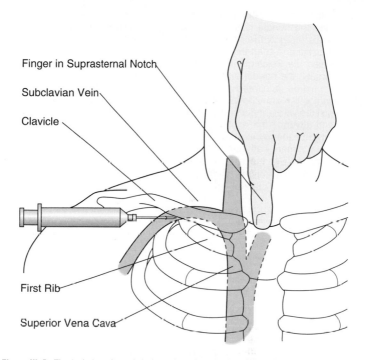

Figure III–2. The technique for subclavian vein catheterization. (*Reproduced, with permission, from Gomella LG (editor):* Clinician's Pocket Reference, *9th ed., McGraw-Hill. Copyright © 2002.*)

6. Apply backpressure while the needle is advanced deep to the clavicle but above the first rib, and watch for a "flash" of blood.

7. A free return of blood indicates entry into the subclavian vein. Remember that occasionally, the vein is punctured through both walls, and a flash of blood may not appear while the needle is advanced. Therefore, when a free return of blood does not occur on needle advancement, the needle should be withdrawn slowly with intermittent pressure. A free return of blood will herald the entry of the end of the needle into the lumen. Bright red blood that forcibly enters the syringe indicates that the subclavian artery has been entered. If the arterial entry occurs, remove the needle. In the majority of patients, the surrounding tissue will tamponade any bleeding from the arterial puncture. Because the artery is under the clavicle, holding pressure has little effect on bleeding.

8a. When an Intracath is being used, remove the syringe, place a finger over the needle hub, and advance the catheter an appropriate distance through the needle. Then withdraw the needle to just outside the skin and snap the protective cap over the tip of the needle.

8b. When the Seldinger wire technique is to be used, advance the wire through the needle and then withdraw the needle. The pulse or ECG should be monitored during the wire passage as the wire can induce ventricular arrhythmias. Arrhythmias will usually resolve if you calmly pull the wire out several centimeters. Nick the skin with a no. 11 blade and advance the dilator approximately 5 cm; remove the dilator and advance the catheter in over the guidewire (use the brown port on the triple lumen catheter). While advancing either the dilator or the catheter over the wire, you should periodically ensure that the wire moves freely in and out. When placing a cordis introducer, the catheter and dilator are advanced over the guide wire as one unit (see section under Pulmonary Artery Catheter Insertion for more details). If the wire does not move freely, it usually has kinked, and the catheter or dilator should be removed and repositioned. Maintain a firm grip on the guidewire at all times. Remove the wire and attach the IV tubing. Note that the wire used to insert a single-lumen catheter is shorter than the wire supplied with the triple-lumen catheter. This is most critical when exchanging a triple lumen for a single-lumen catheter; the clinician must use the longer triple-lumen wire and insert the wire into the brown port. Shiley catheters are placed using the Seldinger wire technique.

9. Attach the catheter to the appropriate IV solution, and place the IV bottle below the level of the deep-line site to ensure a good backflow of blood into the tubing. If there is no backflow, the catheter may be kinked or is not in the proper position.

10. Securely suture the assembly in place with 2-0 or 3-0 silk. Apply an occlusive dressing with povidone-iodine ointment.

11. Obtain a chest radiograph immediately to verify placement of the catheter tip and to rule out pneumothorax. The catheter tip will ideally lie in the superior vena cava at its junction with the right atrium, at about the fifth thoracic vertebra. Catheters that go into the neck may be used only for saline infusion and not for monitoring or total parenteral nutrition infusion. Catheters that cannot be manipulated at the bedside into the chest usually can be positioned properly in the interventional radiology suite with the aid of fluoroscopy.

B. Internal Jugular Technique (Central Approach) (Fig III–3):

1. & 2. Follow steps 1 and 2 for the subclavian technique.

3. Locate the triangle formed by the clavicle and the two heads of the sternocleidomastoid muscle. Use a 25-gauge needle and 1% lidocaine (mixed 1:1 with sodium bicarbonate 1 mEq/L removes the sting) to raise a small skin wheal at the apex of this triangle. Change to a 22-gauge needle to anesthetize the deeper layers, and then use gen-

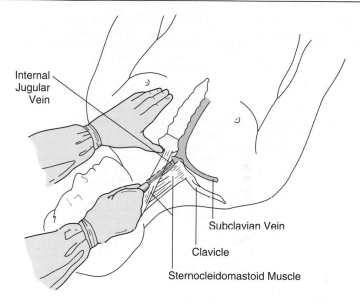

Figure III–3. The technique for internal jugular vein catheterization, central approach. (*Reproduced, with permission, from Gomella LG (editor):* Clinician's Pocket Reference, *9th ed., McGraw-Hill. Copyright © 2002.*)

tle aspiration, with the same needle, to initially locate the internal jugular vein. (Some clinicians prefer to leave this needle and syringe in the vein and place the large-bore needle directly over the smaller needle into the vein. This is commonly called the "finder needle" technique.)

4. Attach a large-bore, deep-line needle (14-gauge needle with a 16-gauge catheter at least 12 in long) to a 10–20-mL syringe. Direct the needle through the skin wheal caudally, directed toward the ipsilateral nipple and at a 30-degree angle to the frontal plane. If the vein is not entered, withdraw the needle slightly and redirect it 5–10 degrees more laterally. Apply intermittent backpressure.
5. If bright red blood forcibly fills the syringe, the carotid artery has been punctured. Remove the needle and apply firm pressure for 10 min.
6. Follow step nos. 8 through 11 as described for the subclavian technique.

C. Femoral Vein Approach: There are several advantages to this procedure. It is safer, because arterial and venous sites are easily compressible, and it is impossible to cause pneumothorax from this site. Placement can be accomplished without interrupting cardiopulmonary resuscitation. This site can be used to place a variety of intravascular appliances, including temporary pacemakers, pulmonary artery catheters (expertise with fluoroscopy is needed), and triple-lumen catheters. The major disadvantage is the somewhat increased risk of sepsis and the immobilization it causes. In addition, fluoroscopy is required for placement of pulmonary artery catheters or transvenous pacemakers.

1. Place the patient in the supine position.
2. Use sterile preparation and appropriate draping. Administer local anesthesia in the area to be explored.
3. Palpate the femoral artery. Use the NAVEL technique (see under Arterial Line, above) to locate the vein.
4. Guard the artery with the fingers of one hand.
5. Explore for the vein just medial to the operator's fingers with a needle and syringe.
6. It may be helpful to have a small amount of anesthetic in the syringe ready for injection during the exploration.
7. The needle is directed cephalad at about a 30-degree angle and should be inserted below the femoral crease.
8. Puncture is heralded by the return of venous, nonpulsatile blood on application of negative pressure to the syringe.
9. Advance the guidewire through the needle.
10. The guidewire should pass with ease into the vein to a depth at which the distal tip of the guidewire is always under the operator's control even when the sheath/dilator or catheter is placed over the guidewire.
11. Remove the needle once the guidewire has advanced into the femoral vein.
12. When the catheter is 6 Fr or larger, a skin incision with a scalpel blade is generally, but not always needed. The catheter can then be advanced in unison with the guidewire into the femoral vein. Be sure always to control the distal end of the guidewire.
13. Follow step nos. 1 through 6 for the internal jugular technique.

Complications: Pneumothorax, hemothorax, hydrothorax, arterial puncture with hematoma, catheter tip embolus, air embolus. When you suspect air embolus, place the patient head down and turned on the left side to keep the air in the right atrium; attempt to aspirate the air through the catheter. Obtain an immediate portable radiograph to see whether air is present in the heart.

IV. Chest Tube Insertion

(See also Section I, Problem 22, page 25).

Indications:

1. Pneumothorax (simple or tension).
2. Hemothorax.
3. Hydrothorax.
4. Empyema.

Materials: Chest tube (28–36 Fr for adults; 18–28 Fr for children).

1. Water-seal drainage system (Pleur-Evac, etc) with connecting tubing, minor procedure tray and instrument tray, silk suture (0 or 2-0), Vaseline gauze.

Procedure:

1. For a pneumothorax, choose a high anterior site, such as the second or third intercostal space, midclavicular line, or subaxillary position (more cosmetic). Place a low lateral chest tube in the fifth or sixth intercostal space in the midaxillary line and directed posteriorly for fluid removal. (In most patients this location corresponds to the inframammary crease.) For a traumatic pneumothorax, use a low lateral tube, because this condition usually is associated with bleeding. Use a 24–28 Fr tube for pneumothorax and a 36 Fr tube for fluid removal.

2. When the procedure is elective, sedation may be helpful. Prepare the area with antiseptic and drape it with towels. Use 1% lidocaine (with or without epinephrine) to anesthetize the skin and periosteum of the rib; start at the center of the rib and gently work over the top. Remember, the neurovascular bundle runs *under* the rib (Fig III–4A).

3. Make a 2–3-cm transverse incision over the center of the rib. Use a hemostat to bluntly dissect over the top of the rib and create a subcutaneous tunnel. Injection of additional lidocaine into the muscle will help ease the discomfort (Fig III–4B).

4. Puncture the parietal pleura with the hemostat and spread the opening. Insert a gloved finger into the pleural cavity to gently clear any clots or adhesions and to ensure that the lung is not accidentally punctured by the tube.

5. Carefully insert the tube superiorly into the desired position with a hemostat or gloved finger. Ensure that all the holes in the tube are in the chest cavity. Rotating the tube away from the patient's body while it is being inserted will assist in posterior placement. Attach the end of the tube to a water-seal or Pleur-Evac suction system.

6. Suture the tube in place. Place a heavy silk (0 or 2-0) suture through the incision next to the tube. Tie the incision together, then tie the ends around the chest tube. Alternatively, a purse string suture can be placed. Ensure that all of the suction holes are beneath the skin before the tube is secured. An alternative technique is to secure the tube with tape and then suture the tape to the skin. This is most useful for smaller chest tubes used in infants and children (Fig III–4C).

7. Wrap the tube with Vaseline gauze and cover with plain gauze. Make the dressing occlusive with tape.

8. Start suction (usually 220 cm in adult; 216 cm in children) and take a chest radiograph immediately to check the placement of the tube and to evaluate for residual pneumothorax or fluid.

9. If a patient manifests signs of a tension pneumothorax (acute shortness of breath, hypotension, distended neck veins, tachypnea, tra-

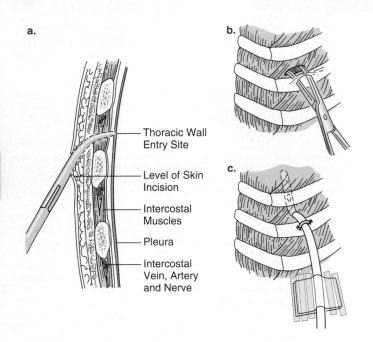

a.

Thoracic Wall
Entry Site

Level of Skin
Incision

Intercostal
Muscles

Pleura

Intercostal
Vein, Artery
and Nerve

b.

c.

Figure III–4. Chest tube technique, demonstrating the location of the neurovascular bundle and the creation of the subcutaneous tunnel. (*Reproduced, with permission, from Gomella TL (editor): Chest Tube Placement. In: Neonatology, 4th ed. Originally published by Appleton & Lange. Copyright © 1999 by The McGraw-Hill Companies, Inc.*)

cheal deviation) before a chest tube is placed, urgent treatment is needed. Insert a 14-gauge needle into the chest in the second intercostal space in the midclavicular line to rapidly decompress the tension pneumothorax and proceed with chest tube insertion.

10. To remove a chest tube, ensure that the pneumothorax or hemothorax is cleared. Check for an air leak by having the patient cough; observe the water-seal system for bubbling that indicates either a system (tubing leak) or persistent pleural air leak.

11. Take the tube off suction but not off water seal and cut the retention suture. Do not cut the suture until the tube is ready to be removed. Have the patient perform the Valsalva maneuver while you apply pressure with Vaseline gauze and 4 × 3 × 4 gauze squares or Tega-

derm. Pull the tube rapidly and make an airtight seal with tape. Check an upright chest radiograph for any residual pneumothorax.

Complications: Infection, bleeding, lung damage, subcutaneous emphysema, persistent pneumothorax or fluid collection, poor tube placement, liver injury, splenic injury, postprocedure shock.

V. Compartment Pressure Measurements

A. The Extremity:

Indication: Rule out compartment syndrome caused by the following conditions:

1. Trauma (fracture/dislocations, vascular injury)
2. Burns
3. Arterial insufficiency
4. Iatrogenic (tight casts, MAST trousers)

Equipment: 18-gauge needle, sterile IV connector tubing, electric transducer as used for measuring central venous pressures or A-line pressures or a Stryker pressure and monitoring kit.

The lower extremity is usually associated with and is prone to the development of compartment syndrome. It has four compartments: anterior, lateral, superficial, and deep posterior. Compartment syndrome is a limb-threatening emergency that requires treatment by fasciotomy.

Procedure:

1. The leg is prepared with Betadine and draped in a sterile fashion.
2. All four compartments may be assessed. The normal contralateral leg can serve as a normal control.
3. When the electronic pressure monitor is used, the 10 gauge needle should be attached to the IV tubing and then attached to the transducer, which should be at the same height as the extremity being measured. The system is appropriately calibrated to zero, and the tubing should be flushed through. The needle is then inserted into the muscle belly of each compartment, and the pressure readings noted. The needle should not be against bone, because this may cause false readings.
4. Normal pressure in the lower leg ranges from 5–10 mm Hg. Levels greater than 30 mm Hg warrant concern and levels more than 40 mm Hg generally indicate an absolute necessity for fasciotomy. For a high-risk patient, it is useful to serially monitor the compartment pressures, because this is a simple procedure. It is often better to have the same person measuring the pressures, because the absolute value of the pressure is not as important as the changes in pressure,

and because different techniques may vary, producing different numbers.
5. The Stryker device may be used, which is a small hand-held monitor, with disposable needles that insert into the device. It is used in a similar fashion.

B. The Abdomen:

An abdominal compartment syndrome may occur secondary to massive ascites, bowel distention, and edema from a bowel obstruction, or it can result from closure of a large hernia with return of abdominal contents under pressure. It may also result after major trauma caused by massive intraabdominal blood loss, bowel edema, third space fluid loss, or after abdominal packing (damage control) in a trauma laparotomy.

Abdominal hypertension occurs, a disorder that can have severe systemic effects, such as shock and difficulty with patient ventilation. Clinically, the abdomen appears tense, and often the patient becomes oliguric.

Equipment: Foley catheter, sterile saline, clamp, 18-gauge needle attached to IV tubing, which is connected to the pressure transducer.

Procedure:

The patient is in the supine position, with the transducer at the same height as the pubis, and the monitor is zeroed.

In a sterile fashion, about 50 cc of sterile saline is instilled via the Foley catheter, filling the patient's bladder and catheter, which is then clamped. The 18-gauge needle, connected to its tubing, is then inserted into the lumen of the Foley catheter, and the pressure reading is observed. It is generally agreed that a measurement of 25–30 mm Hg is consistent with a compartment syndrome, and a measurement greater than 30 mm Hg requires operative intervention, with a laparotomy.

VI. Cricothyrotomy (Needle and Surgical)

Indications: Mechanical ventilation is indicated, but an endotracheal tube cannot be placed (eg, severe maxillofacial trauma, excessive oropharyngeal hemorrhage).

Contraindications: Surgical cricothyrotomy is contraindicated in children younger than 12 years.

Materials:

Needle Cricothyrotomy: 12–14-gauge catheter over needle (Angiocath or Jelco), 6–12-mL syringe, 3-mm pediatric endotracheal tube adapter, oxygen connecting tubing, high-flow oxygen source (tank or wall).

Surgical Cricothyrotomy (Minimum Requirements): Povidone-iodine solution, sterile gauze pads, scalpel handle and blade (No. 10 preferred), hemostat (optional), No. 5 to No. 7 tracheostomy tube, tracheostomy tube adapter to connect to bag-mask ventilator. (Often it is easier to place a 5–7mm endotracheal tube rather than a tracheostomy tube.)

Procedures:

A. Needle Cricothyrotomy:

1. Palpate the cricothyroid membrane, which resembles a notch located between the caudal end of the thyroid cartilage and the first tracheal ring (also called the **cricoid cartilage**).
2. Prepare the area with povidone-iodine solution. Local anesthesia can be used when the patient is awake.
3. Mount the syringe on the 12- or 14-gauge catheter over the needle assembly, and advance through the cricothyroid membrane at a 45-degree angle, applying backpressure on the syringe until air is aspirated.
4. Advance the catheter and remove the needle. Attach the hub to a 3-mm endotracheal tube adapter, which is connected to the oxygen tubing. Allow the oxygen to flow at 15 L/min for 1–2 seconds on, then 4 seconds off by using a "Y-connector" or a hole in the side of the tubing to turn the flow on and off.
5. The needle technique is only useful for about 45 minutes because the exhalation of CO_2 is suboptimal.

B. Surgical Cricothyrotomy:

1. & 2. Follow step nos. 1 and 2 for needle cricothyrotomy.
3. While stabilizing the trachea with the nondominant hand by holding the thyroid cartilage, use a no. 11-blade scalpel to penetrate the skin and membrane in one move. When performing this procedure emergently, a vertical skin incision is optimal. It will allow for better exposure and cause less risk of iatrogenic vascular injury, which may lead to bleeding, obscuring a dry field in which to work.

    Be careful not to injure the posterior wall of the trachea with the blade. Move the blade horizontally, incising the skin and membrane simultaneously for 2 cm. The handle of the knife can then be placed into the wound and turned 90 degrees to dilate the opening.
4. Insert a small (5–7 mm) tracheostomy tube or 5–7mm endotracheal tube, inflate the balloon (if present), and secure in position with the attached cotton tapes.
5. A surgical cricothyrotomy may be left in place for 1–2 weeks with minimal complications. When long-term intubation is contemplated, it may be converted to a formal tracheostomy in the operating theater.

Complications: Bleeding, esophageal perforation, subcutaneous emphysema, pneumomediastinum and thorax, CO_2 retention (especially with the needle procedure).

VII. Cystostomy-Suprapubic Percutaneous

Indications:

1. Urinary/urethral obstruction.
2. Traumatic urethral injury.

Contraindications: (None are truly absolute.) A nonpalpable or nondistended bladder, previous lower abdominal surgery, pregnancy, coagulopathy, bladder cancer.

Materials: Prepackaged suprapubic catheter set (of which there are several types), drainage bag (often not part of the kit), catheter of choice (10– 12–14 Fr in adults.), 22-gauge 1-inch needle, 20-gauge spinal needle, 25-gauge needle, 3-ml and 10-ml syringe, sterile field, and gloves, no. 11 scalpel, 1% lidocaine, 3-0 nylon suture.

Procedure:

1. Place the patient in the supine position in a well-lighted area.
2. Open the kit and put on the gloves. Get all the materials ready before beginning. Open the preparative solution and soak the applicator balls. Shave the midline suprapubic region, then prepare, and apply the sterile drapes.
3. Percuss the lower abdomen to assess level of bladder.
4. Raise a wheal using 1% lidocaine in the midline two fingerbreadths above the symphysis pubis, anesthetizing the skin and deeper tissues.
5. Insert the spinal needle directing it towards the symphysis pubis at a 60-degree angle to the skin. If the patient has had previous lower midline surgery, either perform the procedure 2-cm lateral to the midline scar, or direct the needle in a more caudal fashion with a smaller angle toward the pubis. There should be two "pops" or points of resistance that are punctured, the rectus sheath and the bladder wall. At this point, one should be able to aspirate urine.
6. Make a 1-cm horizontal incision adjacent to the spinal needle.
7. Advance the particular catheter over the enclosed trocar adjacent to the spinal needle and, in the same fashion, short rapid and controlled stabbing motions may be required to puncture the above mentioned layers.
8. Aspirate urine to confirm placement, then advance the catheter, over the trocar 2–3 cm, and remove the trocar.
9. Attach drainage bag.
10. Secure catheter to skin in place with 3-0 nylon suture. Apply sterile dressing.

11. If blood or clots are present, the bladder should be gently irrigated with a catheter-tipped syringe and normal saline.
For the most part, this procedure is done by members of the Urology service.

Complications: Bowel injury (may be evident by aspiration of air. If this occurs, change needles and continue with the procedure). Peritonitis is rare, leakage around catheter, bleeding, major vascular injury.

VIII. Endotracheal Intubation

Indications:

1. Airway management during cardiopulmonary resuscitation.
2. Any indication for using mechanical ventilation (coma, surgery, etc).
3. It has been said, "better to intubate 24 hours too early than 5 minutes too late."

Contraindications: Massive maxillofacial trauma, fractured larynx, suspected cervical spinal cord injury.

Materials: Endotracheal tube (Table III–1), laryngoscope handle and blade (straight or curved, no. 3 for adults, no. 1–1.5 for small children), 10-mL syringe, adhesive tape, suction equipment, malleable stylet (optional).

Procedure:

1. Orotracheal intubation is most commonly used. Orotracheal intubation should be performed with great care in any patient with possible cervical spine trauma. Two people are required, one to intubate, and one to hold constant in-line traction. Some clinicians opt for nasotracheal intubation in such instances.

TABLE III–1. RECOMMENDED ENDOTRACHEAL TUBE SIZES.

Patient	Internal Diameter (mm)
Premature infant	2.5–3.0 (uncuffed)
Newborn infant	3.5 (uncuffed)
3–12 mo	4.0 (uncuffed)
1–8 y	4.0–6.0 (uncuffed)[a]
8–16 y	6.0–7.0 (cuffed)
Adult	7.0–9.0 (cuffed)

[a]Rough estimate is to measure the patient's little finger.

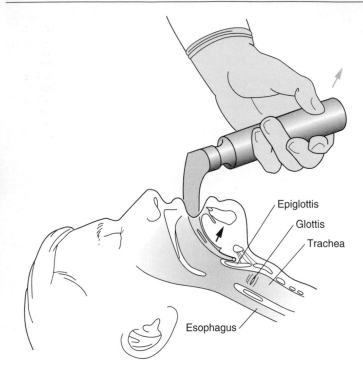

Epiglottis
Glottis
Trachea
Esophagus

Figure III–5. Endotracheal intubation using a curved laryngoscope blade. (*Reproduced, with permission, from Gomella LG (editor):* Clinician's Pocket Reference, *9th ed., McGraw-Hill. Copyright* © 2002.)

2. Any patient who is hypoxic or apneic must be ventilated before attempting endotracheal intubation (bag-mask or mouth-to-mask). Remember to avoid prolonged periods of no ventilation when the intubation is difficult.
3. Extend the laryngoscope blade to 90 degrees to verify that the light is working and check the balloon on the tube (if present) for leaks.
4. Place the patient's head in the "sniffing position" (neck extended anteriorly and the head extended posteriorly). Use suction to clear the upper airway if needed.
5. Hold the laryngoscope in the left hand, hold the patient's mouth open with the right hand, and use the blade to push the tongue to the pa-

tient's left and ensure that the tongue remains anterior to the blade. Advance carefully toward the midline until the epiglottis is seen.

6. When the straight laryngoscope blade is passed under the epiglottis, the blade is then lifted upward, and the vocal cords should be visualized. When a curved blade is used, it is placed anterior to the epiglottis and gently lifted anteriorly. The handle should not be used to pry the epiglottis open, but rather gently lifted in both cases (Fig III–5).

7. While maintaining visualization of the cords, the tube is grasped in the right hand and passed through the cords. With more difficult intubations, the malleable stylet can be used to direct the tube.

8. When using a cuffed tube (adult and older children), gently inflate with a 10–mL syringe until there is an adequate seal (about 5 mL). Ventilate the patient while auscultating and visualizing both sides of the chest to verify positioning. If the left side does not seem to be ventilating, it may signify that the tube has been advanced down the right mainstem bronchus. Withdraw the tube 1–2 cm and recheck the breath sounds. An end-tidal carbon dioxide detector may be attached to the endotracheal tube to further confirm tracheal intubation. Confirm positioning with an immediate chest radiograph. The end of the endotracheal tube should lie approximately 3 cm below the cords and 3 cm above the carina.

9. Tape the tube in position, and insert an oropharyngeal airway to prevent the patient from biting the tube.

Complications: Bleeding, oral or pharyngeal trauma, improper tube positioning (esophageal intubation, right mainstem bronchus), aspiration, tube obstruction or kinking.

IX. Gastrointestinal Tubes

Indications:

1. Gastrointestinal decompression (ileus, obstruction, pancreatitis, post operatively).
2. Lavage of the stomach with gastrointestinal bleeding or drug overdose.
3. Prevention aspiration in an obtunded patient.
4. Feeding a patient who is unable to swallow.

Materials: Gastrointestinal tube of choice (see below), lubricant jelly, catheter tip syringe, glass of water with a straw, stethoscope.

Types of Gastrointestinal Tubes:

A. Nasogastric Tubes:

1. Levin tube: Single-lumen tube that must be placed on intermittent suction to evacuate gastric contents.

2. Salem-sump tube: A double-lumen tube, with the smaller tube acting as an air intake vent. Use 14–18 Fr size in adults—the best tube for continuous suction.
3. Ewald tube: Large (18–36 Fr) double-lumen tube, especially suited for gastric lavage of drug overdose, more often inserted by the orogastric route.

B. Feeding Tubes: Although any small bore nasogastric tube can be used as a feeding tube, certain weighted tubes are designed to pass into the duodenum and decrease the risk of aspiration of gastric contents.

1. Dobbhoff, Entriflex, Keogh tubes: Weighted mercury tip with stylet.
2. Vivonex: Tungsten tipped.

C. Sengstaken-Blakemore Tube: A triple-lumen tube used exclusively for the control of bleeding esophageal varices by tamponade. Be sure to review the instruction sheet that accompanies the device in the package. One lumen is for aspiration, one is for the gastric balloon, and the third is for the esophageal balloon. (Used less today because of improved GI and radiographic interventions: sclerotherapy, transjugular intrahepatic portosystemic shunts). Placement of this tube is via either the nasal or oral route.

The bulkiness of the tube often requires oral placement. Patients are almost always on a ventilator. Upon reaching the stomach, the gastric balloon is inflated to 100 cc, then pulled back till resistance is met, signifying the gastric balloon is at the gastroesophageal junction. At that point 100–150 cc of additional air is injected, and a plain abdominal radiograph may be obtained to verify the tube's position. The stomach is lavaged through the lumen of the tube. If there is no further bleeding the tube is left as is, on traction. When bleeding persists, the esophageal balloon is inflated to a pressure of 24–45 mm Hg, and this is verified by simple manometry. The goal is to use the lowest possible pressure that will stop the bleeding. At this point the tube is placed on traction.

A small nasogastric tube should be placed through the nose proximal to the Blakemore tube to continue to check for bleeding and to aspirate secretions.

The pressure in the esophageal balloon should be checked every 2–4 h, the balloons should be deflated after 24 h to see whether the bleeding has stopped, and the entire tube should not be left in for longer then 48 h.

Complications: Recurrent bleeding after tube removal, esophageal perforation, esophageal or gastric necrosis, and aspiration.

Procedure: (general outline for most nasogastric tubes)

1. Inform the patient about the procedure and encourage cooperation, if the patient is able. Choose the nasal passage that appears most open.

2. Lubricate the distal 3–4 in of the tube with a water-soluble jelly (K-Y jelly or viscous 2% lidocaine), and insert the tube gently along the floor of the nasal passageway. Maintain gentle pressure that will allow the tube to pass into the nasopharynx.

3. When the patient can feel the tube in the back of the throat, ask the patient to swallow small amounts of water through a straw as you advance the tube 2–3 in at a time.

4. To ensure that the tube is in the stomach, aspirate gastric contents or blow air into the tube and listen over the stomach with a stethoscope for a "pop" or "gurgle."

5. Attach one lumen of the dual-lumen sump tube (eg, Salem-sump) to continuous low wall suction and the single-lumen tube (Levin) to intermittent suction.

6. Feeding tubes and pediatric feeding tubes in adults are more difficult to insert because they are more flexible. Many are provided with stylets that make their passage easier. Feeding tubes are best placed into the duodenum or jejunum to decrease the risk of aspiration. Administering 10 mg of metoclopramide intravenously 10 min before insertion of the tube will assist in placing the tube into the duodenum. Once the feeding tube is in the stomach, the bell of the stethoscope can be placed on the right side of the patient's midabdomen. As the tube is advanced, air can be injected to confirm progression of the tube to the right, toward the duodenum. If the sound of the air becomes more faint, the tube is probably curling in the stomach. Pass the tube until a slight resistance is felt, signifying the presence of the tip of the tube at the pylorus. Holding constant pressure and slowly injecting water through the tube is often rewarded with a "give" that signifies passage through the pylorus. The tube often can be advanced far into the duodenum with this method. The duodenum usually provides constant resistance which will yield with slow injection of water. Placing the patient in the right lateral decubitus position may help the tube enter the duodenum. Always confirm the location of the tube with an abdominal radiograph.

7. Tape the tube securely in place but do not allow it to apply pressure to the ala of the nose. Patients have been disfigured because of ischemic necrosis of the nose caused by a poorly positioned tube.

8. A chest radiograph must be obtained before starting any feeding through a tube to check its placement in the stomach.

Complications: Inadvertent passage into the trachea (can be life-threatening if feedings are administered into the lung), coiling of the tube in the mouth or pharynx, bleeding in the mucosa of the nose, pharynx, or stomach.

Contraindication: Nasogastric tubes should not be placed in patients with fractures that may involve the anterior base of the skull.

X. Intra-aortic Balloon Pump (IABP)

Indications:
1. Cardiogenic shock (post-MI, acute mitral regurgitation, ventricular septal defect)
2. Before and after cardiopulmonary bypass
3. Unstable angina
4. Bridge to transplantation

Contraindications:
1. Aortic insufficiency
2. Severe peripheral vascular disease
3. Aortic dissection
4. Abdominal aortic aneurysm

Function:
Improves cardiac output, and decreases myocardial oxygen demand, by increasing coronary artery perfusion pressure, and decreasing left ventricular afterload.

Materials: Continuous monitoring (ECG, arterial pressure), IABP-kit, fluoroscopy (useful but not required), sterile drape, preparation kit.

Procedure: The catheter and balloon are usually inserted through the common femoral artery, either percutaneously, or open, via a synthetic graft anastomosed to the common femoral artery. The left or right groin may be used, with the site of puncture being just below the inguinal ligament. A broad spectrum IV antibiotic should be administered.

After the groin is shaved, prepared, and draped in a sterile fashion, and the surgeon is in a mask, sterile gown, and gloves, the femoral pulse is palpated, and 1% lidocaine is injected to anesthetize the skin and subcutaneous tissue. The Seldinger technique as described earlier is followed, and a no. 11-blade scalpel is used to enlarge the puncture site adjacent to the guidewire. Increasingly sized dilators are passed successively over the guidewire. The IABP catheter is advanced over the guidewire, up the descending aorta to a point where the tip is about 2 cm distal to the left subclavian artery. The guidewire is removed, and the catheter and sheath are sutured in place. To ensure proper position, fluoroscopy may be used, or the catheter may be measured previous to insertion by placing it over the chest wall to the angle of Louis. After insertion obtain a portable chest radiograph to check proper position.

Before beginning, and after catheter placement, it is important to palpate and assess the distal extremity pulses. Once the catheter is inserted, systemic heparinization is instituted.

The balloon, which has a volume of 30–50 cc, is inflated with helium and synchronized to inflate during diastole and deflate during systole.

The technique for removing the catheter involves (1) deflating the balloon, (2) withdrawing the sheath, using manual pressure distal to the puncture site, and (3) allowing the artery to backbleed, for two heart beats, followed by pressure proximally. These steps try to prevent migration of any thrombus. Pressure is then held over the site of puncture for a full 30 min. The patient is kept supine and immobile for the next 6–8 h.

Complications:

1. Lower limb ischemia
2. Aortic dissection
3. Thromboembolism
4. Bleeding
5. Infection
6. Renal injury

XI. Intracranial Pressure (ICP) Monitor (bolt)

Indications: After head injury, in the comatose patient, or in a patient where an accurate neurologic exam is not possible. The intracranial pressure (ICP) may be monitored in many ways as follows:

1. Ventriculostomy, which has the ability to withdraw cerebral spinal fluid and control ICP
2. Subarachnoid bolt
3. Epidural bolt, is the least accurate, has the lowest complication rate
4. Intracerebral fiberoptic sensor

Equipment: Sterile setup, scalpel, hand-held cranial twist drill, device of choice (ventricular catheter, bolt, intraparenchymal device).

Procedure:

1. Prophylactic systemic antibiotic sensitive to *Staphylococcus* and **Streptococcus** should be administered.
2. The patient should be supine with the head of the bed raised, or in reverse Trendelenburg 20–25 degrees.
3. A CT scan of the brain should ideally be obtained, before placing the bolt.
4. The patient should be intubated and sedated on a ventilator, with nasogastric tube decompression.
5. The patient's head should be in a neutral position.
6. The head should be shaved, prepared, and draped in a sterile fashion. Sterile technique should be implemented with gown, mask, and gloves.
7. The right nondominant, side is most commonly used. Kocher's point is identified. It is 1–2 cm anterior to the coronal suture, and 3–4 cm lateral to the midline. It can also be found by finding the point midway between the line formed by the tragus of the right

ear, and the lateral canthus, and heading perpendicular from that line toward the right midpupillary line.

8. 1% lidocaine with epinephrine is injected, at Kocher's point, followed by a 2-cm incision with a scalpel, down to the cranium.

9. Using the twist drill, drill a hole in the skull (be careful not to drill the brain).

10. Puncture the dura with a spinal needle and slightly widen the incision.

11. For a ventriculostomy, the procedure is as follows:

  a. Slowly insert the catheter about 6 cm perpendicular to the surface of the brain.

  b. After about 4–5 cm a pop or give should be felt, signifying that the frontal horn has been entered.

  c. Remove the stylet and advance the catheter another centimeter; there should now be a free flow of CSF. If there is no return of CSF, replace the stylet and advance to a total distance of 9 cm. If there is still no CSF, remove the entire catheter, reassess the trajectory and re-attempt. A review of the head CT scan may often aid in proper placement.

  d. Once proper placement is confirmed by CSF return, bring the distal end of the catheter out of the scalp through a separate lateral small incision.

  e. Close the medial incision with a nylon suture, secure the catheter to the scalp via a nylon stitch, and then attach the catheter to the pressure transducer.

  f. A sterile dressing is then applied.

12. For a subarachnoid bolt, if either planned or if 3 attempts at ventriculostomy have been unsuccessful, the same technique is followed. After piercing the dura, the bolt is inserted, and screwed in until the tip is flush with the skull's inner table. Attach the bolt to a pressure monitor, and apply a sterile dressing. For an intraparenchymal monitor, insert the bolt 1–2 cm into brain parenchyma.

Complications:
1. Bleeding
2. Infection

XII. Lumbar Puncture

Indications:
1. Diagnostic purposes (analysis of cerebrospinal fluid [CSF]).
2. Measurement of CSF pressure.
3. Injection of various agents (contrast media, chemotherapy).

Contraindications: Increased intracranial pressure (papilledema, mass lesion), infection near the puncture site, planned myelography or pneumoencephalography, coagulopathy.

Materials: A sterile, disposable LP kit or minor procedure tray, spinal needles (20–21 gauge for adults, 22-gauge for children), sterile specimen tubes.

Procedure:
1. Examine the visual fields for evidence of papilledema, and review the CT scan of the head if available. Discuss the procedure with the patient to dispel any myths. Some prefer to call the procedure a "subarachnoid analysis" rather than a spinal tap. Obtain informed consent from the patient or legal representative.
2. Place the patient in the lateral decubitus position close to the edge of the bed or table. The patient (held by an assistant, if possible) should be positioned with the knees pulled up toward the abdomen and the head flexed onto the chest. This enhances flexion of the vertebral spine and widens the interspaces between the spinous processes. Place a pillow beneath the patient's side to prevent sagging and ensure alignment of the spinal column. For an obese patient or a patient with arthritis or scoliosis, the sitting position or leaning forward may be preferred.
3. Draw an imaginary line between the iliac crests. This should cross the spine at the L4 vertebral body and assist in locating the L4-L5 interspace.
4. Open the kit, put on sterile gloves, and prepare the area with povidone-iodine solution in a circular fashion, covering several interspaces. Next, drape the patient.
5. With a 25-gauge needle and 1% lidocaine, raise a skin wheal over the L4-L5 interspace. Anesthetize the deeper structures with a 22-gauge needle.
6. Examine the spinal needle with stylet for defects, and then insert it into the skin wheal and into the spinous ligament. Hold the needle between the index and middle fingers, with the thumb holding the stylet in place. Direct the needle cephalad at a 30–45-degree angle in the midline and parallel to the bed.
7. Advance through the major structures and "pop" into the subarachnoid space through the dura. An experienced operator can feel these layers, but an inexperienced one may need to periodically remove the obturator to look for return of fluid. Direct the bevel of the needle parallel to the long axis of the body, so that the dural fibers are separated rather than sheared; this method helps cut down on "spinal headaches."
8. When no fluid returns, it is sometimes helpful to rotate the needle slightly. If still no fluid appears, and you think that you are within the subarachnoid space, 1 mL of air can be injected, because it is not uncommon for a piece of tissue to clog the needle. Never inject saline or distilled water. If no air returns, and if spinal fluid cannot be aspirated, the bevel of the needle probably lies in the epidural space; advance it with the stylet into place.

9. When fluid returns, attach a manometer and stopcock and measure the pressure. Normal opening pressure is 70–180 mm water. Increased pressure may be a result of a tense patient, congestive heart failure, ascites, subarachnoid hemorrhage, infection, or a space-occupying lesion. Decreased pressure may result from needle position or obstructed flow (it may be necessary to leave the needle in for a myelogram, because if it is moved, the subarachnoid space may be lost).

10. Collect 0.5–2.0-mL samples in serial, labeled containers. Send them to the laboratory in the following order:
    a. 1st tube for bacteriology: Gram's stain, routine culture and sensitivity (C&S), acid-fast bacilli (AFB), and fungal cultures and stains.
    b. 2nd tube for glucose and protein.
    c. 3rd tube for cell count: CBC with differential.
    d. 4th tube for special studies: VDRL test, CIEP, etc.
       Note: Some clinicians prefer to send the first and last tubes for CBC, because this procedure permits a better differentiation between a subarachnoid hemorrhage and a traumatic tap. In a traumatic tap, the number of red blood cells in the first tube should be much higher than in the last tube. In a subarachnoid hemorrhage, the cell counts should be equal, and xanthochromia of the fluid should be present, indicating the presence of old blood.

11. Withdraw the needle and place a sterile dressing over the site.

12. Instruct the patient to remain recumbent for 6–12 h and encourage an increased fluid intake to help prevent spinal headaches. Interpret the results based on Table III–2.

Complications: Spinal headache is the most common complication seen in about 20% of the patients. It typically ceases when the patients are lying down and is aggravated when they are sitting up. To help prevent spinal headaches, keep patients recumbent for 6–12 h, encourage the intake of fluids, use the smallest needle possible, and keep the bevel of the needle parallel to the long axis of the body to help prevent a persistent CSF leak. Other complications include trauma to nerve roots, herniation of either the cerebellum or the medulla, and meningitis.

XIII. Paracentesis

Indications:

1. To determine the cause of ascites.
2. To determine whether intra-abdominal bleeding is present, or whether a viscus has ruptured. Diagnostic peritoneal lavage is considered a more accurate test.
3. Therapeutic removal of fluid (eg, respiratory distress).

TABLE III–2. DIFFERENTIAL DIAGNOSIS OF CEREBROSPINAL FLUID.

Condition	Color	Opening Pressure (mm H$_2$O)	Protein (mg/100 mL)	Glucose (mg/100 mL)	Cells (#/mL)
Adult (normal)	Clear	70–180	15–45	45–80	0–5 lymphs
Newborn (normal)	Clear	70–180	20–120	2/3 serum glucose	40–60 lymphs
Viral infection	Clear or opalescent	Normal or slightly increased	Normal or slightly increased	Normal	10–500 lymphs (polys early)
Bacterial infection	Opalescent or yellow, may clot	Increased	50–1500	<, usually <20	25–10,000 polys
Granulomatous (TB, fungal)	Clear or opalescent	Often >	>, but usually <500	<, usually 20–40	10–500 lymphs
Subarachnoid hemorrhage	Bloody or xanthochromic after 2–8 h	Usually >	>	Normal	WBC/RBC[a] ratio same as blood

[a]WBC = white blood cell; RBC = red blood cell.

Contraindications: Abnormal coagulation factors, uncertainly whether distention is due to peritoneal fluid or to a cystic structure (ultrasound can often differentiate these).

Materials: Minor procedure tray, catheter over needle IV set (18–20 gauge with a 1 1\2-inch needle), 20–60 mL syringe, sterile specimen containers.

Procedure:
1. Obtain informed consent. Have the patient empty his or her bladder.
2. The entry site is usually the midline 3–4 cm below the umbilicus. Avoid old surgical scars, because the bowel may be adhered to the abdominal wall. Alternatively, the entry site can be in the left- or right-lower quadrant, midway between the umbilicus and the anterior superior iliac spine or be in the patient's flank, depending on the percussion of the fluid wave.
3. Prepare the skin and drape the patient. Raise a skin wheal with the 1% lidocaine over the proposed entry site.

4. With the Angiocath mounted on the syringe, go through the anes-thetized area carefully while gently aspirating. Some resistance will be met as the fascia is entered. When free return of fluid is obtained, leave the catheter in place, remove the needle, and begin to aspirate. Sometimes it is necessary to reposition the catheter because of abut-ting bowel.
5. Aspirate the amount needed for tests (20–30 mL). For a therapeutic tap, do not remove more than 500 mL in 10 min. A liter is the maxi-mum that should be removed at one time.
6. Quickly remove the needle, apply a sterile 4 × 3 × 4 gauze square, and apply pressure with tape.
7. Depending on the clinical picture of the patient, send samples for total protein, specific gravity, lactate dehydrogenase (LDH), amylase, cy-tology, culture, stains, CBC, or food fibers. See Table III-3 for the dif-ferential diagnosis of the fluid obtained.

Complications: Peritonitis, perforated viscus, hemorrhage, precipitation of hepatic coma if patient has severe liver disease, oliguria, hypotension.

XIV. Pericardiocentesis

Indications: Emergency treatment of cardiac tamponade (Fig III–6), diag-nose pericardial effusion.

Materials: Electrocardiogram machine, procedure and instrument tray, pericardiocentesis needle or 16–18 gauge needle 10-cm long.

TABLE III–3. DIFFERENTIAL DIAGNOSIS OF ASCITIC FLUID. TRANSUDATIVE ASCITES: CIRRHOSIS, NEPHROSIS, CONGESTIVE HEART FAILURE. **EXUDATIVE ASCITES:** MALIGNANCY, PERITONITIS (TB, PERFORATED VISCUS), HYPOALBUMINEMIA.

Lab Value	Transudate	Exudate
Specific gravity	<1.016	>1.016
Protein (ascitic fluid)	<3 g/100 mL	>3 g/100 mL
Protein (ascitic to serum ratio)	<0.5	>0.5
LDH (ascitic to serum ratio)	<0.6	>0.6
Ascitic fluid LDH	<200 IU	>200 IU
Glucose (serum to ascitic ratio)	<1	>1
Fibrinogen (clot)	No	Yes
White blood cells	<500/μL	>1000/μL
Red blood cells		>100 RBC/μL

Food fibers: [Found in most causes of a perforated viscus.]
Cytology: [Bizarre cells with large nuclei may represent reactive mesothelial cells and not a malignancy; malignant cells suggest a tumor.]
TB = tuberculosis; LDH = low-density lipoprotein.

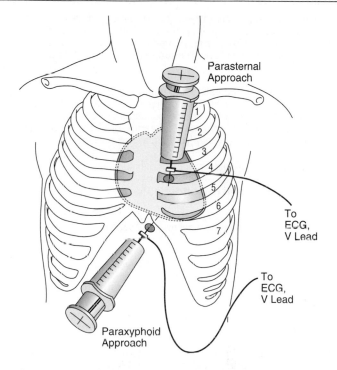

Figure III–6. Techniques for pericardiocentesis. The paraxiphoid approach is the most popular. (*Reproduced, with permission, from Stillman RM (editor):* Surgery, Diagnosis, and Therapy. *Originally published by Appleton & Lange. Copyright © 1989 by The McGraw-Hill Companies, Inc.*)

Procedure:

1. When time permits, use sterile skin preparation and draping with gown, mask, and gloves.
2. The approach to drainage of pericardiocentesis can be either via left paraxiphoid or through a left parasternal fourth intercostal approach. The paraxiphoid is usually used (see Fig III–6).
3. Anesthetize the insertion site with 1% lidocaine. Connect the needle with an alligator clip to lead V on the ECG machine. Attach the limb leads, and monitor the machine.
4. Insert the pericardiocentesis needle just to the left of the xiphoid and direct upward 45 degrees toward the left shoulder.
5. Aspirate while advancing the needle until the pericardium is punctured and the effusion is tapped. If the ventricular wall is felt, withdraw

the needle slightly. In addition, if the needle contacts the myocardium, a pronounced ST segment elevation will be noted on the ECG.

6. If the procedure is being performed for cardiac tamponade, removal of as little as 50 mL of fluid will dramatically improve blood pressure.

7. Blood from a bloody pericardial effusion is usually defibrinated and will not clot, whereas blood from the ventricle will clot.

8. Send fluid to the laboratory for hematocrit level, cell count, or cytology if indicated. Serous fluid is consistent with CHF, bacterial, tuberculous, hypoalbuminemia, or viral pericarditis. Bloody fluid (Hct > 10%) may be traumatic, iatrogenic, MI, uremia, or be caused by coagulopathy or malignancy (usually lymphoma, leukemia, breast, and lung).

Complications: Arrhythmia, ventricular puncture, lung injury.

XV. Peritoneal Lavage (Diagnostic Peritoneal Lavage)

Indications:

1. Evaluation of intra-abdominal trauma (bleeding, perforation).
2. Acute peritoneal dialysis.

Contraindications: None are absolute. Relative contraindications include multiple abdominal procedures, pregnancy, and any coagulopathy. (Perform open tap in pelvic fracture.)

Materials: Prepackaged diagnostic peritoneal lavage or peritoneal dialysis tray.

Procedure:

1. For a diagnostic peritoneal lavage (DPL), a Foley catheter and NG tube must be in place. Prepare the abdomen from above the umbilicus to the pubis. Wear gloves and mask.

2. The site of choice is in the midline 1–2 cm below the umbilicus. Avoid the site of old surgical scars (danger of adherent bowel). When a subumbilical scar or pelvic fracture is present, a supraumbilical approach is preferred.

3. Infiltrate the skin with 1% lidocaine with epinephrine. Incise the skin in the midline vertically and expose the fascia.

4. Pick up the fascia and either incise it or puncture it with the trocar and peritoneal catheter. Caution is needed to avoid puncturing any viscera. Use one hand to hold the catheter near the skin and to control the insertion while the other hand applies pressure to the end of the catheter. After entering the peritoneal cavity, remove the trocar, and direct the catheter inferiorly into the pelvis.

5. For a diagnostic lavage, gross blood indicates a positive tap. If no blood is encountered, instill 10 mL/kg (about 1 L in adults) of lactated Ringer's solution or NS into the abdominal cavity.

6. Gently agitate the abdomen to distribute the fluid and after 5 min, drain off as much fluid as possible into a bag on the floor (minimum fluid for a valid analysis is 200 mL in an adult). Send the fluid for analysis (amylase, bile, bacteria, food fibers, hematocrit, cell count). See Table III–4 for the approach to the diagnosis of the condition resulting in ascites formation.
7. Remove the catheter and suture the skin. When the catheter is inserted for pancreatitis or peritoneal dialysis, suture it in place.
8. A negative diagnostic peritoneal lavage (DPL) does not rule out retroperitoneal trauma. A false-positive DPL can be caused by a pelvic fracture.

Complications: Infection, bleeding, perforated viscus.

XVI. Peripherally Inserted Central Catheters (PICC)

Indications:

1. Home infusion of hypertonic or irritating solutions and drugs.
2. Infusion of a short course of intravenous antibiotics.
3. Total parenteral nutrition.
4. Repetitive venous blood sampling.

TABLE III–4. DIAGNOSTIC PERITONEAL LAVAGE FINDINGS THAT SUGGEST INTRA-ABDOMINAL TRAUMA.

Positive	20 mL gross blood on free aspiration (10 mL in children)
	>100,000 RBC/μL
	>500 WBC/μL (if obtained > 3 h after the injury)
	>175 units amylase/dL
	Bacteria on Gram's stain
	Bile (by inspection or chemical determination of bilirubin contents)
	Food particles (microscopic analysis of strained or spun specimen)
Intermediate	Pink fluid on free aspiration
	50,000–100,000 RBC/μL
	in blunt trauma
	100–500 WBC/μL
	75–175 units amylase/dL
Negative	Clear aspirate
	<100 WBC/μL
	<75 units amylase/dL

RBC = red blood cells; WBC = white blood cells.
Source: (Reproduced, with permission, from Macho JR, Lewis FR Jr, Krupski WC: Management of the Injured Patient. In: Current Surgical Diagnosis & Treatment, 10/e, Way LW (editor). Appleton & Lange, 1994.)

Contraindications: Infection over placement site.

Materials: PICC catheter kit, tourniquet, sterile gauze, dressing, sterile gloves, mask, sterile gown, sterile towels, Betadine, alcohol, 1% lidocaine with epinephrine, heparin flush, 10-ml syringes.

Procedure:

1. Using a measuring tape, determine the length of the catheter required.
2. Wear mask, gown, protective eyewear, and sterile gloves.
3. Carefully wipe any powder off the gloves. Prepare and drape the skin in the standard fashion. Set up an adjacent sterile working area.
4. Anesthetize the skin at the proposed area of insertion. Apply a tourniquet above the proposed IV site. Insert the catheter and introducer needle into the antecubital vein. Once the catheter is in the vein, remove the introducer needle.
5. Flush the PICC and then insert through catheter into the vein. Advance gradually until the catheter has progressed to the requisite length. Remove the inner stiffening wire slowly, once the catheter has been adequately advanced. Flush the catheter with heparin solution. Set up Luer-lock. Apply a sterile dressing over the IV site.
6. Confirm placement in the central circulation with a chest radiograph. Always document the type of PICC, the length inserted, and the site of its radiologically confirmed placement. If vein cannulation is difficult, a surgical cutdown may be necessary to cannulate the vein.
7. Instruct the patient on the maintenance of the PICC. The PICC should be flushed with heparinized saline after each use. Dressing changes should be performed at least every 7 d under sterile conditions. The patient must be instructed to evaluate the PICC site for signs and symptoms of infection. The patient must also be instructed to come to the emergency room for evaluation of any fevers.
8. For venous samples, a specimen of volume at least one and a half times the catheter volume (1–3 cc) must first be withdrawn and then discarded. The PICC must always be flushed with heparinized saline after each blood draw.
9. For PICC removal: Position the patient's arm at a 90-degree angle to his body. Remove the dressing and gently pull the PICC out. Apply pressure to the site for 2–3 min. Always measure the length of the catheter and check prior documentation to ensure that the PICC line has been removed in its entirety. If a piece of a catheter is left behind, an emergency interventional radiology consultation may be required.

Complications: Subclavian thrombosis, infection, broken catheter, embolization.

XVII. Pulmonary Artery Catheterization

(See also Section I, Problem 76, page 222).

Indications:
1. Acute heart failure.
2. Complex circulatory and fluid conditions (burn patients, patients in shock).
3. Diagnosis of cardiac tamponade.
4. Perioperative management (elderly or debilitated patients, patients with severe cardiac or pulmonary diseases).

Materials: Central venous catheter equipment; flow-directed balloon-tipped catheter (Swan-Ganz® catheter); 7 Fr with thermistor or pulse oximetry port is most frequently used in adults (Fig III–7A); sheath, dilator, no. 11 blade, and guide wires for catheter insertion (usually supplied as a kit, such as Cordis or Arrow Introducer Kit); connecting tubing; transducer and oscilloscope; heparin flush solution (1 U heparin per 1-mL NS); pressure bags; ECG monitor; crash cart; and rapid access to 100-mg lidocaine bolus for IV use.

Procedure:
1. Obtain informed consent. The patient must be on an ECG monitor, have a working IV in place, and the crash cart should be nearby, because arrhythmias are a frequent complication. Coagulation profile should ideally be normal.
2. Gown, gloves, mask, and cap along with a wide sterile field are needed.
3. Remove the pulmonary artery catheter from the package, place on a sterile field, and flush all the lumens with heparinized saline. The transducer should be balanced at the reference point of the midaxillary line with the patient supine. All ports should be connected to the monitoring lines. Check the function of the transducer by gently flicking the tip and observing oscillation on the monitor.
4. Check the flow balloon at the end of the catheter by gently inflating the balloon with 1.5 mL of air (for a 7 Fr catheter). Some operators check the balloon in a cup of sterile water for leaks. If there is the possibility of a left-right shunt, carbon dioxide is suggested for inflation. Liquid should not be used to inflate the balloon.
5. Obtain access to a central vein using a guide wire, as described in "Central venous catheter placement," page 323. The subclavian access is usually preferred because of the ease of securing the catheter to the relatively flat upper-chest wall. The internal jugular, antecubital routes are also acceptable. Avoid the femoral vein, if possible, because of the increased risk of infection and embolism.
6. Place the guide wire in the introducer set at least halfway into the vein. Monitor the patient continuously during the procedure, because arrhythmia, usually ventricular, may occur.

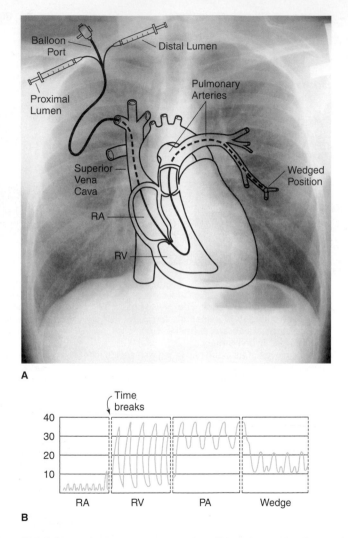

A

B

Figure III–7. A: An example of a pulmonary artery catheter. This one has an oximetric measuring feature. (*Reproduced, with permission, from Gomella LG (editor):* Clinician's Pocket Reference, *8th ed., Appleton & Lange. Copyright © 1997.*) **B:** Positioning and pressure waveforms seen as the pulmonary artery catheter is advanced. (*Reproduced, with permission, from Stillman RM (editor):* Surgery, Diagnosis, and Therapy. *Originally published by Appleton & Lange. Copyright © 1989 by The McGraw-Hill Companies, Inc.*)

7. Mount the dilator inside the introducer, nick the skin with a no. 11 blade, and slowly advance the assembly over the guide wire.

8. Flush the pulmonary artery catheter ports with heparinized saline one more time to remove air bubbles. Remove the guide wire and dilator and leave the introducer in position. Place a finger over the end of the introducer to prevent excessive bleeding or an air embolus. A telescoping clear plastic contamination guard, if used, should be mounted to the hub of the introducer, and a rubber gasket assembly will usually prevent excessive bleeding before the catheter is threaded into the introducer. This guard will allow the catheter to be adjusted over a range of approximately 20 cm under sterile conditions after the catheter has been positioned.

9. Advance the catheter slowly to approximately the right atrium. Follow the characteristic patterns as the catheter is advanced (Fig III–7B). Most catheters have markings every 10 cm. The reference lengths to the right atrium are as follows: right internal jugular or subclavian, 10–20 cm; left internal jugular or subclavian, 20–30 cm; left or right antecubital vein, 40–50 cm; left or right femoral vein, 30 cm.

10. While at the approximate level of the right atrium, slowly inflate the balloon of the 7-Fr catheter with 1.5-mL air (0.8 mL for the 5-Fr catheter). Advance the catheter and observe the pressure tracing (Fig III–7B) on the oscilloscope from the distal port to follow the catheter tip as it flows through the right ventricle and out the pulmonary artery. Do not hesitate if ventricular ectopy is seen. Rapidly pass the catheter through the ventricle and use IV lidocaine (50–100 mg IV bolus) if the ectopy persists. Once at the pulmonary artery, advance the catheter 10–20 cm farther to obtain the wedge pressure. If multiple attempts fail to successfully pass the catheter out of the pulmonary artery, fluoroscopy may be needed.

11. Deflate the balloon, and the pulmonary artery tracing should reappear. Adjust the catheter as needed, so that this pattern is reproduced. Never leave the balloon inflated continuously, as pulmonary infarction or arterial rupture may occur. Never leave the balloon inflated while pulling the catheter back. The pulmonary artery tracing should be observed at all times unless the balloon is inflated.

12. Suture the introducer and pulmonary artery catheter in position with 2-0 silk. If there is a contamination shield, extend it about halfway to allow the catheter to be moved, should repositioning be needed.

13. Dress the site with povidone-iodine and gauze or transparent shield dressing (eg, Op-Site).

14. Obtain an immediate portable chest radiograph to verify the proper catheter position and to rule out a pneumothorax. A properly positioned pulmonary artery catheter should follow a smooth curve, and the tip of the catheter should not be farther than 5 cm from the midline and, most often, in the right pulmonary artery.

15. Normal pulmonary artery parameters are listed in Table III–5, and diagnosis of conditions associated with certain readings are listed in Table III–6.

TABLE III–5. NORMAL PULMONARY ARTERY CATHETER MEASUREMENTS.

Parameter	Range
Right atrial pressure	1–7 mm Hg
Right ventricular systolic pressure	15–25 mm Hg
Right ventricular diastolic pressure	0–8 mm Hg
Pulmonary artery systolic pressure	15–25 mm Hg
Pulmonary artery diastolic pressure	8–15 mm Hg
Pulmonary artery mean pressure	10–20 mm Hg
Pulmonary capillary wedge pressure	6–12 mm Hg
SVR (systemic vascular resistance)[a]	900–1200 dynes/sec/cm[a]
Cardiac output	3.5–5.5 L/min
Cardiac index	2.8–3.2 L/min

[a] $SVR = \dfrac{(\text{mean arterial pressure - central venous pressure}) \times 80}{\text{Cardiac output}}$

Complications: All complications associated with central venous catheter placement (see page 323), arrhythmia, pulmonary artery rupture or pulmonary infarction, knotting of catheter or rupture of the balloon, sepsis, complete heart block.

XVIII. Thoracentesis

Indications:
   1. Diagnosis of pleural effusion.

TABLE III–6. DIFFERENTIAL DIAGNOSIS OF COMMON PULMONARY ARTERY CATHETER READINGS.

Low right atrial pressure: Volume depletion

High right atrial pressure: Volume overload, congestive heart failure, cardiogenic shock, increased pulmonary vascular resistance (hypoxia, ventilator effects of PEEP, pulmonary disease, primary pulmonary hypertension)

Low right ventricular pressures: Volume depletion

High right ventricular pressures: Volume overload, congestive heart failure, cardiogenic shock, increased pulmonary vascular resistance (see above)

High pulmonary artery pressure: Congestive heart failure, increased pulmonary vascular resistance (hypoxia, ventilator effect of PEEP, pulmonary disease), cardiac tamponade

Low wedge pressure: Volume depletion

High wedge pressure: Cardiogenic shock, left ventricular failure, ventricular septal defect, mitral regurgitation and stenosis, severe hypertension, volume overload, cardiac tamponade

PEEP = positive end-expiratory pressure.

  2. Therapeutic removal of pleural fluid.
  3. Instillation of sclerosing compounds (such as tetracycline) to obliter-
     ate the pleural space.

Contraindications: Pneumothorax, hemothorax, or respiratory impairment
in the contralateral side, coagulopathy (relative).

Materials: Prepackaged thoracentesis kit or minor procedure tray (see
page 357) plus 20–60-mL syringe, 20- or 22-gauge, 1 1\2-in needle, three-
way stopcock, specimen containers.

Procedure:

  1. It requires at least 300 mL of fluid to visualize a pleural effusion on a
     standard upright chest radiograph.
  2. Discuss the procedure with the patient and obtain informed consent.
     Teach the patient the Valsalva maneuver or ensure that the patient
     can hum. Some clinicians recommend oxygen supplementation by
     mask while performing thoracentesis.
  3. The usual site for the thoracentesis is the posterolateral back over the
     diaphragm but under the fluid level. Percuss out the fluid level or use
     the chest radiograph and count out the ribs. The site will be above the
     rib to avoid the neurovascular bundle that travels **below** the rib.
  4. Prepare the area with povidone-iodine and drape. The patient should
     be sitting up comfortably, leaning slightly forward. The bed stand is
     helpful for this.
  5. Make a skin wheal over the proposed site with a 25-gauge needle and
     1% lidocaine. Change to a 22-gauge, 1 1/2-in needle, and infiltrate up
     and over the rib; try to anesthetize the deeper structures and the
     pleura. During this time, you should be aspirating back for pleural
     fluid. Once fluid returns, note the depth of the needle and mark it with
     a hemostat. This will provide an approximate depth. Remove the
     needle.
  6. Measure the 15–18 gauge thoracentesis needle to the same depth as
     the first needle with a hemostat. Penetrate through the anesthetized
     area with the thoracentesis needle. A catheter over needle assembly
     (Angiocath) may also be used and the plastic catheter left in position
     to remove the fluid. Always go over the top of the rib to avoid the neu-
     rovascular bundle that runs below the rib. To prevent shearing, **never**
     pull the catheter back over the needle. Attach the three-way stopcock
     and tubing, and aspirate the amount needed. Turn the stopcock
     and evacuate the fluid through the tubing. Never remove more than
     1000 mL per tap!
  7. Have the patient hum or do the Valsalva maneuver while the needle is
     withdrawn. This maneuver increases intrathoracic pressure and de-
     creases the chances of a pneumothorax. Bandage the site.

8. Obtain a chest radiograph to evaluate the fluid level and to rule out a pneumothorax. An expiratory film may be best, because it can help to reveal a small pneumothorax.

9. Distribute specimens in containers, label slips, and send them to the laboratory. Always order pH, specific gravity, protein, LDH, cell count and differential, glucose, Gram's stain and cultures, acid-fast and fungal cultures, and smears. Optional laboratory studies are cytology when a malignancy is suspected, amylase when an effusion secondary to pancreatitis (usually on the left) is suspected, and a Sudan stain and triglycerides when a chylothorax is suspected. See Table III–7 for the differential diagnosis.

Complications: Pneumothorax, hemothorax, infection, pulmonary laceration, hypotension.

XIX. Venous Cutdown

Indication: Venous access when percutaneous puncture is not practical.

Materials: Prepackaged cut-down tray or minor-procedure tray and instrument tray (Table III–8) with silk suture (3-0, 4-0), catheter of choice (eg, Medicut, Angiocath).

TABLE III–7. DIFFERENTIAL DIAGNOSIS OF PLEURAL FLUID.
TRANSUDATE: NEPHROSIS, CONGESTIVE HEART FAILURE (CHF), CIRRHOSIS. **EXUDATE:** INFECTION (PNEUMONIA, TB), MALIGNANCY, EMPYEMA, PERITONEAL DIALYSIS, PANCREATITIS, CHYLOTHORAX.

Lab Value	Transudate	Exudate
Specific gravity	<1.016	>1.016
Protein (pleural fluid)	<2.5 g/100 mL	>3 g/100 mL
Protein ration (pleural fluid to serum ratio)	<0.5	>0.5
LDH ratio (pleural fluid to serum ratio)	<0.5	>0.6
Pleural fluid LDH	<200 IU	>200 IU
Fibrinogen (clot)	No	Yes
Cell count and differential	Very low WBC	Suspect an inflammatory exudate (eary polys, later monos)

Grossly bloody tap: Trauma, pulmonary infarction, tumor, and iatrogenic causes. pH: The pH of pleural fluid is usually > 7.3. If between 7.2 and 7.3, suspect TB or malignancy or both. If < 7.2, suspect an empyema.
Glucose: Normal pleural fluid glucose is 2/3 serum glucose. Pleural fluid glucose is much lower than serum glucose in effusions due to rheumatoid arthritis (0–16 mg/100 mL).
Triglycerides and positive sudan stain: Chylothorax.

TABLE III–8. MOST PROCEDURES CAN BE ACCOMPLISHED WITH COMMERCIALLY AVAILABLE KITS. IN THE EVENT THESE KITS ARE NOT AVAILABLE, THE FOLLOWING GUIDELINES ARE PROVIDED AND REFERRED TO IN EACH PROCEDURE SECTION WHERE APPROPRIATE.

Minor procedure tray

Sterile gloves

Sterile towels/drapes

4×4 gauze sponges

Povidone–iodine (Betadine) prep solution

Syringes 5, 10, 20 mL

Needles 18, 20, 22, 25 gauge

1% lidocaine (with or without epinephrine)

Adhesive tape

Instrument tray

Scissors

Needle holder

Hemostat

Scalpel and blade (No. 10 for adult, No. 15 for children or delicate work)

Suture of choice

Procedure (Fig III–8):

1. The most common site for a cutdown is the greater saphenous vein. The best location for a cutdown is approximately one fingerbreadth anterior and superior to the medial malleolus. Other sites on the foot, hand, or arm can be used.
2. Apply a tourniquet proximal to the site. Children may need to be restrained. Prepare the skin with antiseptic solution, drape the patient, and put on sterile gloves.
3. Infiltrate the skin over the vein with 1% lidocaine. Incise the skin transversely.
4. Spread the incision in the direction of the vein with a hemostat until the excess tissue is cleaned off. Lift the vein off the posterior tissues.
5. Pass two chromic or silk ties (3-0 or 4-0) behind the vein. Tie off the distal vein. The upper tie is used for traction.
6. Make a transverse nick in the vein. A catheter introducer ("banana") may be necessary to hold open the lumen of the vein.
7. Insert the plastic catheter or IV cannula into the vein and tie the proximal suture to secure it in place. The catheter may also be inserted through a separate stab wound and then passed into the vein.
8. Attach the fluid, release the tourniquet, and close the skin with a silk or nylon suture. Apply a sterile dressing.

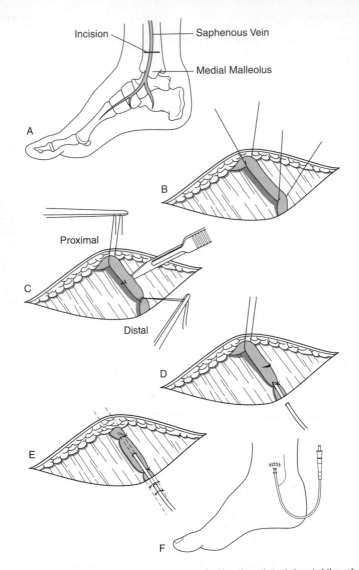

Figure III–8. Venous cutdown using the saphenous vein. Here the catheter is inserted through a separate stab wound. (*Reproduced, with permission, from Gomella LG, ed.: Clinician's Pocket Reference, 5th ed., Appleton-Century-Crofts, 1986.*)

Incision

Saphenous Vein

Medial Malleolus

A

B

Proximal

C

Distal

D

E

F

IV. Fluid and Blood-Product Management

I. BACKGROUND AND BASIC CONCEPTS

The proper management of fluid, blood, and electrolytes in the ICU requires both an understanding of normal physiologic requirements and a knowledge of the factors that can disrupt this homeostasis in critically ill patients.

A. Fluids and Electrolytes

1. Body Composition: Depending on age, gender, and lean body mass, total body water makes up 50–70% of total body weight. Young adult males average 60%, while adult females average 50% because of an average higher body fat index. Adipose tissue contains less water than muscle; therefore a person's percent of body water decreases with increasing age and obesity. Total body water is conceptualized as being divided into two main compartments, the intracellular compartment making up ⅔ and the extracellular compartment making up ⅓. The extracellular compartment is then subdivided into interstitial ⅔ and plasma ⅓ compartments (Fig IV–1).

2. Daily Electrolyte Requirements: Normal daily electrolyte requirements in healthy patients are listed in Table IV–1. Patients in ICU frequently suffer from dysfunctions of various organ systems, which may cause substantial differences from normal electrolyte requirements. Dehydration, renal failure, burns, crush, or ischemic injuries may all cause significant alterations in electrolyte balance. Typically, patients should have electrolyte panels drawn upon arrival to the ICU, and these may be repeated daily, or occasionally, more frequently, depending on the circumstances.

3. Fluid Composition: The composition of the most commonly used crystalloid solutions are listed in Table IV–2. As the table indicates, lactated Ringers (LR) solution most closely resembles normal concentrations of serum electrolytes. Massive resuscitation with normal saline (NS) leads to a hyperchloremic metabolic acidosis. However, it may not be safe to administer LR to patients who are in renal failure or liver failure because of their inability to handle potassium and lactate respectively.

Note: Do not mix blood products with hypotonic crystalloids because this may cause hemolysis; do not mix blood products with LR because the calcium may cause chelation with the anticoagulant citrate.

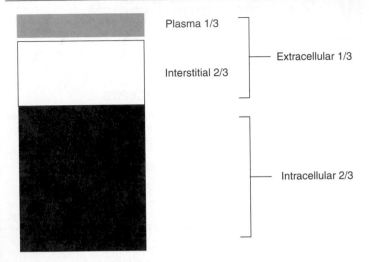

Figure IV–1. Distribution of body water into intracellular and extracellular components.

Colloids differ from crystalloids in that their molecular mass is > 8000 Da. Various studies have come to different conclusions as to the use of colloids in the resuscitation of critically ill patients. Some studies suggest that colloid resuscitation leads to increased morbidity and mortality in patients with leaky capillaries from a systemic inflammatory response (Sepsis, ARDS, etc). In these patients, colloids do not remain in the intravascular system much longer than crystalloids, and once they leak into the interstitium, they tend to draw

TABLE IV–1. AVERAGE DAILY ADULT ELECTROLYTE REQUIREMENTS.

Electrolyte	Daily Requirement in mEq/d
Sodium (Na$^+$)	80–120
Potassium (K$^+$)	50–100
Chloride (Cl$^-$)	80–120
Calcium (Ca^{2+})	6–10
Magnesium (Mg^{2+})	20
Phosphorus (HPO^{2-})	30
Glucose	100–200 g/d

TABLE IV-2. COMPOSITION OF COMMONLY USED CRYSTALLOID SOLUTIONS.

Fluid	Sodium (Na⁺)	Chloride (CL⁻)	Potassium (K⁺)	Calcium (Ca⁺)	Bicarbonate (HCO₃²⁻)	Glucose (g/L)	Kcal/L
3% NS	513	513	—	—	—	—	—
NS (0.9% NaCl)	154	154	—	—	—	—	—
½ NS (0.45%)	77	77	—	—	—	—	—
D5 ½ NS	77	77	—	—	—	50	170
D5 ¼ NS	38	38	—	—	—	50	170
D5W	—	—	—	—	—	50	170
Lactated Ringer's	130	110	4	3	27	—	—

NS = normal saline.
Numbers represent mEq of the components.

more fluid into these areas (such as the lung). Therefore, most ICUs have abandoned their use in all areas except cardiac and liver transplant surgery.

4. Daily Losses & ICU Considerations: Fluid losses in ICU patients who are febrile or on ventilators in addition to those with severe trauma, pancreatitis, sepsis, bleeding, or renal failure may vary drastically from daily fluid losses seen in typical postoperative patients. Predictable sources of daily fluid losses along with some variables encountered in ICU patients are depicted in Table IV-3. Other body fluid sources, daily production and crystalloids typically used to replace these fluid losses are listed in Table IV-4.

TABLE IV-3 AVERAGE ADULT DAILY FLUID LOSSES.

Source	ml Loss/d
Urine	800–2000
Stool	200–500
Insensible (lungs and skin)	600–900
Fever	Increased insensible losses by 15% for every 1°C >37°C
Ventilator	
Humidified	No additional losses
Nonhumidified	May increase insensible losses by 20–50%
Diabetes Insipidus	Up to 1500 mL/h
Pancreatitis	Up to 30 L/d
Sepsis	Up to 30 L/d
Burn	Up to 50 L/d

TABLE IV–4. AVERAGE ADULT PRODUCTION AND COMPOSITION OF BODY FLUIDS
INCLUDING APPROPRIATE REPLACEMENT.

Body Fluid	Average Production (mL/d)	Na+	K+	(mEq) Cl−	HCO₃⁻	Replacement Fluid (cc:cc or ½ cc:cc)
Sweat	Varies	50	5	40	—	
Saliva	700–1500	30	25	15	40	D5 1/4 NS w/20 mEq KCl/L
Gastric	1200–2500	70	10	130	—	D5 1/2 NS w/20 mEq KCl/L
Duodenum	250–2000	130	8	90	5	D5 LR w/10 mEq KCl/L
Bile	100–800	145	5	110	25	D5 LR w/25 mEq/L HCO3⁻
Pancreatic	200–800	130	5	75	110	D5 LR w/50 mEq/L HCO3⁻
Small Intestine	2000–9000	140	5	100	30	D5 LR
Colon	100	80	30	40	—	D5 LR w/20 mEq KCl/L

NS = normal saline; LR = lactated Ringer's.

5. Maintenance Fluid Calculations: Fluid requirements in the ICU often cannot be managed through simple formulas but require an educated, informed assessment of the patient's fluid status, recognition of ongoing losses, and continued reassessment of the patient's response to treatment. (A more detailed discussion of this is presented in part II of this section.) It is important to calculate maintenance fluid requirements for stable patients, and in unstable patients, maintenance fluids should be administered in addition to any overt resuscitative fluid requirements.

Maintenance fluid requirements for adult patients can be calculated using the "kg method" as follows:

100 mL/kg/day for the first 10 kg of body weight
50 mL/kg/day for the second 10 kg of body weight
20 mL/kg/day for the third 10 kg of body weight

B. Basics of Blood Product Replacement in the ICU

There always is at least one patient admitted to the ICU for ongoing active bleeding (ulcer, diverticulum, varices, etc); even more common is the coagulopathic patient who after severe trauma or a damage control operation requires massive transfusion of multiple blood products. Knowledge of the patient's last hemoglobin and hematocrit levels, coagulation profile, and platelet count is paramount to proper blood product administration. It must be remembered that blood products are indicated to replace blood loss and correct coagulation disorders but are not meant as a resuscitative fluid. All blood products should be administered through warming lines.

1. Blood Volume, Indications for Transfusion, and Formulas to Calculate Blood Product Replacement: Total circulating blood volume is equal to approximately 7% of body weight in adults (70 mL/kg).

There are very few indications for transfusing whole blood. This product is frequently unavailable and is not an efficient use of this scarce resource. Historic indications include acute massive bleeding and open heart surgery. Transfusions of packed red blood cells (PRBC), fresh frozen plasma (FFP) or platelets have supplanted the use of whole blood in replacing acute blood loss. Indications for the transfusion of PRBC have changed during the past 10 years. An Hgb level ≤ 10, the classic "transfusion trigger," is no longer a hard and fast rule. Assessing the patient's physiologic status, comorbid conditions (coronary artery disease, hypertension, diabetes mellitus, smoking, age), and ongoing blood loss—all factor into the decision to transfuse. Oxygen-carrying capacity is partially dependent on the Hgb concentration; therefore, an Hgb level < 10 in the presence of risk factors, such as tachycardia, hypotension, a high oxygen extraction ratio, low mixed venous saturation, or ongoing blood loss should cause one to consider transfusing PRBCs. Whereas an Hgb level of 8 appears to be a threshold for patients without symptoms or risk factors, the Hct of PRBC is about 70% and whole blood is about 40%. Transfusion of 1 unit of PRBC typically increases the Hct by approximately 2–3%. Leukocyte poor and washed RBCs are also available for patients who have antileukocyte antibodies. To calculate the volume of whole blood or PRBCs needed to raise the hematocrit to a specific percent, the following formula can be used.

$$\text{Volume of cells} = (\text{Total blood volume of patient}) \times \frac{(\text{Desired Hct} - \text{Actual Hct})}{\text{Hct of transfusion product}}$$

Current indications for the transfusion of platelets (except for certain circumstances such as ITP) include preoperative platelet levels of < 100,000 before major surgical procedures, <50,000 for minor operations, platelet count < 50,000 with ongoing bleeding, to prevent dilutional thrombocytopenia during massive blood product administration (transfusion of > 6 units of PRBC), and to reduce the risk of spontaneous hemorrhage when the platelet count is < 20,000. Transfusion of 1 unit of multiple donor platelets should increase the platelet count by approximately 5,000–8,000/mL within an hour after transfusion, dropping to approximately 4500 by 24 h. Platelets are usually transfused at a dose of 1 U/10 kg of body weight (hence, the term transfuse one "six pack of platelets").

FFP contains many important constituents of the clotting cascade and is critically important in the coagulopathic, oozing patient. Often patients arriving in the ICU are hypothermic and profoundly coagulopathic (PTT > 212 and PT > 40). The most important aspect of these patients' care is to warm them as quickly as possible. Continued "medical oozing" may require that FFP be given; however, until the patient is warm, the coagulopathy will not abate. Rechecking coagulation factors 1–3 h after transfusion will allow you to decide whether more FFP is needed. A massive transfusion of PRBC may also dilute the clotting factors, requiring that FFP be given to avoid a dilutional coagulopathy.

Cryoprecipitate is also useful in coagulopathic patients and is often used to replete fibrinogen in patients with DIC or other consumptive coagulopathies. This product can also be used for patients with von Willebrand's disease (contains factor VIII) and hemophilia A (contains factor VII) when concentrate is not available. Table IV–5 lists the contents and typical volumes of the most commonly used blood products.

2. Complications of Blood Product Administration: Transfusion of blood products carries a small, but not insignificant risk of transfusion reactions or transmitting infectious diseases, the most common of which are listed in Table IV–6.

Massive blood product transfusions may incur other complications, such as hypothermia, hyperkalemia, acidosis, dilutional thrombocytopenia, coagulopathy, and DIC.

II. MANAGEMENT OF FLUID RESUSCITATION IN THE ICU

The basic concepts of fluid, electrolyte, and blood product management are useful in calculating maintenance requirements, while adjusting for some additional losses or minor physiologic abnormalities. Many critically ill patients, however, require acute intensive resuscitation that cannot be determined by a simple formula. Patients with severe traumatic injuries, pancreatitis, sepsis, or peritonitis are often hypothermic, acidotic, and coagulopathic. These patients require all of your clinical skills along with an understanding of the effectiveness of specific monitoring equipment and laboratories to help guide fluid and electrolyte therapy. Some basic concepts to remember include (1) running all fluids and blood products through a warming device; (2) correcting acidosis via resuscitation; (3) recalling that only 20% of infused crystalloid solutions remain in the vascular space; and (4) always looking out for the early signs of shock, renal failure, and CHF.

TABLE IV–5. COMPOSITION OF COMMONLY USED BLOOD PRODUCTS.

Product	Description	Typical Volume
Whole Blood	Erythrocytes, white cells, plasma and platelets	400–500 mL
PRBC	Erythrocytes with most plasma removed	250–300 mL
Platelets	Thrombocytes	1 pack–50 packs
FFP	Factors, II, V, VII, IV, X, XI, XII, XIII	150–200 mL
Cryoprecipitate	Factors VII, VIII, fibrinogen	1U–10 U

PRBC = packed red blood cells; FFP = fresh frozen plasma.

TABLE IV–6. INFECTIOUS AND OTHER COMPLICATIONS OF TRANSFUSIONS.

Complication		Reported Risk[a]
Infectious	HIV	1/200,000–2,000,000
	HTLV I & II	1/50–100,000
	Malaria	1/1,000,000
	Hepatitis A	1/1,000,000
	Hepatitis B	1/30–250,000
	Hepatitis C	1/30–150,000
	CMV[a]	1/2
Bacterial contamination	PRBC	1/500,000
	Platelets	1/12,000
Acute hemolytic reaction		1/250,000–1,000,000
Delayed hemolytic reaction		1/1,000
Transfusion-related acute lung injury		1/5,000

[a]It is possible to request CMV negative blood for immunocompromised patients.
HIV = human immunodeficiency virus; HTLV = human T-cell leukemia virus; CMV = cytomegalovirus.

A. First Priority in Fluid Resuscitation

1. Assess the Patient's Immediate Fluid Requirements Upon Their Arrival to the ICU: The first priority in evaluating a patient being admitted to the surgical ICU is assessing the ABCs. This section will concentrate on the circulation.

When admitting a patient into the surgical ICU it is often difficult but vitally important to assess their fluid status, recognize their deficits, and determine their acute and ongoing fluid requirements. Unlike healthy postoperative patients, fluid resuscitation of critically ill patients often requires that fluids or blood products be given as boluses, with a continued reassessment of the patient's response to therapy.

2. History: It is vitally important to speak directly with the surgeon or resident who participated in the operation, and to the anesthesiologist to find out details about the operation and the patient's physiologic status in the OR. Were there any episodes of hypotension? What was the heart rate? How much fluid or blood was administered during the case? How much blood was lost? (Ask both the surgeon and anesthesiologist this question.) What was the urine output? Were there any other fluid losses, nasogastric tubes, pleural effusion, ascites, etc? (I once admitted a patient after an inguinal hernia repair to the ICU; what everyone neglected to mention is that the surgeon opened the hernia sac and drained 4 L of ascites from the abdomen.)

3. Physical Exam: First ensure that the patient has adequate IV access for resuscitation and possibly the simultaneous infusion of fluids, drugs, and electrolytes.

A physical exam to assess a patient's fluid status should begin with evaluation of the patient's vital signs, and should proceed to a more detailed examination of the patient, looking for signs of hyper- or hypovolemia. Table IV–7 lists some of the common physical findings in hypo- and hypervolemic patients. The importance of looking for the early signs of shock cannot be overemphasized, as proper fluid management to prevent overt hypotension can avoid the dire consequences of inadequate organ perfusion.

The "shock index" Heart Rate/Systolic Blood Pressure (HR/SBP) is a simple formula to remember as part of the bedside assessment of patients who may be in an early shocklike state. Studies have shown that this index correlates well with left ventricular stroke work, and patients with an index > 0.9 are at significant risk for acute circulatory failure. The sensitivity of this index is hindered by the fact that normal vital signs may fall into this index range. Other signs of a shocklike state include a narrowed pulse pressure and relative hypotension in elderly patients. An SBP of 120 mm Hg that would be fine in a young adult may be inadequate in an elderly individual accustomed to an SBP of 150–170 mm Hg. Therefore, any drop in normal SBP of > 30 points may also signal impending hemodynamic collapse.

4. Invasive Monitoring: Some patients are in such a decompensated state, having significant underlying cardiac disease, or taking certain medication (beta-blockers or digoxin) that the physical exam may be unreliable. These patients require invasive monitoring to assess their fluid status and help guide further resuscitation. Monitors, such as arterial lines and Foley catheters provide continuous feedback regarding blood pressure and urine output, while central lines, Swan-Ganz (pulmonary arterial) catheters, and gastric tonometers provide an objective measurement of cardiac filling pressures, cardiac output, and organ perfusion. (See specific sections in this book on how to use these devices.) Data from these monitors can be used

TABLE IV–7. TYPICAL PHYSICAL FINDINGS IN HYPO- AND HYPERVOLEMIC PATIENTS.

Hypovolemic	Hypervolemic
Pallor	S_3 Heart sound
Flat neck veins	Jugular venous distention
Poor capillary refill	Crackles
Dry mucus membranes (unreliable with paralytics)	Foamy or pink ETT secretions
Decreased skin turgor	Edema (unreliable)
Hypothermia	—
Mental status changes (shock)	—

to help assess the adequacy of resuscitation. Table IV–8 lists typical derangements in hemodynamic parameters in hypo- and hypervolemic patients.

5. Laboratory Values: Certain laboratory values can also help determine a patient's fluid status and their overall physiologic state. Baseline laboratory values include sodium, chloride, potassium, bicarbonate, BUN, creatinine, blood glucose, Hgb, Hct, platelet count, coagulation profile, type and screen (on all), type and crossmatch (if there is any possibility that the patient may require blood products in the next 24–48 h). Blood to determine calcium, magnesium, and phosphorus levels should be drawn when patients are having any cardiovascular rhythm disturbances, are malnourished, or have undergone massive volume replacement. The calcium level will also decrease in patients receiving several units of PRBC because of the preservative citrate. The free water deficit (FWD) in a hypernatremic patient can be calculated from the patient's serum sodium as follows:

$$\text{FWD (in liters)} = \frac{(\text{Patient's Na}^+ - 140)}{140} \times 2/3 \ (\text{Patient's weight in kg})$$

Other laboratory studies provide more specific information about the patient's physiologic state and the need for further resuscitation. These include values of arterial blood gas, mixed venous gas, arteriovenous oxygen content difference ($AVDO_2$), and lactate.

Table IV–9 lists some laboratory parameters that may suggest hyper- or hypovolemia. Occasionally these laboratory values can be misleading (patients in renal failure, receiving hypertonic solutions or certain medications); therefore, the results of laboratory values should be used in conjunction with the physical exam findings and hemodynamic parameters to decide on a treatment strategy.

TABLE IV–8. TYPICAL ADULT HEMODYNAMIC PARAMETERS IN HYPO- AND HYPERVOLEMIC PATIENTS.

	HR (bpm)	RR (breaths/ min)	BP (mm Hg)	MBP (mm Hg)	SVR (dynes/ s/cm²)	CVP	PCWP
Hypervolemic	↔ or ↑	↔ or ↑	↔	↔	↓	↑	↑
Euvolemic	50–90	10–15	100–150/ 40–90	90	900–1200	4–10	6–12
Hypovolemic	↑	↑	↓/↓	↓	↑	↓	↓

HR = heart rate; RR = respiration rate; BP = blood pressure; MBP = mean blood pressure; SVR = systemic vascular resistance; CVP = central venous pressure; PCWP = pulmonary capillary wedge pressure; ↑ = increased; ↓ = decreased; ↔ = no change.

TABLE IV–9. TYPICAL LABORATORY VALUES IN HYPO- AND HYPERVOLEMIC PATIENTS.[a]

	Na$^+$ (mmol/L)	Cl$^-$ (mmol/L)	Serum Osmolality (mOsm/kg)	BUN/Cr ratio	FENa$^+$	UNa$^+$ (mEq/L)	Urine Osmolality (mOsm/kg)
Hypervolemic	↓	↓	↓	↔ or ↓	>1.5%	↔	↓
Euvolemic	135–145	95–105	280–295	6–20:1	varies	20–40	250–500
Hypovolemic	↑	↑	↑	>20	<1%	<20	↑

[a]Note these values and alterations represent typical changes. There are circumstances where laboratory values do not accurately reflect a patient's volume status. These patients may have adrenal, pituitary, or renal abnormalities (especially acute tabular necrosis), which may alter electrolyte profiles.

↓ = decreased; ↑ = increased; ↔ = no change; FENa$^+$ = fraction of excreted sodium; UNa$^+$ = urinary sodium.

6. Decide on a Plan Using All of the Data: Once the patient has been assessed, adequate access has been ensured, appropriate adjuvant invasive monitoring devices have been placed, and useful laboratory tests have been sent, then this information must be combined to decide on a therapeutic plan. When hypovolemia is suspected, a bolus of crystalloid, such as D$_5$LR can help confirm the patient's fluid status. A bolus of 25% (for adults, 15 mL/kg) of the circulating blood volume can be given to a patient who is euvolemic without dire consequences. Another bedside test that can be performed for a patient with a pulmonary arterial catheter involves measuring the cardiac output before and immediately after the administration of a rapid bolus of 250-cc NS. This test will help indicate the patient's fluid status, because an improved cardiac output (starling curve) suggests hypovolemia and provides evidence that an additional preload will improve cardiac output. Formulating a plan for resuscitation may also include using the formulas mentioned previously for transfusion of blood products or replacing a free water deficit.

7. Closely Monitor the Patient's Response to Treatment: The administration of fluid or blood products should be directed by a continual reassessment of the patient's response through normalization of vital signs: increasing BP, decreasing HR, improving urine output, and correcting acidosis. Studies have shown that improvements in these parameters provide valuable guidelines for assessing resuscitation during its early stages. However, these measures can be unreliable in patients with abnormal baseline cardiac function, and they frequently underestimate the fluid status of patients after the initial stages of resuscitation.

Other parameters should also be examined to assess the patient's response to treatment including improvement in pulmonary capillary wedge pressure (PCWP), CO, arterial blood gas, mixed venous gas, arteriovenous oxygen content difference ($AVDO_2$), and lactate.

B. Second Priority in Fluid Resuscitation

Attempt to correct electrolyte abnormalities: Electrolyte abnormalities, such as hyper- and hyponatremia, hyper- and hypokalemia, and hyper- and hypochloremia are common in ICU patients. It usually is not necessary to administer exogenous K^+ during the first 24–48 h in patients who have received multiple units of PRBC or have sustained major crush or ischemic injuries, because these patients frequently become hyperkalemic. Refer to the specific sections in this book, which discuss the various electrolyte disorders and treatment options.

C. Third Priority in Fluid Resuscitation

Recognize and attempt to correct acid-base abnormalities: The most common scenario for acid-base abnormalities in the ICU is metabolic acidosis (usually lactic acid) from hypoperfusion. Other texts discuss differential diagnoses for the various acid-base disorders and provide formulas to recognize mixed disorders and the limits of compensation. On a ventilated patient, a useful temporary aid to partially compensate for a metabolic acidosis is mild hyperventilation. However, adequate resuscitation and determining the cause of the acid-base disorder is paramount, and, when dealt with properly, will often reverse the condition. Beware of renal tubular acidosis, contraction alkalosis, loss of H^+ ions via NGT drainage, medications, drugs, or alcohol, which may still be in the patient's system. Most intensivists discourage the administration of bicarbonate, as it does not treat the cause of the acidosis and may have deleterious effects, such as hyperosmolarity, reduction in cardiac output, and possibly, even the induction of hypotension. Only after prolonged cardiopulmonary resuscitation or when the pH is < 7.2 is it considered acceptable to administer bicarbonate. In this situation, the bicarbonate level must be measured directly in a chemistry panel and not taken from an arterial blood gas estimate. The formula used to calculate the bicarbonate deficit is as follows:

$$HCO_3 \text{ deficit} = 0.5 \times (\text{weight in kg}) \times (\text{desired } HCO_3 - \text{Serum } HCO_3)$$

Administer ½ of this as a bolus, and the other ½ over 4–8 h.

D. Burns

Treatment of burn patients begins with as assessment of the ABCs. After this, the patient's body surface area of 2nd- and 3rd-degree burns should determine. This can be estimated with the "rule of nines" (9% head, 18% for each anterior and posterior trunk, 9% for each arm, 18% for each leg, and 1% for the perineum). However, a body surface area chart should ideally be used to accurately determine the percent of body surface area burned. Once the burn area is known, the Parkland formula given below is used to calculate the patient's fluid requirements for the first 24 h.

Patient's fluid requirements for the first 24 h

$$= (\% \text{ Body burn}) \times (\text{weight in kg}) \times 4 \text{ mL})$$

This fluid requirement is administered as lactated Ringer's solution as follows:

½ over the first 8 h (starting at the time of the initial burn)
½ over the remaining 16 h to equal a total of 24 h

After the initial resuscitation, fluid requirements are adjusted on the basis of the patient's vital signs and urine output.

REFERENCES

Goodnough LT et al: Transfusion medicine. First of two parts–blood transfusion [see comments]. N Engl J Med 1999;340: 438.

Dabrowski GP et al: A critical assessment of endpoints of shock resuscitation. Surg Clin North Am 2000;80:825.

Graf H, Arieff AI: The use of sodium bicarbonate in the therapy of organic acidosis. Intensive Care Med 1986;12:285.

Graf H, Leach W, Arieff AI: Evidence for a detrimental effect of bicarbonate therapy in hypoxic lactic acidosis. Science 1985;227:754.

Marino P: Lactic acid, ketoacids, and alkali therapy. In Marino P (editor): The ICU Book, p 427, Williams & Wilkins, 1991.

V. Nutritional Management of the Critically Ill Patient

Adequate nutritional support is one of the most important goals in the care of the critically ill patient. Severely malnourished patients are prone to developing complications, such as poor wound healing, impaired organ function, and compromised immunity. It has now been clearly established that many hospitalized patients are malnourished. To optimize the patient's nutritional status, both the primary diagnosis and the metabolic status must be considered. Nutritional support, whether enteral or parenteral, when used appropriately, can help to prevent nutrition-related morbidity in the surgical patient. However, the approach to specialized nutritional support may not always be clear. No data are available to support the use of routine nutritional support in the preoperative period except for the severely malnourished patient.

Assessment

Differentiation of acute and chronic malnutrition is helpful in the decision of when to initiate specialized nutritional support. Acute malnutrition, also called **kwashiorkor** or **acute hypoalbuminemia,** is defined as starvation occurring during a catabolic stress, such as surgery, infection, burn, or trauma and is a more aggressive nutritional insult than simple starvation for a brief period. Chronic malnutrition, also called **marasmus,** is characterized by growth retardation and wasting of muscle and subcutaneous fat. In the surgical patient, these two nutritional insults may be superimposed. The most recent guidelines from the American Society for Parenteral and Enteral Nutrition state, "patients should be considered malnourished or at risk of developing malnutrition if they have inadequate nutrient intake for 7 d or more or if they have a weight loss of 10% or more of their pre-illness body weight."

Formal evaluation is important to identify patients at nutritional risk and to provide a baseline to assess the achievement of therapeutic goals with the specialized nutritional support. The patient's history is useful to evaluate weight loss and dietary intolerance (eg, glucose or lactose and disease states that may influence nutritional tolerance). Anthropometric evaluations, such as midarm muscle circumference (MAMC) and triceps skin fold (TSF) have much interobserver variability and are generally not useful unless performed by an experienced evaluator. Absolute lymphocyte count and response to skin test antigens provide insight to the patient's immune function.

Visceral protein markers, such as albumin, prealbumin, transferrin, and retinol binding protein may be helpful in evaluating nutritional status and catabolic stress. However, their concentration often reflects the patient's hydration status and metabolic response to injury (ie, the acute phase response) more than the nutritional state of the patient. Serum concentrations of visceral proteins increase with dehydration and decrease with overhydration. The liver manufactures all of these proteins, and their levels may be altered by hepatic insufficiency. In addition to disease states, the proteins half-life also accounts for serum concentration. For example, the level of albumin may be normal in malnourished patients because of its relatively long half-life of 20 d. Because of its shorter half-life, transferrin may be more useful as a marker for malnutrition in the surgical patient. The half life of some commonly measured serum proteins are as follows:

Albumin   20 d
Transferrin   8 d
Prealbumin   2 d
Retinol binding protein   12 h

Nitrogen balance is an important tool to evaluate the adequacy of the patient's nutritional regimen if the specimen is collected accurately. A 24-h urine collection for urinary nitrogen is required to calculate the nitrogen balance

- Nitrogen balance = Nitrogen input – nitrogen output
- Nitrogen input = Protein in grams/6.25 (6.25 g protein contains 1 g nitrogen)
- Nitrogen output = 24-h urinary urea nitrogen (UUN) + 4 g/d (nonurinary loss)

Fecal nitrogen accounts for the majority of nonurinary nitrogen loss. Measurements of fecal nitrogen are difficult to obtain and are therefore estimated at 4 g/d. Certain disease states, including high-output fistulas or massive diarrhea, will increase the amount of nonurinary losses for nitrogen and may necessitate an adjustment to the estimated loss.

A positive nitrogen balance ensures that the amount of protein being administered is sufficient to cover the losses of endogenous protein, which occur secondary to catabolism. Once positive balance has been achieved, protein replacement has been optimized. This may not be possible in the acute phase of injury, or in patients with severe trauma or burns. Thus, a minimization of loss (between 2 and 4 g/d) may be the goal during this period.

A negative nitrogen balance indicates insufficient protein replacement for the degree of skeletal muscle loss. In most circumstances, an attempt to achieve positive balance should be made.

There are a number of disorders including preexisting illnesses and coexisting metabolic abnormalities usually present in the critically ill patient. Preexisting conditions, such as hepatic insufficiency, congestive heart failure, and renal impairment must be taken into consideration when instituting nutritional support. For example, a high carbohydrate load in patients with respiratory failure can lead to a significant increase in CO_2 production. In general, it is important to correct coexisting metabolic abnormalities, such as hypophosphatemia or hyperglycemia before instituting nutritional support, particularly parenteral nutrition.

The decision to begin nutritional support is not an "On-Call Problem" in the literal sense. It is never a decision that must be made late at night by the house officer. Instead, it should be a considered decision made by the team responsible for the care of the patient. Clear indications for nutritional support include

- Weight loss >10% or more of body weight (or weight < 85% of ideal body weight).
- Expected > 7 d of no oral intake.
- Inadequate nutrient intake for 7 d or more.
- Albumin < 3.5 g/dL, transferrin < 200 mg/dL.

Hospital Diets

There are a number of standard dietary formulations available in the hospital. Most hospitals have a manual available for reference that provides details of the available diets. In addition, registered dietitians are available for consultation. This service should be used when questions arise about the use of specialized diets and dietary supplements in the care of individual patients.

Regular. Used for adult patients without dietary restrictions. The composition is based on Recommended Dietary Allowances.

Soft. Calorically and nutritionally similar to a regular diet, but tender foods are used (this is not a ground or pureed diet). Useful for patients with oral or dental problems preventing the chewing of food.

Mechanical Soft. Uses ground foods, also useful for those with chewing difficulties (eg, edentulous patients).

Pureed. Foods are ground finely, also useful for patients with difficulty chewing or swallowing.

Clear Liquids. Usually used in the immediate preoperative or postoperative period, particularly in the transition from NPO to the start of oral feedings. This diet leaves little residue and requires minimal digestive activity for absorption. In general, this diet should not be used for more than 3 d without supplementation.

Full Liquids. Includes foods that are liquid at room temperature, such as milk or milk-products (eg, puddings, ice cream, etc). In the past, this diet was used widely as a transition diet from clear liquids to regular, but it is used less often now. This diet can be difficult for many patients because it contains high-fat, lactose-containing ingredients.

Low Fiber (Residue). Indicated for patients with colitis, ileitis, or diarrhea. Decreases fecal volume.

High Fiber. Useful for atonic constipation, diverticular disease, irritable bowel syndrome, and diabetes.

Diabetic (ADA). Used for patients with IDDM or NIDDM. These diets are prescribed at a specified number of calories per day (eg, 2000 calories ADA, 2400 calories ADA, etc). Assessment by a clinical dietitian helps to determine the appropriate energy level, and helps the patient maintain the correct diet after leaving the hospital.

Reduction. Used to assist in weight loss to achieve ideal body weight. Assessment by a clinical dietitian is helpful in determining the appropriate energy level.

Pediatric. Usually ordered as "Diet for age."

Hyperlipidemia. Used for patients with lipid abnormalities. Diet is written as type I, IIa, IIb, III, IV, or V, depending on the diagnosis of each individual patient.

Low Fat. Designed to limit fat intake to approximately 50 g/d. Indicated for some diseases of the gallbladder, liver, or pancreas.

Protein Restricted. Useful for patients with renal failure or hepatic disorders. Specify number of grams of protein to be given.

Sodium Restricted. Used for the management of patients with congestive heart failure (CHF), hypertension, or other diseases resulting in fluid retention. Specify amount of sodium in milligrams or grams. Sodium restriction at levels < 1000 mg/d is not recommended because of the poor palatability of such diets. The average person in the United States consumes 12.5–15 g of salt per day.

Potassium Restricted. Used mostly for patients with renal failure. Specify in grams or milliequivalents. A typical renal diet is limited to 40 mEq of potassium daily.

Nutritional Requirements

Overall, nutritional requirements are the same whether feeding the patient enterally or parenterally. Appropriate calculations of calories and protein are important to achieve optimal anabolism while avoiding the metabolic complications associated with overfeeding.

Caloric Requirements: Caloric requirements are dictated by the patient's needs for energy to support metabolic processes and activity. Catabolic patients with stresses from infections, burns, surgery, or trauma require additional energy to allow for the increased basal metabolic rate and increased metabolic demands associated with these conditions. Using the appropriate weight to predict energy needs is important for the patient who is not at ideal body weight. For an underweight patient, it is important to use the actual weight to avoid the complications associated with overfeeding. Similarly, for the overweight patient, it is important to estimate the amount of mass that is metabolically active to avoid unnecessary metabolic stress. This weight is 25% of the difference between the ideal weight and the actual weight added to the ideal weight.

Ideal body weight:

Males: 50 kg + 2.3 kg/in > 5 feet.
Females: 45.5 kg + 2.3 kg/in > 5 feet.

Metabolically active weight for obese patients:
(Actual weight − ideal body weight) × 0.25 + ideal body weight.

The amount of energy to support the metabolic process can be estimated from a number of equations or a nomogram. The Harris-Benedict equation is frequently used to provide an estimation of basal energy expenditure (BEE). The formula follows:

Men:

$$BEE \ (kcal/24h) = 66 + (13.7 \times wt) + (5.0 \times ht) - (6.7 \times age)$$

Women:

$$BEE \ (kcal/24h) = 655 + (9.6 \times wt) + (1.8 \times ht) - (4.7 \times age)$$

The predicted basal energy expenditure should be approximately 22 kcal/kg when calculated correctly. To estimate a patient's caloric requirement, the basal energy expenditure is multiplied by a factor for activity and injury, the so-called stress level. Factors used to adjust the basal energy expenditure are less than originally published, as the risks of overfeeding became apparent. The stress level is determined by the patient's disease. Burn and trauma patients tend to have the highest energy requirements. Overall, total energy provision (protein + nonprotein calories) should not exceed 105–126 kJ/kg (25–30 kcal/kg) for the nonstressed patient and 126–147 kJ/kg (30–35 kcal/kg) for the catabolically stressed patient.

Protein Requirements: Protein intake is required to minimize breakdown of endogenous proteins. As opposed to carbohydrates and fat, no protein stores are present in the body. Daily maintenance protein requirements are 0.8–1 g/kg. Patients with mild-to-moderate physiologic stress require 1.2–1.5 g/kg/d. Those with severe injuries may require as much as 2.5 g/kg/d. Protein administration may be limited by relative hepatic or renal insufficiency. For patients with a history of hepatic encephalopathy, protein doses greater than 0.8 g/kg are rarely tolerated. Such patients may benefit from amino acid formulations with higher concentrations of branched chain amino acids.

Carbohydrates & Fat: Generally, the caloric goal is achieved using carbohydrate and fat when feeding a patient parenterally. The protein is not counted as energy intake in the acutely stressed patient. Conceptually, this is to provide adequate energy for nitrogen incorporation and to allow adequate protein for tissue anabolism, although this practice differs in various medical centers. Optimal calorie to nitrogen ratios to achieve nutritional anabolism are estimated to 150:1 for the nonstressed patient and 100:1 for the catabolic patient. On the average, protein is composed of 16% nitrogen.

The majority of energy requirements are provided as carbohydrate. This is consistent with the typical diet. Carbohydrate administration, either enterally or parenterally may be limited owing to hyperglycemia, increased CO_2 production, or fatty liver infiltration. Generally, the maximal glucose administration tolerated is 4–5 mg/kg/min or 20–25 kcal/kg/d.

A minimum amount of lipid must be given to patients receiving parenteral nutrition to prevent the development of essential fatty acid deficiency (EFAD). This minimum is 4% of the total energy requirement in the form of linoleic acid. However, additional energy from fat is used to decrease the amount of glucose given to patients. Maximal intravenous lipid administration is between 1 and 2.5 g/kg/d. Fat emulsions should not be infused in patients with triglyceride values > 300–400 mg/dL. Although at one time, practitioners considered intravenous fat emulsion contraindicated in pancreatitis, IV lipids may be a better-tolerated fuel source for patients with pancreatitis without hypertriglyceridemia. Intravenous fat emulsion has been associated with impaired immune function in animal studies. For this reason, IV lipid emulsion should not be administered to acutely septic patients or to patients during the immediate perioperative period.

Determining the Route of Nutritional Support

Having determined that nutritional support is indicated, select the route to be used. Clinical and laboratory studies demonstrate that the intestinal tract plays a critical role in the progress of many disease states. Enteral nutrition helps to preserve gut morphology, is better tolerated metabolically, and is less expensive. In addition, in animal studies, enteral nutrition has been shown to prevent translocation of bacteria across the gut mucosa; therefore, enteral nutrition may have a role in preventing septicemia. Furthermore, there is no advantage to parenteral nutrition for the patient with a functioning gastrointestinal tract. Parenteral nutrition does not achieve greater anabolism nor provide greater control over a patient's nutritional regimen. Thus, parenteral nutrition is indicated only when the enteral route is not usable. In other words, **"If the gut works, use it."**

The factors involved in choosing the route for enteral nutrition include the duration, gastrointestinal tract pathophysiology, and the risk for aspiration. Nasally placed tubes are the most frequently used. Patient comfort is maximized when a small-bore flexible tube is used. However, such tubes do not allow monitoring of residual volumes that may be significant if gastric emptying is questionable. Although no specific number exists for a safe gastric residual volume, in general, residuals less than 200 cc for low-rate tube feeds and 4 times the hourly rate for high-rate tube feeds are considered safe. In addition to the absolute number, the trend in gastric residuals may be more important in determining whether a patient is tolerating tube feeds. Stable residual volumes indicate that a patient is tolerating tube feeds. Increasing residual volumes may require that tube feeds be stopped. Patients at risk of aspiration require that feeding tubes be placed into the jejunum or duodenum with a port for gastric decompression. When long-term feeding is anticipated, an indwelling tube may be required. Percutaneous endoscopic gastrostomy tubes (PEG) are usually placed without general anesthesia. However, patients with tumors, gastrointestinal obstruction, adhesions from prior upper-abdominal surgery, or abnormal anatomy may require open surgical placement. A jejunal feeding tube may be threaded through a PEG for small-bowel feeding. The placement of a needle catheter or Witzel jejunostomy during surgery generally will allow earlier postoperative feeding with an elemental formulation than if one waited for the return of gastric emptying and colonic function.

Some patients, because of their disease states, are unable to be fed enterally and require parenteral feedings. Enteral nutrition is to be avoided for patients with active, massive gastrointestinal bleeding, obstruction, high-output fistulas, or short-gut syndrome. Other contraindications for enteric feeding include severe diarrhea of small-bowel origin, peritonitis, severe acute pancreatitis, shock, or intestinal hypomotility.

1. ENTERAL NUTRITION

Enteral nutrition is best tolerated when instilled into the stomach, because there are fewer problems with osmolarity or feeding volumes. Remember that the stomach serves as a barrier to hyperosmolarity; thus, the use of isotonic feedings is mandated only when instilling nutrients directly into the small intestine. The use of gastric feedings is thus preferable and should be used whenever possible and safe. Patients at risk of aspiration and patients with impaired gastric emptying may need to be fed past the pylorus into the jejunum or the duodenum. Feedings via a jejunostomy placed at the time of surgery can be initiated on the first postoperative day obviating the need for parenteral nutrition. Jejunal feedings must be isotonic.

Although enteral nutrition is generally safer than parenteral nutrition, aspiration can be a significant morbid event in the care of a patient. Appropriate monitoring for residual volumes in addition to keeping the head of the bed elevated can help to prevent this complication. A significant residual may be defined as 4 times the instillation rate. This can be managed in a number of ways. There may be a transient postoperative ileus managed best by waiting. Metoclopramide, erythromycin, or cisapride may be useful pharmacologic therapy. Patients who have been tolerating feedings and develop a new high residual should be carefully assessed for the cause, concentrating on intra-abdominal infections.

The question of when to start enteral feedings in the postoperative patient must be clarified. Often, the presence of bowel sounds is used as the single criterion. It is important to realize that the presence of bowel sounds may not be a reliable indicator of gastrointestinal motility. The passage of flatus indicates colonic motility, and because the colon is the last part of the gastrointestinal tract to regain motility after laparotomy in most cases, flatus may be a more useful indicator.

However, a more global approach to assessment of the gastrointestinal tract is warranted. If feeding into the stomach, gastric emptying should be evaluated. Generally, if an adult patient drains 600 mL per 24-h shift on nasogastric suction, the pylorus is functioning appropriately. Clamping of the nasogastric tube to evaluate gastric emptying may be dangerous, as it exposes the patient to the risk of aspiration unnecessarily. Tolerance to enteral feeding can be assessed with the instillation of an isotonic diet given for 24 h at 30 mL/h as a trial. Feeding intolerance is characterized by vomiting, abdominal distention, diarrhea, or high gastric residual volumes.

The nutritional components and osmolality of the enteral product help classify the formulations to simplify selection. The protein component can be supplied as intact proteins, partially digested hydrolyzed proteins, or crystalline amino acids. Each gram of protein provides 4 cal when oxidized. The carbohydrate source may be intact complex starches, glucose polymers, or simpler disaccharides, such as sucrose. Carbohydrates provide 4 cal/g. Fat in enteral products usually is supplied as long-chain fatty acids. However, some enteral products contain medium-chain triglycerides (MCT), which are transported directly in the portal circulation rather than via chyle production. Because MCT oil does not contain essential fatty acids, it cannot be used as the sole fat source. Long-chain fatty acids provide 9 cal/g and MCT provide 8 cal/g.

The osmolality of an enteral product is determined primarily by the concentration of carbohydrates, electrolytes, amino acids, or small peptides. The clinical importance of osmolality is often debated. Hyperosmolar formulations with osmolalities exceeding 450 mOsm/L may contribute to diarrhea by acting in a manner similar to osmotic cathartics. Hyperosmolar feedings are well tolerated when delivered into the stomach (as opposed to the small bowel), because gastric secretions dilute the feeding before it leaves the pylorus to traverse the small bowel. Thus, feedings administered directly to the small bowel (eg, via feeding jejunostomy) should not exceed 450 mOsm/L.

On the basis of osmolality and macronutrient content, the clinician can classify enteral products into several categories. Low osmolality formulas are isotonic and contain intact macronutrients. They usually provide 1 cal/mL and require approximately 2 L to provide the RDA for vitamins. These products are appropriate for the general patient population. Two examples are Ensure and Isocal.

High-density formulas may provide up to 2 cal/mL. These concentrated solutions are hyperosmolar and also contain intact nutrients. The RDA for vitamins can be met with volumes of 1500 mL or less. These products are used for volume-restricted patients. Examples are Deliver 2.0 and Ensure Plus HN Liquid.

Chemically defined or elemental formulas provide the macronutrients in the predigested state. These formulations are usually hyperosmolar and have poor palatability. Patients with compromised nutrient absorptive abilities or gastrointestinal function may benefit from elemental type feedings. Vivonex TEN and Peptamen are two such products.

Several enteral formulas have been developed that have been altered for various disease states. Products for pulmonary patients, such as Pulmocare, contain a higher percent of energy from fat to decrease the carbon dioxide load from the metabolism of excess glucose. A low carbohydrate, high-fat product for persons with diabetes, is available that also contains fiber that may help regulate glucose control. Other fiber-containing enteral feedings are available to help regulate bowel function, eg, Enrich. Patients with hepatic insufficiency may benefit from formulations containing a higher concentration of the branched-chain amino acids and less aromatic amino acids in an attempt to correct their altered serum amino acid profile, eg, Hepatic-Aid II. Formulas containing only essential amino acids have been marketed for the renal failure patient. The clinical usefulness of many specialty products remains controversial.

Oral supplements differ from other enteral feedings by design, so that they are more palatable to improve compliance. Furthermore, oral supplements contain lactose, which is inappropriate for patients with lactase deficiency, whereas, most enteral products do not contain lactose.

Guidelines for ordering enteral feedings are

- Determine nutritional needs.
- Assess gastrointestinal tract function and appropriateness of enteral feedings.
- Determine fluid requirements and volume tolerance based on overall status and concurrent disease states.
- Select an appropriate enteral feeding product.
- Verify that the regimen selected satisfies micronutrient requirements.
- Monitor and assess nutritional status to evaluate the need for changes in the selected regimen.

COMPLICATIONS OF ENTERAL NUTRITION

Gastroesophageal Reflux: Surgical patients that are placed in a supine position are prone to gastroesophageal reflux. In addition, large-bore feeding tubes function as a stent to open the gastroesophageal junction and place patients at higher risk of reflux. Reflux can be minimized by elevating the head of the bed, monitoring gastric residuals, and using agents that increase lower-esophageal sphincter pressure.

Diarrhea: A common complication of enteral feeding is diarrhea. It occurs in about 10–60% of patients receiving enteral feedings. The clinician must evaluate the patient for infectious causes, such as *Clostridium difficile* before initiating antimotility agents, because increased gastrointestinal motility is one of the primary methods for eliminating infectious organisms from the bowel. Formula-related causes include contamination, excessive cold temperature, lactose intolerance, osmolality, and the method and/or route of delivery. Before using antidiarrheal medications, eliminate potential causes as follows:

- Check medication profile for possible drug-induced cause.
- Rule out *C difficile* colitis for patients receiving antibiotics.
- Attempt to decrease rate.
- Change formulation: Limit lactose, reduce osmolality, and increase fiber.
- Use pharmacologic therapy only after eliminating treatable causes.

Constipation: Although less common than diarrhea, constipation can occur in the enterally fed patient. Check to ensure that adequate fluid volume is being given. Patients with additional requirements may benefit from water boluses or dilution of the enteral formulation. Fiber can be added to help regulate bowel function.

Aspiration: Aspiration is a serious complication of enteral feedings and is more likely to occur in the patient with diminished mental status. The best approach here is prevention, accomplished by elevating the patient's head and carefully monitoring residual fluid volume. Any patient suspected of possible aspiration or assessed to be at increased risk of aspiration should be further evaluated before enteral feedings are instituted. They may not be a candidate for gastric feedings and may necessitate small-bowel feedings.

Drug Interactions: The vitamin K content of various enteral products varies from 22 mg to 156 mg per 1000 cal. This can significantly affect the anticoagulation profile of a patient receiving warfarin. Tetracycline products should not be administered 1 h before or 2 h after enteral feedings to avoid the inhibition of absorption. Similarly, enteral feedings should be stopped 2 h before and after the administration of phenytoin.

2. PARENTERAL NUTRITION

Peripheral Versus Central Parenteral Nutrition: The use of total parenteral nutrition (TPN) necessitates a central venous catheter with its concomitant risks. Although some patients require parenteral nutrition, they have additional nutritional needs that can be met better with the use of peripherally administered parenteral nutrition (PPN).

The limiting factor in the use of PPN is the osmolality of the solution. Because centrally administered fluids are rapidly diluted at the catheter tip, osmolality is not a concern, whereas peripherally administered fluids of high osmolality rapidly result in venous sclerosis owing to the relatively low flow and slow dilution of these fluids. Thus, only patients with modest nutritional requirements will be able to meet these criteria for the necessarily low-energy-containing solutions that can be administered peripherally.

PPN can be up to 900 mOsm/kg and can be prepared from amino acid mixtures (5%), dextrose solutions (10%), and fat emulsions (20%). They have a low energy density of about 1.26–2.52 kJ/mL (0.3–0.6 kcal/mL) compared with TPN solutions and can thus only provide about 5000–9600 kJ/d (1200–2300 kcal/d) in 2000–3500 mL of solution. Thus, with PPN, the ability to provide energy needs in relatively small volumes is lost; this may be clinically significant for patients requiring fluid restriction.

In general, the largest-bore intravenous catheter should be used. The site should be changed frequently, usually every 72 h. Fat emulsion can be given through a Y-connector or using a three-in-one bag as is commonly used for centrally administered parenteral nutrition. Septic complications are uncommon, but thrombophlebitis can occur at the infusion site.

While peripherally administered parenteral nutrition alleviates some of the complications associated with central TPN, its use is limited by the inability to provide the level of nutritional support frequently needed in the surgical patient. Patients with large nutritional requirements owing to stress or chronic malnutrition, high electrolyte needs, fluid restrictions, or prolonged intravenous feeding are inappropriate candidates for PPN.

PRESCRIBING TOTAL PARENTERAL NUTRITION (CENTRAL TPN)

Central vein infusions allow greater concentrations of both macronutrients and electrolytes. Therefore, central TPN is more flexible in meeting a patient's requirements. With the use of permanent types of catheters (eg, the tunneled subclavian catheter, the implantable port, or a peripherally inserted central line), TPN can be administered in the hospital or home setting, depending on the patient's overall clinical condition.

When calculating caloric provision of parenteral nutrition, intravenous fat emulsion 10% provides about 4.6 kJ/mL (1.1 kcal/mL), and 20% provides about 0.4 kJ/mL (2 kcal/mL). Intravenous dextrose provides about 14.3 kJ/g (3.4 kcal/g) rather than 16.8 kJ/g (4 kcal/g) because it is a monohydrate and therefore less calorically dense.

Centrally administered TPN is given through a central venous catheter (placed percutaneously or an operatively placed tunneled catheter). The solutions are usually > 1900 mOsm/kg and contain at least 4.2 kJ/mL (1 kcal/mL). Thus the usual infusion of 2000-2500 L/d provides at least 8400–10,500 kJ/d (2000–2500 kcal/d). This is sufficient to meet the nutritional needs of most surgical patients.

The solutions are formulated in the hospital pharmacy and are typically ordered using a standard "check-list" available in most hospitals. A typical 1-l bag will contain amino acids (5%) and dextrose (20%). Lipids are given in a separate emulsion in a 10 or 20% concentration. Carbohydrate concentrations may be increased to 35% to limit volume in fluid-overloaded patients.

Electrolytes and vitamins to create a solution containing all nutrient requirements are as follows:

Sodium	40 mEq/L
Potassium	30 mEq/L
Phosphate	20 mmol/L
Magnesium	5 mEq/L
Calcium	4.5 mEq/L
Chloride	35 mEq/L
Acetate	29.5 mEq/L

The values given here represent commonly used amounts, but must be adapted to the nutritional and electrolyte needs of individual patients and must consider concurrent disease states, such as renal or hepatic failure.

Electrolyte administration must be changed to also reflect losses. Salts are usually administered as chloride or acetate, usually in similar amounts.

However, patients losing fluid by nasogastric suction require increased amounts of chloride. Similarly, patients with high-output pancreatic or small-bowel fistulas will require more acetate.

Trace elements are added daily. Commercially available mixtures are usually adequate to provide needed amounts. Similarly, vitamins are usually added as pre-made mixtures. In addition to these mixtures (eg, MVI–12), the clinician must administer vitamin K, 5–10 mg IM weekly. Increased amounts of zinc are necessary with small bowel losses.

Trace element	Parenteral daily dose
Zinc	2.5–6 mg
Copper	0.3–0.5 mg
Selenium	20–50 mg
Chromium	10–15 mg
Manganese	0.4–8 mg

Starting TPN: TPN is usually begun at 25–50 mL/h, with increases of 25 mL/h until the precalculated final rate is achieved. Glucose is carefully monitored, especially in the early phase of TPN administration, because glucose intolerance is very common. Ensure that serum electrolytes (especially PO_4) and glucose are checked before starting TPN. Remember that new glucose intolerance in a patient who initially had normal glucose levels while on TPN may be an early sign of sepsis. If a patient is undergoing surgery, the TPN is usually tapered to help prevent stress-related hyperglycemia and assist in fluid administration.

Stopping TPN: Although commonly practiced, weaning is generally not necessary. Most patients tolerate cessation of TPN, especially when they are taking oral nutrition at the time TPN is stopped. If there are concerns about hypoglycemia, the TPN rate can be halved for 1 h and then stopped completely. Similarly, a 10%-dextrose solution can be used to prevent hypoglycemia. For the majority of patients, TPN can be stopped without weaning or the use of 10%-dextrose solution.

Complications: Complications associated with parenteral nutrition are generally divided into mechanical, infectious, and metabolic problems.

A.   Mechanical Complications: After placement of the central venous catheter, a chest radiograph is obtained to evaluate the catheter tip position and the presence of a pneumothorax. The tip should be at the atrial-caval junction. A catheter tip deep into the right ventricle can cause arrhythmias and may damage the tricuspid valve. Pneumo- and hydrothorax should be treated with appropriate chest tube drainage.

B.   Infectious Complications: The use of central lines always has the potential for infectious problems. Always consider infection in a patient with new glucose intolerance on TPN. The line is usually the source of infection. Once suspected, the line should be removed. If TPN is still necessary, then a new site should be used. The catheter tip should be carefully removed and cultured. A secondary infection of the catheter and seeding from another septic site are also possibilities and also may necessitate catheter removal.

C.   Hyperglycemia: The most frequently occurring metabolic complication is hyperglycemia. Hyperglycemia for the patient receiving TPN is defined as a glucose level > 200 mg/dL. The approach to hyperglycemia should be dictated by first determining its cause. The initial step in this process is to assess the appropriateness of overall energy provisions and to clarify the fuel sources. Energy from carbohydrate in excess of 126–147 kJ/kg (30–35 kcal/kg) should be decreased. For patients who are diabetic, on steroids, or otherwise glucose intolerant, glucose in excess of 150–200 g/d may be tolerated poorly. Energy from fat should be increased to approximately 30% of the nonprotein energy in the nonseptic patient. If after adjustments, hyperglycemia persists, a review of the patient's clinical condition and medications is warranted.

Patients with new onset hyperglycemia should always be evaluated for an infection. Corticosteroids are the leading cause of hyperglycemia. For patients with infections or changing steroid doses, management of hyperglycemia can be achieved with sliding scale insulin or insulin infusions when the patient is in the ICU. Insulin should not be incorporated in the TPN of patients with new-onset hyperglycemia, because their hyperglycemia is due to increased hepatic gluconeogenesis and a relative insulin resistance, not to a lack of endogenously released insulin. Hyperglycemia associated with parenteral nutrition generally requires aggressive sliding scale coverage. Only regular insulin should be used to manage hyperglycemia in TPN patients. Patients who are stable on a given dose of insulin may have the insulin placed in the TPN bag.

Insulin infusions are typically compounded by adding 150 U of regular insulin to 150 mL of 0.9% sodium chloride. The infusion is started at 1–2 U/h and titrated upward to control the glucose at 200 mg/dL. When insulin infusions exceed 8–10 U/h, insulin resistance is occurring. At this point, it is often best to discontinue the TPN and to correct the hyperglycemia.

D.   Refeeding Syndrome: Often when malnutrition is recognized, the inclination is to rapidly and aggressively initiate specialized nutritional support. Unfortunately, this approach is associated with more hazards than the underlying malnutrition. The refeeding syndrome and morbidity associated with overfeeding are real clinical hazards associated with both parenteral and enteral nutrition. The refeeding syndrome is a constellation of severe fluid and electrolyte shifts associated with initiating nutrition in the chronically malnourished individual.

Typically, hypophosphatemia, hypomagnesemia, and hypokalemia are the electrolyte abnormalities that can result in cardiac and respiratory dysfunction and failure. Thiamine deficiency, hyperglycemia, and volume overload have also occurred. The best approach to the refeeding syndrome is prevention. TPN should be started at no more than 4200 kJ (1000 kcal) or about 84 kJ/kg (20 kcal/kg) on the first day and titrated on the basis of patient tolerance, as defined by glucose monitoring and electrolyte values. Empiric replacement of vitamins, phosphorus, magnesium, and potassium is appropriate in the patient at risk.

E.   Electrolyte Abnormalities: In general, when electrolyte deficiencies are present in the patient before initiating TPN, it is best to correct the problems and delay intravenous feeding. Electrolyte deficiencies that occur once the patient is receiving parenteral nutrition should be corrected with runs outside of the parenteral nutrition. If the patient has increased maintenance requirements because of chronic gastrointestinal losses or other reasons, the maintenance requirements should be incorporated into the parenteral nutrition mixture. The use of inadequate or excessive amounts of any additive results in the corresponding electrolyte abnormality. The amount of the corresponding electrolyte must be adjusted to correct the abnormality.

F.   Acid-Base Disturbances: Hyperchloremic metabolic acidosis is fairly common in patients receiving TPN and may result from bicarbonate loss, which can be caused by severe diarrhea, pancreatic fistulas, or small-bowel losses. The treatment is to administer more Na and K as acetate salts (instead of the Cl salt).

G.   Impaired Liver Function Tests: Hepatic and biliary complications associated with parenteral nutrition are generally characterized by the duration of parenteral nutrition. Abnormal liver function tests are common in both short-term and long-term patient populations. The most common hepatic complication associated with short-term TPN administration is hepatic steatosis. This fatty liver infiltration is thought to be a result of overfeeding, especially of carbohydrate energy. The incidence of hepatic steatosis has decreased with the introduction of IV fat emulsion and the growing consideration of conservative energy feeding. Biliary sludge formation and cholelithiasis with its associated complications have been noted in patients receiving TPN for 3 weeks or longer. Biliary stasis caused by the lack of stimulation resulting from bowel rest or short-gut is thought to be the primary mechanism. Long-term TPN administration is associated with hepatic steatonecrosis. Its pathogenesis is unclear at this time.

The diagnosis of TPN-associated hepatotoxicity is a diagnosis of exclusion. Once other causes have been ruled out, management of hepatotoxicity includes reformulation of the caloric regimen, cyclic administration of TPN, and metronidazole.

H.   Prerenal Azotemia: Excessive amino acid infusion with inadequate energy administration can result in prerenal azotemia. A rising BUN should be monitored, but probably not treated until it is greater than 100 mg/dL. This is treated by reducing the amino acid intake and increasing energy input administered as glucose. Prerenal azotemia resulting from intravascular volume depletion should be ruled out.

I.   Bleeding Abnormalities: These can be caused by inadequate amounts of vitamin K, iron deficiency, folate deficiency, or vitamin B_{12} deficiency. Adjust the nutrient administration to the required amount.

J.   Overfeeding: It is imperative to nutritionally support a patient on a rational and measured basis. To do this, the clinician must know the requirements for each nutritional component. Energy requirements are dependent on gender, weight, height, age, energy expenditure, and seriousness of the injury. Overfeeding places patients at risk for hepatic complications, increased carbon dioxide production, and hyperglycemia.

TPN in Specific Disease States: The administration of TPN must be changed for patients with the following diseases.

    A.   Cardiac Failure: Fluid administration must be limited in these patients. Therefore, a concentrated dextrose solution up to 35% can be used to limit the amount of fluid administered while providing adequate energy. The remainder of the energy is given as lipids. Protein can be limited to 0.8–1 g/kg, and sodium limited to 0.5–1.5 g/d.

    B.   Diabetes: Use increased energy from fat for these patients to limit the energy from carbohydrate while providing sufficient energy for protein anabolism. Insulin can be added to the bag in a patient with stable insulin requirements. In general, fat should provide no more than 50% of total energy intake and no more than 2.5 g/kg/d.

    C.   Hepatic Dysfunction: Patients with hepatic dysfunction usually benefit from increased amounts of branched-chain amino acids (leucine, valine, and isoleucine) and reduced amounts of aromatic amino acids, which are precursors to centrally active amines and thus, contribute to hepatic encephalopathy. Specialized mixtures of amino acids are available and should be used only for patients with hepatic encephalopathy. Lipid emulsions should be limited for those with severe hepatic dysfunction.

    D.   Renal Disease: These patients have a number of specific restrictions that must be carefully considered in the administration of TPN, including fluid, protein, potassium, magnesium, and sodium. Protein must be restricted to 0.6–0.8 g/kg/d for patients not undergoing dialysis. Patients receiving hemodialysis generally require 1.2 g/kg of protein per day, and patients undergoing peritoneal dialysis need 1.5 g/kg/d. The latter patient also absorbs approximately 2100 kJ/d (500 kcals/d) of dextrose from the dialysate, which needs to be considered when designing their nutritional regimen. Patients on hemodialysis may receive the usual protein load of 1–1.5 g/kg/d. Specially formulated amino acid mixtures are used for these patients, which contain higher amounts of essential amino acids. In general, TPN should not contain potassium or magnesium in patients with renal failure. Reduced sodium for these patients may also be necessary.

    E.   Pulmonary Dysfunction: Carbohydrate metabolism (including overfeeding) results in production of CO_2. Thus, patients with impaired ventilation, who already may retain CO_2, are further stressed when high carbohydrate loads are administered. This problem may be treated by increasing the energy fraction from fat (up to 50%). Overall, the total energy should not exceed 126–147 kJ/kg (30–35 kcal/kg). These patients also may be sensitive to phosphate depletion and should be monitored carefully for the development of hypophosphatemia. Once identified, this condition is treated with phosphate supplementation.

RECOMMENDED LITERATURE

ASPEN Board of Directors. Guidelines for the use of parenteral and enteral nutrition in adult and pediatric patients. J Parenter Enteral Nutr 1998.

Gomella LG (editor): Total parenteral nutrition. In Clinician's Pocket Reference, 8th ed. Appleton & Lange, 1998.

McCarthy MC: Nutritional support in the critically ill surgical patient. Surg Clin North Am 1991;71:831.

Rombeau JL, Rolandelli RH, Wilmore DW: Nutritional support. In Wilmore DW et al (editors): Care of the Surgical Patient, Scientific American, 1989.

Rosen GH: An overview of enteral nutrition. Pharmacy Times, Sept 1991:33.

VI. Ventilator Management

INDICATIONS AND SETUP

I. Indications for Ventilatory Support

Respiratory failure can be divided into two categories: failure to oxygenate and failure to ventilate. Ventilatory support is indicated when patients are unable to achieve or maintain adequate gas exchange on their own.

A. **Failure to Oxygenate.** Oxygenation takes place at the alveolar-capillary membrane, where equilibrium of oxygen concentration is achieved between the oxygen in the inflated alveolus and in the pulmonary capillary blood. The partial pressure of oxygen gradient between alveolus (PAO_2) and capillary (PaO_2) favors transfer of oxygen into the blood. It is measured by pulse oximetry or by measuring PaO_2 in the arterial blood at a known inspired fraction of oxygen (FiO_2). Oxygenation, however, depends less on good alveolar ventilation than on adequate matching of pulmonary blood flow to ventilated alveoli, the so-called "ventilation-perfusion matching."

B. **Failure to Ventilate.** Ventilation has the main function to excrete carbon dioxide (CO_2). Criteria of ventilatory failure are listed in Table VI–1. The minute ventilation (MV) is defined as the total amount of gas exhaled per minute, the product of the respiratory rate (RR) and the tidal volume (V_T). Two thirds of MV promotes gas exchange in the alveoli (alveolar ventilation, V_A); one third of MV is in the conducting airways and nonperfused alveoli and constitutes dead space ventilation(V_D). The ratio V_D/V_T normally is 0.33. CO_2 excretion correlates directly with the amount of V_A. Regulation takes place in the respiratory center in the brainstem, with input from three sources: chemoreceptors in the carotid body and aortic arch that sense PaO_2 pressure, central chemoreceptors in the brainstem that sense CO_2 pressure, and pH values, and stretch receptors in the lung parenchyma. In general, hypercapnia is the stronger stimulus for increasing ventilation. In some chronic forms of lung disease, hypoxia becomes the dominant stimulus in the presence of chronically elevated $PaCO_2$. Ventilation is monitored via end-tidal CO_2 monitor or via blood gas measurement of $PaCO_2$. A $PaCO_2 > 50$ mm Hg generally indicates ventilatory failure; however, patients with chronic ventilatory failure with renal compensation (eg, COPD) retain HCO_3 to adjust the pH toward normal. Thus, absolute pH is often a better guide than $PaCO_2$ to determine the need for ventilatory assistance. A respiratory acidosis with a rapidly falling pH or an absolute pH ≤ 7.25 is an indication for ventilatory support.

The main indication for ventilatory support overall is hypoxemia. Three main categories of nonpulmonary causes of hypoxemia have to be considered:

TABLE VI–1. CRITERIA FOR DIAGNOSIS OF ACUTE RESPIRATORY FAILURE.

Parameter	Normal	Respiratory Failure
Respiratory rate (BPM)	12–20	>35
Vital capacity (mL/kg body wt)	65–75	<15
FEV$_1$ (mL/kg body wt)	50–60	≤10
Inspiratory force (cm H$_2$O)	75–100	≤20–25
Compliance (mL/cm H$_2$O)	100	<20
Pao$_2$ (mm/cm H$_2$O)	80–90 on room air	<70
Aa$_{DO_2}$ on FIo$_2$ 100%	25–65	>450
QS/QT	5–8	>20
Paco2	35–45	>55
V$_D$/V$_T$	0.2–0.3	>0.6

FEV$_1$ = forced expiratory volume in 1 second; Pao$_2$ = partial pressure of oxygen in arterial blood; Aa$_{DO_2}$ = alveolar-arterial oxygen gradient; FIo$_2$ = fraction of inspired oxygen; Paco$_2$ = partial pressure of carbon dioxide in arterial blood; V$_D$/V$_T$ = ratio of dead space to tidal volume. *Source: Reproduced, with permission, from Demling RH, Goodwin CW: Pulmonary dysfunction. In Wilmore DW (editor): Care of the Surgical Patient. Scientific American, 1989.*

1. Decrease in cardiac index
2. Decrease in oxygen-carrying capacity (hemoglobin/red blood cells)
3. Increase in oxygen consumption (VO$_2$).
   Pulmonary causes of hypoxemia can be divided into four categories:
1. *Absolute shunt:* blood passes from the right to the left heart without being exposed to alveolar O$_2$. No response is shown to increase FIo$_2$.
   a. Capillary shunting: ARDS, pneumonia, atelectasis, cardiogenic pulmonary edema
   b. Anatomic shunting: congenital heart defects, arterio-venous malformations
2. *Relative shunt:* ventilation-perfusion (V̇/Q̇) mismatch: perfusion in excess of ventilation, eg, COPD, nitrate, Nipride, or bronchodilator administration
3. *Hypoventilation:* Carbon dioxide replaces O$_2$ in the lungs (see: alveolar gas equation, appendix)
4. *Diffusion defects:* The alveolar-capillary membrane can be widened significantly without resultant hypoxemia. If it thickens (eg, fibrosis), diffusion may be reduced to the extent of resulting hypoxemia. This is unusual, however, because normally at rest the hemoglobin molecule in the pulmonary circulation is fully saturated after one third of it is far past the alveolus. In most interstitial lung diseases (eg, sarcoidosis, interstitial pneumonitis), hypoxemia is due to V̇/Q̇ mismatch rather than diffusion defects.

C. **Endotracheal Intubation.** There are four indications for endotracheal intubation (rule of 4 *P*'s):

1. Impaired airway **p**atency
2. Inadequate airway **p**rotection
3. Inadequate **p**ulmonary toilet
4. Requirement for **p**ositive pressure ventilation

The safest route in most situations is **orotracheal intubation** (see Procedures page 335); if necessary, with in-line traction of the head to maintain cervical spine precautions. **Nasotracheal intubation** requires a spontaneously breathing patient. It is usually not indicated in an emergency situation. Emergency tracheostomy or cricoidotomy is indicated, when an airway cannot be obtained safely and in timely fashion by other routes. Elective tracheostomy is performed if a patient's respiratory dysfunction is estimated to last several weeks; it can be done early in the clinical course once the patient is stabilized.

Key factors for successful intubation are complete preparation of all supplies before attempting intubation. This includes appropriate IV access; ECG and pulse oximetry monitoring; availability of medications, oxygen, and ventilator; and, if possible, additional personnel in the room to help with suction, cricoid pressure, and administration of medications. Proper placement should be confirmed immediately by an adequate pulse oximetry saturation, bilateral breath sounds, and chest movement on auscultation, with no breath sounds in the epigastrium, and a color change of the attached end-tidal CO_2 monitor (between the endotracheal tube (ETT) and the Ambu bag). Right mainstem bronchus intubation is avoided by verifying tube placement on an immediately obtained portable chest radiograph and the subsequent documentation of the level of the ETT at the lip (in centimeters).

II. Ventilator Setup

A. **The Ventilator.** The majority of adult ventilator models currently used in the operating room, recovery room, and ICU are volume-controlled ventilators. The operator sets the tidal volume, respiratory rate, and the inspiratory gas flow. The ventilator will deliver the set volume of gas, regardless of the airway pressure (unless a pressure limit is set). In a pressure-controlled ventilator, the operator sets the respiratory rate, the inspiratory gas flow, and the peak airway pressure. The ventilator will deliver inspired gas until the desired pressure is reached, regardless of the tidal volume. The set pressure is maintained for the duration of inspiration, and the tidal volume is measured. It will vary, depending on the lung compliance: in stiff lungs, the same pressure will achieve a much smaller V_T than in normal, compliant lungs.

Become thoroughly familiar with the ventilator models used in the hospital. Most conventional and microprocessor-driven ventilators can be further classified by the mechanism used to produce the change-over from mechanical inhalation to the exhalation phase ("cycle off").

1. **Time-cycled mechanical ventilation:** The inhalation is terminated after a preselected inspiratory time (I-time). The timing mechanism is electronic (eg, in the commonly used Hamilton Veolar), or pneumatic (eg, in the IMV Bird). The V_T delivered is the product of inspiratory time (seconds) and inspiratory flow (mL/s). It is controlled by the operator and is not influenced by the peak inflation pressure (PIP) generated or by the patient's lung and chest-wall compliance. When the compliance decreases, the PIP increases (as they are generally inversely proportional); the I-time is unaffected (as it is set), but the inspiratory flow rate may decrease as a result of increased backpressure. Thus, the V_T decreases. For its restoration, either I-time or inspiratory flow rate has to be increased.

2. **Pressure-limited, time cycled mechanical ventilation:** A specific value for pressure limit is selected. Once this pressure limit is reached upon inspiration, the airway pressure is held at this level until the ventilator time-cycles "off." Active gas flow is present from the ventilator during this pressure plateau phase. This mechanism is believed by some clinicians to decrease mechanical trauma to the lung by limiting peak pressure. It is also suggested that oxygenation and distribution of ventilation are improved by prolonged alveolar distention during the inspiration phase.

3. **Volume-cycled mechanical ventilation:** The inhalation is terminated after a set V_T has been delivered by the ventilator, regardless of PIP, I-time, or inspiratory flow rate (eg, Puritan Bennett MA-1). Upon delivery of the selected V_T, PIP increases when compliance decreases. The V_T at high PIP varies, because it is distributed between the ventilator breathing circuit tubing and the patient's lungs. The more compliant the tubing and the less compliant the lungs, the greater the fraction of V_T will be compressed in the circuit and will not contribute to gas exchange. Thus, exhaled V_T should be measured between the Y-piece of the breathing circuit and the ETT to confirm the actual V_T the patient receives. The Hamilton Veolar measures the delivered V_T at the patient's Y-piece. Because of compression loss, the delivered volume is frequently less than the set volume. The Puritan Bennett 7200 measures volume delivered at the machine; thus, delivered volume closely approximates set volume. The volume loss in the tubing is only calculated, not measured, and then added to the set V_T. A decrease in the patient's compliance with increased PIP and increased compression volume will not be sensed by the 7200 model.

4. **Flow-cycled mechanical ventilation:** In flow-cycled ventilation, the inhalation phase of ventilation continues until the inspiratory

flow rate decays to a certain percentage (~25%) of the initial peak value. Then the flow ceases, the ventilator cycles "off," and the exhalation valve opens for passive exhalation, irrespective of delivered V_T and inspiratory time. This mechanism is used by microprocessor-controlled ventilators in the pressure-support ventilation (PSV) mode: when the ventilator is patient-triggered "on," it senses a pressure change of −2 to −3-cm water (from patient's effort, inspiratory work) and immediately increases airway pressure, delivering a high inspiratory flow rate. The response time or the delay between demand (generation of negative pressure to cycle "on") and supply is approximately 50 ms. Thus, the work imposed on a patient to trigger a breath is dramatically improved with the current microprocessor-controlled triggering system, minimizing the work of breathing for the patient to initiate a breath. The "flow-by" function decreases response time even more and decreases pressure sensitivity to even less than −2-cm water (see below).

B. Ventilator Modes

1. **Controlled Mechanical Ventilation:** In the controlled mechanical ventilation (CMV) mode, the ventilator is time triggered and either volume- or pressure-limited. Its function is determined by the settings of the primary controls (see below), regardless of what the patient does. No gas flows when the patient makes a spontaneous inspiratory effort. This mode is appropriate for a patient who is heavily sedated or paralyzed or has severe brain stem injury. It is rarely used.

2. **Assist-Control:** In the assist-control (AC) mode, the ventilator is time- or effort-triggered "on" and either volume- or pressure-controlled. Used as a full-support mode ("control") in a sedated patient, the respiratory rate is set high enough to provide the desired MV as determined by the primary controls. Used as a supportive mode ("assist") the respiratory rate is set at half the spontaneous rate. This gives the patient time to generate negative inspiratory effort to trigger the ventilator; then a full V_T is delivered (as preselected) each time a spontaneous trigger is sensed. The set V_T is automatically delivered, if the patient does not initiate a spontaneous breath within an appropriate period. The only difference between an "assist" and a "control" breath in this mode is the manner in which it is triggered; the V_T is the same.

3. **Synchronized Intermittent Mandatory Ventilation** (SIMV): In this mode, ventilation also is time-triggered and either volume- or pressure-limited at the rate and volume determined by the primary controls. Additional gas is made available if the patient generates a spontaneous negative inspiratory force. The volume of the gas provided is proportional to the patient's effort and is usually small unless it is augmented by the feature of "pressure support" (PS).

SIMV can be used as a full-support mode when the respiratory rate is set sufficiently high that it can provide the entire desired MV. Used as a partial ventilatory support mode, the set rate is decreased to less than half the spontaneous respiratory rate. A negative inspiratory force generated by the patient is sensed, additional gas is provided, and the spontaneous breath is augmented by the PS up to (or greater than) the set V_T.

In distinction to AC, the spontaneous V_T in SIMV mode varies in proportion to the patient effort and amount of PS added, whereas in AC the V_T set at the primary controls is delivered whenever patient effort is sensed. In both modes, the work of breathing for the patient is determined by the trigger sensitivity, the response time of the ventilator, and the inspiratory flow rate of the gas provided. In SIMV, breath "stacking" is avoided by correctly timing, or synchronizing, the mandatory breaths with the patient-generated inspiratory effort (which is not possible in AC). This is thought to be of advantage by preserving the coordination of respiratory muscles and breathing pattern. It is also more comfortable for the patient and avoids respiratory alkalosis with all its resultant negative consequences. During spontaneous respiration, the distribution of ventilation is improved because spontaneous breaths tend to go to the more dependent areas of the lung, improving $\dot{V}/\dot{Q}$ matching, whereas mechanical breaths distribute to the less dependent areas, which are usually more compliant. Proponents of AC state as its advantages the decreased work of breathing and "letting the patient rest," thereby decreasing oxygen consumption. In AC, only a small inspiratory force needs to be generated, then the ventilator takes over the rest of the inspiratory phase. In practice, however, no major benefit accrues to AC if the trigger sensitivity is decreased, making the patient draw −5 cm water pressure or more, or if the inspiratory flow rate is decreased when the patient needs a high flow rate, or if the pattern of gas flow does not meet the patient's inspiratory effort after triggering the ventilator. Instead, the energy expenditure can be increased by as much as 30–50%. The patient does not cease inspiratory effort after triggering the ventilator, because he still experiences "hunger for air."

4. **Pressure-Support Ventilation:** The ventilator triggers "on" when a sub-baseline pressure is detected near the proximal airway. A positive pressure flow is immediately activated and continues until a predetermined inspiratory airway pressure is reached. This constant inspiratory plateau is maintained until the inspiratory flow rate decreases below a set level (usually a fraction of the initial flow rate) or until a set time has passed. The ventilator continually monitors the airway pressure and adjusts flow. The V_T is determined by the set level of pressure support and the patient effort. At a high level of PS, this mode can function as a full-support mode, with minimal work of breathing (only the negative inspira-

tory force to trigger the ventilator) and optimal comfort in an awake, spontaneously breathing patient.

5. **Continuous Positive Airway Pressure:** A continuous positive airway pressure (CPAP) is maintained in a spontaneously breathing patient. No mechanical breaths are provided. A CPAP level of 5 is similar to positive end-expiratory pressure (PEEP) level of 5 in the setting of, for example, SIMV mode. In both modes, SIMV and CPAP, a PS can be added to the spontaneous V_T. The difference is that in SIMV (eg, rate of 10), ten mechanical breaths are given when the patient does not generate a spontaneous effort. CPAP has this feature only as a backup, when the apnea alarm is triggered. CPAP is used as a weaning mode.

6. **Pressure-Control Ventilation (PCV):** In this mode, the inspiratory time and the inspiratory (peak) pressure is controlled; the V_T depends on flow rate, airway resistance, and lung or chest wall compliance. The ventilator is time-triggered "on" and provides initially rapid gas flow to a set maximum level, then maintains a plateau inspiratory pressure, during which the V_T is distributed to the less compliant areas of the lung with a slower, more gentle flow. This prolonged inspiratory pressure is thought to recruit alveoli and benefit oxygenation of injured lung areas, while minimizing barotrauma and stretch injury.

III. Ventilator Settings

A. **Primary Controls:** The initial ventilator settings should be determined by the clinical situation and the underlying condition. The 5 primary controls are mode of ventilation, tidal volume, rate, FiO_2, and level of PEEP. In most situations in surgical patients, the initial mode will be either SIMV or AC, depending on the clinical situation, especially, the neurologic status, and the hemodynamic stability of the patient. The V_T is chosen on the basis of body weight (BW); recommended are 5–10 mL/kg BW. Data from recent prospective randomized controlled studies support a V_T of 5–8 mL/kg. This is thought to limit stretch injury to diseased alveoli and decrease secondary lung damage. The rate is set to provide adequate MV, again depending on the patient's hemodynamic and neurologic status and prior arterial blood gas (ABG) values. As initial FiO_2 it is safest to choose 100%, and after stabilization of the patient, to rapidly wean to a "nontoxic" FiO_2 value of ≤60% on the basis of pulse oximetry and ABG. At 1 atm, general guidelines are the following:

FiO_2	Duration before symptoms
100%	12 h
70%	48 h
60%	3 d
50%	6 d

Little evidence exists that $FIO_2 < 50\%$ is associated with O_2-toxicity in humans. Oxygen toxicity has been documented and studied extensively but is always difficult to distinguish from the natural progression of disease, except in experiments with animals or healthy human lungs. It varies with amount and duration of exposure, atmospheric pressure, and with each individual.

PEEP increases volume at end-expiration, preventing or decreasing airway collapse. This restores functional residual capacity (FRC) and decreases closing volume (CV). People are subject to about 5-cm water of PEEP in a normal nonintubated condition. Because the normal closing of the glottis at the end of respiration is lost with an intubated patient, PEEP maintains the FRC above the critical closing volume. It recruits collapsed alveoli. PEEP does not decrease extravascular lung water (EVLW) but does not cause any change. Whether it may increase EVLW by inhibiting lymphatic outflow is controversial and would take place only at high levels of PEEP. PEEP is not contraindicated for patients with COPD who have a high FRC and expiratory reserve volume preoperatively; their FRC decreases postoperatively with atelectasis, pain, and an elevated diaphragm like it does in normal lungs, and they may benefit from PEEP to restore FRC. The main advantage of PEEP is the improvement in oxygenation and distribution of ventilation, making the lungs responsive to lower levels of FIO_2. The maximal level of PEEP depends on the ventilator capability, the PEEP valve used, and the hemodynamic status of the patient. Historically, when PEEP was introduced, a high incidence of barotrauma and cardiovascular compromise was reported because of inadequacies in setup, equipment, and use. An arbitrary maximal level of PEEP was set at 15-cm water. A study in 1975 including 28 patients with severe ARDS showed that the use of PEEP > 25-cm water and as high as 44-cm water in conjunction with the lowest rate IMV that the patients could tolerate did not result in high complication rates. Pneumothorax occurred in 4 patients (14%), and there was no hemodynamic compromise as long as intravascular volume was maintained. Prerequisites for using high PEEP appropriately are as follows:

1. Maintain adequate cardiovascular monitoring (Swan-Ganz pulmonary artery catheter), intravascular volume, and cardiac support.
2. Use the correct equipment (ie, true threshold resistor PEEP systems (not flow resistor types, which can increase barotrauma and work of breathing), and the lowest rate of mechanical breaths that can be tolerated should be used. The less mechanical breaths, the lower the mean airway pressure and, secondarily, the mean intrathoracic pressure.
1. **Complications of PEEP:** Side effects of PEEP are many and are interrelated with the effects of positive-pressure mechanical ventilation per se on other organ systems.

a. **Pulmonary:** Barotrauma incidence is lower than believed in the past. Most damage in this regard is thought to occur at peak inspiration. As PEEP is increased, compliance may improve, resulting in minimal change in peak pressure. More susceptible to barotrauma are patients with COPD/emphysema and trauma patients.

b. **Cardiac:** PEEP above a level of 5–10-cm H_2O may decrease preload, that is, decrease venous return by increasing intrathoracic pressure. Positive-pressure mechanical ventilation alone and elevated mean airway pressures may have this effect also, regardless of PEEP. PEEP can lead to a decrease in the size of the left ventricle (LV) with decreased distensibility (compliance) from a right-to-left septal shift. It may increase the right ventricular (RV) size and increase the RV afterload because of increasing pulmonary vascular resistance by compressing pulmonary capillaries. On the other hand, the failing heart may be supported by surrounding positive pressure and reduction of pre- and afterload. Because of mechanical and pressure shifts, atrial tachyarrhythmias may arise.

c. **Renal:** The mechanisms of fluid retention and decrease in urine output are the result of a complex interaction of neurohumoral and cardiovascular responses, especially in the postoperative or trauma patient. Receptor mechanisms of the atria, carotid bodies, and aortic arch interact with the hypothalamus and the renovascular response, producing antidiuretic hormone, renin, and other hormones. It is unclear whether PEEP is the major factor in this response. If mean airway and mean intrathoracic pressure are the major determinants, then the number of mechanical breaths per minute may play a role. Mechanical ventilation per se redistributes renal blood flow from cortical to medullary areas, leading to decreased filtration rate and urine output.

d. **Neurologic:** PEEP more than 5–10-cm H_2O may increase intracranial pressure; the mechanism is thought to be decreased venous return with "back-up" venous congestion. There appears to be high individual variation.

B. **Secondary Controls:** These are used to optimize mechanical ventilation. The inspiratory flow-rate control determines the rate of gas delivery to the patient in the inspiration phase. A low flow rate results in a longer inspiration time, a gradual pressure buildup, and smoother ventilation with more time for V_T distribution to less compliant areas. On the other hand, patients may feel dyspneic, if they have a higher flow demand and are generating negative inspiratory effort to increase the flow, which increases the energy expenditure. A high gas flow leads to a sudden attainment of peak airway pressure, an increased mean airway pressure, a short inspiratory time, and less well-distributed ventilation to areas of poor compliance. The "blast" of gas may stimulate cough; however, a patient with high flow demand will not feel "hungry" for air.

At a set respiratory rate, a high inspiratory flow rate will shorten the I/E ratio. This favors exhalation and CO_2 excretion. A normal I/E ratio is 1:3. Lengthening the I-time and thus increasing the I/E ratio, or even inverting the I/E ratio (in severe respiratory failure with failure to oxygenate) favors alveolar inflation. The advantage of increasing the I/E ratio over increasing PEEP is proposed to be the generation of the same PEEP at the level of the alveoli without increase in PIP. The disadvantage is the possibility of hemodynamic compromise; therefore comprehensive cardiovascular monitoring is indicated when using inverse I/E ratio ventilation.

Various inspiratory flow wave patterns are available. With the "descending ramp" pattern, the flow quickly reaches a peak and then decelerates but is maintained until the ventilator cycles "off," and passive exhalation occurs. This allows better distribution of V_T, gives the lowest peak airway pressure, but gives higher mean airway pressure than the "square-wave" pattern. With the square wave, the V_T is delivered as a constant linear drive of gas flow into the patient without acceleration or deceleration. It results in the lowest mean airway pressure. When switching from the decelerating ramp pattern to the square wave, the flow rate has to be decreased to prevent the volume from being pushed too hard into the patient. "Accelerating" and sine wave forms do not have the peak flow at the beginning of inspiration, when the patient seems to need it most. These forms mimic the gas flow pattern of spontaneously breathing healthy patients but cannot meet the patient's initial fast-flow demand. The patient then has to generate negative inspiratory effort and work. Therefore, they should not be used.

The trigger sensitivity has to be adjusted astutely in all "assist" modes of ventilation to minimize work and discomfort for the patient. Historically, in a demand valve setup (ie, MA-1), the patient has to generate a certain negative pressure to open the valve and get the gas necessary for inspiration. The trigger is a sensor that detects a change in pressure (negative deflection). In a continuous-flow ventilator system (ie, Emerson), the ventilator was triggered when it sensed a change in flow. This effect decreased the work of breathing by half. The current microprocessor-controlled ventilators constitute a discontinuous, synchronized system with a significantly improved triggering system. They sense pressure change generated by the patient at an average level of -2 to -3-cm H_2O, decreasing work for the patient markedly.

The pressure sensitivity may be decreased to less than -2-cm H_2O by the flow-by function, setting a continuous basal flow rate. The sensing flow rate may then be set at, for example, 3 L/min, which means that every time the patient generates a flow of 3 L/min, the machine detects a decrease in basal flow and supplies inspiratory gas flow by opening a valve. The gas flow is almost immediately available at the patient's mouthpiece.

IV. Further Considerations at Initiation of Mechanical Ventilation

A. After intubation, the correct endotracheal tube (ETT) placement is confirmed by auscultation, color change of the end tidal CO_2 monitor probe, and by chest radiograph. The ETT is secured with tape and the level at the lips in cm should be documented.

1. A naso- or orogastric tube should be placed on all intubated patients unless there are contraindications (eg, esophageal surgery).

2. Adequate sedation for stress minimization and patient comfort needs to be individualized.

3. Restraints for patient safety may be indicated.

4. For most surgical patients, an arterial catheter is indicated for blood pressure and ABG monitoring during ventilation. Suitable sites are radial, dorsalis pedis and femoral arteries. Axillary lines are a second choice. Brachial catheters should be avoided because of poor collateral flow.

5. Additional pulmonary therapy should be ordered as indicated. This includes chest physiotherapy, bronchodilators, frequent suctioning, secretolytic agents (eg, Mucomyst), and head-of-bed elevation. If there are copious secretions or a new infiltrate on chest radiograph, sputum per tracheal aspirate should be sent as soon as possible for cultures.

6. Peptic ulcer prophylaxis should be instituted with either sucralfate, H_2 blockade, or proton pump inhibitors, depending on the clinical situation.

7. Deep vein thromboembolism prophylaxis with sequential pneumatic compression boots, thigh high, or placed on the arms, if not otherwise possible, should be started immediately. Further measures, including subcutaneous heparin, LMWH, low continuous intravenous heparin, or low-dose warfarin should be instituted as indicated clinically.

8. Decubitus prophylaxis with change of position, padding, and special beds must be started as soon as possible and monitored closely.

9. Any ventilated patient, whether in the acute phase of respiratory failure or during recovery, needs adequate energy supplies to meet the increased demands. The nutritional status, therefore, must be optimized. Whenever possible, and as soon as possible, enteral feedings should be started.

10. Electrolyte imbalances, especially the acid-base status, should be corrected, as this may interact with the respiratory drive and interfere with weaning.

V. Modification of Ventilator Settings

A. Checklist for the daily assessment of ventilated patients
  1. Observe:
     a. Respiratory rate and trend in rate
     b. Breathing pattern: chest expansion, abdominal breathing, use of accessory muscles, discoordinated breathing, "stacking" of breaths, paradoxic movements of the chest wall in relation to respiratory phase, "fighting" the ventilator
     c. Amount color, and consistency of secretions, and any change over 24 h
     d. Protection of airway: mental status, level of sedation, gag or cough reflex, and strength
  2. Listen for:
     a. Decreased breath sounds: Differential Diagnosis: (DD): atelectasis versus infiltrate versus effusion versus pneumothorax
     b. Rales DD: secretions in tracheobronchial tree versus pulmonary edema
     c. Wheezing DD: bronchospasm versus secretions versus obstruction of airway
  3. Check ventilator for the following items:
     a. ETT: Is the ETT secured? Check tape level on ETT at lip
     b. Tubing: Is the tubing intact? Is there any condensation, trapped secretions, or a leak?
     c. Humidifier: Is the humidifier functioning? Is the temperature set at 37 °C?
     d. Ventilator settings: Confirm on ventilator:
        • Mode and rate
        • FIO_2
        • V_T
        • PEEP setting
        • flow rate
        • PIP: observe trend: If high (> 50 cm H_2O):
        • DD: Airway obstruction versus lung stiffness versus chest wall stiffness
        • MV: normal 5–10 L/min. If higher, look at PCO_2 or acid-base status to assess whether a higher MV is necessary to correct PCO_2 and is generated by the patient (increased work of breathing) or by inappropriate vent settings (correct V_T, rate, mode, assess sedation, or mental status)
  4. Assess:
     1. Is the patient better or worse?
     2. Is he/she ready to wean?
     3. Adjust individual parameters.

VI. Trouble Shooting

Arterial blood gases should be monitored and adjusted to a normal pH (7.35–7.45) and a PaO_2 > 60 mm Hg on <60% O_2. Once correlation of the oxygen saturation by pulse oximeter and the blood gas has been established, the arterial blood gases for oxygenation can be minimized.

A. Adjusting Pa_{O_2}

1. To Decrease: FI_{O_2} should be decreased in increments of 10–20% with either ABGs or oximetry control between adjustments. The "rule of 7's" states that there will be a 7-mm Hg decrease in Pa_{O_2} for each 1% decrease in FI_{O_2}.

2. To Increase:
   a. Ventilation has some effect on Pa_{O_2} (as shown by the alveolar gas equation, see Appendix); therefore, correction of the respiratory acidosis will improve oxygenation.
   b. Positive-end expiratory pressure (PEEP) can be added in increments from 2–4 cm H_2O. It counteracts pulmonary shunts and raises Pa_{O_2}. If PEEP levels > 10–12 cm H_2O are needed, the placement of a Swan-Ganz catheter is recommended to monitor preload, mixed venous oxygen levels, shunt, and cardiac output. The effects of PEEP have a slower onset than changes in FI_{O_2} and can require 1–4 h to become apparent.
   c. Increase I:E ratio. This can be used supplemental or alternative to an increase in PEEP (see Paragraph III B).

B. Adjusting Pa_{CO_2}

1. To Decrease:
   a. Increase the rate
   b. Increase the tidal volume
   c. Check for leaks in the system

2. To Increase:
   a. Decrease the rate
   b. Decrease the tidal volume
   c. Determine the cause of hyperventilation: desaturation, anxiety, new-onset sepsis, acid base disturbance, pain, and treat appropriately.
   d. Rule out artificial causes of increased respiratory rate, such as condensation or secretions within the tubing causing movement that is sensed as respiratory effort by the ventilator; trigger sensitivity set too low.
   Auto-PEEP: arises from
1. Increase in expiratory resistance
2. Decrease in compliance
3. Increase in MV
4. Increase in inspiratory time
5. Increase in expiratory time
   Its effect on left ventricular filling is more variable, overall less than exogenous PEEP. Correct by
1. Adjusting I/E ratio, V_T, respiratory rate to decrease auto-PEEP
2. Increasing external (set) PEEP to level of auto-PEEP

Institute treatment and workup simultaneously. Remember: hypoxia kills. Take patient off the ventilator and ventilate by Ambu bag on 100% FIO_2 if there are any suspicions regarding the ventilator function. Call for additional personnel to help you. Suction and lavage and administer bronchodilator treatment as needed. Obtain ABG, monitor pulse oximetry reading, and correlate with ABG. Obtain chest radiograph and check ETT placement while you go through your differential diagnosis for each patient individually according to the clinical situation.

VII. Weaning

    A. Criteria. The following criteria should be fulfilled:

        1. The underlying disease should be significantly improved or resolved. Hemodynamic stability and no major acid base disturbance should be present.

        2. The patient should be able to maintain airway patency. The mental status should be appropriate; if obtunded, special attention should be given to the presence of cough, gag, and swallow reflexes. The amount of secretions, the frequency of suctioning, and the strength of the patient should be considered.

        3. Oxygenation and ventilation should be adequate.

        4. Additional criteria, which correlate to variable degrees with predictability of successful extubation are

RR < 35/min	(normal 12–20/min)
VC > 15 mL/kg	(normal 65–75 mL/kg)
NIF > –25-cm H_2O	(normal 75–100-cm H_2O)
V_D/V_T < 0.6	(normal 0.25–0.40)
Compliance > 30 mL/cm H_2O	(normal 50–100 mL/cm H_2O)
QS/QT < 20 %	(normal < 5%)
Pco_2 < 55 mm Hg with pH > 7.25	
Pao_2/FIO_2 > 300	

        5. Work of breathing can be measured with a flowmeter and esophageal probes (eg, "Bicore") and was found to be a useful criterion in some studies. Patients were found extubatable if work was < 1.34 kg-m/min.

        6. CPAP/room air trial (Civetta): Extubatable if tolerating 30 min.

        7. Trial of spontaneous breathing of room air via disconnected ETT: Extubatable if tolerated for 2 min. Vital signs, saturation, respiratory rate, breathing pattern, and strength of cough are observed by clinician after disconnecting the ventilator while leaving the ETT in place. Saturation should remain ≥90% with respiratory rate <28 bpm and no distress or change in vital signs for success.

        8. Cuff test: In patients with concerns about upper-airway patency (laryngeal edema, swelling), the ETT cuff is deflated and the patient auscultated for air movement (ie, leak) around the ETT, signifying enough space.

B. **Weaning Techniques**

1. **T-Piece (or T-tube bypass).** The patient is taken off the respirator for a limited period, and the ETT is connected to a constant flow of O_2 (usually 40–50%). If the patient tolerates breathing independently, the length of time off the respirator is progressively increased. It can be used for patients with no underlying lung disease (eg, a patient recovering from a drug overdose). Drawbacks to this technique are (1) no alarms are available because the patient is totally disconnected from the ventilator; (2) it is time consuming for the respiratory therapists and nurses; and (3) it is much more work than breathing spontaneously without an ETT. This is due to the relatively small diameter of the tube. Remember, resistance increases by the fourth power of the radius. Therefore, patients are usually placed on a T-piece for intervals of <2 h at a time. This method is commonly used by anesthesiologists and is safe when used in settings in which T-pieces are commonly used. The same effect can be achieved by placing the patient on CPAP with zero pressure support and either zero or minimal PEEP (5 mm Hg). The latter has the advantage of safety: The connection to the alarms of a ventilator is maintained.

2. **Synchronized Intermittent Mandatory Ventilation.** In this method, fewer and fewer machine breaths are given as the patient begins taking spontaneous breaths in between. For example, a patient breathing at a rate of 14 breaths/min in AC mode is switched to SIMV mode, rate 14. The rate is then stepwise decreased to 4 or 2. Most physicians either place the patient on continuous positive airway pressure mode at this point or observe the patient briefly on a T-piece. The theoretical advantages over T-piece weaning are (1) back-up alarms including automatic rates in case of apnea are in place; (2) a graded assumption of work allows respiratory muscle "retraining;" and (3) the extra work of breathing caused by the ETT resistance and the inherent resistance of the SIMV circuit valves and vent tubing can be decreased by applying PS.

3. **Continuous Positive Airway Pressure and Pressure Support Ventilation.** The patient is switched to the spontaneous breathing mode, which in most ventilators today is the CPAP mode. In current usage, CPAP is equivalent to PEEP, except it is used exclusively in spontaneously breathing mode. If the patient had PEEP of 5 mm Hg in the "assist" mode, a CPAP of 5 is set. Then, pressure support starting at 10 or 15 mm Hg is added, if the patient's prior ventilator settings did not include this. Pre-extubation ventilator settings, for example, are CPAP, 5; PS, 8; and Fio_2, 40%. Some physicians accept PS 10 as a minimal setting before extubation. This method requires an alert, cooperative patient who is spontaneously breathing. The advantage of this method is a smooth transition and a comfortable patient; machine back-up

functions remain in place in case of apnea or other inadequate parameters.

VIII. Special Modes of Ventilation

A. Pressure Control/Inverse Ratio Ventilation (PCV/IRV). This mode can be used with or without inverse I/E ratio (see item II, 6). With a normal I/E ratio, this mode provides lower PIP (especially in the "descending ramp" inspiratory flow wave pattern) and higher mean airway pressures. Often one sees higher V_T being delivered at the same or lower PIP. This may be due to the higher inspiratory flow generated in this PCV mode compared with volume-controlled ventilation. IRV is thought to generate the same PEEP at the alveolar level without an increase in the PIP. Longer I-time will open up less compliant lung areas, after initial distribution of the tidal volume to more compliant regions. A short E-time may help in prevention of end-expiratory alveolar collapse. Inverse I/E ratio is generated by turning down PEEP, then slowly prolonging I-time, monitoring saturation, V_T, hemodynamic parameters, and the flow volume curves to prevent auto-PEEP. The disadvantage of an inverse I/E ratio is patient discomfort: it requires total control of the breathing pattern, thus, patients usually have to be heavily sedated or paralyzed to benefit.

B. Permissive Hypercapnia. This ventilation strategy was developed to minimize distribution or stretch-induced lung injury. In severe disease, (eg. acute respiratory distress syndrome) the lung is inhomogeneous; that is, more healthy, compliant areas are distended at pressures (volumes) that cannot even inflate other, noncompliant alveolar regions. In such severely diseased lungs, to achieve oxygenation alone would cause secondary injury to the more distensible, healthier areas. To also achieve normoventilation, additional stress has to be exerted on the lungs, eg, by increasing MV via an increase in RR or by an increase in V_T to normalize P_{CO_2} after having barely accomplished adequate oxygenation. The concept of allowing CO_2 to increase weighs the risk of hypercapnia against the risk of overdistention-induced lung damage. The risks of hypercapnia are minimal, as long as the pH is maintained >7.20 or 7.25 with administration of $NaHCO_3$ or Tris buffer and allowing renal compensation to take place.

C. High Frequency Ventilation (HFV). This ventilation strategy achieves oxygenation by continuous positive airway pressure with O_2 supplementation and ventilation with "shaking" the airway: very small V_T at a very rapid rate (200–300/min) are supplied. The mechanism by which CO_2 diffusion and excretion of a normal (or even high) CO_2-load is achieved is actually still unclear. Traditionally, gas has to be transported by bulk flow to the alveolar zone for exchange to take place; therefore, volume has to be greater than dead space. With HFV, V_T is much smaller than V_D. One theory is that convection is a major mechanism; gas flow is proportional to both frequency and pressure.

1. **High frequency positive pressure ventilation (HFPPV)** cycles 60–150 breaths per minute (BPM) at volumes of 2–5 mL/kg with flow rates of 175–250 L/min. The delivered V_T equals V_D. It can be used on a conventional ventilator with a modified breathing circuit. Inspiration is active and exhalation passive.

2. **High frequency jet ventilation (HFJV)** gives short gas jets via a small-bore cannula of <2-mm diameter with V_T 3–6 mL/kg at rates of 100–300 bpm and flow rates of 175–250 L/min. The gas is delivered to a rapidly cycling valve; the jet entrains supplemental gas before entering the airway. Inspiration is active, the gas moves through the center of the tubes. Simultaneously, passive exhalation occurs along the tube walls.

3. **High frequency oscillation (HFO)** can deliver 60–900 BPM with even smaller V_T of 1.5–2.5 mL/kg at flow rates of 5–10 L/min. Oscillation occurs during both phases of the respiration. Various HF machines can be used combined with conventional ventilators in IMV or CPAP mode.

   Disadvantages of HFV are
   - Poor humidification with frequent development of thick, dried secretions and crusts at ETT
   - Inability to measure V_T
   - Airway pressure at the mouth may not reflect the distal airway pressure: a sophisticated monitor with an adequately high frequency response needs to be placed inside the ETT
   - Increased PEEP (similar to Auto-PEEP) and CO_2-retention can occur at > 200 bpm
   - Requires special equipment and expertise to administer and to troubleshoot

   Advantages are
   - Smaller V_T with less increase in airway pressure can be delivered
   - A presumption of less hemodynamic effect, less elevation of ICP, and decreased risk of barotrauma

   Examples of indications are (1) noncompliant lung with bronchopleural fistula and large air leak; (2) multiple pneumothoraces with high airway pressures; (3) failure to oxygenate and ventilate on conventional modes; (4) high ICP combined with high airway pressures; (5) high airway pressures S/P lung resection with bronchial anastomosis or pneumonectomy; and (6) inhalation injury.

D. **Tracheal Insufflation.** Gas is insufflated near the carina through a small catheter. This removes CO_2 from the major airway, lowers V_D/V_T and allows CO2 clearance without hyperventilation of overdistention. This technique, also called **intratracheal pulmonary venti-**

lation, uses the Bernoulli effect and can be applied in conjunction with conventional methods of ventilation.

E. **Extracorporeal Life Support (ECLS).** Extracorporeal membrane oxygenation (ECMO) uses a modified heart-lung machine for gas exchange via membranes and pumps while resting the diseased lungs. This can be sustained for days to weeks and is indicated if the mortality rate from conventional ventilation is estimated to be >90%, and the primary process is reversible. Specific indications usually include a shunt of >30%, and compliance of less than 0.5 mL/cm H_2O per kg despite optimal conventional therapy. It is commonly used in infants with diaphragmatic hernia pre- and perioperatively and in adults as a bridge to transplant.

IX. Ventilator Equations

A. Acidosis/alkalosis

1. Metabolic acidosis:

Expected $Paco_2 = 1.5 \times (HCO_3) + 8 \ (\pm 2)$

2. Metabolic alkalosis:

Expected $Paco_2 = 0.7 \times (HCO_3) + 21 \ (\pm 2)$

3. Respiratory acidosis/alkalosis: For each 10 mm Hg change in CO_2, HCO_3 changes by 2 if acute, by 4 ± 1 if chronic.
4. pH: Acute change: every 10 mm Hg change in Pco_2, pH changes 0.08.
   Chronic change: every 10 mm Hg change in Pco_2, pH changes 0.03.

B. Alveolar gas equation

1. $Pao_2 = [Fio_2 \times (PB - PH_2O)] - Paco_2 / RQ$

   Example:

   PB (barometric pressure) = 760 mm Hg

   PH_2O (water pressure) = 47 mm Hg

   RQ (respiratory quotient) = 0.8 (with mixed fuel)

   If: $Fio_2 = 0.21$ (room air) and $Paco_2 = 40$ mm Hg, then Pao_2 {~/=} 105 mm Hg.
   If: $Fio_2 = 0.21$ mm Hg and $Paco_2 = 80$ mm Hg, then Pao_2 {~/=} 49 mm Hg.
   Apnea (definition): $Paco_2$ increased by {~/=} 3 mm Hg/min

   C. **ARDS/ALI:** Definition (by the American-European Consensus Committee on ARDS)
   1. ALI: $Pao_2/Fio_2 \leq 300$ mm Hg
   2. ARDS: $Pao_2/Fio_2 \leq 200$ mm Hg
      a. Acute onset
      b. Bilateral infiltrates on chest radiograph
      c. Hypoxemia
      d. No evidence of left atrial hypertension/pulmonary artery occlusion pressure ≤ 18 mm Hg

      "ALI–ARDS is a continuum, the technical difference is the degree of hypoxemia."

D. **Arterial content of O_2 = Cao_2**

   $$CAO_2(mL/dL) = (PAO_2 \times 0.0031) + (l\ lb \times 1.39 \times Sao_2)$$

E. **Capillary content of O_2 = Cco_2** (measured on 100% Fio_2, as it is assumed that PAO_2 equals the O_2 content of pulmonary capillary blood at full saturation, which itself is inaccessible to measurement).

   $$Cco_2(mL/dL) = [(Fio_2 \times 713) - Paco_2 / 0.8] \times 0.0031 + (Hb \times 1.39)$$

F. **Compliance (C) = change in volume/change in pressure ($\Delta V/\Delta P$)**
   Normal $\{\sim\!\!\backslash\!\!=\} 200$ mL/cm H_2O; $\{\sim\!\!\backslash\!\!=\} 100$ mL/cm H_2O in ventilated patients.

   $$C_{dyn} = V_T / (PIP - PEEP) \qquad \text{dynamic compliance}$$

   $$C_{stat} = V_T / PPLAT - PEEP) \qquad \text{static compliance}$$

G. **Dead space (Bohr equation):** measures physiologic (anatomical and alveolar) dead space. Normal = 33%.

   $$V_D / V_T = Paco_2 - Peco_2 / Paco_2$$

   where $Peco_2$ = end-expiratory pressure of CO_2 and anatomic deadspace = 2 mL/kg

H. **Mixed venous oxygen saturation: Svo_2**

   $$Svo_2 = Sao_2 - VO_2 / (CO \times Hb \times 1.39)$$

   where Sao_2 = arterial blood O_2 saturation; VO_2 = O_2 consumption; CO = cardiac output; and Hb = hemoglobin

I. **Shunt equation**
   Definition: the fraction of the cardiac output (QT) that perfuses unventilated alveoli (QS).

   $$QS / QT \text{ (no units)} = (Cco_2 - Cao_2) / (Cco_2 - Cvo_2)$$

Note: This equation includes all pulmonary factors affecting oxygenation except PEEP.

J. West zones of the lung
  Definition: Distribution of blood flow in relation to ventilation depending on gravity.

Zone I: $P_A > Pa > Pv$, where P_A = alveolar pressure
Zone II: $Pa > P_A > Pv$, where Pa = arterial pressure
Zone III: $Pa > Pv > P_A$, where Pv = venous pressure

RECOMMENDED LITERATURE

The ARDS Network: Ventilation with lower tidal volumes as compared with traditional tidal volumes for acute lung injury and the acute respiratory distress syndrome. N Engl J Med 2000;342(18):1301.

Civetta JM: Nosocomial respiratory failure or iatrogenic ventilator dependency. Crit Care Med 1993;21: 171.

Esteban A, et al: A comparison of 4 methods of weaning patients from mechanical ventilation. N Engl J Med 1995;332(6):345.

Hickling KG, Henderson SJ, Jackson R. Low mortality associated with low-volume pressure-limited ventilation with permissive hypercapnia in severe ARDS. Intensive Care Med 1990;16:372.

Lefor AT, Gomella LG (editors): Surgery on Call, 3rd ed. McGraw-Hill, 2001.

Mehta S, et al: Prediction of post-extubation work of breathing. Crit Care Med 2000;28 (5):1341.

Operator Handbooks on your hospital's ventilator models.

Scientific American Surgery: II. Care in the ICU, 4, Pulmonary Dysfunction; 5, Use of the Mechanical Ventilator, 2000.

Shoemaker WC, et al: Textbook of Critical Care, 4th ed. VII. Pulmonary Care. WB Saunders, 2000.

Stock MC, Perel A: Handbook of Mechanical Ventilatory Support. Williams and Wilkins, 2nd ed. 1997.

Tobin MJ (editor): Principles and Practice of Mechanical Ventilation. McGraw-Hill, 1994.

VII. Transplantation: Special Considerations in Critical Care

With the advent of modern surgical techniques and advances in immuno-suppression, transplantation has become the treatment of choice for end-stage diseases of several major organ systems. Organ transplantation, combined with careful patient selection and sound clinical judgment, provides a therapeutic alternative with an acceptable quality of life for many patients who would not otherwise survive their disease process. To care for these patients successfully requires the integration of surgical technique, critical care, and principles of transplant immunology. Fundamental principles and organ specific considerations will be addressed in this section.

LIVER

Introduction

First described in the 1950s, orthotopic liver transplantation (OLT) became a reality in 1967 when Dr. Thomas Starzl performed the first successful liver transplant. Since then, liver transplantation has blossomed into a therapeutic option limited only by the supply of donor organs. In the United States, in 1999, 4698 liver transplants were performed with 1-year and 4-year survival rates of 82% and 73%, respectively. After transplantation, up to 90% of all transplanted patients will ultimately achieve an improved quality of life.

Indications and Contraindications

Liver transplantation is indicated for patients with demonstrable end-stage liver disease and an expected survival of less than 1 year. Signs and symptoms include progressive hyperbilirubinemia and jaundice, portal hypertension, uncontrolled encephalopathy, poor synthetic function, and an inability to function or to maintain normal activity. Severe portal hypertension may lead to intractable ascites, hypersplenism, and variceal bleeding. In patients with poor synthetic function, the prothrombin time will be increased, and the albumin and fibrinogen will be decreased. Liver transplantation may also be performed in select patients with resectable hepatic malignancy confined to the liver. In patients who have had prolonged hepatorenal syndrome, simultaneous renal transplantation may be necessary if the patient has been dialysis dependent for 4 or more weeks.

Frequently, candidates for liver transplantation are in critical condition in the ICU. Several contraindications however, should be noted concerning transplantation. Exclusionary criteria include advanced cardiopulmonary disease, defined as an oxygen requirement greater than 50% and positive end-expiratory pressure (PEEP) greater than 5 mm Hg, or hypotension requiring two pressors (renal dose dopamine excluded), or poor cardiac function. Uncontrolled sepsis and acquired immune deficiency syndrome (AIDS) are also contraindications to transplantation. Because of the psychologic support and disciplined care needed postoperatively, patients who either lack an appropriate social support system or have abused alcohol or other substances in the last 6 months are not suitable for transplantation. Careful evaluation of the neurologic status of patients with encephalopathy is mandatory because irreversible brain damage or neurologic impairment is a contraindication for transplantation. Neurologic or neurosurgical consultation is appropriate in these situations.

Causes of Liver Failure

Any number of diseases may culminate in liver failure requiring transplantation. They can be divided into several broad categories. In the most acute situation, fulminant hepatic failure (see the following for definition) may necessitate urgent transplantation. The most common entities that result in transplantation in the United States are cirrhosis (Laennec, cryptogenic, primary biliary) or chronic hepatitis (autoimmune, types B, C, and non-B or C). Other causes leading to transplantation are Budd-Chiari disease, neoplasm, primary sclerosing cholangitis, and biliary atresia.

Evaluation

Certain criteria are used for the evaluation of patients with liver failure. The most recognized classification system is the Child-Pugh criteria. The Child's criteria were initially described for operative mortality and long-term prognosis after portosystemic shunts. For transplantation, it is the current system used to estimate hepatic reserve and prognosis. It separates into three classes (A/B/C) six criteria of hepatic function: bilirubin, albumin, ascites, encephalopathy, nutrition, and PT prolongation (Table VII–1). The operating room mortality rate for the three classes is as follows: class A, 0–5%; class B, 10–15%; and class C, >25%.

Beyond the synthetic capability of the liver, other considerations are also important during the evaluation of a liver transplant patient or candidate. Many patients with end-stage liver disease have some degree of hepatic encephalopathy. This can vary from mild to profound. Encephalopathy is categorized into four stages. In stage I, the patient has altered sleep habits, loss of spatial orientation, slowed mentation, and slight asterixis. This progresses to stage II where the patient demonstrates inappropriate behavior, incontinence, marked asterixis, and drowsiness but continues to respond to simple commands. In stage III hepatic encephalopathy, the patient is stuporous with marked confusion and slurred speech. Patients in stage IV are comatose with no response to pain. Patients in stage III or IV hepatic en-

TABLE VII–1. CHILD-PUGH CRITERIA.

Class	A	B	C
Criteria			
Bilirubin	<2.0	2.0–3.0	>3.0
Albumin	>3.5	3.0–3.5	<3.0
Ascites	none	controlled	refractory
Encephalopathy	none	I–II	III–IV
Nutrition	good	fair	poor
PT prolongation	<4 sec	4–6 sec	>6 sec
OR mortality	0–5%	10–15%	>25%

cephalopathy have severely altered mentation, and intubation should be considered for airway management.

Primary management for patients with hepatic encephalopathy is enteral lactulose, a poorly absorbed disaccharide that works as an osmotic laxative and prevents ammonia absorption by acidification of colonic contents. Therapy is titrated to approximately four bowel movements a day. Oral nonabsorbed antibiotics, such as neomycin, may be used to alter the colonic flora. Patients are typically placed on protein restriction and given L-carnitine and sodium benzoate.

Hepatorenal syndrome (HRS) may be seen in patients with liver disease. HRS is a functional abnormality of the kidneys that decreases the glomerular filtration rate (GFR). The pathogenesis is thought to involve vasoconstriction of the renal circulation associated with systemic vasodilatation, leading to decreased renal perfusion and, subsequently, decreased GFR. The kidneys have a normal histologic appearance and regain normal or near-normal function after liver transplantation. Two types of HRS are known. Type I has a rapid and progressive impairment of renal function (GFR) with a doubling of the creatinine to greater than 2.5 mg/dL or a 50% reduction in creatinine clearance to less than 20 cc/min within 2 weeks. Type II has a less severe GFR reduction and is associated with intense sodium retention and ascites that is diuretic resistant. HRS may be exacerbated by spontaneous bacterial peritonitis, gastrointestinal bleeding, and diuretics.

The physiologic abnormality of HRS includes increased cardiac output and decreased mean arterial pressure and systemic vascular resistance. A functional renal impairment is present in which the kidney avidly retains sodium, resulting in low urinary sodium and a low (<1) fractional excretion of sodium (FENA). The diagnosis of HRS is established when the Cr exceeds 1.5 mg/dL in the absence of other causes (shock, infection, or nephrotoxic drugs) and fails to improve with plasma expansion and withdrawal of diuretics. Ultrasound can be used to exclude intrinsic or postrenal abnormalities. The urine is characteristically of low volume (< 500 cc/d), low sodium (< 10 mEq/L), and devoid of sediment. The only treatment for HRS is transplantation.

Fulminant Hepatic Failure

Fulminant hepatic failure (FHF) is defined as the acute onset of hepatic dysfunction without prior liver disease, resulting in encephalopathy within 8 weeks of onset. Usually, there is concurrent jaundice and coagulopathy. Patients with FHF require careful and aggressive management as their clinical situation and mental status can deteriorate rapidly, requiring intubation, intracranial pressure monitoring, central venous access, and pulmonary artery catheterization.

Stage III or IV hepatic encephalopathy is commonly associated with cerebral edema. Although the precise cause of cerebral edema is unclear, both vasogenic and cytotoxic mechanisms have been implicated. A breakdown of the blood-brain barrier occurs with an increase in capillary permeability. In addition, inhibition of neuronal Na-K ATPase activity, glutamine accumulation, and primary injury to astrocytes ensue. Cerebral edema leads to increases in intracranial pressure (ICP) and decreased cerebral blood flow (CBF). ICP monitoring is crucial toward preserving CBF because persistent cerebral perfusion pressures (mean arterial pressure minus ICP) less than 50 mm Hg predict a poor outcome after liver transplantation. Although a CT scan is helpful, a negative scan does not exclude intracranial hypertension, and positive radiologic findings are often delayed.

Fulminant hepatic failure can result in multisystem organ dysfunction, including acute respiratory distress syndrome, hepatopulmonary syndrome, hepatorenal syndrome, coagulopathy, and infection. In the United States, the most common causes of FHF are from acetaminophen, viral hepatitis, and idiosyncratic drug reactions. Of the cases, 10–15% are indeterminate. Patients with FHF have an 80% mortality rate without transplantation. Those patients with viral and acetaminophen-induced FHF have a better chance of recovery, whereas those patients with indeterminate hepatitis, drug-induced disease, and Wilson's disease have worse prognoses.

Certain indicators can be used to predict prognosis. Upon arrival to the ICU, Factor V and VII blood levels should be drawn. A Factor V level less than 20% (age < 30 years) or less than 30% (age > 30 years) is associated with a poor prognosis. This level should be obtained before correction of any coagulopathy with fresh frozen plasma. A poor prognosis is also associated with a level V:VII ratio < 10% and INR > 3.5. Patients with stage III or IV hepatic encephalopathy or hyperbilirubinemia for greater than 1 week also have a poor prognosis.

Transplantation Procedure

The orthotopic liver transplantation (OLT) operation can be divided into three phases. Transplantation begins with the **recipient hepatectomy** and back table preparation of the donor organ. During the hepatectomy, the abdominal wall is opened with a standard chevron incision and the peritoneal cavity is entered. The attachments and pedicles of the liver are dissected and isolated. These include the porta hepatis, the inferior vena cava (supra- and infra hepatic), and both hepatic ligaments (retroperitoneal and diaphragmatic). On the back table, the donor organ is prepared with reconstruction of the vascular system. The Carrel patch is inspected, the tributaries are ligated (gastroduodenal, gastric, and splenic), and any aberrant arteries are reconstructed.

The **anhepatic phase** begins with the establishment of venovenous bypass and cannulation of the portal, femoral, and axillary veins. After this is done, the major vascular structures and common bile duct are clamped and divided. The recipient liver is then removed and sent to the pathology laboratory for analysis.

Transplantation begins with the insertion of the donor organ. The venous anastomoses are performed first. In a running fashion, the suprahepatic and infrahepatic inferior vena cava (IVC) are sutured to the donor organ. Flushing of the portal vein is performed before the completion of the infrahepatic IVC anastomosis to wash out air bubbles and residual preservation solution. The portal vein cannula is then removed, and the portal vein anastomosis is performed. The crossclamps are then removed in the following order: (1) suprahepatic, (2) infrahepatic, and (3) portal. The reperfusion and establishment of caval flow then begins. Large volumes of acidic products return to the heart during reperfusion, and temporary hypotension, hypothermia, and cardiac arrhythmias are possible.

After reperfusion, the arterial anastomosis is performed. A patch is created from the left and right hepatic arteries of the recipient and anastomosed to the donor Carrel patch. The variability of hepatic arterial anatomy requires creativity and flexibility during this portion of the operation to create a durable arterial anastomosis. Therefore, variation from a standard technique may be necessary. Following the arterial reconstruction, a duct-to-duct or Roux-en-Y-choledochojejunostomy biliary anastomosis is performed, depending on the clinical situation. Hemostasis is obtained and three Jackson-Pratt drains are placed in the following locations: (1) right lobe extending toward suprahepatic cava, (2) biliary anastomosis, and (3) left lobe traversing the retrohepatic cava. The abdominal wall and skin incision are closed, and the intubated patient is transported from the operating room to the ICU.

Post-transplant Care

Meticulous and specialized care is required for post-transplant patients. A specialized ICU is desirable to optimize postoperative management. Evaluation of graft function is possible immediately after surgery. A functioning graft demonstrates immediate postoperative bile production. Resolution of acidemia and normalization of the INR will occur. If the patient had preoperative hepatorenal syndrome, the renal function should improve after transplantation. Finally, the patient's encephalopathy will clear.

Liver transplant patients and candidates have a characteristic pattern of high cardiac output and cardiac index with a low systemic vascular resistance. Pressor selection should be based upon Swan-Ganz catheter numbers and may include renal-dose dopamine, norepinephrine (Levophed), and phenylephrine (Neo-Synephrine). Norepinephrine and phenylephrine provide high alpha tone to increase SVR with minimal beta effect. Dobutamine is rarely indicated except in cases of poor cardiac function or concurrent cardiac disease.

Standard intensive care protocols of each institution should be followed for liver transplant patients. These include protocols for nutrition, central venous access, ulcer or gastritis, deep venous thrombosis prophylaxis, fluid and electrolyte repletion, and ventilation management.

Complications

After liver transplantation, a variety of complications are possible. These may be divided into four categories: biliary, vascular, primary nonfunction (PNF), and other. Early recognition and treatment is essential, because delayed diagnosis increases morbidity and mortality rates.

Biliary complications are the most common with an incidence ranging from 6% to 27%. Biliary strictures usually occur at the choledochocholedochostomy anastomosis and are ischemic, mechanical, or technical in nature. During the operation, the terminal donor duct is trimmed until bleeding is noted from the cut edge, indicating adequate blood flow. Because the transplanted terminal duct derives its blood supply from the hepatic artery, a stricture should prompt examination of the hepatic artery. Intrahepatic biliary strictures may occur from ischemia or preservation damage of the liver allograft. Other causes of biliary obstruction and stricture include organ rejection, cytomegalovirus infection, and recurrence of sclerosing cholangitis. Biliary leaks are associated with a 50% mortality rate and are usually caused by necrosis of the bile duct. Leaks are most common in the 3rd or 4th postoperative week and may be accompanied by hepatic artery thrombosis, bile peritonitis, or infected biloma.

Vascular complications may involve the hepatic artery or the portal vein. Hepatic artery thrombosis (HAT) has an incidence of 5%. Several items may contribute to the development of this complication, including technical factors, high hematocrit (hematocrit > 30% increases viscosity), and a posttransplant hypercoagulable state (earlier production of clotting factors V and VIII rather than protein clinical status and antithrombin III). In addition, a greater risk of HAT exists with complex interposition grafts or intraoperative revision of the arterial anastomosis. HAT is diagnosed by a marked increase in the prothrombin time and liver transaminases (AST/ALT) and an abnormal Doppler ultrasound. Urgent thrombectomy and revision of the arterial anastomosis is required. Portal vein thrombosis (PVT) is a rare complication with an incidence of 1–4%. PVT may cause acute portal hypertension and gastrointestinal bleeding in addition to coagulopathy and elevation of the liver enzymes. Doppler ultrasound observation of the portal vein is helpful in the diagnosis. As with HAT, urgent thrombectomy and reconstruction of the portal vein is required for graft salvage.

Primary nonfunction (PNF) has an incidence of 2–10% and represents acute allograft failure. Essential criteria for diagnosis are its occurrence within the first 96 h and a normal flow in the hepatic artery and portal vein. Also, three of the following findings must be present: (1) bile production < 20 cc for 12 h, bilirubin > 10 mg/dL or increasing more than 5 mg/dL per day, international normalization ratio (INR) of 1.5 or greater, and factors V and VIII < 25%. Liver enzymes will be elevated in the 5000–10,000 U/L range. The treatment for PNF is urgent retransplantation.

Postoperative hemorrhage occurs in approximately 10–15% of patients. Treatment includes correction of coagulopathy, correction of hypothermia, and transfusion. Urgent reoperation demonstrates a specific bleeding point in only 50% of the cases. These cases are associated with a better prognosis. Diffuse bleeding is associated with a poor prognosis, because coagulopathy is likely related to poor graft function. For patients with postoperative bleeding not requiring urgent exploration, a return to the OR is appropriate after 1–3 d for evacuation of the intra-abdominal hematoma and relief of intra-abdominal pressure. Such explorations can often improve coagulopathy by interrupting the primary fibrinolysis caused by the presence of intra-abdominal blood.

Peritoneal sepsis occurs in approximately 5% of patients. This complication has a high mortality rate and may approach 50–60% because of patient frailty and immunosuppression. Sepsis occurs secondary to leakage of bile or enteric contents or infection of ascitic fluid. When the infection is localized to an abscess cavity, percutaneous drainage or surgical drainage may be performed.

Rejection

Two main types of rejection are seen after liver transplantation. Acute cell-mediated rejection occurs frequently but is easily treated with immunosuppression. Acute rejection is most common within the first 2 months after transplantation. Diagnosis is based on clinical and histologic examinations. Typical laboratory findings include increases in liver transaminases, alkaline phosphatase, and bilirubin. A decrease in bile output and a change in bile quality from thick dark to a watery light-green will be noted. Biopsy will demonstrate a characteristic triad of portal lymphocytosis, subendothelial mononuclear cells, and biliary destruction. Bile duct epithelial cells express large amounts of class II HLA antigens, and therefore, they are the prime targets of immune attack.

Chronic rejection has an incidence ranging from 8%–15%. Because of the persistent attack by the immune system, the small bile ducts gradually obliterate, resulting in a clinical presentation similar to obstruction. A biopsy demonstrates obliteration and absence of small bile ducts. Chronic rejection responds poorly to immunosuppression and usually requires retransplantation. Hyperacute rejection from preformed antibodies is rarely seen in liver transplantation.

KIDNEY

Introduction

In 1954, at the Peter Bent Brigham Hospital in Boston, the first successful kidney transplant between monozygotic twins was performed, resulting in the award of the Nobel Prize to Dr. Joseph Murray. Almost 50,000 patients are currently on the waiting list for kidney transplantation, making up about 65% of all patients on transplant waiting lists. In 1999, almost 12,500 kidney transplants alone and 1000 simultaneous kidney-pancreas transplants were performed. One- and 4-year graft survival rates for kidney transplants are 92% and 81% (living donor) and 83% and 67% (cadaveric donor). The immense success of renal transplantation has not only changed the face of end-stage renal disease but has also spurred on the development of transplantation of other major organs.

Indications and Contraindications

Patients with end-stage renal disease who are currently using dialysis therapy and patients with chronic renal disease and impending failure are candidates for renal transplantation. Because of the scarcity of donor organs, potential kidney transplant recipients undergo extensive medical and psychosocial evaluation. Once the need for renal replacement therapy is established, the candidate undergoes testing for other comorbidities that would preclude a major operation and the life-long use of immunosuppression. These include any history of incurable malignancy or infections, significant cardiovascular or pulmonary disease, the presence of any psychiatric illness or history of noncompliance, and blood and tissue typing. Cardiac disease remains a major cause of morbidity and mortality after renal transplantation; and potential transplant recipients are carefully screened for any history of ischemic heart disease. A history of bladder dysfunction or genitourinary abnormalities warrants a more extensive urologic workup to ascertain whether the patient's native bladder can be used. Pretransplant native nephrectomy should be considered for patients with chronic renal parenchymal infections, infected stones, heavy proteinuria, intractable hypertension, polycystic kidney disease, acquired renal cystic disease, and infected reflux nephropathy. Those patients with type I diabetes mellitus without significant comorbid disease should be considered for simultaneous kidney-pancreas transplantation.

Those patients with incurable malignancies or metastatic disease should not be considered for kidney transplantation. Theoretically, the lack of a fully functioning immune system favors the growth of malignancies. A history of previous malignancy does not necessarily exclude a patient from consideration for transplantation. However, most centers require a waiting period to screen for those patients who might otherwise develop tumor recurrence.

Any patient with an ongoing active infection or who is infected with the human immunodeficiency virus (HIV) is generally excluded from transplantation. In addition, all patients are screened for other infections, such as cytomegalovirus (CMV), tuberculosis, hepatitis B, and hepatitis C. CMV continues to be an important cause of morbidity in the transplant population. Although most of the population has been exposed to CMV at some point during their lives, those patients who have never been exposed are at greater risk of posttransplant CMV infections, particularly if their donor was exposed to the virus. These patients are at risk of primary disease and, therefore, should receive prophylaxis with acyclovir or ganciclovir.

Recurrent disease affecting the transplanted kidney is generally not a contraindication to transplantation. Other than Alport's syndrome, polycystic kidney disease, chronic pyelonephritis, and chronic interstitial nephritis, most kidney diseases will affect the graft; however, less than 5% of all graft loss can be attributed to recurrent disease. Those patients with higher risks of recurrent disease should be counseled, particularly if a living donor graft is being considered. Certain individuals with focal and segmental glomerulosclerosis (FSGS) have greater than a 50% risk of recurrence, and those individuals who have lost a prior transplanted graft to this disease have as great as an 80% risk of losing a subsequent graft. An inherited familial prostacyclin synthesis abnormality has been described in hemolytic uremic syndrome (HUS), thus making living related transplantation fraught with slightly more risk.

Most transplant centers also offer transplant candidates the option of a living donation. Patients who receive grafts from living donors instead of cadaveric donors not only have better long-term graft survival, less-delayed graft function, and less acute rejection, but also require less overall immunosuppression. Moreover, with the shortage of donor organs, the use of a living donor can decrease waiting time by several years and may even avoid dialysis altogether with preemptive transplantation. While HLA-identical living donor grafts fare best, even those living donation grafts that are not as well matched fare better than the best-matched cadaveric kidney grafts.

Living donors must also undergo extensive evaluation. The advent of laparoscopic donor nephrectomies has minimized hospital stay and postoperative recovery. However, to preserve the health and function of the donor, a detailed evaluation is performed. Factors that may contribute to perioperative morbidity are assessed, and donors are also screened for any history of glucose intolerance, obesity, hypertension, or renal disease. Reduced creatinine clearance, proteinuria > 300 mg per 24 h, and hematuria are generally contraindications to living donation. Nephrolithiasis, renal cysts, and abnormal or variant renal arterial anatomy may also preclude donation.

Operation

Donors between the ages of 5 and 60 years and without evidence of sepsis, malignancy, diabetes mellitus, and renal disease are generally considered for kidney procurement. Given the relative shortage of organs, many "marginal" donors are now being considered also. Marginal donors are those with evidence of hypertension; diabetes; age < 5 or > 60 years; premortem complications, such as acute tubular necrosis (ATN), disseminated intravascular coagulopathy (DIC), severe atherosclerosis, or anatomical abnormalities; procurement injury; sepsis; positive hepatitis C serology; or cold ischemia time > 36 h. Biopsies are recommended for these marginal organs; those with greater than 20–30% glomerulosclerosis or glomerular thrombi, severe ATN, interstitial infiltrates, or fibrosis are generally not used. As would be expected, these grafts tend to have delayed graft function after transplantation.

In the recipient, a curved "hockey stick" incision is made over the iliac fossa. The incision is brought down to the retroperitoneal space, and the peritoneal contents are retracted medially to expose the iliac vessels. The inferior epigastric artery and veins are ligated. In the female, the round ligament is divided; in the male, the spermatic cord is protected. Peri-iliac lymphatics are meticulously ligated to reduce the incidence of posttransplant lymphoceles. The iliac vessels are dissected cephalad to the bifurcation of the internal and external iliac and distally to the level of the inguinal ligament. When transplanting a right donor kidney, it may be necessary to divide the hypogastric veins to fully mobilize the external iliac vein and facilitate anastomosis to the shorter right donor renal vein.

The donor kidney is then brought to the field. Intravenous heparin is administered, and the vascular anastomoses are performed. An end-to-side anastomosis is made between the donor renal vein and the recipient external iliac vein. Although historically described as an end-to-end anastomosis, the donor renal artery and the recipient external iliac artery are now usually connected using an end-to-side anastomosis. When multiple renal arteries are present, a single arterial anastomosis can often be performed by creating a Carrel patch by using the donor aorta. Reperfusion is accomplished through release of the venous clamp first and then the arterial clamp. After reperfusion, the kidney should become firm and pink. Urine output should begin soon thereafter. Papaverine or intra-arterial verapamil is sometimes used to relieve arterial spasm.

Urinary tract reconstruction is then performed. The bladder is distended with an antibiotic irrigation solution. The ureter is shortened to minimize redundancy and to prevent ischemia of the distal portion. The distal tip is spatulated. The bladder detrusor muscle is incised over a length of approximately 3–4 cm down to the mucosal layer. A small cystotomy is performed at the distal end of the incision, and a mucosa-to-mucosa ureterocystostomy is performed. The detrusor muscle is then closed over the ureter, creating a submucosal antireflux tunnel.

The wound is then closed. Drains are not usually left in the wound. In some transplant centers, a duplex ultrasound is performed in the recovery room to assess blood flow in the graft. The Foley catheter is left in place for 3–5 d postoperatively to protect the uretero-cystostomy.

Post-transplant Care

Early postoperative care of the kidney transplant recipient encompasses not only routine postoperative matters but also issues related to volume management and surgery in the end-stage renal patient. These patients often have poor nutritional status, hypoproteinemia, platelet dysfunction, anemia, and electrolyte disturbances. Moreover, many of these patients' courses are further complicated by the administration of immunosuppressive drugs, particularly high-dose corticosteroids.

Although each center has a unique regimen for immunosuppression, most patients are placed on "triple therapy" immunosuppression. All patients are placed on prednisone in combination with cyclosporine or tacrolimus, in addition to azathioprine or mycophenolate mofetil. Antibody therapy may also be used in the initial postoperative period in selected patients with a high immunologic risk secondary to preformed anti-HLA antibodies, in those patients with a previous graft, or in those patients who are at risk of delayed graft function.

Volume management requires frequent monitoring in the early postoperative phase, because brisk diuresis helps to avoid delayed graft function. The central venous pressure is used to determine the intravascular volume status, and urine output is monitored hourly. Volume is usually replaced intravenously using D5 0.45% NS according to urinary output until the creatinine level decreases to < 3.0 mg/dL.

Complications

The kidney transplant recipient is at risk for many of the postoperative complications related to having had a major operation, initiation of immunosuppression, and renal failure. However, most early complications are manifested by oliguria or anuria. These symptoms demand a prompt workup, because rapid treatment can often reverse renal dysfunction without permanent effects on the graft. The differential diagnosis includes hypovolemia, ATN, mechanical obstruction, renal artery or venous thrombosis, or hyperacute rejection.

Initial workup should include assessment of the central venous pressure, the patency of the Foley catheter, and a hematocrit assessment. Next, an ultrasound of the transplanted kidney should be obtained to evaluate for perinephric fluid secondary to bleeding, lymphatic fluid, urine, or seroma. Urine leaks should be addressed urgently with re-exploration and possible nephrostomy tube drainage. Postoperative bleeding also necessitates re-exploration.

In addition, the ultrasound can be used to observe the patency of the renal vessels. Increased resistance, and thus a reduction in diastolic flow, has been associated with parenchymal edema, oftentimes secondary to ATN, or less-often, external compression. If the vessels are thrombosed, the patient will require transplant nephrectomy.

Currently, the incidence of hyperacute rejection is exceedingly low; advances in crossmatching techniques have nearly eliminated this complication. Usually manifested by poor reperfusion and a failure to achieve normal color and turgor, this complication is treated by transplant nephrectomy.

The most common cause of poor renal function in the immediate postoperative period is ATN. This ischemic injury is generally a diagnosis of exclusion and is usually reversible. However, the time to recovery varies and may take anywhere from a few days to several weeks. Common histopathologic findings range from mild tubular changes to frank tubular necrosis. During recovery, patients may require dialysis support.

Beyond the first postoperative week, acute allograft rejection becomes a more likely cause of graft dysfunction. Other differential diagnoses include drug-related nephrotoxicity from cyclosporine or tacrolimus, prerenal azotemia, vascular complications, ureteral obstruction, and lymphoceles. Acute allograft rejection is generally diagnosed on clinical criteria and is confirmed by percutaneous biopsy. It occurs in up to 60% of renal transplant patients and is most common during the second and third weeks after transplantation. Although initially asymptomatic, acute rejection can occasionally manifest as oliguria, fever, hypertension, and graft tenderness and swelling.

Up to 70% of those patients diagnosed with acute rejection can be successfully treated with the administration of pulsed high-dose corticosteroids. Steroids are usually the first-line treatment for renal transplant patients with acute rejection. Some centers, however, are using antithymocyte or antilymphocyte globulin and monoclonal antibodies as a first-line treatment against rejection. Most centers, however, reserve these modalities for those patients with rejection refractory to steroid pulsing.

Late vascular complications include renal artery stenosis, usually manifested by the development of hypertension. These complications can be treated operatively or with balloon angioplasty. Ureteral obstruction is usually managed acutely with the placement of percutaneous nephrostomy drainage; reoperation is then performed. Lymphocele formation is treated with drainage of the lymphocele into the peritoneal cavity. This procedure can be performed either laparoscopically or using an open approach.

HEART

Introduction

The field of cardiac transplantation has grown significantly since its beginning in 1967. 2184 heart transplants were performed in the United States in 1999. After transplantation, most patients achieve New York Heart Association (NYHA) functional Class I status. The 1-year and 4-year survival rates after transplantation are 84% and 72%, respectively.

Indications, Contraindications, and Evaluation

Cardiac transplantation is indicated in end-stage cardiac disease where residual life expectancy is 6 months to 1 year, despite maximization of medical therapy. With the exception of cardiac disease, candidates should be otherwise healthy. Most patients are NYHA class III or IV before transplantation.

The NYHA classifications are as follows:

Class I: No limitation of physical activity. Ordinary physical activity does not cause undue fatigue or dyspnea.
Class II: Slight limitation of physical activity. Comfortable at rest, but ordinary physical activity results in fatigue or dyspnea.
Class III: Marked limitation of physical activity. Comfortable at rest, but less than ordinary activity causes fatigue or dyspnea.

Class IV: Unable to carry on any physical activity without symptoms. Symptoms are present even at rest. If any physical activity is undertaken, symptoms are increased.

As with other forms of transplantation, the postoperative care is extremely rigorous and requires dedication and strict compliance. Consequently, candidates must be emotionally stable without a history of medical noncompliance. In the past, an upper age limit of 60 years was placed upon candidates, but recent studies have shown that older patients have survival rates and benefits similar to younger patients.

Despite the lethality of end-stage cardiac disease, cardiac transplantation does have contraindications. Significant systemic infection, multisystem disease, and irreversible pulmonary, hepatic, or renal dysfunction are contraindications to transplantation. Severe pulmonary hypertension increases early posttransplant mortality threefold, especially when the preoperative pulmonary vascular resistance is > 5 Wood's units or when the transpulmonary pressure gradient is > 15 mm Hg. Patients with severe pulmonary hypertension should be evaluated for combined heart and lung transplant. Ongoing tobacco, alcohol, or illicit drug use precludes cardiac transplantation, as does the presence of an incurable malignancy. Patients should be carefully evaluated by the transplant team (cardiologist, transplant surgeon, pulmonologist, clinical psychologist, and social worker) to determine candidacy.

Additional information is necessary to provide a suitable organ for the recipient. The patient's clinical status affects priority for receiving an organ. Status I (ICU with inotropic or mechanical support) patients are given priority over status II (all others) patients. ABO blood group match is essential because of the possibility of hyperacute rejection. Optimally, the donor should not be less than 80% of the recipient's body weight, and the ischemia time of the organ should be < 2 h. Although it is preferable for the recipient to have an ejection fraction of > 20%, it is more important to tailor medical therapy to decrease the pulmonary capillary wedge pressure.

Indications for Heart Transplantation

The most common causes accounting for approximately 75% of heart transplants are end-stage coronary artery disease (ischemic cardiomyopathy) and idiopathic cardiomyopathy. The remainder of patients awaiting cardiac transplantation have diagnoses of congenital heart disease, valvular heart disease, and defined cardiomyopathies (viral, post-partum, familial, and drug-induced).

Transplantation Procedure

An orthotopic heart transplant (OHT) begins with excision of the recipient heart. After a median sternotomy, the pericardium is opened, and the aorta and both vena cavae are cannulated. The patient is placed on cardiopulmonary bypass. The snares on the vena cavae are secured, and the aorta and pulmonary artery are crossclamped. Cardioplegic solution is infused into the aortic root, causing arrest of the recipient heart. The great vessels are isolated and divided at the level of the valve commissures, just above the sinuses of Valsalva. Excision of the recipient heart is continued along the atrioventricular groove leaving two recipient atrial cuffs. The recipient heart is then passed from the field.

The donor heart is carefully examined for any abnormalities, including a patent foramen ovale and unconventional coronary anatomy. The right atrium is opened carefully with a curvilinear incision extending from the inferior vena cava to the right atrial appendage. The sinus node is identified, and avoided. The left atrial anastomosis is performed first in a running fashion using 3-0 monofilament suture. After this is done, the right atrial anastomosis is performed in similar fashion, taking care to avoid encroachment on the sinus node or the coronary sinus. Alternatively, a bicaval anastomosis may be performed. Just before completion, the oximetric thermodilution pulmonary artery catheter is passed through the right ventricle into the pulmonary artery.

End-to-end anastomosis of the pulmonary artery is performed with running 4-0 monofilament suture. Systemic rewarming is initiated at this time, and the caval snares are released, permitting blood to flow into the heart and lungs and displacing any residual air. The recipient aortic trunk and donor aortic root are anastomosed with running 4-0 monofilament suture. Just before completion, additional venting is performed to release trapped air. The aortic crossclamp is removed, and a needle vent is placed. Electrical activity of the heart is resumed and defibrillation is performed, if necessary.

Careful hemostasis is obtained, and all suture lines are inspected. Cardiopulmonary bypass is slowly weaned and isoproterenol infusion (0.005–0.01 µg/kg/min) is initiated for inotropic and chronotropic support. Bypass cannulas are removed with closure of the arteriotomy and venotomy. Atrial and ventricular pacing wires are placed. Chest tubes are placed in the mediastinum and both pleural spaces. The sternum, fascia, and skin are closed in the usual fashion. The intubated patient is then transported to the ICU.

Posttransplant Care

The primary objective in the immediate posttransplant period is to maintain perfusion while minimizing cardiac work. Most patients demonstrate transient cardiac dysfunction secondary to prolonged ischemia, preservation, and catechol depletion. Additionally, the new heart is working against the elevated pulmonary vascular resistance of the recipient as a result of the previous congestive heart failure. Consequently, inotropic support is usually required for the first 72 h. This entails the use of dopamine, dobutamine, and isoproterenol infusions.

About 10–20% of patients experience transient sinus node dysfunction manifest by sinus bradycardia. Because the cardiac output of the transplanted organ (especially the right ventricle) is initially primarily dependent upon rate, pacing and chronotropic support with isoproterenol may be necessary. Posttransplant right ventricular dysfunction accounts for 15–20% of the early mortality rate of heart transplantation. This is related to recipient pulmonary hypertension (mean pulmonary artery pressure greater than 25 mm Hg), high pulmonary vascular resistance, warm ischemia during implantation, and potential air embolization of the right coronary artery. The heart rate should be maintained between 90–110 bpm to prevent heart failure. After the initiation of oral intake, terbutaline may be started for chronotropic support.

The systolic blood pressure is optimized to 90–110 mm Hg by afterload reduction with nitroglycerin or nitroprusside infusion. Urinary output should be at least 0.5 cc/kg/h, and renal-dose dopamine may be used to facilitate renal perfusion. The ventilatory parameters include maintaining $Pao_2 > 75$ mm Hg, $Paco_2$ between 30 and 40 mm Hg, and pH between 7.35 and 7.45.

During organ procurement, the donor heart is denervated with loss of sympathetic and parasympathetic fibers from the cardiac plexus resting between the tracheal bifurcation and aortic arch. This plexus normally regulates cardiac rate and contractility. The transplanted organ thus becomes dependent upon circulating catecholamines to increase cardiac output. Its sensitivity to catechols is increased because of an increased receptor density on transplanted myocardial cells.

Standard intensive care conventions of each institution should be followed for cardiac transplant patients. These would incorporate protocols for nutrition, central venous access, ulcer, gastritis, deep venous thrombosis prophylaxis, fluid and electrolyte repletion, and ventilation management.

Complications

The most acute complication after cardiac transplantation is bleeding with resultant tamponade. Chest tube output must be carefully monitored immediately after the operation. Persistent bloody output should be emergently addressed. Tamponade is manifest by decreased cardiac output and index, elevated central venous pressure, and equalization of the left- and right-heart pressures. Classically, pulsus paradoxus is present. Therapy is emergent subxyphoidectomy and drainage of mediastinal hematoma.

The leading cause of morbidity and mortality after cardiac transplantation is infection. Infections peak within the first few months and decline subsequently. Early infections tend to be bacterial and include pneumonia, mediastinitis, catheter sepsis, and urinary tract infections. Treatment is with appropriate antibiotic coverage and control of the source. Late infections tend to be opportunistic, viral, fungal, and protozoan. Treatment of these infections is more difficult and centers on the use of prophylactic antibiotics and immunizations. The most common post transplant infection is from cytomegalovirus (CMV) and may result in pneumonia, gastroenteritis, hepatitis, and retinitis. CMV pneumonitis has a mortality rate of 13%. CMV is best treated with ganciclovir and hyperimmune globulin.

Rejection of the organ is a major cause of death after cardiac transplantation. The incidence is highest during the first 3 months and falls to one episode per patient-year afterwards. Surveillance for rejection is performed by endomyocardial biopsy of the right ventricular septum, starting 7–10 d posttransplant and occurring at regular intervals afterwards. Rejection can be divided into acute and chronic rejection.

Acute rejection is characterized by a lymphocytic infiltration and myocytic necrosis. The severity is assessed on the basis of the International Grading System as follows:

Grade 0: No rejection
Grade 1A: Focal infiltrate without necrosis
Grade 1B: Diffuse but sparse infiltrate without necrosis
Grade 2: One focus with aggressive infiltration or focal myocyte damage
Grade 3A: Multifocal aggressive infiltrates or myocyte damage
Grade 3B: Diffuse inflammatory process with necrosis
Grade 4: Diffuse aggressive polymorphous with or without infiltrate, edema, hemorrhage, or vasculitis, necrosis present

Treatment is based on the severity of rejection and may entail increased oral prednisone in mild cases and pulsed steroid in severe cases. Refractory rejection can be treated with antithymocyte globulin (ATG) or OKT3 monoclonal antibody. Repeat biopsy should be performed in 10–14 d to assess treatment effectiveness. Close collaboration with the transplant cardiologist and coordinator is mandatory.

Chronic rejection is manifested by accelerated graft coronary artery disease. Patients typically do not have anginal symptoms because the transplanted heart is denervated. The mechanism is speculated to be chronic immunologically mediated damage to coronary vascular endothelium. Diffuse narrowing of the coronary arteries is present and extends to the distal branches. If focal narrowing is present, angioplasty or coronary artery bypass grafting can be performed. Generally, the only definite therapy is retransplantation.

PANCREAS

Introduction

In 1966, Kelly and Lillehei first attempted whole-organ pancreas transplantation at the University of Minnesota. Since that time, pancreas transplantation has become a viable therapeutic option for those patients with brittle diabetes. Compared with other major organ transplants, however, pancreas transplantation still remains a relatively risky procedure. One- and 5-year graft survival rates are 80% and 60% (simultaneous pancreas and kidney), 60% and 32% (pancreas after kidney), and 55% and 28% (pancreas transplant alone). Moreover, the morbidity rate remains higher for this organ than for kidney transplantation alone.

Indications and Contraindications

Insulin-dependent diabetes mellitus (IDDM) remains the leading cause of end-stage renal disease (ESRD) and accounts for approximately one third of new ESRD patients each year. The dismal 5-year survival rate of diabetic patients on dialysis makes kidney transplantation the treatment of choice for patients with end-stage diabetic nephropathy. Increasingly, these patients are offered the option of whole-organ pancreas transplantation. The addition of successful pancreas transplantation can enhance quality of life, improve certain diabetic complications, most notably neuropathy and nephropathy, normalize glycosylated hemoglobin levels, and achieve an insulin-independent euglycemic state.

Although the general criteria for recipients of pancreas transplantation and kidney transplantation are similar, the higher morbidity and mortality rates of pancreas transplantation require more specific criteria. The ideal pancreas transplant candidate is usually between the ages of 20 and 40 years, with minimal or limited secondary complications of diabetes, and impending or established ESRD. Patients usually are those with type I diabetes with renal failure, although patients with type II diabetes are considered if their beta-cell insulin secretion is exhausted.

Although a major contraindication to pancreas transplantation is significant cardiovascular disease, other relative contraindications include severe peripheral vascular disease, the lack of clearly defined complications from diabetes, and obesity. Other general contraindications are similar to those for other major organ transplants: severe cardiac or pulmonary disease that would preclude a major operation, inability to tolerate the immunosuppressive regimen required posttransplant, the presence of ongoing infection, recent or metastatic malignancy, substance abuse or dependence, noncompliance, and psychiatric illness.

Select patients may qualify for pancreas transplant alone. These patients usually have early diabetic complications or exogenous insulin failure with hyperlabile diabetes. For patients who also qualify for kidney transplant, choosing between simultaneous pancreas-kidney transplant (SPK) or pancreas-after-kidney transplant (PAK) can be somewhat of a problem. This difficulty is exacerbated by the potential option of using living related kidney donors. These patients historically fare better than those who receive cadaveric kidney transplants alone. Although additional morbidity is associated with pancreas transplantation, patients who undergo SPK fare better than those who receive a kidney transplant alone unless the donor is HLA-identical. Thus, patients with a living-related HLA-identical donor are usually encouraged to undergo kidney transplant first. Otherwise, patients who are acceptable candidates for SPK are generally encouraged to wait for dual organ transplantation.

Operation

Meticulous donor selection and procurement are important factors in recipient outcome. Blood sugar and serum amylase results are screened to determine the integrity of the donor islet cell function and pancreas gland. Donors with a history of diabetes, obesity, hyperglycemia, previous pancreatic surgery or trauma, alcohol abuse, pancreatitis, intravenous drug use, and previous splenectomy are generally not retrieved.

During procurement, care is taken to identify pancreatic disease and vascular anatomy, with particular attention to the superior mesenteric artery, splenic artery, and portal vein. After crossclamping of the aorta and infusion of preservation solution, the donor pancreas is removed en bloc with the spleen and the povidone-iodine flushed duodenum. Although the pancreas can tolerate up to 24 h of cold ischemia, it is preferred that not more than 16 h pass before reperfusion to minimize ischemia reperfusion injury.

Back-table preparation includes careful skeletonization of extra tissue, shortening of redundant duodenal tissue, oversewing the mesentery containing branches of the superior mesenteric artery (SMA), and the creation of an arterial Y graft by anastomosing the bifurcation of the donor iliac vessels to the SMA and splenic arteries of the pancreas.

A "hockey stick" incision is made over the iliac fossa of the recipient, and, unlike the kidney graft, the pancreas graft is placed intraperitoneally. The iliac vessels are mobilized from the level of the inferior vena cava to the level of the inguinal ligament. The internal iliac vein and all tributaries of the external iliac vein are carefully ligated and divided to allow complete mobilization of the external iliac vein. The donor portal vein is anastomosed to the recipient external iliac vein; the Y graft is anastomosed to the recipient iliac artery.

Exocrine secretions are drained via the donor duodenal segment anastomosed to the bladder, a Roux limb, or an end-to-side enteric anastomosis. Although most centers currently drain via the bladder, enteric drainage is gaining favor. Although a higher initial complication rate is associated with enteric anastomoses, enteric drainage decreases the metabolic and urologic complications associated with bladder drainage.

Posttransplant Care

After pancreas transplantation, patients are monitored in an ICU setting, where particular care is placed on insulin requirements, adequate hydration, and fluid resuscitation. Some form of anticoagulation, often low-molecular weight dextran, is started to prevent graft thrombosis. Graft perfusion is assessed with Doppler ultrasound, and fingerstick blood sugar and urinary amylase levels in patients requiring bladder drainage are monitored closely.

Most transplant centers use a quadruple-drug immunosuppressive regimen. Induction therapy is started either intraoperatively or in the immediate postoperative period to maintain an immunosuppressed state until serum levels of other agents are adequate. Induction therapy usually consists of monoclonal anti-T-cell agents, such as OKT3, and is maintained until 7–12 d after transplant.

Complications

The morbidity rate associated with SPK transplantation is higher than for kidney transplantation alone. Pancreas transplantation is also associated with complications involving exocrine function, vascular flow, bladder or enteric anastomosis, and rejection. Poor functioning of the beta cells in the early postoperative period may require the temporary use of exogenous insulin.

The earliest complications are generally related to exocrine function. Ischemia reperfusion of the donor graft can lead to serum hyperamylasemia and, occasionally, to frank pancreatitis. Development of graft pancreatic pseudocysts may necessitate percutaneous drainage. Occasionally, the clinical picture will progress to severe hemorrhagic pancreatitis, leading to vascular thrombosis and necessitating allograft pancreatectomy. Thrombosis more commonly occurs in the portal vein rather than in the arterial Y graft. Many centers institute some form of anticoagulation postoperatively as a prophylactic measure against graft thrombosis. Diagnosis is usually confirmed by duplex ultrasound or angiography.

For those patients with anastomoses to the bladder for exocrine drainage, metabolic derangements can be severe. Bicarbonate-rich secretions excreted through the urine can lead to acidemia when bicarbonate losses are not repleted. Moreover, this metabolic acidosis can be further exacerbated by renal tubular acidosis caused by tacrolimus or cyclosporine. The irritation to the bladder caused by the pancreatic enzymes can result in cystitis, at times hemorrhagic, which can persist for weeks after transplantation. The anastomosis may be at risk because of the constant irritation of the pancreatic enzymes. Extended use of a Foley catheter and alkalinization of the urine is recommended.

Enteric anastomoses can also be associated with leaks. Unlike bladder leaks that are usually treated with prolonged use of the Foley catheter, enteric anastomotic leaks necessitate reexploration. Additionally, patients with enteric anastomoses also carry the risk of prolonged postoperative ileus, small bowel obstruction, and reflux pancreatitis.

Because of an increased rate of acute rejection, pancreas transplant patients generally require increased levels of immunosuppression. However, rejection remains an extremely difficult diagnosis in this patient group, and accounts for up to 40% of graft failures. Usually, the diagnosis of rejection is based on a constellation of clinical findings. The patient may be febrile or have allograft tenderness and swelling, vague abdominal pain, or leukocytosis. When bladder drainage is used, a drop in the 8-h urine amylase can be an early sign of graft dysfunction. Hematuria also occasionally occurs. Unfortunately, hyperglycemia is a late sign of rejection and often indicates that partial or complete graft loss has already occurred.

For those patients with SPK, renal allograft function can often serve as a guide to pancreas allograft function. Manifestations of renal allograft rejection often parallel or precede pancreas allograft rejection. Ultrasound-guided fine needle biopsies of the pancreas allograft can be used to aid in diagnosing rejection, but the utility of this procedure may be center-specific. Once rejection is diagnosed, the mainstay of therapy remains increased immunosuppression, often in the form of pulsed corticosteroids, anti-lymphocyte preparations, or both.

IMMUNOSUPPRESSION

Immunosuppression regimens vary by institution and organ system. A variety of medications are available for immunosuppression. The common medications along with their mechanism of action and side effects are described here. Refer to your institution's regimen before instituting immunosuppression.

Corticosteroids

Steroids have multiple roles in the transplant patient. The two most commonly used forms are methylprednisolone (Solu-medrol) and prednisone. Their roles include pretransplant immunosuppression, postoperative taper, acute rejection therapy, and chronic oral therapy. The metabolic side effects of steroids are varied and well described and include hypertension, hyperglycemia, osteoporosis, decreased wound healing, and blunting of the inflammatory response. Steroid regimens may be extremely varied depending upon the organ system and the institution.

Tacrolimus (Prograf; FK-506)

Derived from the fungus *Streptomyces tsukabaensis,* Tacrolimus is a macrolide immunosuppressant that suppresses both humoral and cellular immune responses. Tacrolimus inhibits calcineurin, a calcium/calmodulin dependent phosphatase enzyme, preventing activation of T-cell specific transcription factors involved in lymphokine expression. Inhibition of interleukin-2 (IL-2) transcription leads to a reduction in T-cell proliferation. In addition, tacrolimus also inhibits the expression of IL-2 receptors. Tacrolimus is metabolized by the liver and is approximately 100 times more potent than cyclosporine.

In adults, blood trough levels between 5 and 15 ng/mL are therapeutic. The most common adverse effects are nephrotoxicity and neurotoxicity. Tacrolimus causes constriction of the afferent arteriole and may lead to decreased glomerular filtration rate (GFR), increased serum creatinine, and hyperkalemia. Toxic levels of tacrolimus may cause headache, tingling, tremors, and, in severe cases, coma.

Cyclosporine (Neoral)

Cyclosporine, derived from the fungus *Tolypocladium inflatum Gams,* blocks the activation and proliferation of T-lymphocytes. Cyclosporine binds to the cyclophilin family of molecules. The bimolecular complex then inhibits the enzymatic function of calcineurin, similar to the mechanism of tacrolimus, leading to inhibition of IL-2 transcription and receptor expression. Neoral is a microemulsion formulation of cyclosporin A with improved oral bioavailability and more consistent gastrointestinal absorption. Cyclosporin A is metabolized by the liver and is not dialyzable.

Cyclosporine may have a variety of adverse effects. The most concerning side effect is nephrotoxicity, leading to increased serum creatinine and hyperkalemia. In addition, cyclosporin A may cause hepatotoxicity, hypertension, leukopenia, headache, tremor, and seizures.

Mycophenolate Mofetil (Cellcept)

Mycophenolate Mofetil (MMF) is an antimetabolite that inhibits both cell-mediated and humoral immunity. After oral administration, MMF is rapidly absorbed and hydrolyzed to its active form, mycophenolic acid (MPA). MPA is a potent, selective inhibitor of inosine monophosphate dehydrogenase (IMPDH) and inhibits the de novo pathway of guanosine nucleotide synthesis. Whereas other cell types can use salvage pathways for purine synthesis, lymphocytes are dependent on de novo purine synthesis for proliferation. Consequently, lymphocytes are selectively inhibited by MPA. Cellcept is more potent and more selective than azathioprine.

General dosing ranges from 0.5–1 g BID, with reduction for renal dysfunction. The principal adverse reactions are gastrointestinal and include nausea, vomiting, diarrhea, and abdominal pain. Patients may also experience leukopenia and an increased incidence of sepsis and infections.

Azathioprine (Imuran)

Azathioprine is an antimetabolite that interferes with the precursors of purine synthesis and suppresses de novo purine synthesis. Consequently, azathioprine inhibits T- and B-cell proliferation by blocking cellular DNA and RNA synthesis. Azathioprine is metabolized by the liver, and the metabolites are excreted in the urine. Adverse effects include bone marrow suppression, hepatotoxicity, and gastrointestinal disturbances. Cellcept, a less toxic and more potent antimetabolite, may eventually supplant Imuran.

Monoclonal Antibodies

Monoclonal antibodies may be used for induction therapy or for steroid-resistant rejection. OKT3 is a purified murine monoclonal antibody that binds to the CD3 T-cell receptor and causes cell lysis and opsonization by the reticuloendothelial system. Because OKT3 may lead to life-threatening adverse reactions from cytokine release, patients require premedication with methylprednisolone (Solu-Medrol) and acetaminophen. Daclizumab (Zenapax) is a monoclonal antibody that binds to the α-chain of the IL-2 receptor causing a rapid depletion of cells expressing the IL-2 receptor. Possible serious side effects include pulmonary edema, renal tubular necrosis, and renal dysfunction.

RECOMMENDED LITERATURE

Busuttil RW, Klintmalm GB (editors): Transplantation of the Liver. WB Saunders, 1996.
Danovitch G (editor): Handbook of Kidney Transplantation, 3rd ed. Lippincott, 2001.
Ginns LC, Cosimi AB, Morris PJ (editors): Transplantation, Blackwell Science, 1999.
Norman DJ, Suki WN (editors): Primer on Transplantation, American Society of Transplant Physicians, 1998.
UNOS Website: www.unos.org

VIII.   Commonly Used Medications

This section is a quick reference to commonly used medications. You should be familiar with all of the dosages, indications, contraindications, side effects, and drug interactions of the medications that you prescribe. Such detailed information is beyond the scope of this book and can be found in the package insert, *Physicians' Desk Reference* (PDR), or the American Hospital Formulary Service.

Drugs in this section are listed in alphabetical order by generic names. Common uses are listed that include both labeled indications and common off-label uses based on recommendations of our editorial board. Some of the more common trade names are listed for each medication. Where no pediatric dose is provided, the implication is that the use of the agent is not well established in this age group or is infrequently used. Drugs under the control of the Drug Enforcement Agency (Schedule 2–5 controlled substances) are indicated by the symbol [C].

CLASSIFICATION

Allergic Disorders

Antihistamines

Cetirizine	Cyproheptadine	Hydroxyzine
Chlorpheniramine	Diphenhydramine	Loratadine
Clemastine Fumarate	Fexofenadine	

Miscellanous Agents

Budesonide	Cromolyn

Antidotes

Acetylcysteine	Digoxin Immune FAB	Methylene Blue
Charcoal	Flumazenil	Naloxone
Dantrolene Sodium	Ipecac Syrup	Physostigmine
Deferoxamine	Mesna	Protamin

Antimicrobial Agents

Antibiotics

AMINOGLYCOSIDES

Amikacin	Neomycin	Tobramycin
Gentamicin	Streptomycin	

CEPHALOSPORINS, FIRST GENERATION

Cefadroxil	Cephalexin	Cephradine
Cefazolin	Cephapirin	

CEPHALOSPORINS, SECOND GENERATION

Cefaclor	Cefotetan	Cefprozil
Cefmetazole	Cefoxitin	Loracarbef
Cefonicid	Cefuroxime	

CEPHALOSPORINS, THIRD GENERATION

Cefdinir	Cefotaxime	Ceftibuten
Cefixime	Cefpodoxime	Ceftizoxime
Cefoperazone	Ceftazidime	Ceftriaxone

CEPHALOSPORINS, FOURTH GENERATION

Cefepime

FLUOROQUINOLONES

Ciprofloxacin	Gatifloxacin	Moxifloxacin
Ciprofloxacin and	Levofloxacin	Norfloxacin
Hydrocortisone Otic	Lomefloxacin	Ofloxacin

MACROLIDES

Azithromycin	Dirithromycin	Erythromycin
Clarithromycin		

PENICILLINS

Amoxicillin	Mezlocillin	Penicillin V
Amoxicillin-Clavulanate	Nafcillin	Piperacillin
Ampicillin	Oxacillin	Piperacillin-Tazobactam
Ampicillin-Sulbactam	Penicillin G Aqueous	Ticarcillin
Cloxacillin	Penicillin G Benzathine	Ticarcillin-Clavulanate
Dicloxacillin	Penicillin G Procaine	

TETRACYCLINES

Doxycycline	Tetracycline

MISCELLANEOUS AGENTS

Aztreonam	Linezolid	Quinupristin/Dalfopristin
Clindamycin	Meropenem	Silver Nitrate
Colistimethate/Colistin	Metronidazole	Silver Sulfadiazine
Cortisporin, Otic	Mupirocin	Trimethoprim-
Fosfomycin	Nitrofurantoin	Sulfamethoxazole
Imipenem-Cilastatin	Pentamidine	Vancomycin

Antifungals

Amphotericin B	Clotrimazole	Ketoconazole
Amphotericin B Cholesteryl	Econazole	Miconazole
Amphotericin B Lipid Complex	Fluconazole	Nystatin
Amphotericin B Liposomal	Itraconazole	

Antimycobacterials

Ethambutol	Pyrazinamide	Rifapentine
Isoniazid	Rifampin	

Antiretrovirals

Abacavir	Indinavir	Saquinavir
Amprenavir	Lamivudine	Stavudine
Delavirdine	Nelfinavir	Zalcitabine
Didanosine	Nevirapine	Zidovudine
Efavirenz	Ritonavir	

Antivirals

Acyclovir	Interferon alpha 2B	Ribavirin
Amantadine	and Ribavirin	Rimantadine
Famciclovir	Interferon Alfacon-1	Valacyclovir

Foscarnet
Ganciclovir

Oseltamivir

Zanamivir

Antineoplastic Agents

Alkylating Agents

Altretamine
Carboplatin

Cisplatin

Triethyline-
Triphosphamide

NITROGEN MUSTARDS
Chlorambucil
Cyclophosphamide

Ifosfamide

Melphalan

NITROSOUREAS
Carmustine

Antibiotics

Bleomycin Sulfate
Dactinomycin

Daunorubicin
Doxorubicin

Idarubicin
Plicamycin

Antimetabolites

Cytarabine
Cytarabine Liposomal
Fludarabine

Fluorouracil
Mercaptopurine

Methotrexate
6-Thioguanine

Hormones

Anastrozole
Bicalutamide
Goserelin

Leuprolide Acetate
Megestrol Acetate

Nilutamide
Tamoxifen Acetate

Mitotic Inhibitors

Etoposide
Teniposide

Vinblastine
Vincristine

Vinorelbine

Miscellaneous Agents

Aldesleukin
Aminoglutothimido
BCG
Dacarbazine

Docetaxel
Hydroxyurea
Levamisole
Mitoxantrone

Paclitaxel
Porfimer
Thiotepa

Cardiovascular Agents

Alpha-1 Adrenergic Blockers

Doxazosin

Prazosin

Terazosin

Angiotensin-Converting Enzyme Inhibitors

Benazepril
Captopril
Enalapril and Enalaprilat
Fosinopril

Lisinopril
Moexipril
Perindopril

Quinapril
Ramipril
Trandolapril

Angiotensin II Receptor Antagonist

Candesartan
Eprosartan

Irbesartan
Losartan

Telmisartan
Valsartan

Antiarrhythmic Agents

Adenosine
Amiodarone
Atropine
Digoxin
Disopyramide
Esmolol

Flecainide
Ibutilide
Lidocaine
Mexiletine
Moricizine

Procainamide
Propafenone
Quinidine
Sotalol
Tocainide

Beta-Blockers

Acebutolol
Atenolol
Betaxolol
Bisoprolol
Carteolol

Carvedilol
Labetalol
Metoprolol
Nadolol
Penbutolol

Pindolol
Propranolol
Timolol

Calcium Channel Antagonists

DIHYDROPYRIDINES
Bepridil

Diltiazem

Verapamil

NON-DIHYDROPYRIDINES
Amlodipine
Felodipine
Isradipine

Nicardipine
Nifedipine

Nimodipine
Nisoldipine

Centrally Acting Antihypertensive Agents

Clonidine
Guanabenz

Guanadrel
Guanethidine

Guanfacine
Methyldopa

Diuretics

Acetazolamide
Amiloride
Bumetanide
Chlorothiazide
Chlorthalidone
Ethacrynic acid

Furosemide
Hydrochlorothiazide
Hydrochlorothiazide plus
    Triamterene
Indapamide
Mannitol

Metolazone
Spironolactone
Torsemide
Triamterene

Inotropic Agents

Amrinone
Digoxin
Dobutamine

Dopamine
Epinephrine
Isoproterenol

Milrinone
Norepinephrine
Phenylephrine

Lipid-Lowering Agents

Atorvastatin
Cholestyramine
Colestipol

Colesevelam
Fluvastatin
Gemfibrozil

Lovastatin
Pravastatin
Simvastatin

Vasodilators

Epoprostenol
Fenoldopam
Hydralazine

Isosorbide Dinitrate
Isosorbide Mononitrate
Minoxidil

Nitroglycerin
Nitroprusside
Tolazoline

Central Nervous System

Antianxiety

Alprazolam
Buspirone
Chlordiazepoxide

Clorazepate
Diazepam
Lorazepam

Meprobamate
Oxazepam

Anticonvulsants

Carbamazepine (see Table VIII–9, page 527)
Clonazepam
Diazepam
Ethosuximide
Fosphenytoin
Gabapentin
Lamotrigine
Levetiracetam
Lorazepam
Oxcarbazepine
Pentobarbital
Phenobarbital
Phenytoin
Tiagabine
Topiramate
Valproic acid
Zonisamide

Antidepressants

Amitriptyline
Amoxapine
Bupropion
Citalopram
Desipramine
Doxepin
Fluoxetine
Fluvoxamine
Imipramine
Maprotiline
Mirtazapine
Nefazodone
Nortriptyline
Paroxetine
Phenelzine
Sertraline
Trazodone
Trimipramine
Venlafaxine

Antiparkinson Agents

Amantadine
Benztropine
Bromocriptine
Carbidopa/Levodopa
Entacapone
Pergolide
Pramipexole
Procyclidine
Selegiline
Trihexyphenidyl

Antipsychotics

Chlorpromazine
Clozapine
Fluphenazine
Haloperidol
Lithium Carbonate
Mesoridazine
Molindone
Olanzapine
Perphenazine
Prochlorperazine
Risperidone
Thioridazine
Thiothixene
Trifluoperazine

Sedative Hypnotics

Chloral Hydrate
Diphenhydramine
Estazolam
Flurazepam
Hydroxyzine
Midazolam
Pentobarbital
Phenobarbital
Propofol
Quazepam
Secobarbital
Temazepam
Triazolam
Zaleplon
Zolpidem

Miscellaneous Agents

Nimodipine
Tacrine

Endocrine System

Antidiabetic Agents

Acarbose
Acetohexamide
Chlorpropamide
Glimepiride
Glipizide
Glyburide
Insulin
Metformin
Miglitol
Pioglitazone
Repaglinide
Rosiglitazone
Tolazamide
Tolbutamide

Hormone & Synthetic Substitutes

Cortisone
Desmopressin
Desoxycorticosterone
Dexamethasone
Fludrocortisone Acetate
Glucagon
Hydrocortisone
Methylprednisolone
Metyrapone
Prednisolone
Prednisone
Vasopressin

Hypercalcemia Agents

Calcitonin
Etidronate
Gallium Nitrate
Plicamycin

Osteoporosis Agents

Alendronate
Calcitonin
Raloxifene
Risedronate

Thyroid/Antithyroid

Levothyroxine
Liothyronine
Methimazole
Potassium Iodide
Propylthiouracil
Thyroid

Miscellanous Agents

Demeclocycline
Diazoxide

Gastrointestinal Tract

Antacids

Alginic Acid
Aluminum Carbonate
Aluminum Hydroxide
Aluminum Hydroxide with
  Magnesium Carbonate
Aluminum Hydroxide with
  Magnesium Hydroxide
Aluminum Hydroxide with
  Magnesium Hydroxide
  and Simethicone
Calcium Carbonate
Magaldrate
Simethicone

Antidiarrheal

Bismuth Subsalicylate
Diphenoxylate
  with Atropine
Kaolin/Pectin
Lactobacillus
Loperamide
Octreotide

Antiemetic

Buclizine
Chlorpromazine
Dimenhydrinate
Dolasetron
Dronabinol
Droperidol
Granisetron
Meclizine
Metoclopramide
Ondansetron
Prochlorperazine
Promethazine
Scopolamine
Thiethylperazine
Trimethobenzamide

Antiulcer

H_2-ANTAGONIST
Cimetidine
Famotidine
Nizatidine
Ranitidine
Proton Pump Inhibitor:
Lansoprazole
Omeprazole
Pantoprazole
Rabeprazole

MISCELLANEOUS AGENTS
Sucralfate

Cathartics/Laxatives

Bisacodyl
Docusate Calcium
Docusate Potassium
Docusate Sodium
Glycerin Suppositories
Lactulose
Magnesium Citrate
Magnesium Hydroxide
Mineral Oil
Polyethylene Glycol-
  Electrolyte Solution
Psyllium
Sorbitol

Enzymes

Pancreatin
Pancrelipase

Miscellaneous Agents

Dexpanthenol
Dicyclomine
Hyoscyamine
Hyoscyamine, Atropine,
  Scopolamine and
  Phenobarbital
Infliximab
Mesalamine
Metoclopramide
Misoprostol
Olsalazine
Propantheline
Sulfasalazine
Vasopressin

Hematologic Modifiers

Anticoagulants

Ardeparin
Dalteparin

Enoxaparin
Heparin

Warfarin

Antiplatelet

Abciximab
Aspirin
Clopidogrel

Eptifibatide
Reteplase

Ticlopidine
Tirofiban

Antithrombic Agents

Alteplase, Recombinant
(TPA)
Aminocaproic Acid
Anistreplase

Aprotinin
Dextran 40
Reteplase

Streptokinase
Tenecteplase
Urokinase

Hemopoietic Stimulants

Epoetin alfa (Erythropoietin)

Filgrastim (G-CSF)

Sargramostim (GM CSF)

Volume Expanders

Albumin
Dextran 40

Hetastarch

Plasma Protein Fraction

Miscellaneous Agents

Antihemophilic Factor VIII
Argatroban

Desmopressin
Lepirudin

Pentoxifylline

Immune System

Immunomodulators

Interferon alfa

Interferon Alfacon

Immunosuppressive Agents

Antithymocyte
Globulin (ATG)
Azathloprlne
Basiliximab

Cyclosporine
Dacliximab
Muromonab-CD3
Mycophenolate Mofetil

Sirolimus
Steroids
Tacrolimus

Vaccine/Serums/Toxoids

CMV Immune Globulin
Haemophilus B Conjugate
Hepatitis A Vaccine
Hepatitis B Immune
Globulin

Hepatitis B Vaccine
Immune Globulin,
Intravenous
Pneumococcal Vaccine,
Polyvalent

Pneumococcal 7-Valent
Conjugate
Tetanus Immune
Globulin
Tetanus Toxoid

Musculoskeletal Disorders

Antigout Agents

Allopurinol
Colchicine

Probenecid

Sulfinpyrazone

Muscle Relaxants

Aspirin and Meprobamate
Baclofen
Carisoprodol
Chlorzoxazone

Cyclobenzaprine
Dantrolene
Diazepam

Metaxalone
Methocarbamol
Orphenadrine

Neuromuscular Blockers

Atracurium	Pancuronium	Succinylcholine
Mivacurium	Pipecuronium	Vecuronium

Miscellaneous Agents

Edrophonium	Leflunomide	Methotrexate

OB/GYN

Contraceptives

Levonorgestrel Implants	Norgestrel

Estrogen Supplementation

Esterified Estrogens	Estradiol	Estrogen, Conjugated
Esterified Estrogens with	Estradiol Transdermal	with Methyltestos-
Methyltestosterone	Estrogen, Conjugated	terone
		Ethinyl estradiol

Vaginal Preparations

Amino-Cerv pH 5.5 Cream	Nystatin	Tioconazole
Miconazole	Terconazole	

Miscellaneous Agents

Gonadorelin	Medroxyprogesterone	Oxytocin
Leuprolide	Methylergonovine	Terbutaline
Magnesium Sulfate		

Opthalmic Agents

Acetazolamide	Fomivirsen	Norfloxacin
Apraclonidine	Gentamicin	Ofloxacin
Artificial Tears	Ketorolac	Phenylephrine
Atropine	Latanoprost	Pilocarpine
Bacitracin and Polymixin B	Levobunolol	Prednisolone
(Polysporin)	Levocabastine	Rimexolone
Betaxolol	Lodoxamide	Sulfacetamide
Brimonidine	Naphazoline and Antazoline	Timolol
Brinzolamide	Naphazoline and Pheniramine	Tobramycin
Carteolol	Neomycin, Bacitracin and	Tobramycin and Dexa-
Ciprofloxacin	Polymyxin-B (Neosporin)	methasone
Cromolyn	Neomycin, Polymyxin-B and	(TobraDex)
Cyclopentolate	Dexamethasone, (Maxitrol)	Tropicamide
Diclofenac	Neomycin, Polymyxin-B and	Trifluridine
Dipivefrin	Hydrocortisone (Cortico-	Vidarabine
Dorzolamide	tropin Ophthalmic)	
Dorzolamide and Timolol	Neomycin, Polymyxin-B and	
Echothiophate Iodine	Prednisolone (Poly-Pred)	
Erythromycin		

Pain Relievers

Local Anesthetics

Antipyrine and Benzocaine	Cocaine	Lidocaine
Anusol	Bupivacaine	Lidocaine/Prilocaine
Capsaicin	Dibucaine	

Narcotics

Alfentanil
Buprenorphine
Butalbital and Acetamino-
  phen
Butalbital and Aspirin
Butalbital, Aspirin and
  Codeine
Butorphanol
Codeine
Fentanyl
Fentanyl Transdermal
Fentanyl Transmucosal

Hydrocodone
Hydrocodone and
  Acetaminophen
Hydrocodone and Aspirin
Levorphanol
Meperidine
Methadone
Morphine
Nalbuphine
Oxycodone and
  Acetaminophen
Oxycodone and Aspirin

Oxymorphone
Pentazocine
Propoxyphene
Propoxyphene and
  Acetaminophen
Propoxyphene
  and Aspirin
Sufentanil

Non-Narcotic Agents

Acetaminophen
Acetaminophen
  with Codeine

Aspirin
Aspirin with Codeine

Tramadol

Nonsteroidal Anti-Inflammatory Agents

Celecoxib
Diclofenac
Diflunisal
Etodolac
Fenoprofen
Flurbiprofen
Ibuprofen

Indomethacin
Ketoprofen
Ketorolac
Meloxicam
Nabumetone
Naproxen

Naproxen Sodium
Oxaprozin
Piroxicam
Rofecoxib
Sulindac
Tolmetin

Respiratory Tract

Antitussives and Decongestants

Acetylcysteine
Benzonatate
Codeine
Dextromethorphan
Guaifenesin

Guaifenesin and Codeine
Guaifenesin and
  Dextromethorphan
Hydrocodone and
  Homatropine

Hydrocodone and
  Pseudoephedrine
Hydromorphone and
  Guaifenesin
Pseudoephedrine

Bronchodilators

Albuterol
Aminophylline
Bitolterol
Epinephrine

Isoetharine
Isoproterenol
Levalbuterol
Metaproterenol

Pirbuterol
Salmeterol
Terbutaline
Theophylline

Respiratory Inhalants

Acetylcysteine
Beclomethasone
Cromolyn Sodium

Flunisolide
Fluticasone

Ipratropium
Nedocromil

Miscellanous Agents

Beractant
Montelukast

Zafirlukast

Zileuton

Steroids

Systemic

Betamethasone
Cortisone
Dexamethasone
Hydrocortisone

Methylprednisolone
  Acetate
Methylprednisolone
  Succinate

Prednisolone
Prednisone

Topical (see Table VIII–7, page 525)

Alclometasone Dipropionate
Amcinonide
Betamethasone
Clobetasol Propionate
Clocortolone Pivalate
Desonide

Desoximetasone
Dexamethasone Base
Diflorasone Diacetate
Fluocinolone
Flurandrenolide
Fluticasone Propionate

Halcinonide
Halobetasol
Hydrocortisone
Mometasone Furoate
Prednicarbate
Triamcinolone

Supplements

Calcium Chloride
Calcium Acetate
Calcitrol
Cholecalciferol
Cyanocobalamin
  (Vitamin B_{12})

Ferrous Sulfate
Folic Acid
Iron Dextran
Leucovorin
Magnesium Oxide
Magnesium Sulfate

Phytonadione (Vitamin K)
Potassium Supplements
Pyridoxine (Vitamin B_6)
Sodium Bicarbonate
Sodium Ferric Gluconate
Thiamine (Vitamin B_1)

Urinary Tract Agents

Ammonium Aluminum Sulfate
Belladonna and Opium
  Suppositories
Bethanechol
DMSO
Flavoxate
Hyoscyamine

Methenamine Mandelate
Nalidixic Acid
Neomycin-Polymyxin
  Bladder Irrigant
Nitrofurantoin
Oxybutynin
Pentosan polysulfate

Phenazopyridine
Potassium Citrate
Potassium Citrate
  and Citric Acid
Sodium Citrate
Trimethoprim

Benign Prostatic Hyperplasia

Doxazosin
Finasteride

Tamsulosin

Terazosin

Miscellaneous Agents

Megestrol Acetate
Metyrosine
Naltrexone

Sodium Polystyrene
  Sulfonate

Witch hazel

GENERIC DRUGS

Abacavir (Ziagen)

COMMON USES: HIV-1 infections in combination therapy.
DOSAGE: *Adults:* 300 mg PO bid. *Peds:* 8 mg/kg (maximum 300 mg) PO bid.

Abciximab (ReoPro)

COMMON USES: Prevention of acute ischemic complications in patients undergoing percutaneous transluminal coronary angioplasty (PTCA).
DOSAGE: 0.25 mg/kg administered 10–60 min before PTCA, then 0.125 µg/kg/min (10 mg/min) continuous infusion for 12 h.

NOTES: Used concomitantly with heparin; may cause allergic reactions.

Acarbose (Precose)

COMMON USES: Type 2 diabetes mellitus.
DOSAGE: 25–100 mg PO tid with meals.
NOTES: May be taken concomitantly with sulfonylureas.

Acebutolol (Sectral)

COMMON USES: Hypertension; ventricular arrhythmias, angina
DOSAGE: 200–400 mg, PO bid.

Acetaminophen (Tylenol, others)

COMMON USES: Mild pain, headache, fever.
DOSAGE: *Adults:* 650–1000 mg PO or PR q4–6h. *Peds:* 10 mg/kg/dose PO or PR q4–6h.
NOTES: Overdose causes hepatotoxicity and treated with *N*-acetylcysteine; charcoal is not usually recommended; has no anti-inflammatory or platelet-inhibiting action.

Acetaminophen with Codeine (Tylenol No. 1, No. 2, No. 3, No. 4; others) [C]

COMMON USES: No. 1, No. 2, No. 3 for mild to moderate pain; No. 4 for moderate-to-severe pain; antitussive.
DOSAGE: *Adults:* 1–2 tablets q3–4h prn. **Peds:** Acetaminophen 10–15 mg/kg/dose; codeine 0.5–1.0 mg/kg dose q4–6h (useful elixir dosing guide: 3–6 y, 5 mL/dose; 7–12 y, 10 mL/dose).
NOTES: Capsules contain 325-mg acetaminophen, tablets, 300 mg; Codeine in No.1. 7.5 mg, No. 2: 15 mg, No. 3: 30 mg, No. 4: 60 mg; 5-mL elixir contains 120-mg acetaminophen, 12-mg codeine plus alcohol.

Acetazolamide (Diamox)

COMMON USES: Diuresis, glaucoma, alkalinization of urine, refractory epilepsy.
DOSAGE: *Adults:* Diuretic: 250–375 mg IV or PO q24h in divided doses. Glaucoma: 250–1000 mg PO QD in divided doses. *Peds:* Epilepsy: 8–30 mg/kg/24h PO in 4 divided doses.
Diuretic: 5 mg/kg/24h PO or IV. Alkalinization of urine: 5 mg/kg/dose PO bid–tid. Glaucoma: 20–40 mg/kg/24h PO in 4 divided doses.
NOTES: Contraindicated in renal failure, sulfa hypersensitivity; follow Na^+ and K^+; watch for metabolic acidosis.

Acetohexamide (Dymelor)

COMMON USES: Management of non-insulin-dependent diabetes mellitus.
DOSAGE: 250–1500 mg QD.

Acetylcysteine (Mucomyst)

COMMON USES: Mucolytic agent as adjuvant therapy of chronic bronchopulmonary diseases and cystic fibrosis; as antidote to acetaminophen hepatotoxicity within 24 h of ingestion.
DOSAGE: *Adults* and *Peds:* Nebulizer: 3–5 mL of 20% solution diluted with equal volume of water or normal saline administered tid–qid. Antidote: PO or NG; 140 mg/kg diluted 1:4 in carbonated beverage as loading dose, then 70 mg/kg q4h for 17 doses.
NOTES: Watch for bronchospasm when used by inhalation in asthmatics; activated charcoal adsorbs acetylcysteine when given PO for acute APAP ingestion.

Acyclovir (Zovirax)

COMMON USES: Herpes simplex and herpes zoster viral infections.
DOSAGE: *Adults:* Topical: Apply 0.5-inch ribbon q3h. Oral: Initial genital herpes: 200 mg PO q4h while awake; 5 caps/d for 10 d. Chronic suppression: 400 mg PO bid–tid.
Intermittent therapy: The same as for initial treatment, except treat for 5 d at the earliest prodrome. Herpes zoster: 800 mg PO 5 times/d. Intravenous: 5–10 mg/kg/dose IV q8h. *Peds:* 5–10 mg/kg/dose IV or PO q8h or 750 mg/m^2/24h divided q8h.
NOTES: Adjust dose in renal insufficiency.

Adenosine (Adenocard)

COMMON USES: Paroxysmal supraventricular tachycardia, including that associated with Wolff-Parkinson-White syndrome.
DOSAGE: *Adults:* 6 mg rapid IV, repeated in 1–2 min at 12-mg IV if no response. *Peds:* 0.03–0.25 mg/kg IV bolus; repeat higher dose in 1–2 min if no response.
NOTES: Doses > 2 mg are NOT recommended; caffeine and theophylline antagonize the effects of adenosine.

Argatroban (Novostan)

COMMON USES: Prevention or treatment of thrombosis in heparin-induced thrombocytopenia.
DOSAGE: Initial dose of 2 µg/kg/min IV, NOT to exceed 10 µg/kg/min.
NOTES: Monitor aPTT 2 h after initial infusion, adjust dose based on aPTT ratio, maintain a ratio of 1.5:3.

Albumin (Albuminar, Buminate, Albutein, others)

COMMON USES: Plasma volume expansion for shock resulting from burns, surgery, hemorrhage, or other trauma.
DOSAGE: *Adults:* 25 g IV initially; subsequent infusions should depend on clinical situation and response. *Peds:* 0.5–1.0 g/kg/dose; infuse at 0.05–0.1 g/min.
NOTES: Contains 130–160 mEq Na$^+$/L.

Albuterol (Proventil, Ventolin)

COMMON USES: Treatment of bronchospasm in reversible obstructive airway disease, prevention of exercise-induced bronchospasm.
DOSAGE: *Adults:* 2–4 inhalations q4–6h; 1 Rotacaps inhaled q4–6h; 2–4 mg PO tid–qid. *Peds:* 2 inhalations q4–6h; 0.1–0.2 mg/kg/dose PO to maximum dose of 2–4 mg PO tid.

Aldesleukin [IL-2] (Proleukin)

COMMON USES: Treatment of metastatic renal cell carcinoma, melanoma, and colorectal cancer.
DOSAGE: 600,000 IU/kg (0.037 mg/kg) administered every 8 h by a 15-min infusion for 14 doses. Following 9 d of rest, repeat schedule for another 14 doses, for a maximum of 28 doses per cycle.
NOTES: Only administer in a hospital with an intensive care unit and specialist available; may cause severe hypotension and capillary leaking, resulting in reduced organ perfusion.

Alendronate (Fosamax)

COMMON USES: Treatment and prevention of osteoporosis and Paget's disease.
DOSAGE: Osteoporosis treatment: 10 mg PO once daily. Prevention: 5 mg PO once daily. Paget's disease: 40 mg PO once daily.
NOTES: Should take 30 min before meals to avoid GI upset.

Alfentanil (Alfenta) [C]

COMMON USES: Adjunct in the maintenance of anesthesia.
DOSAGE: *Adults* and *Peds* > 12 y: 8–75 mg/kg IV infusion, total dose depends on the duration of the procedure.

Alginic Acid with Aluminum Hydroxide and Magnesium Trisilicate (Gaviscon)

COMMON USES: Symptomatic relief of heartburn, GE reflux.
DOSAGE: 2–4 tablets or 15–30 mL PO qid followed by water.

Allopurinol (Zyloprim, Lopurin)

COMMON USES: Gout, treatment of hyperuricemia of malignancy, uric acid urolithiasis.
DOSAGE: *Adults:* Initial 100 mg PO qd; usual 300 mg PO qd. *Peds:* Use only for treating hyperuricemia of malignancy in children; 10 mg/kg/24h divided q6–8h (maximum 600 mg/24h).
NOTES: Aggravates acute gouty attack, do NOT begin until acute attack resolves.

Alprazolam (Xanax) [C]

COMMON USES: Anxiety and panic disorders and anxiety associated with depression.
DOSAGE: 0.25–2 mg PO tid.
NOTES: Reduce dose in elderly and debilitated patients.

Alteplase, Recombinant [TPA] (Activase)

COMMON USES: Acute MI and pulmonary embolism.
DOSAGE: 100 mg IV over 3 h.
NOTES: May cause bleeding.

Altretamine (Hexalen)

COMMON USES: Palliative treatment of ovarian cancer.
DOSAGE: 260 mg/m^2/d PO divided q6h, for 14–21 consecutive days of a 28-d cycle.
NOTES: May cause neurologic and hematologic toxicity.

Aluminum Carbonate (Basaljel)

COMMON USES: Hyperacidity (peptic ulcer, hiatal hernia, etc); supplement to management of hyperphosphatemia in renal disease.
DOSAGE: *Adults:* 2 capsules or tablets or 10 mL (in water) q2h prn. *Peds:* 50–150 mg/kg/24h PO divided q4–6h.

Aluminum Hydroxide (Amphojel, ALTernaGEL, Alu-Cap, Alu-Tab)

COMMON USES: See Aluminum Carbonate.
DOSAGE: *Adults:* 10–30 mL or 2 tablets or capsules PO q4–6h. *Peds:* 5–15 mL PO q4–6h.
NOTES: Can be used in renal failure; may cause constipation.

Aluminum Hydroxide with Magnesium Carbonate (Gaviscon)

COMMON USES: Hyperacidity (peptic ulcer, hiatal hernia, etc).
DOSAGE: *Adults:* 15–30 mL PO pc and hs. *Peds:* 5–15 mL PO qid or prn.
NOTES: Doses qid are best given after meals and at bedtime; may cause hypermagnesemia.

Aluminum Hydroxide with Magnesium Hydroxide (Maalox)

COMMON USES: Hyperacidity (peptic ulcer, hiatal hernia, etc).
DOSAGE: *Adults:* 10–60 mL or 2–4 tablets PO qid or prn. *Peds:* 5–15 mL PO qid or prn.
NOTES: Doses qid are best given after meals and at bedtime; may cause hypermagnesemia in renal insufficiency.

Aluminum Hydroxide with Magnesium Trisilicate (Gaviscon-2)

COMMON USES: Hyperacidity.
DOSAGE: Chew 2–4 tablets qid and hs.

Aluminum Hydroxide with Magnesium Hydroxide and Simethicone (Mylanta, Mylanta II, Maalox Plus)

COMMON USES: Hyperacidity with bloating.
DOSAGE: *Adults:* 10–60 mL or 2–4 tablets PO qid or prn. *Peds:* 5–15 mL PO qid or prn.
NOTES: May cause hypermagnesemia in renal insufficiency; Mylanta II contains twice the amount of aluminum and magnesium hydroxide as Mylanta.

Amantadine (Symmetrel)

COMMON USES: Treatment or prophylaxis of influenza A viral infections; Parkinsonism.
DOSAGE: Influenza A: 200 mg PO qd or 100 mg PO bid. Parkinsonism: 100 mg PO qd–bid. *Peds:* 1–9 y: 4.4–8.8 mg/kg/24h to a maximum of 150 mg/24h divided qd–bid; *Peds > 9 y:* same as adults.
NOTES: Reduce dose in renal insufficiency.

Amikacin (Amikin)

COMMON USES: Treatment of serious infections caused by gram-negative bacteria.
DOSAGE: *Adults* and *Peds:* 15 mg/kg/24h divided q8–12h or based on renal function; refer to Aminoglycoside dosing (see Table VIII–1, page 518).

NOTES: May be effective against gram-negative bacteria resistant to gentamicin and tobramycin; monitor renal function carefully for dose adjustments; monitor serum levels (see Table VIII–2, page 519).

Amiloride (Midamor)

COMMON USES: Hypertension and congestive heart failure.
DOSAGE: 5–10 mg PO qd.
NOTES: Hyperkalemia may occur; monitor serum potassium levels.

Aminocaproic Acid (Amicar)

COMMON USES: Excessive bleeding resulting from systemic hyperfibrinolysis and urinary fibrinolysis.
DOSAGE: *Adults* and *Peds:* 100 mg/kg IV, then 1 g/m^2/h to maximum of 18 g/m^2/d or 100mg/kg/dose q8h.
NOTES: Administer for 8 h or until bleeding is controlled; contraindicated in disseminated intravascular coagulation; NOT for upper urinary tract bleeding; oral form rarely used.

Aminoglutethimide (Cytadren)

COMMON USES: Adrenal cortex carcinoma, Cushing's syndrome, and prostate cancer.
DOSAGE: 750–1500 mg/d in divided doses plus dexamethasone 2–5 mg/d or hydrocortisone 20–40 mg/d.
NOTES: Toxicity includes adrenal insufficiency ("medical adrenalectomy"), hypothyroidism, masculinization, hypotension, vomiting, rare hepatotoxicity, rash, myalgia, and fever.

Amino-Cerv pH 5.5 Cream

COMMON USES: Mild cervicitis, postpartum cervicitis or cervical tears, postcauterization, postcryosurgery, and postconization.
DOSAGE: 1 applicator intravaginally qhs for 2–4 wk.
NOTES: Contains 8.34% urea, 0.5% sodium propionate, 0.83% methionine, 0.35% cystine, 0.83% inositol, benzalkonium chloride.

Aminophylline

COMMON USES: Asthma and bronchospasm; apnea of prematurity.
DOSAGE: *Adults:* Acute asthma: Load 6 mg/kg IV, then 0.4–0.9 mg/kg/h IV continuous infusion. Chronic asthma: 24 mg/kg/24h PO or PR divided q6h. *Peds:* Load 6 mg/kg IV, then 1.0 mg/kg/h IV continuous infusion.
NOTES: Individualize dose; signs of toxicity include nausea, vomiting, irritability, tachycardia, ventricular arrhythmias, and seizures; follow serum levels carefully (see Table VIII–3, page 520); aminophylline is about 85% theophylline; erratic absorption with rectal doses.

Amiodarone (Cordarone)

COMMON USES: Recurrent ventricular fibrillation or hemodynamically unstable ventricular tachycardia.
DOSAGE: *Adults:* Load: 800–1600 mg/d PO for 1–3 wk. Maintenance: 600–800 mg/d PO for 1 month, then 200–400 mg/d. Intravenous: 15 mg/min for 10 min, then 1 mg/min for 6 h; maintenance dose of 0.5 mg/min continuous infusion. *Peds:* 10–15 mg/kg/24h divided q12h PO for 7–10 d, then 5 mg/kg/24h divided q12h or qd (infants and neonates may require a higher loading dose).
NOTES: Average half-life is 53 d; potentially toxic effects leading to pulmonary fibrosis, liver failure, and ocular opacities, as well as exacerbation of arrhythmias; IV concentrations of > 0.2 mg/mL should be administered via a central catheter.

Amitriptyline (Elavil)

COMMON USES: Depression, peripheral neuropathy, chronic pain, cluster and migraine headaches.
DOSAGE: *Adults:* Initially, 50–100 mg PO qhs; may increase to 300 mg qhs. *Peds:* Not recommended if aged < 12 y unless for chronic pain: 0.1 mg/kg qhs initially, then advance over 2–3 wk to 0.5–2 mg/kg qhs.

NOTES: Strong anticholinergic side effects; may cause urinary retention and sedation.

Amlodipine (Norvasc)

COMMON USES: Hypertension, chronic stable angina, and vasospastic angina.
DOSAGE: 2.5–10 mg PO qd.

Ammonium Aluminum Sulfate (Alum)

COMMON USES: Hemorrhagic cystitis.
DOSAGE: 1–2% solution used with constant bladder irrigation with NSS.
NOTES: Can be used safely without anesthesia and in the presence of vesicoureteral reflux. Encephalopathy reported, obtain aluminum levels especially in patients with renal insufficiency. Alum solution often precipitates and clogs catheters.

Amoxapine (Asendin)

COMMON USES: Depression and anxiety.
DOSAGE: Initially, 150 mg PO qhs or 50 mg PO tid; increase to 300 mg daily.
NOTES: Reduce dose in elderly patients; taper slowly when discontinuing therapy.

Amoxicillin (Amoxil, Larotid, Polymox, Others)

COMMON USES: Treatment of susceptible gram-positive bacteria (streptococci), and gram-negative bacteria (*Haemophilus influenzae, Escherichia coli, Proteus mirabilis*) (ie, SBE prophylaxis, otitis media, respiratory, skin and urinary tract infections.
DOSAGE: *Adults:* 250–500 mg PO tid. *Peds:* 25–100 mg/kg/24h PO divided q8h. 200–400 mg PO bid (equivalent to 125–250 mg tid).
NOTES: Cross-hypersensitivity with penicillin; may cause diarrhea; skin rash is common; many hospital strains of *E coli* are resistant.

Amoxicillin/Potassium Clavulanate (Augmentin)

COMMON USES: Treatment of infections caused by beta-lactamase producing strains of *H influenzae, Staphylococcus aureus,* and *E coli.*
DOSAGE: *Adults:* 250–500 mg as amoxicillin PO q8h or 875 mg q12h. *Peds:* 20–40 mg/kg/d as amoxicillin PO divided q8h.
NOTES: Do NOT substitute two 250-mg tablets for one 500-mg tablet or an overdose of clavulanic acid will occur; may cause diarrhea and gastrointestinal intolerance. Combination of a beta-lactamase antibiotic and a beta-lactamase inhibitor.

Amphotericin B (Fungizone)

COMMON USES: Severe, systemic fungal infections (eg, *Candida* spp., histoplasmosis, etc); bladder irrigation for fungal infections.
DOSAGE: *Adults* and *Peds:* Test dose of 1 mg, then 0.25–1.5 mg/kg/24h IV over 4–6 h. Doses often range from 25–50 mg qd or every other day. Total dose varies with indication.
  Bladder Irrigation: 50 mg in 1-L sterile water irrigated over 24 h; used for 2–7 d or until culture is negative.
NOTES: Severe side effects with IV infusion; monitor renal function; hypokalemia and hypomagnesemia may be seen from renal wasting; pretreatment with acetaminophen and antihistamines (Benadryl) to help minimize adverse effects such as fever; topical and oral forms available.

Amphotericin B Cholesteryl (Amphotec)

COMMON USES: Invasive fungal infection in persons refractory or intolerant to conventional amphotericin B.
DOSAGE: *Adults* and *Peds:* Test dose of 1.6 mg–8.3 mg, over 15 to 20 min, followed by a dose of 3–4 mg/kg/d. Infuse at a rate of 1 mg/kg/h.
NOTES: Do NOT use in-line filter, final concentration 0.6 mg/mL.

Amphotericin B Lipid Complex (Abelcet)

COMMON USES: Invasive fungal infection in persons refractory or intolerant to conventional amphotericin B.
DOSAGE: 5 mg/kg/d IV administered as a single daily dose; infuse at a rate of 2.5 mg/kg/h.

NOTES: Filter solution with a 5-mm filter needle; do NOT mix in electrolyte-containing solutions. If infusion exceeds 2 h, mix content of the bag.

Amphotericin B Liposomal (Ambisome)

COMMON USES: Invasive fungal infection in persons refractory or intolerant to conventional amphotericin B.
DOSAGE: *Adults* and *Peds:* 3–5 mg/kg/d, infused over 60–120 min.

Ampicillin (Amcill, Omnipen)

COMMON USES: Treatment of susceptible gram-negative (*Shigella, Salmonella, E coli, H influenzae, P mirabilis*) and gram-positive (streptococci) bacteria.
DOSAGE: *Adults:* Between 500 mg and 2 g PO, IM, or IV q6h. *Peds:* Neonates < 7 d: 50–100 mg/kg/24h IV divided q8h. Term infants: 75–150 mg/kg/24h divided q6–8h IV or PO.
Infants > 1 month and children: 100–200 mg/kg/24h divided q4–6h IM or IV; 50–100 mg/kg/24h divided q6h PO up to 250 mg/dose. Meningitis: 200–400 mg/kg/24h divided q4–6h IV.
NOTES: Cross-hypersensitivity with penicillin; can cause diarrhea and skin rash; many hospital strains of *E coli* are now resistant.

Ampicillin/Sulbactam (Unasyn)

COMMON USES: Treatment of infections caused by beta-lactamase-producing organisms of *S aureus, Enterococcus, H influenzae, P mirabilis,* and *Bacteroides* spp.
DOSAGE: *Adults:* 1.5–3.0 g IM or IV q6h.
Peds: Dosed by ampicillin content 100–200 mg ampicillin/kg/d (150–300 mg Unasyn) divided q6h; max daily dose 8 g ampicillin (12 g Unasyn) per day.
NOTES: 2:1 ratio of ampicillin/sulbactam; adjust dose in renal failure; observe for hypersensitivity reactions.

Amprenavir (Agenerase)

COMMON USES: HIV-1 in combination therapy.
DOSAGE: *Adults:* 1200 mg PO bid. *Peds:* (weighing < 50 kg): 20 mg/kg bid or 15 mg/kg tid, NOT to exceed doses > 2.4 g/d.

Amrinone (Inocor)

COMMON USES: Short-term management of congestive heart failure.
DOSAGE: *Adults* and *Peds:* Initially, give IV bolus of 0.75 mg/kg over 2–3 min followed by maintenance dose of 5–10 mg/kg/min.
NOTES: Not to exceed 10 mg/kg/d; incompatible with dextrose-containing solutions; monitor for fluid and electrolyte changes and renal function during therapy.

Anastrozole (Arimidex)

COMMON USES: Treatment of breast cancer following tamoxifen.
DOSAGE: 1 mg once daily.
NOTES: No detectable effect on adrenal corticosteroids or aldosterone; may increase cholesterol levels.

Anistreplase (Eminase)

COMMON USES: Treatment of acute MI.
DOSAGE: 30 units IV over 2–5 min.
NOTES: May not be effective if readministered more than 5 d after anistreplase, streptokinase, or streptococcal infection caused by production of antistreptokinase antibody.

Antihemophilic Factor [factor VIII] (Monoclate, others)

COMMON USES: Treatment of classic hemophilia A with factor VIII deficiency.
DOSAGE: *Adults* and *Peds:* 1 AHF U/kg increases factor VIII concentration in the body by approximately 2%. Units required = Body weight (kg) × (desired factor VIII increase as % normal) × (0.5). Prophylaxis of spontaneous hemorrhage: 5% normal. Hemostasis following trauma or surgery: 30% normal. Head injuries, major surgery or bleeding: 80–100% normal.

Patient's percentage of normal level of factor VIII concentration must be ascertained before dosing for these calculations. Typical dosing is 20–50 U/kg/dose given q12–24h.
NOTES: Not effective in controlling bleeding of patients with von Willebrand's disease; derived form pooled human plasma.

Antipyrine and benzocaine (Auralgan)
COMMON USES: Temporary relief of painful inflammatory conditions of the ear (serous otitis media, swimmers ear, otitis externa); aid to cerumen removal.
DOSAGE: *Adults* and *Peds:* Fill ear canal and place cotton plug to retain; repeat q1–2h prn; cerumen: apply tid–qid for 2–3 d.

Antithymocyte Globulin [ATG] (Atgam)
COMMON USES: Management of allograft rejection in renal transplant patients.
DOSAGE: *Adults:* 10–30 mg/kg/d. *Peds:* 5–25 mg/kg/d.
NOTES: Do NOT administer to a patient with a history of severe systemic reaction to any other equine gamma globulin preparation; discontinue treatment if severe unremitting thrombocytopenia or leukopenia occurs.

Apraclonidine (Iopidine)
COMMON USES: Glaucoma.
DOSAGE: 1–2 drops of 0.5% tid.

Aprotinin (Trasylol)
COMMON USES: Reduction or prevention of blood loss in patients undergoing coronary artery bypass grafting.
DOSAGE: High-dose: 2 million KIU load, 2 million KIU for the pump prime dose, followed by 500,000 KIU/h until surgery ends. Low-dose: 1 million KIU load, 1 million KIU for the pump prime dose, followed by 250,000 KIU/h until surgery ends. Maximum total dose of 7 million KIU.
NOTES: 10,000 KIU = 1.4 mg of aprotinin.

Ardeparin (Normiflo)
COMMON USES: Prevention of deep venous thrombosis and pulmonary embolism after knee replacement.
DOSAGE: 35–50 U/kg SC q12h. Begin the day of surgery and continue for < 14 d.
NOTES: Laboratory monitoring is not necessary.

Artificial Tears [OTC] (Tears Naturale, others)
COMMON USES: Dry eyes.
DOSAGE: 1–2 drops tid–qid.

Aspirin (Bayer, Ecotrin, St. Joseph, ASA, others)
COMMON USES: Mild pain, headache, fever, inflammation, prevention of emboli, myocardial infarction, and transient Ischemic attack (TIA).
DOSAGE: *Adults:* Pain, fever: 325–650 mg q4-6h PO or PR. Rheumatoid arthritis: 3–6 g/d PO in divided doses.
Platelet inhibitory action: 325 mg PO qd. Prevention of MI: 160–325 mg PO qd. TIA: 1.3 g/d PO divided bid–qid. *Peds:* Caution: Use linked to Reye's syndrome; avoid use with viral illness in children. Antipyretic: 10–15 mg/kg/dose PO or PR q4h up to 80 mg/kg/24h. Rheumatoid arthritis: 60–100 mg/kg/24h PO divided q4–6h (monitor serum levels to maintain between 15 and 30 mg/dL).
NOTES: Gastrointestinal upset and erosion are common adverse reactions; discontinue use 1 wk before surgery to avoid postoperative bleeding complications.

Aspirin with Codeine (Empirin No. 1, No. 2, No. 3, No. 4) [C]
COMMON USES: Relief of mild-to-moderate pain.
DOSAGE: *Adults:* 1–2 tablets PO q3-4h prn. *Peds:* Aspirin 10 mg/kg/dose; codeine 0.5–1.0 mg/kg/dose q4h.
NOTES: Codeine in No. 1: 7.5 mg, No. 2: 15 mg, No. 3: 30 mg, No. 4: 60 mg.

Aspirin with meprobamate (Equagesic) [C]

COMMON USES: Treatment of musculoskeletal disease in patients with signs of tension or anxiety.
DOSAGE: *Adults:* 1 tablet PO tid–qid.

Atenolol (Tenormin)

COMMON USES: Hypertension, angina, post MI, antiarrhythmic, acute alcoholic withdrawal.
DOSAGE: *Adults:* Hypertension and angina: 50–100 mg PO qd. AMI: 5 mg IV × 2 doses, then 50 mg PO bid.

Atorvastatin (Lipitor)

COMMON USES: Elevated cholesterol and triglycerides along with dietary modifications.
DOSAGE: Initial dose 10 mg daily, may be increased to 80 mg/d.
NOTES: May cause myopathy, monitor liver function test regularly.

Atracurium (Tracrium)

COMMON USES: Adjunct to anesthesia to facilitate endotracheal intubation.
DOSAGE: *Adults* and *Peds:* 0.4–0.5 mg/kg IV bolus, then 0.08–0.1 mg/kg every 20–45 min prn.
NOTES: Patient must be intubated and on controlled ventilation. Use adequate amounts of sedation and analgesia.

Atropine

COMMON USES: Preanesthetic, symptomatic bradycardia, asystole. Organophosphate poisoning, bronchodilator, mydriatic and cycloplegic for eye exam, uveitis, reversal of neuromuscular blockade with neostigmine or edrophonium.
DOSAGE: *Adults:* Emergency cardiac care, bradycardia: 0.5 mg IV q5min up to 2.0 mg total. Asystole: 1.0 mg IV, repeat in 5 min. Preanesthetic: 0.3–0.6 mg IM/IV/SC. Ophthalmic: 1–2 drops qid or 1/4 in of 1% ointment; refraction: administer 1 h before exam. *Peds:* Emergency cardiac care: 0.01–0.03 mg/kg IV q2–5 min up to 1.0 mg total dose; minimum dose of 0.1 mg. Preanesthetic: 0.01 mg/kg/dose SC/IM/IV (maximum 0.4 mg).
NOTES: Can cause blurred vision, urinary retention, dried mucous membranes.

Azathioprine (Imuran)

COMMON USES: Adjunct for the prevention of rejection after organ transplantation; rheumatoid arthritis; systemic lupus erythematosus.
DOSAGE: *Adults* and *Peds:* 1–3 mg/kg IV or PO daily.
NOTES: May cause gastrointestinal intolerance; injection should be handled with cytotoxic precautions.

Azithromycin (Zithromax)

COMMON USES: Treatment of acute bacterial exacerbations of chronic obstructive pulmonary disease (COPD), mild community-acquired pneumonia, pharyngitis, otitis media, skin and skin structure infections, nongonococcal urethritis, and PID. Treatment and prevention of mycobacterium avium complex (MAC) infections in HIV-infected persons.
DOSAGE: *Adults:* PO: Respiratory tract: 500 mg on the first day, followed by 250 mg PO qd for 4 more days. Nongonococcal urethritis: 1 g as a single dose. Prevention of MAC: 1200 mg PO once a week. Intravenous: 500 mg for at least 2 d, followed by 500 mg PO for total of 7–10 d. *Peds:* Otitis media: 10 mg/kg PO on day 1, then 5 mg/kg/d on days 2–5. Pharyngitis: 12 mg/kg/d PO for 5 d.
NOTES: Should be taken on an empty stomach.

Aztreonam (Azactam)

COMMON USES: Infections caused by aerobic gram-negative bacteria where beta-lactam may not be useful; including *Enterobacter, H influenzae, Pseudomonas;* sepsis, UTI, skin infections, intra-abdominal and gynecologic infections.
DOSAGE: *Adults:* 1–2 g IV/IM q6–12h. *Peds:* Premature infants: 30 mg/kg/dose IV q12h. Term infants, children: 30–50 mg/kg/dose q6–8h.

NOTES: Not effective against gram-positive or anaerobic bacteria; may be given to penicillin-allergic patients.

Bacitracin and polymixin B (Polysporin)

COMMON USES: Blepharitis, conjunctivitis, and prophylactic treatment of corneal abrasions.
DOSAGE: Apply q3–4h.

Baclofen (Lioresal)

COMMON USES: Spasticity secondary to severe chronic disorders, such as multiple sclerosis or spinal cord lesions.
DOSAGE: 5 mg PO tid initially, increase every 3 d to maximum effect; maximum 80 mg/d.
NOTES: Caution in epileptics and neuropsychiatric disturbances.

BCG (TheraCys, TICE, Pacis)

COMMON USES: Treatment and prophylaxis of superficial bladder cancer.
DOSAGE: 1 ampule in 30–50-mL NS instilled into bladder by catheter and held for 2 h (standard induction treatment weekly for 6 wk); maintenance schedules recommended include three weekly doses 3, 6, 12, 18, 24 or single monthly dose for 12 mo.
NOTES: Do NOT give within 10 d of bladder biopsy, if catheterization is traumatic or if patient is immunosuppressed.

Basiliximab (Simulect)

COMMON USES: Prevention of acute organ transplant rejections.
DOSAGE: *Adults:* 20 mg IV 2 h before transplant, then 20 mg IV 4 d posttransplant. *Peds:* 12 mg/m² up to a maximum of 20 mg 2 h before transplant, then the same dose IV 4 d post transplant.
NOTES: Murine/human monoclonal antibody.

Beclomethasone (Beconase, Vancenase Nasal Inhalers)

COMMON USES: Allergic rhinitis refractory to conventional therapy with antihistamines and decongestants.
DOSAGE: *Adults:* 1 spray intranasally bid–qid.
  Peds: 6–11 y: 1 spray intranasally tid.
NOTES: Nasal spray delivers 42 mg/dose.

Beclomethasone (Beclovent Inhaler, Vanceril Inhaler)

COMMON USES: Chronic asthma
DOSAGE: *Adults:* 2–4 inhalations tid–qid (maximum 20/d). *Peds:* 1–2 inhalations tid–qid (maximum 10/d).
NOTES: Not effective for acute asthmatic attacks, may cause oral candidiasis.

Belladonna and Opium Suppositories (B & O Supprettes) [C]

COMMON USES: Treatment of bladder or rectal spasms; moderate-to-severe pain.
DOSAGE: Insert 1 suppository rectally q4–6h prn. (15A = 30-mg powdered opium; 16.2-mg belladonna extract. 16A = 60 mg-powdered opium; 16.2-mg belladonna extract.
NOTES: Anticholinergic side effects; caution subjects about sedation, urinary retention, constipation.

Benazepril (Lotensin)

COMMON USES: Hypertension.
DOSAGE: 10–40 mg PO qd.
NOTES: May cause symptomatic hypotension in patients taking diuretics; may cause a nonproductive cough.

Benzonatate (Tessalon Perles)

COMMON USES: Symptomatic relief of nonproductive cough.
DOSAGE: 100 mg PO tid.
NOTES: May cause sedation.

Benztropine (Cogentin)

COMMON USES: Treatment of Parkinson's disease and drug-induced extrapyramidal disorders.
DOSAGE: 1–6 mg PO, IM, or IV in divided doses.
NOTES: Anticholinergic side effects.

Bepridil (Vascor)

COMMON USES: Treatment of chronic stable angina, hypertension, and congestive heart failure.
DOSAGE: 200–400 mg PO daily (adjust dose after 10 d).
NOTES: May cause serious ventricular arrhythmias, including torsades de pointes and agranulocytosis.

Beractant (Survanta)

COMMON USES: Prevention and treatment of respiratory distress syndrome (RDS) in premature infants.
DOSAGE: 4 mL/kg intratracheally; up to 4 doses in the first 48 h of life at least 6 h apart; additional therapy based on clinical response.

Betamethasone and clotrimazole, topical (Lotrisone)

COMMON USES: Topical treatment of fungal skin infections.
DOSAGE: Apply bid. Topical: Apply twice daily.
NOTES: Combination antifungal and anti-inflammatory.

Betamethasone, systemic (Celestone, others)

COMMON USES: Steroid replacement, anti-inflammatory, immunosuppressive.
DOSAGE: 0.6–7.2 mg/d PO divided bid–tid; up to 9 mg/d IM; intra-articular 0.5–2.0 mL.

Betamethasone, topical (Diprolene, Diprolene AF, Valisone, others)

COMMON USES: Topical steroid therapy of dermatosis (psoriasis, seborrhea, atopic, allergic and neurodermatitis)
DOSAGE: Apply to lesion up to tid.
NOTES: Betamethasone dipropionate and augmented (Diprolene) available in 0.05% gel, ointment, or lotion; betamethasone valerate (Valisone) available as cream 0.01, 0.1%, lotion and ointment 0.1%.

Betaxolol (Kerlone)

COMMON USES: Hypertension, ocular for glaucoma.
DOSAGE: 10–20 mg PO, qd; ophthalmic 1–2 drops of solution or suspension bid.

Bethanechol (Urecholine, Duvoid, various)

COMMON USES: Neurogenic atony of the bladder with urinary retention, acute postoperative and postpartum functional (nonobstructive) urinary retention.
DOSAGE: *Adults:* 10–50 mg PO tid–qid or 5 mg SC tid–qid and prn. *Peds:* 0.3–0.6 mg/kg/24h PO divided tid–qid or 1/2 the oral dose SC.
NOTES: Contraindicated in bladder outlet obstruction, asthma, coronary artery disease; do NOT administer IM or IV.

Bicalutamide (Casodex)

COMMON USES: Treatment of advanced prostate cancer in combination with LHRH analogue.
DOSAGE: 50 mg PO qd.
NOTES: Monitor LFTs; can cause gynecomastia.

Bicarbonate, see Sodium Bicarbonate

Bisacodyl (Dulcolax, others)

COMMON USES: Constipation, bowel preparation.
DOSAGE: *Adults:* 5–10 mg PO or 10 mg rectally prn. *Peds < 2 y:* 5 mg rectally prn; *> 2 y:* 5 mg PO or 10 mg rectally prn.

NOTES: Do NOT use with an acute abdomen or bowel obstruction; do NOT chew tablets; do NOT give within 1 h of antacids or milk.

Bismuth Subsalicylate (Pepto-Bismol, others)

COMMON USES: Indigestion, nausea, and diarrhea.
DOSAGE: *Adults:* 2 tablets or 30 mL PO prn. *Peds:* 3–6 y: 1/3 tablet or 5 mL PO prn; 6–9 y: 2/3 tablet or 10 mL PO prn; 9–12 y: 1 tablet or 15 mL PO prn.

Bisoprolol (Zebeta)

COMMON USES: Hypertension.
DOSAGE: 5–10 mg qd.

Bitolterol (Tornalate)

COMMON USES: Prophylaxis and treatment of asthma and reversible bronchospasm.
DOSAGE: *Adults* and *children* > 12 y: 2 inhalations q8h.

Bleomycin (Blenoxane)

COMMON USES: Treatment of corvical, ovarian, squamous cell, testicular cancer, and lymphoma; sclerotherapy of malignant effusion.
DOSAGE: 0.25–0.5 U/kg/dose IV, IM, or SC once or twice weekly.
NOTES: Pulmonary toxicity is increased with total doses of > 400 U.

Brimonidine (Alphagan)

COMMON USES: Glaucoma.
DOSAGE: 1 drop bid.
NOTES: DO NOT APPLY with soft contacts in place.

Brinzolamide (Azopt)

COMMON USES: Glaucoma.
DOSAGE: 1 drop in eye(s) tid.

Bromocriptine (Parlodel)

COMMON USES: Parkinsonian syndrome.
DOSAGE: Parkinson's: 1.25 mg PO bid initially, titrated to effect.
NOTES: Nausea and vertigo are common side effects.

Budesonide (Rhinocort, Pulmicort)

COMMON USES: Management of allergic and nonallergic rhinitis, management of asthma.
DOSAGE: Intranasal: 2 sprays in each nostril bid. Oral inhaled: 1–4 inhalations twice daily. *Peds:* 1–2 inhalations twice daily.

Bumetanide (Bumex)

COMMON USES: Edema from congestive heart failure, hepatic cirrhosis, and renal disease.
DOSAGE: *Adults:* 0.5–2.0 mg PO daily; 0.5–1.0 mg IV q8–24h. *Peds:* 0.015–0.1 mg/kg/dose PO, IV, IM q6–24h.
NOTES: Monitor fluid and electrolyte status during treatment.

Bupivacaine (Marcaine, Sensorcaine)

COMMON USES: Local infiltration anesthesia, lumbar epidural.
DOSAGE: Dependent on the procedure, vascularity of the tissues, depth of anesthesia, and degree of muscle relaxation required. Maximum infiltration dose in 70-kg adult is 70 mL of 0.25%.

Buprenorphine (Buprenex) [C]

COMMON USES: Relief of moderate-to-severe pain.
DOSAGE: 0.3 mg IM or slow IV push every 6 h prn.
NOTES: May induce withdrawal syndrome in opioid-dependent subjects.

Bupropion (Wellbutrin, Zyban)

COMMON USES: Treatment of depression, adjunct to smoking cessation.

DOSAGE: Depression: 100–450 mg/d divided bid–tid. Smoking: 150 mg daily for 3 d, then 150 mg twice daily.
NOTES: Has been associated with seizures; avoid use of alcohol and other CNS depressants.

Buspirone (BuSpar)

COMMON USES: Short-term relief of anxiety.
DOSAGE: 5–10 mg PO tid.
NOTES: No abuse potential. No physical or psychological dependence.

Butalbital and Acetaminophen (Fioricet, Medigesic, Phrenilin, Phrenilin Forte, Sedapap-10, others) [C]

COMMON USES: Tension headache, pain.
DOSAGE: 1–2 tabs PO q4h prn, max 6 tabs/d.
NOTES: Butalbital habit forming; Medigesic caps: butalbital 50 mg, caffeine 40 mg, and acetaminophen 325 mg; Phrenilin Forte caps: butalbital 50 mg and acetaminophen 650 mg; Fioricet Tabs: butalbital 50 mg, caffeine 40 mg, and acetaminophen 325 mg; Phrenilin Tabs: butalbital 50 mg and acetaminophen 325 mg; Sedapap-10: butalbital 50 mg and acetaminophen 650 mg.

Butalbital and Aspirin (Fiorinal, Lanorinal, Marnal, others) [C]

COMMON USES: Tension headache, pain
DOSAGE: 1–2 PO q4h prn, max 6 tabs/d.
NOTES: Butalbital habit forming; Fiorinal, Lanorinal, Marnal Caps and Tabs: Butalbital 50 mg, caffeine 40 mg, and aspirin 325 mg.

Butalbital, Aspirin and Codeine (Fiorinal with codeine) [C]

COMMON USES: Moderate pain.
DOSAGE: 1–2 PO q4h prn, maximum 6/d.
NOTES: Butalbital may be habit forming; may cause sedation; contains butalbital 50 mg, caffeine 40 mg, aspirin 325 mg, codeine 30 mg.

Butorphanol (Stadol) [C]

COMMON USES: Analgesic for moderate-to-severe pain; migraine headache.
DOSAGE: 1–4 mg IM or 0.5–2 mg IV every 3–4 h prn; 1 spray in 1 nostril (1 mg), reevaluate in 60–90 min and repeat if needed; repeat 2 dose sequence prn in 3–4 h.
NOTES: May induce withdrawal syndrome in opioid-dependent patients.

Calcitriol (Rocaltrol)

COMMON USES: Reduction of elevated parathyroid levels, hypocalcemia associated with dialysis.
DOSAGE: **Adults:** renal failure 0.25 µg PO, qd increase 0.25 µg/d every 4–6 wk prn; 0.5 µg 3 times a week IV, increase as needed. Hyperparathyroidism:0.5–2.0 µg/d. **Peds:** renal failure 15 ng/kg/d, increase prn typical maintenance 30-60 ng/kg/d. Hyperparathyroidism: < 5 y, 0.25–0.75 µg/d; > 6 y, 0.5–2.0 µg/d.
NOTES: 1,25 dihydroxycholecalciferol, a vitamin D analogue; monitor dosing to keep calcium levels within normal range.

Calcitonin (Cibacalcin, Miacalcin)

COMMON USES: Paget's disease of bone; hypercalcemia; osteogenesis imperfecta, postmenopausal osteoporosis.
DOSAGE: Paget's salmon form:100 U/d IM/SC initially, 50 U/d or 50–100 U q1–3d maintenance. Paget's human form: 0.5 mg/d initially; maintenance: 0.5 mg 2–3 times/week or 0.25 mg/d, maximum: 0.5 mg bid. Hypercalcemia salmon calcitonin: 4 U/kg IM/SC q12h; increase to 8 U/kg q12h, maximum q6h. Osteoporosis salmon calcitonin: 100 U/d IM/SC; Intranasal: 200 U = 1 nasal spray/d.
NOTES: Human (Cibacalcin) and salmon forms; only human form approved for Paget's' bone disease.

Calcium Acetate (PhosLo)

COMMON USES: ESRD-associated hyperphosphatemia.
DOSAGE: 2–4 tabs PO with meals.
NOTES: Can cause hypercalcemia, monitor levels.

Calcium Carbonate (Alka-Mints, Caltrate, Tums, Os-Cal, others)

COMMON USES: Hyperacidity associated with peptic ulcer disease, hiatal hernia, etc; calcium supplementation, management of hyperphosphatemia in ESRD.
DOSAGE: From 500 mg–2.0 g PO prn.

Calcium Salts (chloride, gluconate)

COMMON USES: Calcium replacement, ventricular fibrillation, electromechanical dissociation, management of hyperphosphatemia in ESRD.
DOSAGE: *Adults:* Replacement: 1–2 g PO qd. Cardiac emergencies: Calcium chloride 0.5–1.0 g IV every 10 min or calcium gluconate 1–2 g IV every 10 min. *Peds:* Replacement: 200–500 mg/kg/24h PO or IV divided qid. Cardiac emergency: 100 mg/kg/dose IV every 10 min of gluconate salt.
NOTES: Calcium chloride contains 270 mg (13.6 mEq) elemental calcium per gram, and calcium gluconate contains 90 mg (4.5 mEq) elemental calcium per gram.

Candesartan (Atacand)

COMMON USES: Treatment of hypertension.
DOSAGE: 2–32 mg/d, usual dose is 16 mg once daily
NOTES: Monitor BP and titrate to effect; maximum BP response within 2 wk.

Capsaicin (Zostrix, others)

COMMON USES: Topical analgesic (postherpetic neuralgia, arthritis, postoperative pain).
DOSAGE: OTC form, apply tid–qid.

Captopril (Capoten)

COMMON USES: Treatment of hypertension, congestive heart failure, and diabetic nephropathy.
DOSAGE: *Adults;* Hypertension: Initially, 25 mg PO bid–tid; titrate to a maintenance dose every 1–2 wk by 25 mg increments per dose (maximum 450 mg/d) to desired effect. Congestive heart failure: Initially, 6.25–12.5 mg PO tid; titrate to desired effect. *Peds:* Infants < 2 mo: 0.05–0.1 mg/kg/dose PO tid–qid. Children: Initially, 0.15 mg/kg/dose PO; double q2h until blood pressure is controlled, to maximum of 6 mg/kg/d; maintenance, 0.5–0.6 mg/kg/d PO divided bid–qid.
NOTES: Use with caution in renal failure. Give 1 h before meals; can cause rash, proteinuria, and cough.

Carbamazepine (Tegretol)

COMMON USES: Epilepsy; trigeminal neuralgia.
DOSAGE: *Adults:* 200 mg PO bid initially; increase by 200 mg/d; usual 800–1200 mg/d. *Peds 6–12 y:* 100 mg/dose PO bid or 10 mg/kg/24h PO divided qd–bid initially; increase to a maintenance dose of 20–30 mg/kg/24h divided tid–qid.
NOTES: Can cause severe hematologic side effects; monitor CBC and serum levels, see Tables VIII–3 and VIII–9 pages 520 and 527; generic products are NOT interchangeable.

Carbidopa/Levodopa (Sinemet)

COMMON USES: Parkinson's disease.
DOSAGE: Start at 10/100 PO bid–tid; titrate as needed.
NOTES: May cause psychiatric disturbances, orthostatic hypotension, dyskinesias, and cardiac arrhythmias.

Carboplatin (Paraplatin)

COMMON USES: Treatment of cervical, ovarian, and lung cancer.
DOSAGE: Varies with treatment protocol; 300–360 mg/m^2 on day 1 every 4 wk.

NOTES: May cause bone marrow suppression, vomiting, and anaphylaxis; monitor platelet and neutrophil counts.

Carisoprodol (Soma)

COMMON USES: Adjunct to sleep and physical therapy for the relief of painful musculoskeletal conditions.

DOSAGE: 350 mg PO qid.

NOTES: Avoid alcohol and other CNS depressants; also available with 16 mg codeine/tablet [C].

Carteolol (Cartrol, Ocupress Ophthalmic)

COMMON USES: Treatment of hypertension; phthalic solution for increased intraocular pressure.

DOSAGE: 2.5–5 mg PO qd; ophthalmic 1 drop eye(s) bid.

Carvedilol (Coreg)

COMMON USES: Treatment of hypertension and CHF.

DOSAGE: HTN: 6.25–12.5 mg twice daily. CHF: 3.125–25 mg twice daily.

NOTES: Take with food to slow absorption and reduce incidence of orthostatic hypotension.

Cefaclor (Ceclor)

COMMON USES: Treatment of infections caused by susceptible bacteria involving the upper and lower respiratory tract, skin, bone, urinary tract, abdomen, and gynecologic system (*S aureus, S pneumoniae, H influenzae*).

DOSAGE: *Adults:* 250–500 mg PO tid. *Peds:* 20–40 mg/kg/d PO divided tid.

NOTES: Second generation cephalosporin; more gram-negative activity than first generation cephalosporins.

Cefadroxil (Duricef, Ultracef)

COMMON USES: Treatment of infections caused by susceptible strains of *Streptococcus, Staphylococcus, E coli, Proteus* and *Klebsiella* involving the skin, bone, upper and lower respiratory tract, and urinary tract.

DOSAGE: *Adults:* 500–1000 mg PO bid-qd. *Peds:* 30 mg/kg/d divided bid.

NOTES: First generation cephalosporin.

Cefazolin (Ancef, Kefzol)

COMMON USES: Treatment of infections caused by susceptible strains of *Streptococcus, Staphylococcus, E coli, Proteus* and *Klebsiella* involving the skin, bone, upper and lower respiratory tract, and urinary tract.

DOSAGE: *Adults:* 1–2 g IV q8h. *Peds:* 50–100 mg/kg/d IV divided q8h.

NOTES: Widely used for surgical prophylaxis; first generation cephalosporin.

Cefdinir (Omnicef)

COMMON USES: Treatment of infections caused by susceptible bacteria involving the respiratory tract, skin, bone, urinary tract, meningitis, and septicemia.

DOSAGE: *Adults:* 300 mg PO bid or 600 mg PO qd.
Peds: 7 mg/kg PO bid or 14 mg/kg PO qd.

NOTES: Third generation cephalosporin.

Cefepime (Maxipime)

COMMON USES: Treatment of urinary tract infections and pneumonia caused by susceptible *S pneumoniae, S aureus, K pneumoniae, E coli, P aeruginosa,* and *Enterobacter* spp.

DOSAGE: 1–2 g IV q12h for 5–10 d; UTI: 500 mg IV q12h.

NOTES: Fourth generation cephalosporin; improved gram-positive coverage over third generation.

Cefixime (Suprax)

COMMON USES: Treatment of infections caused by susceptible bacteria involving the respiratory tract, skin, bone, urinary tract, meningitis, and septicemia; single dose to treat gonorrhea.

DOSAGE: *Adults:* 200–400 mg PO bid–qd. *Peds:* 8 mg/kg/d PO divided bid–qd, 400 mg/max/d.
NOTES: Third generation cephalosporin; use suspension to treat otitis media.

Cefmetazole (Zefazone)

COMMON USES: Treatment of infections caused by susceptible bacteria involving the upper and lower respiratory tract, skin, bone, urinary tract, abdomen, and gynecologic system.
DOSAGE: *Adults:* treatment of infection: 1–2 g IV 8 h; surgical prophylaxis: 2 g IV 30–90 min preoperatively.
NOTES: Second-generation cephalosporin with more gram-negative activity than first generation cephalosporins; has anaerobic activity.

Cefonicid (Monocid)

COMMON USES: Treatment of infections caused by susceptible bacteria: respiratory, skin, bone and joint, urinary, gynecologic, and septicemia.
DOSAGE: 1 g IM/IV every 24 h.
NOTES: Second-generation cephalosporin.

Cefoperazone (Cefobid)

COMMON USES: Treatment of infections caused by susceptible bacteria: respiratory, skin, urinary tract, sepsis; as a third generation cephalosporin, cefoperazone has activity against gram-negative bacilli (eg, *E coli, Klebsiella,* and *Haemophilus*) but variable activity against *Streptococcus* and *Staphylococcus* spp.; it has activity against *Pseudomonas aeruginosa,* but less than ceftazidime.
DOSAGE: *Adults:* 2–4 g/d, divided q12h IM/IV; 12 g/d maximum. Children: 100–150 mg/kg/d divided q8–12h IM/IV.
NOTES: Third-generation cephalosporin; active against gram-negatives but variable activity against *Staphylococcus* and *Streptococcus* spp.; some activity against *Pseudomonas* spp.

Cefotaxime (Claforan)

COMMON USES: Treatment of infections caused by susceptible bacteria involving the respiratory tract, skin, bone, urinary tract, and septicemia.
DOSAGE: *Adults:* 1–2 g IV q4–12h. *Peds:* 100–200 mg/kg/d IV divided q6–8h.
NOTES: Third-generation cephalosporin.

Cefotetan (Cefotan)

COMMON USES: Treatment of infections caused by susceptible bacteria involving the upper and lower respiratory tract, skin, bone, urinary tract, abdomen, and gynecologic system.
DOSAGE: *Adults:* 1–2 g IV q12h. *Peds:* 40–80 mg/kg/d IV divided q12h.
NOTES: Second-generation cephalosporin; more gram-negative activity then first-generation cephalosporins; has anaerobic activity.

Cefoxitin (Mefoxin)

COMMON USES: Treatment of infections caused by susceptible bacteria involving the upper and lower respiratory tract, skin, bone, urinary tract, abdomen, and gynecologic system.
DOSAGE: *Adults:* 1–2 mg IV q6h. *Peds:* 80–160 mg/kg/d divided q4–6h.
NOTES: Second-generation cephalosporin; more gram-negative activity then first-generation cephalosporins; has anaerobic activity.

Cefpodoxime (Vantin)

COMMON USES: Treatment of infections caused by susceptible bacteria involving the respiratory tract (community-acquired pneumonia due to *S pneumonia* or non-beta-lactamase *H influenzae*), otitis media, pharyngitis, tonsillitis, skin, bone, urinary tract, gonorrhea, meningitis, and septicemia.
DOSAGE: *Adults:* 200–400 mg PO q12h. *Peds:* > 6 mo: 10 mg/kg/d PO divided bid.
NOTES: Second-generation cephalosporin; drug interactions with agents increasing gastric pH.

Cefprozil (Cefzil)

COMMON USES: Treatment of infections caused by susceptible bacteria involving the upper and lower respiratory tract, skin, bone, urinary tract, abdomen, and gynecologic system.
DOSAGE: *Adults:* 250–500 mg PO qd-bid. *Peds:* 6 mo: 7.5–15 mg/kg/d PO divided bid.
NOTES: Second-generation cephalosporin; more gram-negative activity than first-generation cephalosporins; use higher doses for otitis and pneumonia.

Ceftazidime (Fortaz, Ceptaz, Tazidime, Tazicef)

COMMON USES: Treatment of infections caused by susceptible bacteria involving the respiratory tract, skin, bone, urinary tract, meningitis, and septicemia.
DOSAGE: *Adults:* 1–2 g IV q8h. *Peds:* 30–50 mg/kg/d IV divided q8h.
NOTES: Third generation cephalosporin; useful in patients with pseudomonal infections at risk for nephrotoxicity; empiric therapy in febrile granulocytopenic patients.

Ceftibuten (Cedax)

COMMON USES: Treatment of infections caused by susceptible bacteria involving the respiratory tract (bronchitis), skin, bone, urinary tract, and septicemia.
DOSAGE: *Adults:* 400 mg PO once daily. *Peds:* 9 mg/kg PO once daily (400 mg max).
NOTES: Third-generation cephalosporin; take on an empty stomach; little activity against *Streptococcus* spp.

Ceftizoxime (Cefizox)

COMMON USES: Treatment of infections caused by susceptible bacteria involving the respiratory tract, skin, bone, urinary tract, meningitis, and septicemia.
DOSAGE: *Adults:* 1–2 g IV q12–8h. *Peds:* 150–200 mg/kg/d IV divided q6–8h.
NOTES: Third-generation cephalosporin.

Ceftriaxone (Rocephin)

COMMON USES: Treatment of infections caused by susceptible bacteria involving the respiratory tract, skin, bone, urinary tract, meningitis, chancroid, uncomplicated gonorrhea, and septicemia.
DOSAGE: *Adults:* 1–2 g IV q12-24h; GC and chancroid: < 45 kg, 125 mg IM; > 45 kg, 250 mg IM single dose. *Peds:* 50–100 mg/kg/d IV divided q12–24h.
NOTES: Third-generation cephalosporin.

Cefuroxime (Ceftin [oral], Zinacef [parenteral])

COMMON USES: Treatment of infections caused by susceptible bacteria involving the upper and lower respiratory tract, skin, bone, urinary tract, abdomen, and gynecologic system.
DOSAGE: *Adults:* 750 mg–1.5 g IV q8h or 250–500 mg PO bid. *Peds:* 100–150 mg/kg/d IV divided q8h or 20–30 mg/kg/d PO divided bid.
NOTES: Second-generation cephalosporin; more gram-negative activity than first-generation cephalosporins; IV crosses the blood-brain barrier.

Celecoxib (Celebrex)

COMMON USES: Osteoarthritis and rheumatoid arthritis.
DOSAGE: 100–200 mg once or twice daily.
NOTES: May increase bleeding time.

Cephalexin (Keflex, Keftab)

COMMON USES: Treatment of infections caused by susceptible strains of *Streptococcus*, *Staphylococcus*, *E coli*, *Proteus* and *Klebsiella* spp. involving the skin, bone, upper and lower respiratory tract, and urinary tract.
DOSAGE: *Adults:* 250–500 mg PO qid. *Peds:* 25–100 mg/kg/d PO divided qid.
NOTES: First-generation cephalosporin.

Cephapirin (Cefadyl)

COMMON USES: Treatment of infections caused by susceptible strains of respiratory tract, skin, urinary tract, bone and joint, endocarditis and sepsis (but NOT *Enterococcus* spp.); some gram-negatives.

DOSAGE: *Adults:* 1 g IM/IV q6h (12 g/d max). *Peds:* 10–20 mg/kg IM/IV q6h (4 g/d max).
NOTES: First-generation cephalosporin.

Cephradine (Velosef)

COMMON USES: Treatment of susceptible bacterial infections, including group A beta-hemolytic *Streptococcus* spp.
DOSAGE: *Adults:* 2–4 g/d in 4 divided doses (8 g/d max). *Peds > 9 mo:* 25–100 mg/kg/d divided q6–12h (4 g/d max).
NOTES: First-generation cephalosporin.

Cetirizine (Zyrtec)

COMMON USES: Allergic rhinitis and chronic urticaria.
DOSAGE: *Adults* and *Peds > 6 y:* 5–10 mg/d.

Charcoal, Activated (SuperChar, Actidose, Liqui-Char)

COMMON USES: Emergency treatment for poisoning by most drugs and chemicals.
DOSAGE: *Adults:* Acute intoxication: 30–100 g/dose. Gastrointestinal dialysis: 25–50 g q4–6h. *Peds:* Acute intoxication: 1–2 g/kg/dose. Gastrointestinal dialysis: 5–10 g/dose q4–8h.
NOTES: Administer with a cathartic; liquid dosage forms are in sorbitol base; powder mixed with water; protect airway in lethargic or comatose patient.

Chloral Hydrate (Noctec) [C]

COMMON USES: Nocturnal and preoperative sedation.
DOSAGE: *Adults:* Hypnotic: Between 500 mg and 1 g PO or PR 30 min hs or procedure. Sedative: 250 mg PO or PR tid. *Peds:* Hypnotic: 50 mg/kg/24h PO or PR 30 min hs or procedure. Sedative: 25 mg/kg/24h PO or PR tid.
NOTES: Mix syrup in a glass of water or fruit juice.

Chlorambucil (Leukeran)

COMMON USES: Treatment of ovarian cancer, leukemia, and lymphoma.
DOSAGE: Initially, 0.1–0.2 mg/kg/d PO for 3–6 wk, then maintenance therapy with no more than 0.1 mg/kg/d.

Chlordiazepoxide (Librium) [C]

COMMON USES: Anxiety, tension, alcohol withdrawal.
DOSAGE: *Adults:* Mild anxiety, tension: 5–10 mg PO tid–qid or prn. Severe anxiety, tension: 25–50 mg IM or IV tid–qid or prn. Alcohol withdrawal: 50–100 mg IM or IV; repeat in 2–4 h if needed, up to 300 mg in 24 h; gradually taper daily. *Peds:* 0.5 mg/kg/24h PO or IM divided q6–8h.
NOTES: Reduce dose in elderly patients; absorption of IM doses can be erratic.

Chlorothiazide (Diuril)

COMMON USES: Hypertension, edema, congestive heart failure.
DOSAGE: *Adults:* Between 500 mg and 1.0 g PO or IV qd–bid. *Peds:* 20–30 mg/kg/24h PO divided bid.
NOTES: Contraindicated in anuria.

Chlorpheniramine (Chlor-Trimeton, others)

COMMON USES: Seasonal rhinitis, allergic reactions.
DOSAGE: *Adults:* 4 mg PO or IV q4–6h or 8–12 mg PO bid of sustained release. *Peds:* 0.35 mg/kg/24h PO divided q4–6h or 0.2 mg/kg/24h sustained release.
NOTES: Anticholinergic side effects and sedation are common. Available in many OTC combinations (eg, acetaminophen, phenylephrine, pseudoephedrine).

Chlorpromazine (Thorazine)

COMMON USES: Psychotic disorders, apprehension, intractable hiccups, control of nausea and vomiting.
DOSAGE: *Adults:* Acute anxiety, agitation: 10–25 mg PO or PR bid–tid. Severe symptoms: 25 mg IM, can repeat in 1 h, then 25–50 mg PO or PR tid. Hiccups: 25–50 mg PO bid–tid. *Peds:* 2.5–6.0 mg/kg/24h PO, PR or IM divided q4–8h.
NOTES: Beware of extrapyramidal side effects, sedation, has alpha-adrenergic blocking properties.

Chlorpropamide (Diabinese)

COMMON USES: Management of non–insulin-dependent diabetes mellitus.
DOSAGE: 100–500 mg qd.
NOTES: Use with caution in renal insufficiency.

Chlorthalidone (Hygroton)

COMMON USES: Hypertension, edema associated with congestive heart failure, steroid and estrogen therapy.
DOSAGE: *Adults:* 50–100 mg PO qd. *Peds:* 2 mg/kg/dose PO 3 times weekly or 1–2 mg/kg PO daily.
NOTES: Contraindicated in anuric patients.

Chlorzoxazone (Paraflex, Parafon Forte DSC)

COMMON USES: Adjunct to rest and physical therapy for the relief of discomfort associated with acute, painful musculoskeletal conditions.
DOSAGE: *Adults:* 250–500 mg PO tid–qid. *Peds:* 20 mg/kg/d or 600 mg/m^2/d divided in 3–4 doses.

Cholecalciferol [Vitamin D3] (Delta D)

COMMON USES: Dietary supplement for treatment of vitamin D deficiency.
DOSAGE: 400–1000 IU PO daily.
NOTES: 1-mg cholecalciferol = 40,000 IU of vitamin D activity.

Cholestyramine (Questran)

COMMON USES: Adjunctive therapy for the reduction of serum cholesterol in patients with primary hypercholesterolemia; relief of pruritus associated with partial biliary obstruction.
DOSAGE: Individualize dose to 4 g 1–6 times a day.
NOTES: Mix 4-g cholestyramine in 2–6 oz of noncarbonated beverages.

Cimetidine (Tagamet)

COMMON USES: Duodenal ulcer; ulcer prophylaxis in hypersecretory states, such as trauma, burns, surgery, Zollinger-Ellison syndrome; and gastroesophageal reflux disease (GERD).
DOSAGE: *Adults:* Active ulcer: 2400 mg/d IV continuous infusion or 300 mg IV q6–4h; 400 mg PO bid or 800 mg qhs. Maintenance therapy: 400 mg PO qhs. GERD: 800 mg PO bid; maintenance 800 mg PO hs. *Peds:* Neonates: 10–20 mg/kg/24h PO or IV divided q4–6h. Children: 20–40 mg/kg/24h PO or IV divided q4–6h.
NOTES: Extend dosing interval with renal insufficiency; decrease dose in elderly patients.

Ciprofloxacin (Cipro, Ciloxan Ophthalmic)

COMMON USES: Broad-spectrum activity against a variety of gram-positive and gram-negative aerobic bacteria (urinary tract infection, prostatitis, sinusitis, skin, infectious diarrhea, osteomyelitis, ocular infections).
DOSAGE: *Adults:* 250–750 mg PO q12h or 200–400 mg IV q12h. Opthalmic: 1–2 drops in eye(s) q2h while awake. *Peds:* Not recommended for use in children < 18 y, because of cartilage effects.
NOTES: Little activity against streptococci; drug interactions with theophylline, caffeine, sucralfate, and antacids. Nausea, vomiting, and abdominal discomfort are common side effects. Contraindicated in pregnancy.

Ciprofloxacin and hydrocortisone (Cipro HC Otic)

COMMON USES: Otitis externa (swimmers ear)
DOSAGE: 3 drops in ear bid–tid for 1 wk.

Cisplatin (Platinol)

COMMON USES: Treatment of cervical, ovarian, testicular, and other solid tumors.
DOSAGE: 20–70 mg/m^2 IV. Dose and duration of therapy is dependent on individual treatment protocols.
NOTES: Agent is nephrotoxic; hydrate patients with 1–2 L of fluid before infusion.

Citalopram (Celexa)

COMMON USES: Treatment of depression.
DOSAGE: Initial 20 mg/d, may be increased to 40 mg/d.

Clarithromycin (Biaxin)

COMMON USES: Treatment of upper and lower respiratory tract infections, skin, *H pylori* infections, and infections caused by nontuberculosis (atypical) *Mycobacterium*. Prevention of MAC infections in HIV-infected individuals.
DOSAGE: *Adults:* 250–500 mg PO bid. *Mycobacterium:* 500–1000 mg PO bid. *Peds:* 7.5 mg/kg/dose PO bid.
NOTES: Increases theophylline and carbamazepine levels; avoid concurrent use with cisapride; causes metallic taste.

Clemastine (Tavist [OTC])

COMMON USES: Allergic rhinitis.
DOSAGE: 1.34–2.68 mg (1–2 tabs) tid, maximum 8.04 mg/d.

Clindamycin (Cleocin)

COMMON USES: Susceptible strains of streptococci, pneumococci, staphylococci, and gram-positive and gram-negative anaerobes, no activity against gram-negative aerobes. Topical agent for severe acne, vaginal infections.
DOSAGE: *Adults:* 150–450 mg PO qid; 300–600 mg IV q6h or 900 mg IV q8h. Topical: apply bid. Vaginal: 1 applicatorful instilled at bedtime for 1 wk. *Peds:* Neonates: 15–20 mg/kg/24h divided q6–8h. Children > 1 month: 15–40 mg/kg/24h divided q6–8h (4 g/d).
NOTES: Beware of diarrhea that may represent pseudomembranous colitis caused by *Clostridium difficile.*

Clonazepam (Klonopin) [C]

COMMON USES: Lennox-Gastaut syndrome, akinetic and myoclonic seizures, absence seizures.
DOSAGE: *Adults:* 1.5 mg/d PO in 3 divided doses; increase by 0.5–1.0 mg/d every 3 d prn up to 20 mg/d. *Peds:* 0.01–0.05 mg/kg/24h PO divided tid; increase to 0.1–0.2 mg/kg/24h divided tid.
NOTES: CNS side effects including sedation.

Clonidine (Catapres)

COMMON USES: Hypertension, opioid and tobacco withdrawal.
DOSAGE: *Adults:* 0.10 mg PO bid adjusted daily by 0.1–0.2 mg increments (maximum 2.4 mg/d). *Peds:* 5–25 mg/kg/24h divided q6h.
NOTES: Dry mouth, drowsiness, sedation occur frequently; more effective for hypertension when combined with diuretics; rebound hypertension can occur with abrupt cessation of doses greater than 0.2 mg bid.

Clonidine Transdermal (Catapres TTS)

COMMON USES: Hypertension.
DOSAGE: Apply one patch every 7 d to a hairless area on the upper arm or torso; titrate according to individual therapeutic requirements.

NOTES: TTS-1, TTS-2, TTS-3 (delivers 0.1, 0.2, 0.3 mg respectively of clonidine per day, for 1 wk). Doses greater than two TTS-3 are usually not associated with increased efficacy.

Clopidogrel (Plavix)

COMMON USES: Reduction of atherosclerotic events.
DOSAGE: 75 mg once daily.
NOTES: Prolongs bleeding time, use with caution in persons at risk of bleeding from trauma, etc.

Clorazepate (Tranxene) [C]

COMMON USES: Acute anxiety disorders, acute alcohol withdrawal symptoms, and adjunctive therapy in partial seizures.
DOSAGE: *Adults:* 15–60 mg/d PO in single or divided doses. Elderly and debilitated patients: initiate therapy at 7.5–15 mg/d in divided doses. Alcohol withdrawal: Day 1: Initially, 30 mg; followed by 30–60 mg in divided doses. Day 2: 45–90 mg in divided doses. Day 3: 22.5–45 mg in divided doses. Day 4: 15–30 mg in divided doses. *Peds:* 3.75–7.5 mg/dose bid, to a maximum of 60 mg/d divided bid–tid.
NOTES: Monitor patients with renal and hepatic impairment, since drug may accumulate; CNS depressant effects.

Clotrimazole (Lotrimin, Mycelex)

COMMON USES: Treatment of candidiasis and tinea infections.
DOSAGE: Orally: One troche dissolved slowly in mouth 5 times a day for 14 d. Vaginal: Cream: One applicator qhs for 7–14 d; Tablets: 100 mg vaginally qhs for 7 d or 200 mg (2 tablets) vaginally qhs for 3 d or 500 mg tablet vaginally hs for 1 d. Topical: Apply 3–4 times daily for 10–14 d.
NOTES: Oral prophylaxis commonly used in immunosuppressed patients.

Cloxacillin (Cloxapen)

COMMON USES: Treatment of respiratory, skin, bone, joint infections caused by susceptible strains of penicillinase-producing *Staphylococcus*.
DOSAGE: *Adults:* 250–500 mg PO qid. *Peds:* 50–100 mg/kg/d divided qid.
NOTES: Take on an empty stomach.

Clozapine (Clozaril)

COMMON USES: Severe schizophrenia that does NOT respond to standard therapy.
DOSAGE: Initial 25 mg qd–bid, increase dose to 300–450 mg/d over 2 wk. Maintain patient at lowest dose possible.
NOTES: Has limited distribution. Contact local pharmacy for drug availability. Monitor blood counts frequently because of the risk of agranulocytosis. May cause drowsiness and seizures.

Cocaine [C]

COMMON USES: Topical anesthetic for mucous membranes.
DOSAGE: Apply topically lowest amount of solution that provides relief; 1 mg/kg maximum.

Codeine [C]

COMMON USES: Mild-to-moderate pain; symptomatic relief of cough.
DOSAGE: *Adults:* Analgesic: 15–60 mg PO, SC/IM qid prn. Antitussive: 5–15 mg PO or SC q4h prn. *Peds:* Analgesic: 0.5–1.0 mg/kg/dose PO or SC q4–6h prn. Antitussive: 1.0–1.5 mg/kg/24h divided q4h, max 30 mg/24h.
NOTES: Most often used in combination with acetaminophen for pain or with agents such as terpin hydrate as an antitussive; 120 mg IM equivalent to 10 mg morphine IM.

Colesevelam (Welchol)

COMMON USES: Reduction of LDL cholesterol.
DOSAGE: 3 tablets PO twice daily with meals.

Colistimethate sodium (Coly-Mycin)

COMMON USES: Treatment of infections caused by gram-negative bacteria.

DOSAGE: *Adults* and *Peds:* 2.5–5mg/kg daily in 2–4 divided doses.
NOTES: Adjust dose based on renal function.

Colchicine

COMMON USES: Acute gout.
DOSAGE: Initially, 0.5–1.2 mg PO or IV, then 0.5–1.2 mg every 1–2 h until gastrointestinal side effects develop (maximum of 8 mg/d).
NOTES: Caution in elderly patients and patients with renal impairment. Colchicine 1–2 mg IV within 24–48 h of an acute attack can be diagnostic and therapeutic in a monoarticular arthritis.

Colestipol (Colestid)

COMMON USES: Adjunctive therapy for the reduction of serum cholesterol in patients with primary hypercholesterolemia.
DOSAGE: 15–30 g/d divided into 2–4 doses.
NOTES: Do NOT use dry powder; mix with beverages, soups, cereals, etc.

Cortisone

(See Table VIII–4, page 521)

Cromolyn Sodium (Intal, Nasalcrom, Opticrom)

COMMON USES: Adjunct to the prophylaxis of asthma; prevention of exercise-induced asthma; allergic rhinitis; ophthalmic allergic manifestations.
DOSAGE: *Adults* and *Peds > 12 y:* Inhalation: 20 mg (as powder in capsule) inhaled qid or metered-dose inhaler 2 puffs qid. Oral: 200 mg 4 times a day 15–20 min before meals, up to 400 mg 4 times a day. Nasal instillation: Spray once in each nostril 2–6 times daily. Ophthalmic: 1–2 drops in each eye 4–6 times daily. *Peds:* Inhalation: 2 puffs qid of metered-dose inhaler. Oral: Infants < 2 y: 20 mg/kg/d in 4 divided doses. 2–12 y: 100 mg 4 times per day before meals.
NOTES: Has no benefit in acute situations, may require 2–4 wk for maximal effect in perennial allergic disorders.

Cyanocobalamin/Vitamin B$_{12}$

COMMON USES: Pernicious anemia and other vitamin B$_{12}$ deficiency states.
DOSAGE: *Adults:* 100 mg, IM or SC qd for 5–10 d then 100 mg IM twice a week for 1 month, then 100 mg IM monthly. *Peds:* 100 mg qd IM or SC for 5–10 d, then 30–50 mg IM every 4 wk.
NOTES: Oral absorption highly erratic, altered by many drugs and NOT recommended; for use with hyperalimentation see Section V, page 380.

Cyclobenzaprine (Flexeril)

COMMON USES: Adjunct to rest and physical therapy for the relief of muscle spasm associated with acute painful musculoskeletal conditions.
DOSAGE: 10 mg PO tid.
NOTES: Do NOT use for longer than 2–3 wk; has sedative and anticholinergic properties.

Cylopentolate (Cyclogyl)

COMMON USES: Mydriasis and cycloplegia; useful before ocular exam; treatment of iritis.
DOSAGE: 1 drop 1% in eye(s), followed by a second application 5 min later; use 30–45 min before exam; iritis: apply tid.

Cyclophosphamide (Cytoxan, Neosar)

COMMON USES: Hodgkin's and non-Hodgkin's lymphomas, multiple myeloma, breast cancer, ovarian cancer, mycosis fungoides, neuroblastoma, retinoblastoma, acute leukemias, small cell lung cancer, and allogeneic and autologous transplantation in high doses; severe rheumatologic disorders.
DOSAGE: 500–1500 mg/m² as a single dose at 2- to 4-wk intervals; 1.8 g/m² to 160 mg/kg (or approximately 12 g/m² in a 75-kg individual) in the bone marrow transplantation setting.
NOTES: Toxicity includes myelosuppression (leukopenia and thrombocytopenia), sterile hemorrhagic cystitis, SIADH, alopecia, and anorexia; nausea and vomiting are common. Hepato-

toxicity and rarely interstitial pneumonitis may occur. Irreversible testicular atrophy may occur. Cardiotoxicity is rare. Second malignancies (bladder cancer and acute leukemias) have been reported; cumulative risk of 3.5% at 8 y, 10.7% at 12 y. Preventive measures to avoid hemorrhagic cystitis: continuous bladder irrigation and MESNA uroprotection.

Cyclosporine (Sandimmune, Neoral)

COMMON USES: Prophylaxis of organ rejection in kidney, liver, heart, and bone marrow transplants in conjunction with adrenal corticosteroids; other autoimmune diseases.

DOSAGE: *Adults* and *Peds:* Oral: 15 mg/kg/d beginning 12 h before transplant; after 2 wk, taper the dose by 5 mg/wk to 5–10 mg/kg/d. IV: 5–6 mg/kg/d divided q12–24 h. If the patient is unable to take the drug orally, give 1/2 of the oral dose IV, switch to PO as soon as possible.

NOTES: May elevate blood urea nitrogen and creatinine, which may be confused with renal transplant rejection; should be administered in glass containers; has many drug interactions; Neoral and Sandimmune are NOT interchangeable. See Table VIII–3, page 520 for drug levels.

Cyproheptadine (Periactin)

COMMON USES: Allergic reactions; especially good for itching.

DOSAGE: *Adults:* 4 mg PO tid, maximum of 0.5 mg/kg/d. *Peds:* 2–6 y-0.25/kg/24h divided tid–qid (maximum 12 mg/24h); 7–14 y: 0.25 mg/kg/24h divided tid–qid (maximum of 16 mg/24h).

NOTES: Anticholinergic side effects and drowsiness common; may stimulate appetite in some patients.

Cytomegalovirus Immune Globulin [CMV-IVIG] (Cytogam)

COMMON USES: Attenuation of primary CMV disease associated with transplantation.

DOSAGE: Administered for 16 wk posttransplant. See product information for dosing schedule.

Dacarbazine (DTIC-Dome)

COMMON USES: Treatment of soft tissue and uterine sarcoma, melanoma, and Hodgkin's disease.

DOSAGE: Dependent on individual protocol.

NOTES: May cause myelosuppression.

Daclizumab (Zenapax)

COMMON USES: Prevention of acute organ rejection.

DOSAGE: *Adults* and *Peds:* 1 mg/kg IV per dose; first dose prior to transplant followed by 4 doses 14 d apart posttransplant.

Dactinomycin (Cosmegen)

COMMON USES: Treatment of Wilm's tumor, rhabdomyosarcoma, choriocarcinoma, testicular carcinoma, Ewing's sarcoma, and sarcoma botryoides.

DOSAGE: *Adults:* 0.5 mg/d IV for 5 d. *Peds:* 0.015 mg/kg/d IV for 5 d.

NOTES: Severe soft-tissue damage may occur with extravasation.

Dalteparin (Fragmin)

COMMON USES: Unstable angina, non-Q-wave MI, prevention of ischemic complications caused by clot formation in patients on concurrent aspirin, prevention of DVT after surgery.

DOSAGE: Angina/MI: 120 IU/kg (maximum 10,000 IU) SC q12h with aspirin. DVT prophylaxis: 2500–5000 IU SC 1–2 h before surgery, then once daily for 5–10 d. Systemic anticoagulation: 200 IU/kg SC once daily or 100 IU/kg SC twice daily.

NOTES: Predictable antithrombotic effects eliminate need for laboratory monitoring.

Dantrolene Sodium (Dantrium)

COMMON USES: Treatment of clinical spasticity resulting from upper motor neuron disorders, such as spinal cord injuries, strokes, cerebral palsy, or multiple sclerosis; treatment of malignant hyperthermic crisis.

DOSAGE: *Adults:* Spasticity: Initially, 25 mg PO qd, titrate to effect by 25 mg up to maximum dose of 100 mg PO qid prn. *Peds:* Initially, 0.5 mg/kg/dose bid, titrate by 0.5 mg/kg to effec-

tiveness up to max dose of 3 mg/kg/dose qid prn. **Adults** and **Peds:** Malignant hyperthermia treatment: Continuous rapid IV push beginning at 1 mg/kg until symptoms subside or 10 mg/kg is reached. Postcrisis follow-up: 4–8 mg/kg/d in 3–4 divided doses for 1–3 d to prevent recurrence.
NOTES: Monitor ALT and AST closely.

Daunorubicin (Cerubidine)

COMMON USES: Leukemia.
DOSAGE: Varies with individual protocol.
NOTES: Severe tissue necrosis if extravasation occurs.

Deferoxamine (Desferal)

COMMON USES: Acute iron intoxication, chronic iron overload due to multiple transfusions, aluminum toxicity.
DOSAGE: **Adults** and **Peds:** acute iron intoxication: IM or IV 1 g, then 500 mg 4 h later, dependent on clinical response 400 mg every 4–12 h (max dose, 6g/24h).
NOTE: May have orange-red urine.

Delavirdine (Rescriptor)

COMMON USES: HIV-1 infection in combination therapy.
DOSAGE: **Adults:** 400 mg PO tid.

Demeclocycline (Declomycin)

COMMON USES: Treatment of SIADH.
DOSAGE: SIADH: 300–600 mg PO q12h; antimicrobial: 150–300 mg PO q12h.
NOTES: Reduce dose in renal failure. May cause diabetes insipidus.

Desipramine (Norpramin)

COMMON USES: Endogenous depression.
DOSAGE: 25–200 mg/d in single or divided doses; usually as a single bedtime dose.
NOTES: Many anticholinergic side effects, including blurred vision, urinary retention, and dry mouth.

Desmopressin (DDAVP, Stimate)

COMMON USES: Diabetes insipidus; bleeding due to hemophilia A and type I von Willebrand's disease (parenteral), nocturnal enuresis.
DOSAGE: Diabetes Insipidus: **Adults:** intranasal, 0.1–0.4 mL (10–40 µg) daily in 2–3 divided doses. 0.5–1 mL (2–4 µg) IV/SC daily in 2 divided doses. If converting from intranasal to parenteral dosing, use 1/10 of intranasal dose. **Peds:** 3 mo and 12 y: intranasal 0.05–0.3 mL daily in single or 2 doses. Hemophilia A and von Willebrand's disease (type I): **Adults** and **Peds > 10 kg:** 0.3 mg/kg diluted to 50 mL with NSS infuse over 15–30 min. **Peds < 10 kg:** Same as above with dilution to 10 mL with NSS. Nocturnal enuresis: **Peds > 6 y:** 20 µg (0.2 mL) qhs, adjust as needed 10–40 µg.
NOTES: In very young and elderly patients, adjust fluid intake to avoid water intoxication and hyponatremia.

Desoxycorticosterone Acetate (DOCA, Percorten)

COMMON USES: Partial treatment for adrenocortical insufficiency.
DOSAGE: Injection: 2–5 mg/d IM into upper outer quadrant of gluteal region. Pellets: by surgical implantation after 2–3 mo of IM maintenance to determine dosing requirement.
NOTES: Must be used in conjunction with a glucocorticoid.

Dexamethasone, systemic (Decadron, Dexasone, others)

See Steroids, page 509.

Dexpanthenol (Ilopan-Choline, Ilopan)

COMMON USES: Minimize paralytic ileus, treat postoperative distention.

DOSAGE: *Adults:* Relief of gas: 2–3 tablets PO tid. Prevention of postoperative ileus: 250–500 mg IM stat, repeat in 2 h, then q6h as needed. Ileus: IM: 500 mg stat, repeat in 2 h, followed by doses every 6 h, if needed.

NOTES: Do NOT use if obstruction is suspected.

Dextran 40 (Macrodex, Rheomacrodex)

COMMON USES: Plasma expander for adjunctive therapy in shock; prophylaxis of DVT and thromboembolism; adjunct in peripheral vascular surgery.

DOSAGE: Shock: 10 mL/kg infused rapidly with maximum dose of 20 mL/kg in the first 24 h; total daily dose beyond 24 h should NOT exceed 10 mL/kg and should be discontinued after 5 d. Prophylaxis of DVT and thromboembolism: 10 mL/kg IV on day of surgery followed by 500 mL IV daily for 2–3 d; then 500 mL IV every 2–3 days based on patient's risk factors for up to 2 wk.

NOTES: Observe for hypersensitivity reactions; monitor renal function and electrolytes.

Dextromethorphan (Vicks Formula 44, many others)

COMMON USES: To control nonproductive cough.

DOSAGE: *Adults:* 10–20 mg PO q4h prn. *Peds:* 1–2 mg/kg/24h divided tid–qid.

NOTES: May be found in many OTC combination products with guaifenesin, acetaminophen, and pseudoephedrine.

Diazepam (Valium) [C]

COMMON USES: Anxiety, alcohol withdrawal, muscle spasm, status epilepticus, and preoperative sedation.

DOSAGE: *Adults:* Status epilepticus: 0.2–0.5 mg/kg/dose IV q15–30min to 30 mg maximum. Anxiety, muscle spasm: 2–10 mg PO or IM q3–4h prn. Preoperative: 5–10 mg PO or IM 20–30 min before procedure; can be given IV just before procedure. Alcohol withdrawal: Initially, 2–5 mg IV, may require up to 1000–2000 mg in 24-h period for severe withdrawal symptoms. *Peds:* Status epilepticus: < 5 y: 0.2–0.5 mg/kg/dose IV q15–30min up to maximum of 5 mg; > 5 y: may administer up to maximum of 10 mg. Sedation, muscle relaxation: 0.04–0.2 mg/kg/dose q2–4h IM or IV up to maximum of 0.6 mg/kg in 8 h, or 0.12–0.8 mg/kg/24h PO divided tid–qid.

NOTES: Do NOT exceed 5 mg/min IV as respiratory arrest can occur; absorption of IM dose may be erratic.

Diazoxide (Hyperstat, Proglycem)

COMMON USES: Hypertensive emergencies; management of hypoglycemia owing to hyperinsulinism.

DOSAGE: *Adults* and *Peds:* Hypertensive crisis: 1–3 mg/kg/dose IV up to maximum of 150 mg IV; may repeat at 15-min intervals until desired effect is achieved. Hypoglycemia: 3–8 mg/kg/24h PO divided q8–12h. Neonates: Hypoglycemia: 10 mg/kg/24h divided in 3 equal doses; maintenance: 3–8 mg/kg/24h PO in 2 or 3 equal doses.

NOTES: Sodium retention and hyperglycemia frequently occur; possible thiazide diuretic cross-hypersensitivity; cannot be titrated.

Dibucaine (Nupercainal, [OTC])

COMMON USES: Hemorrhoids and minor skin conditions.

DOSAGE: Insert into rectum with applicator bid and after each bowel movement.

Diclofenac (Cataflam, Voltaren)

COMMON USES: Treatment of arthritis (rheumatoid, osteoarthritis) and pain; ophthalmic as an adjunct to cataract surgery.

DOSAGE: 50–75 mg PO bid; ophthalmic 1 drop in eye qid 24 h postoperatively for up to 2 wk.

Dicloxacillin (Dynapen, Dycill)

COMMON USES: Treatment of infections caused by susceptible strains of *S aureus* and *Streptococcus.*

DOSAGE: *Adults:* 250–500 mg qid. *Peds:* 12.5–25 mg/kg/d divided qid.

NOTES: Take on an empty stomach.

Dicyclomine (Bentyl)

COMMON USES: Treatment of functional irritable bowel syndromes.
DOSAGE: *Adults:* 20 mg PO qid titrated to a maximum dose of 160 mg/d or 20 mg IM q6h. *Peds:* > 6 mo: 5 mg/dose tid–qid; children: 10 mg/dose tid–qid.
NOTES: Anticholinergic side effects may limit dose.

Didanosine [ddl] (Videx)

COMMON USES: Treatment of HIV infection in patients who are zidovudine intolerant.
DOSAGE: *Adults:* >60 kg: 400 mg PO qd or 200 mg PO bid. < 60 kg: 250 mg PO qd or 125 mg PO bid. *Peds:* Dose by BSA (see package insert).
NOTES: Reconstitute powder with water; side effects include pancreatitis, peripheral neuropathy, diarrhea, and headache; adults should take 2 tablets for each administration.

Diflunisal (Dolobid)

DOSAGE: Pain: 500 mg PO bid. Osteoarthritis: 500–1500 mg PO in 2–3 divided doses. Supplied: Tablets 250, 500 mg
NOTES: May prolong prothrombin time.

Digoxin (Lanoxin, Lanoxicaps)

Used for emergency cardiac care.
COMMON USES: CHF, atrial fibrillation and flutter, and paroxysmal atrial tachycardia.
DOSAGE: *Adults:* PO digitalization: 0.50–0.75 mg PO, then 0.25 mg PO q6–8h to a total dose between 1.0 and 1.5 mg. IV/IM digitalization: 0.25–0.50 mg IM/IV, then 0.25 mg q4–6h, total dose of about 1 mg. Maintenance: 0.125–0.500 mg PO/IM/IV qd (average daily dose 0.125–0.250 mg). *Peds:* Preterm infants: Digitalization: 30 mg/kg PO or 25 mg/kg IV; give 1/2 of dose initially, then 1/4 of dose at 8–12-h intervals for 2 doses. Maintenance: 10 mg/kg/24h PO or 6–8 mg/kg/24h IV divided q12h. Term infants to 2 y: Digitalization: 65–75 mg/kg PO or 50 mg/kg IV; give 1/2 of the dose initially, then 1/4 of the dose at 8–12-h intervals for 2 doses. Maintenance: 15–20 mg/kg/24h PO or 12–15 mg/kg/24h IV divided q12h. 2–10 y: Digitalization: 30–40 mg/kg PO or 25 mg/kg IV; give 1/2 dose initially, then 1/4 of the dose at 8–12-h intervals for 2 doses. Maintenance: 8–10 mg/kg/24h PO or 6–8 mg/kg/24h IV divided q12h. > 10 y: Same as for adults.
NOTES: Can cause heart block; low potassium can potentiate toxicity, reduce dose in renal failure; symptoms of toxicity include nausea and vomiting, headache, fatigue, visual disturbances (yellow-green halos around lights), and cardiac arrhythmias (see Table VIII–3, page 520); IM injection can be painful and has erratic absorption.

Digoxin Immune FAB (Digibind)

COMMON USES: Treatment of life-threatening digoxin intoxication.
DOSAGE: *Adults* and *Peds:* Based on serum level and patient's body weight. See dosing charts provided with the drug. Empiric where overdose is not known 20 vials (760 mg) IV in adults.
NOTES: Each vial will bind approximately 0.6 mg of digoxin; in renal failure may require redosing in several days due to breakdown of the immune complex.

Diltiazem (Cardizem, Dilacor)

COMMON USES: Treatment of angina pectoris, prevention of reinfarction, hypertension; atrial fibrillation or flutter, and paroxysmal SVT.
DOSAGE: Oral: 30 mg PO qid initially; titrate to 180–360 mg/d in divided doses as needed. Sustained release: 60–120 mg PO bid, titrate to effect, maximum dose 360 mg/d. Continuous dose: 180–300 mg PO qd. Intravenous: 0.25 mg/kg IV bolus over 2 min; may repeat dose in 15 min at 0.35 mg/kg. May begin continuous infusion of 5–15 mg/h.
NOTES: Contraindicated in sick-sinus syndrome, AV block, and hypotension. Cardizem CD and Dilacor XR are NOT interchangeable.

Dimenhydrinate (Dramamine)

COMMON USES: Prevention and treatment of nausea, vomiting, dizziness, or vertigo of motion sickness.

DOSAGE: *Adults:* 50–100 mg PO q4–6h, maximum of 400 mg/d; 50 mg IM/IV prn. *Peds:* 5 mg/kg/24h PO or IV divided qid.
NOTES: Anticholinergic side effects.

Dimethyl sulfoxide DMSO (Rimso 50)

COMMON USES: Interstitial cystitis.
DOSAGE: Intravesical, 50 mL, retain for 15 min; repeat q2wk until relief.

Diphenhydramine (Benadryl, others)

COMMON USES: Allergic reactions, motion sickness, potentiate narcotics, sedation, cough suppression, treatment of extrapyramidal reactions.
DOSAGE: *Adults:* 25–50 mg PO, IV or IM bid–tid.
Peds: 5 mg/kg/24h PO or IM divided q6h (maximum of 300 mg/d).
NOTES: Anticholinergic side effects including dry mouth, urinary retention; causes sedation; increase dosing interval in moderate-to-severe renal failure.

Diphenoxylate with Atropine (Lomotil) [C]

COMMON USES: Diarrhea.
DOSAGE: *Adults:* Initially, 5 mg PO tid or qid until under control, then 2.5–5.0 mg PO bid. *Peds > 2 y:* 0.3–0.4 mg/kg/24h divided bid–qid.
NOTES: Atropine-type side effects.

Dipivefrin (Propine)

COMMON USES: Open angle glaucoma.
DOSAGE: 1 drop into eye every 12 h.

Dirithromycin (Dynabac)

COMMON USES: Treatment of bronchitis, community-acquired pneumonia, and skin and skin structure infections.
DOSAGE: 500 mg PO qd for 7–14 d.
NOTES: Absorption is enhanced when taken with food.

Disopyramide (Norpace, NAPAmide)

COMMON USES: Suppression and prevention of premature ventricular contractions.
DOSAGE: *Adults:* 400–800 mg/d divided q6h for regular release products and q12h for sustained release products. *Peds < 1 y:* 10–30 mg/kg/24h PO; 1–4 y: 10–20 mg/kg/24h PO; 4–12 y: 10–15 mg/kg/24h PO; 12–18 y: 6–15 mg/kg/24h PO.
NOTES: Has anticholinergic side effects (urinary retention); negative inotropic properties may induce CHF; decrease dose in impaired hepatic function.

Dobutamine (Dobutrex)

COMMON USES: Short-term use in patients with cardiac decompensation secondary to depressed contractility.
DOSAGE: *Adults* and *Peds:* Continuous IV infusion of 2.5–15 mg/kg/min; rarely, 40 mg/kg/min may be required; titrate according to response (see Table VIII–8, page 526).
NOTES: Monitor ECG for increase in heart rate, blood pressure, and increased ectopic activity; monitor pulmonary wedge pressure and cardiac output if possible.

Docetaxel (Taxotere)

COMMON USES: Breast and other cancers.
DOSAGE: 60–100 mg/m^2 IV every 3 wk based on protocol.

Docusate Calcium (Surfak, others)

Docusate Potassium (Dialose)

Docusate Sodium (DOSS, Colace, others)

COMMON USES: Constipation-prone patient; adjunct to painful anorectal conditions (hemorrhoids).

DOSAGE: *Adults:* 50–500 mg PO qd. *Peds:* Infants to 3 y: 10–40 mg/24h divided qd–qid; 3–6 y: 20–60 mg/24h divided qd–qid; 6–12 y: 40–120 mg/24h divided qd–qid.
NOTES: No significant side effects, no laxative action.

Dolasetron (Anzemet)

COMMON USES: Prevention of nausea and vomiting associated with chemotherapy.
DOSAGE: *Adults* and *Peds:* 1.8 mg/kg IV as a single dose. *Adults:* 100 mg PO as a single dose. *Peds:* 1.8 mg/kg PO up to 100 mg as a single dose.
NOTES: May cause prolongation of the QT interval.

Dopamine (Intropin, Dopastat)

COMMON USES: Short-term use in patients with cardiac decompensation secondary to decreased contractility; increases organ perfusion.
DOSAGE: *Adults* and *Peds:* 5 mg/kg/min by continuous infusion titrated by increments of 5 mg/kg/min to maximum of 50 mg/kg/min based on effect (see Table VIII–8, page 526).
NOTES: Dose > 10 mg/kg/min may decrease renal perfusion; monitor urinary output; monitor ECG for increase in heart rate, blood pressure, and increased ectopic activity; monitor PCWP and CO if possible.

Dorzolamide (Trusopt)

COMMON USES: Glaucoma.
DOSAGE: 1 drop in eye(s) tid.

Dorzolamide and timolol (Cosopt)

COMMON USES: Glaucoma.
DOSAGE: 1 drop in eye(s) bid.

Doxazosin (Cardura)

COMMON USES: Treatment of hypertension and benign prostatic hypertrophy.
DOSAGE: Hypertension: Initially, 1 mg PO qd; may be increased to 16 mg PO qd. BPH: Initially, 1 mg PO qd, may be increased to 8 mg PO qd.
NOTES: Doses > 4 mg increase the likelihood of excessive postural hypotension; use qhs dosing to limit.

Doxepin (Sinequan, Adapin)

COMMON USES: Depression or anxiety.
DOSAGE: 50–150 mg PO qd; usually qhs but can be in divided doses.
NOTES: Anticholinergic, central nervous system, and cardiovascular side effects. Also, a potent antihistamine available in a 5% topical cream, for short-term relief of severe pruritus associated with various forms of eczematous dermatitis.

Doxorubicin (Adriamycin)

COMMON USES: Treatment of breast, endometrial, and ovarian cancer, and leukemia.
DOSAGE: 60–75 mg/m^2 IV as a single dose, at 21-d intervals.
NOTES: May cause myelosuppression and cardiotoxicity.

Doxycycline (Vibramycin)

COMMON USES: Broad-spectrum antibiotic including activity against *Rickettsiae*, *Chlamydia*, and *Mycoplasma pneumoniae*.
DOSAGE: *Adults:* 100 mg PO q12h first day, then 100 mg PO qd or bid or 100 mg IV q12h. *Peds > 8 y:* 5 mg/kg/24h PO up to a maximum of 200 mg/d, divided qd or bid.
NOTES: Useful for chronic bronchitis; tetracycline of choice for patients with renal impairment.

Dronabinol (Marinol) [C]

COMMON USES: Nausea and vomiting associated with cancer chemotherapy; appetite stimulation.
DOSAGE: *Adults* and *Peds:* Antiemetic: 5–15 mg/m^2/dose q4–6h prn. *Adults:* Appetite: 2.5 mg PO before lunch and supper.

NOTES: Principal psychoactive substance present in marijuana; many CNS side effects.

Droperidol (Inapsine)

COMMON USES: Nausea and vomiting, premedication for anesthesia.
DOSAGE: *Adults:* Nausea: 1.25–2.5 mg IV prn; premedication: 2.5–10 mg IV. *Peds:* 0.1–0.15 mg/kg/dose.
NOTES: May cause drowsiness, moderate hypotension and occasionally tachycardia.

Echothiophate iodide (Phospholine Ophthalmic)

COMMON USES: Glaucoma.
DOSAGE: 1 drop eye(s) bid with one dose at bed time.

Econazole (Spectazole)

COMMON USES: Treatment of most tinea, cutaneous *Candida,* and tinea versicolor infections.
DOSAGE: Apply to affected areas bid (qd for tinea versicolor) for 2–4 wk.
NOTES: Relief of symptoms and clinical improvement may be seen early in treatment, but course of therapy should be carried out to avoid recurrence.

Edrophonium (Tensilon)

COMMON USES: Diagnosis of myasthenia gravis; acute myasthenic crisis; curare antagonist; paroxysmal atrial tachycardia.
DOSAGE: *Adults:* Test for myasthenia gravis: 2 mg IV in 1 min; if tolerated, give 8 mg IV; a positive test is a brief increase in strength. PAT: 10 mg IV to a maximum of 40 mg. *Peds:* Test for myasthenia gravis: total dose of 0.2 mg/kg. Give 0.04 mg/kg as a test dose. If no reaction occurs, give the remainder of the dose in 1-mg increments to a maximum of 10 mg.
NOTES: Can cause severe cholinergic effects; keep atropine available.

Efavirenz (Sustiva)

COMMON USES: HIV-1 infections in combination with at least two other agents.
DOSAGE: *Adults:* 600 mg qd at bedtime. *Peds:* see insert, based on body weight.

Enalapril (Vasotec)

COMMON USES: Hypertension, CHF.
DOSAGE: *Adults:* 2.5–5 mg PO titrated by effect to 10–40 mg/d as 1–2 divided doses, or 1.25 mg IV q6h. *Peds:* 0.05–0.08 mg/kg/dose PO q12–24h.
NOTES: Initial dose can produce symptomatic hypotension, especially with concomitant diuretics; discontinue diuretic for 2–3 d before initiation if possible; monitor closely for increases in serum potassium; may cause a nonproductive cough.

Enoxaparin (Lovenox)

COMMON USES: Prevention of DVT.
DOSAGE: 30 mg SC twice daily.
NOTES: Does not significantly affect bleeding time, platelet function, PT or APTT.

Entacapone (Comtan)

COMMON USES: Treatment of Parkinson disease.
DOSAGE: 200 mg administered concurrently with each levodopa/carbidopa dose to a maximum of 8 times per day.

Epinephrine (Adrenalin, Sus-Phrine, others)

COMMON USES: Cardiac arrest, anaphylactic reactions, acute asthma.
DOSAGE: *Adults:* Emergency cardiac care: 0.5–1.0 mg (5–10 mL of 1:10,000) IV every 5 min to response (see Table VIII–8, page 526). Anaphylaxis: 0.3–0.5 mL of 1:1000 dilution SC; may repeat q10–15 min to maximum of 1 mg/dose and 5 mg/d. Asthma: 0.3–0.5 mL of 1:1000 dilution SC repeated at 20-min to 4-h intervals or 1 inhalation (metered dose) repeated in 1–2 min or suspension 0.1–0.3 mL SC for extended effect. *Peds:* Emergency cardiac care: 0.1 mL/kg of 1:10,000 dilution IV q3–5min to response.
NOTES: Sus-Phrine offers sustained action; in acute cardiac settings can be given via endotracheal tube if a central line is not available.

Epoetin alfa (Epogen, Procrit)

COMMON USES: Treatment of anemia associated with chronic renal failure, zidovudine treatment in HIV-infected patients, and patients receiving cancer chemotherapy; reduction in transfusions associated with surgery.

DOSAGE: *Adults* and *Peds:* 50–150 U/kg 3 times weekly; adjust the dose every 4–6 wk as needed. Surgery: 300 U/kg/d for 10 d before surgery.

NOTES: May cause hypertension, headache, tachycardia, nausea, and vomiting; store in refrigerator.

Epoprostenol (Flolan)

COMMON USES: Treatment of pulmonary hypertension.

DOSAGE: 4 ng/kg/min IV continuous infusion; make dosing adjustments based on clinical status and package insert guidelines.

NOTES: Availability through a pharmacy benefit manager (PBM).

Eprosartan (Teveten)

COMMON USES: Treatment of hypertension.

DOSAGE: 400–800 mg daily as single dose or twice daily.

NOTES: Avoid use during pregnancy.

Eptifibatide (Integrilin)

COMMON USES: Treatment of acute coronary syndrome.

DOSAGE: 180 μg/kg IV bolus, followed by 2 μg/kg/min continuous infusion.

Erythromycin (E-Mycin, Ilosone, Erythrocin, ERYC, others)

COMMON USES: Infections caused by Group A streptococci (*S pyogenes*), alpha-hemolytic streptococci and *N gonorrhoeae* infections in penicillin allergic patients, *S pneumoniae*, *M pneumoniae*, and *Legionella*.

DOSAGE: *Adults:* 250–500 mg PO qid or between 500 mg and 1 g IV qid. *Peds:* 30–50 mg/kg/24h PO or IV divided q6h, to a maximum of 2 g/d.

NOTES: Frequent mild gastrointestinal disturbances; estolate salt is associated with cholestatic jaundice; erythromycin base not well absorbed from the gastrointestinal tract; some forms such as ERYC are better tolerated with respect to gastrointestinal irritation; lactobionate salt contains benzyl alcohol; therefore, use with caution in neonates; base formulation not absorbed and used as part of the "Condon Bowel Prep."

Erythromycin, ophthalmic (Ilotycin)

COMMON USES: Conjunctival infections.

DOSAGE: 0.5% ointment, apply q6h.

Esmolol (Brevibloc)

COMMON USES: Supraventricular tachycardia, noncompensatory sinus tachycardia.

DOSAGE: Initial 500 mg/kg load over 1 min, then 50 mg/kg/min for 4 min; if inadequate response, repeat loading dose and follow with maintenance infusion of 100 mg/kg/min for 4 min; continue titration process by repeating loading dose followed by incremental increases in the maintenance dose of 50 mg/kg/min for 4 min until desired heart rate is reached or a decrease in blood pressure occurs; average dose is 100 mg/kg/min.

NOTES: Monitor closely for hypotension; decreasing or discontinuing infusion will reverse hypotension in approximately 30 min.

Estazolam (ProSom) [C]

COMMON USES: Insomnia.

DOSAGE: 1–2 mg PO qhs prn.

Esterified Estrogens (Estratab, Menest)

COMMON USES: Vasomotor symptoms, atrophic vaginitis, or kraurosis vulvae associated with menopause, female hypogonadism.

DOSAGE: Menopause: 0.3–1.25 mg daily; hypogonadism: 2.5 mg PO qd–tid.

Esterified Estrogens with Methyltestosterone (Estratest)

COMMON USES: Moderate-to-severe vasomotor symptoms associated with menopause, postpartum breast engorgement.
DOSAGE: 1 tablet qd for 3 wk, then 1 wk off.

Estradiol Topical (Estrace)

COMMON USES: Atrophic vaginitis and kraurosis vulvae associated with menopause.
DOSAGE: 2–4 g daily 1–2 wk, then 1 g 1–3 times a week.

Estradiol Transdermal (Estraderm)

COMMON USES: Severe vasomotor symptoms associated with menopause; female hypogonadism.
DOSAGE: 0.05 system twice weekly, adjust dose as necessary to control symptoms. Transdermal patches 0.05 mg, 0.1 mg (delivers 0.05 mg or 0.1 mg/24h).

Estramustine (Emcyt)

COMMON USES: Advanced prostate cancer.
DOSAGE: 1 capsule per 22 lb of body weight, divided tid–qid.

Estrogen, Conjugated (Premarin)

COMMON USES: Moderate-to-severe vasomotor symptoms associated with menopause; atrophic vaginitis; palliative therapy of advanced prostatic carcinoma; prevention of estrogen deficiency-induced osteoporosis.
DOSAGE: 0.3–1.25 mg/d PO cyclically; prostatic carcinoma requires 1.25–2.5 mg PO tid.
NOTES: Do NOT use in pregnancy; associated with an increased risk of endometrial carcinoma, gallbladder disease, and thromboembolism and possibly breast cancer; generic products are NOT equivalent.

Estrogen, Conjugated with Methyltestosterone (Premarin with methyltestosterone)

COMMON USES: Moderate-to-severe vasomotor symptoms associated with menopause, postpartum breast engorgement.
DOSAGE: 1 tablet every day for 3 wk, then 1 wk off.

Ethacrynic Acid (Edecrin)

COMMON USES: Edema, CHF, ascites, any time rapid diuresis is desired.
DOSAGE: *Adults:* 50–200 mg PO qd or 50 mg IV prn. *Peds:* 1 mg/kg/dose IV. Repeated doses are NOT recommended.
NOTES: Contraindicated in anuria; many severe side effects.

Ethambutol (Myambutol)

COMMON USES: Pulmonary tuberculosis and other mycobacterial infections.
DOSAGE: *Adults* and *Peds > 12 y:* 15–25 mg/kg PO daily as single dose.
NOTES: May cause vision changes and gastrointestinal upset.

Ethinyl Estradiol (Estinyl, Feminone)

COMMON USES: Vasomotor symptoms associated with menopause, female hypogonadism.
DOSAGE: 0.02–1.5 mg/d divided qd–tid.

Ethosuximide (Zarontin)

COMMON USES: Absence seizures.
DOSAGE: *Adults:* 500 mg qd PO initially; increase by 250 mg/d every 4–7 d as needed. *Peds:* 20–40 mg/kg/24h PO qd to a maximum of 1500 mg/d.
NOTES: Blood dyscrasias, CNS and gastrointestinal side effects may occur; use caution in patients with renal or hepatic impairment.

Etidronate (Didronel)

COMMON USES: Hypercalcemia of malignancy, hypertropic ossification associated with spinal cord injury, Paget's disease, postmenopausal osteoporosis.

DOSAGE: Hypercalcemia: 7.5 mg/kg IV in NS over 2 h daily for 3 d, then 20 mg/kg/d PO for 1 month. Ossification: 20 mg/kg/d for 2 wk, then 10 mg/kg/d for 10 wk.

Etodolac (Lodine)

COMMON USES: Treatment of arthritis and pain.
DOSAGE: 200–400 mg PO bid–qid.

Etoposide (VePesid)

COMMON USES: Treatment of gestational trophoblastic disease, ovarian, testicular, and lung cancer.
DOSAGE: 35–100 mg/m^2/d IV. Number of doses and duration of therapy is dependent on individual protocols.
NOTES: May cause bone marrow suppression; has low stability in concentrated solutions.

Famciclovir (Famvir)

COMMON USES: Management of acute herpes zoster (shingles) and genital herpes infections.
DOSAGE: Zoster: 500 mg PO q8h. Simplex: 125–250 mg PO bid.

Famotidine (Pepcid)

COMMON USES: Short-term treatment of active duodenal ulcer and benign gastric ulcer; maintenance therapy for duodenal ulcer, hypersecretory conditions, GERD, and heartburn.
DOSAGE: *Adults:* Ulcer: 20–40 mg PO hs or 20 mg IV q12h. Hypersecretory: 20–160 mg PO q6h. GERD: 20 mg PO bid; maintenance 20 mg PO hs. Heartburn: 10 mg PO prn. *Peds:* 1–2 mg/kg/d.
NOTES: Decrease dose in severe renal insufficiency.

Felodipine (Plendil)

COMMON USES: Treatment of hypertension.
DOSAGE: 5–20 mg PO qd.
NOTES: Closely monitor blood pressure in elderly patients and patients with impaired hepatic function; doses of 10 mg should NOT be used in these patients.

Fenofibrate (Tricor)

COMMON USES: Treatment of hypertriglyceridemia.
DOSAGE: Initial dose 67 mg once daily. May be increased to 67 mg 3 times daily.
NOTES: Take with meals to increase bioavailability; may cause pancreatitis.

Fenoldopam (Corlopam)

COMMON USES: Treatment of hypertensive emergency.
DOSAGE: Initial dose 0.03–0.1 µg/kg/min IV continuous infusion, titrate to effect every 15 min with 0.05–0.1 µg/kg/min increments.
NOTES: Avoid concurrent use with beta-blockers.

Fenoprofen (Nalfon)

COMMON USES: Treatment of arthritis and pain.
DOSAGE: 200–600 mg q4–8h, to a maximum of 3200 mg/d.

Fentanyl (Sublimaze) [C]

COMMON USES: Short-acting analgesic used in conjunction with anesthesia.
DOSAGE: *Adults* and *Peds:* 0.025–0.15 mg/kg IV/IM titrated to effect.
NOTES: Causes significant sedation.

Fentanyl Transdermal System (Duragesic) [C]

COMMON USES: Management of chronic pain.
DOSAGE: Apply patch to upper torso every 72 h. Dose is calculated from the narcotic requirements for the previous 24 h. Transdermal patches deliver 25 mg/h, 50 mg/h, 75 mg/h, 100 mg/h.
NOTES: 0.1 mg of fentanyl is equivalent to 10 mg of morphine IM.

Fentanyl Transmucosal System (Actiq, Fentanyl Oralet) [C]

COMMON USES: Induction of anesthesia and breakthrough cancer pain.
DOSAGE: *Adults* and *Peds:* Anesthesia: 5–15 µg/kg. Pain: 200 µg consumed over 15 min, titrate to appropriate effect.

Ferrous Sulfate

COMMON USES: Iron deficiency anemia; iron supplementation.
DOSAGE: *Adults:* 100–200 mg/d of elemental iron divided tid–qid. *Peds:* 1–2 mg/kg/24h divided qd–bid.
NOTES: May turn stools and urine dark; can cause gastrointestinal upset, constipation; vitamin C taken with ferrous sulfate increases the absorption of iron especially in patients with atrophic gastritis.

Fexofenadine (Allegra)

COMMON USES: Relief of allergic rhinitis.
DOSAGE: *Adults* and *Peds > 12 y:* 60 mg twice daily.

Filgrastim [G-CSF] (Neupogen)

COMMON USES: To decrease the incidence of infection in febrile neutropenic patients, and treatment of chronic neutropenia.
DOSAGE: *Adults* and *Peds:* 5 µg/kg/d SC or IV as a single daily dose.
NOTES: May cause bone pain. Discontinue therapy when ANC > 10,000.

Finasteride (Proscar, Propecia)

COMMON USES: Treatment of benign prostatic hyperplasia and androgenetic alopecia.
DOSAGE: BPH (Proscar): 5 mg PO qd. Alopecia (Propecia): 1 mg PO qd.
NOTES: Will decrease prostate-specific antigen levels; may take 3–6 mo to see effect on urinary symptoms.

Flavoxate (Urispas)

COMMON USES: Symptomatic relief of dysuria, urgency, nocturia, suprapubic pain, urinary frequency, and incontinence.
DOSAGE: 100–200 mg PO tid–qid.
NOTES: May cause drowsiness, blurred vision, and dry mouth.

Flecainide (Tambocor)

COMMON USES: Life-threatening ventricular arrhythmias.
DOSAGE: 100 mg PO q12h; increase in increments of 50 mg q12h every 4 d to maximum of 400 mg/d.
NOTES: May cause new or worsened arrhythmias; therapy should be initiated in the hospital; may dose q8h if patient intolerant or uncontrolled at q12h interval; drug interactions with propranolol, digoxin, verapamil, and disopyramide; may cause CHF.

Fluconazole (Diflucan)

COMMON USES: Oropharyngeal and esophageal candidiasis; cryptococcal meningitis; *Candida* infections of the lungs, peritoneum, and urinary tract; prevention of candidiasis in bone marrow transplant patients on chemotherapy or radiation; and candidal vaginitis.
DOSAGE: *Adults:* 100–400 mg PO or IV qd. Vaginitis: 150 mg PO as a single dose. *Peds:* 3–6 mg/kg PO or IV qd.
NOTES: Adjust dose in renal insufficiency; oral dosing produces the same blood levels as IV dosing, so the oral route should be used whenever possible.

Fludarabine Phosphate (Fludara)

COMMON USES: Treatment of leukemia.
DOSAGE: 25 mg/m^2 IV for 5 consecutive days. Give every 28 d.
NOTES: May cause severe bone marrow suppression and neurologic toxicity.

Fludrocortisone Acetate (Florinef)

COMMON USES: Partial treatment for adrenocortical insufficiency.
DOSAGE: *Adults* and *Peds > 1 y:* 0.05–0.1 mg PO qd. Infants: 0.1–0.2 mg PO qd.
NOTES: For adrenal insufficiency, must be used in conjunction with a glucocorticoid supplement; dosing changes based on plasma renin activity.

Flumazenil (Romazicon)

COMMON USES: For complete or partial reversal of the sedative effects of benzodiazepines.
DOSAGE: 0.2 mg IV over 15 s, dose may be repeated if the desired level of consciousness is not obtained to a maximum dose of 1 mg.

Flunisolide (AeroBid)

COMMON USES: Control of bronchial asthma in patients requiring chronic corticosteroid therapy.
DOSAGE: *Adults:* 2–4 inhalations bid. *Peds:* 2 inhalations bid.
NOTES: May cause oral candidiasis; NOT for acute asthma attack.

Fluorouracil (Adrucil)

COMMON USES: Management of carcinoma of the colon, rectum, breast, stomach, and pancreas.
DOSAGE: Varies with individual protocol.

Fluoxetine (Prozac)

COMMON USES: Treatment of depression, obsessive-compulsive disorders, and bulimia.
DOSAGE: Initially, 20 mg PO qd; titrate to a maximum of 80 mg/24h; doses of > 20 mg/d should be divided.
Bulimia: 60 mg once daily in the morning.
NOTES: May cause nausea, nervousness, and weight loss.

Fluphenazine (Prolixin, Permitil)

COMMON USES: Psychotic disorders.
DOSAGE: 0.5–10 mg/d in divided doses PO q6–8h; average maintenance 5.0 mg/d or 1.25 mg IM initially, then 2.5–10 mg/d in divided doses q6–8h prn.
NOTES: Reduce dose in elderly patients; monitor liver functions; may cause drowsiness; do NOT administer concentrate with caffeine, tannic acid, or pectin-containing products.

Flurazepam (Dalmane) [C]

COMMON USES: Insomnia.
DOSAGE: *Adults* and *Peds > 15 y:* 15–30 mg PO qhs prn.
NOTES: Reduce dose in elderly patients.

Flurbiprofen (Ansaid)

COMMON USES: Treatment of arthritis.
DOSAGE: 50–100 mg bid–qid, to a maximum of 300 mg/d.

Flutamide (Eulexin)

COMMON USES: Prostate cancer in combination with LHRH analogue.
DOSAGE: 3 (125 mg) capsules PO q8h.
NOTES: Monitor LFTs.

Fluticasone nasal (Flonase)

COMMON USES: Seasonal allergic rhinitis.
DOSAGE: 2 sprays per nostril qd; may reduce to 1 spray/d; max 4 sprays/d.

Fluticasone oral (Flovent, Flovent Rotadisk)

COMMON USES: Chronic treatment of asthma.
DOSAGE: *Adults* and *adolescents:* 2–4 puffs bid. *Peds 4–11 y:* 50 μg twice daily.
NOTES: Counsel patients carefully on use of device multidose inhaler 44,110 or 220 μg/activation; Rotadisk dry powder 50, 100, and 250 μg/activation; risk of thrush.

Fluvastatin (Lescol)

COMMON USES: Adjunct to diet in the treatment of elevated total cholesterol.
DOSAGE: 20–40 mg PO qhs.

Folic Acid

COMMON USES: Macrocytic anemia.
DOSAGE: *Adults:* Supplement: 0.4 mg PO qd; pregnancy: 0.8 mg PO qd; folate deficiency: 1.0 mg PO qd–tid. *Peds:* Supplement: 0.04–0.4 mg/24h PO, IM, IV, or SC; folate deficiency: 0.5–1.0 mg/24h PO, IM, IV or SC.

Fomivirsen (Vitravene)

COMMON USES: CMV retinitis in AIDS patients who do not respond to other therapies.
DOSAGE: 6.6-mg intraocular injection every other week for 2 wk followed by one injection once every 4 wk.

Foscarnet (Foscavir)

COMMON USES: Treatment of cytomegalovirus; acyclovir-resistant herpes infections.
DOSAGE: Induction: 60 mg/kg IV q8h for 14–21 d. Maintenance: 90–120 mg/kg IV qd (Monday–Friday).
NOTES: Dose must be adjusted for renal function; nephrotoxic; monitor ionized calcium closely (causes electrolyte abnormalities); administer through a central line.

Fosfomycin (Monurol)

COMMON USES: Uncomplicated urinary tract infection in women.
DOSAGE: 3 g in water (one dose).

Fosinopril (Monopril)

COMMON USES: Hypertension.
DOSAGE: Initially, 10 mg PO qd; may be increased to a maximum of 80 mg/d PO divided qd–bid.
NOTES: Decrease dose in elderly patients, no need to adjust dose for renal insufficiency, may cause a nonproductive cough and dizziness.

Fosphenytoin (Cerebyx)

COMMON USES: Treatment of status epilepticus.
DOSAGE: Loading 15–20-mg PE/kg, maintenance 4–6 mg PE/kg/d.
NOTES: Dosed as Phenytoin Equivalents (PE); administer at < 150-mg PE/min to prevent hypotension.

Furosemide (Lasix)

COMMON USES: Edema, hypertension, congestive heart failure.
DOSAGE: *Adults:* 20–80 mg PO or IV qd or bid. *Peds:* 1 mg/kg/dose IV q6–12h; 2 mg/kg/dose PO q12–24h.
NOTES: Monitor for hypokalemia; use with caution in hepatic disease; high doses of the IV form may cause ototoxicity.

Gabapentin (Neurontin)

COMMON USES: Adjunctive therapy in the treatment of partial seizures.
DOSAGE: 900–1800 mg/d PO in 3 divided doses.
NOTES: It is not necessary to monitor serum gabapentin levels.

Gallium nitrate (Ganite)

COMMON USES: Treatment of hypercalcemia of malignancy.
DOSAGE: 100–200 mg/m^2/d for 5 d.
NOTES: Can cause renal insufficiency; 1% acute optic neuritis.

Ganciclovir (Cytovene, Vitrasert)

COMMON USES: Treatment and prevention of cytomegalovirus (CMV) retinitis and prevention of CMV disease in transplant recipients.

DOSAGE: *Adults* and *Peds:* IV: 5 mg/kg IV q12h for 14–21 d, then maintenance of 5 mg/kg IV qd for 7 d/wk or 6 mg/kg IV qd for 5 d/wk. *Adults:* PO: Following induction, 1000 mg PO tid. Prevention: 1000 mg PO tid.

NOTES: Not a cure for CMV; granulocytopenia and thrombocytopenia are the major toxicities; injection should be handled with cytotoxic precautions; take capsules with food.

Gatifloxacin (Tequin)

COMMON USES: Treatment of acute exacerbation of chronic bronchitis, sinusitis, community-acquired pneumonia, urinary tract infections.

DOSAGE: 400 mg PO or IV once daily.

NOTES: Avoid use with antacids; do NOT use in children < 18 y, pregnant or lactating women; reliable activity against *S pneumoniae*.

Gemfibrozil (Lopid)

COMMON USES: Hypertriglyceridemia (types IV and V hyperlipoproteinemia).

DOSAGE: 1200 mg/d PO in 2 divided doses 30 min before the morning and evening meals.

NOTES: Monitor liver function test and serum lipids during therapy; cholelithiasis may occur secondary to treatment; may enhance the effect of warfarin.

Gentamicin (Garamycin)

COMMON USES: Serious infections caused by susceptible *Pseudomonas, Proteus, Escherichia coli, Klebsiella, Enterobacter, Serratia,* and for initial treatment of gram-negative sepsis.

DOSAGE: *Adults:* 3–5 mg/kg/24h IV divided q8–24h. *Peds:* Infants > 7 d: 2.5 mg/kg/dose IV q12–24h; children: 2.5 mg/kg/d IV q8h.

NOTES: Nephrotoxic and ototoxic; decrease dose with renal insufficiency; monitor creatinine clearance and serum concentration for dosing adjustments; see Table VIII–2, page 519.

Gentamicin, Ophthalmic (Garamycin Ophthalmic)

COMMON USES: Conjunctival infections.

DOSAGE: 0.3% ointment apply bid or tid.

Glimepiride (Amaryl)

COMMON USES: Non-Insulin-dependent diabetes mellitus.

DOSAGE: 1–4 mg once daily.

Glipizide (Glucotrol)

COMMON USES: Non-Insulin-dependent diabetes mellitus.

DOSAGE: 5–15 mg qd–bid.

Glucagon

COMMON USES: Treatment of severe hypoglycemia in diabetic patients with sufficient liver glycogen stores.

DOSAGE: *Adults:* 0.5–1.0 mg SC, IM, or IV repeated after 20 min as needed. *Peds:* Neonates: 0.3 mg/kg/dose SC, IM, or IV q4h prn; children: 0.03–0.1 mg/kg/dose SC, IM, or IV repeated after 20 min prn.

NOTES: Administration of glucose IV is necessary; ineffective in states of starvation, adrenal insufficiency, or chronic hypoglycemia.

Glyburide (DiaBeta, Micronase)

COMMON USES: Management of non-insulin-dependent diabetes mellitus.

DOSAGE: Nonmicronized: 1.25–10 mg qd–bid. Micronized: 1.5–6 mg qd–bid.

Glycerin Suppository

COMMON USES: Constipation.

DOSAGE: *Adults:* 1 adult suppository PR, prn. *Peds:* 1 infant suppository PR, qd–bid prn.

Gonadorelin (Lutrepulse)

COMMON USES: Primary hypothalamic amenorrhea.

DOSAGE: 5 µg IV q90min for 21 d using a Lutrepulse reservoir and pump.
NOTES: Risk of multiple pregnancies.

Goserelin (Zoladex)

COMMON USES: Treatment of advanced prostate cancer and endometriosis.
DOSAGE: 3.6 mg SC every 28 d into the abdominal wall.

Granisetron (Kytril)

COMMON USES: Prevention of nausea and vomiting associated with emetogenic cancer therapy.
DOSAGE: *Adults* and *Peds:* 10 mg/kg IV 30 min before initiation of chemotherapy. *Adults:* 1 mg PO 1 h before chemotherapy, then q12h.

Guaifenesin (Robitussin, others)

COMMON USES: Symptomatic relief of dry nonproductive cough; expectorant.
DOSAGE: *Adults:* 200–400 mg (10–20 mL) PO q4h. *Peds:* 2–5 y: 50–100 mg (2.5–5 mL) PO q4h; 6–11 y: 100–200 mg (5–10 mL) PO q4h.

Guaifenesin and Codeine (Robitussin AC, Brontex, others) [C]

COMMON USES: Antitussive with expectorant.
DOSAGE: *Adults:* 10 mL or 1 tab PO q6–8h. *Peds:* 2–6 y: 1–1.5 kg/kg codeine/d divided dose q4–6h; 6–12 y: 5 mL q4h; > 12 y: 10 mL q4h, maximum 60 mL/24h.
NOTES: Brontex tab contains 10-mg codeine; Brontex liquid, 2.5-mg codeine/5 mL; others, 10-mg codeine/5 mL.

Guaifenesin and Dextromethorphan (many OTC brands)

COMMON USES: Cough due to upper respiratory irritation.
DOSAGE: *Adults* and *Peds > 12:* 10 mL PO q6h. *Peds:* 2–6 y: 2.5 mL q6–8h, 10 mL/d maximum; 6–12 y: 5 mL q6–8h, 20 mL max/d.

Guanabenz (Wytensin)

COMMON USES: Hypertension.
DOSAGE: *Adults:* Initially, 4 mg PO bid, increase by 4 mg/d increments at 1–2 wk intervals up to 32 mg bid. *Peds > 12 y:* 0.5–4 mg/d initially, increase by 0.5–2 mg/d at 1-wk intervals up to 24 mg/d divided bid.
NOTES: Sedation, dry mouth, dizziness, and headache common.

Guanadrel (Hylorel)

COMMON USES: Hypertension.
DOSAGE: 5 mg PO bid initially, increase up to 10 mg/d weekly up to 75 mg PO bid.
NOTES: Interactions with tricyclic antidepressants; less orthostatic changes and impotence than guanethidine.

Guanethidine (Ismelin)

COMMON USES: Hypertension.
DOSAGE: *Adults:* Initially, 10–25 mg PO qd, increase dose based on response. *Peds:* 0.2 mg/kg/24h PO initially, increase by 0.2 mg/kg/24h increments q7–10d up to maximum dose of 3 mg/kg/24h.
NOTES: May produce orthostatic hypotension especially with diuretic use; may potentiate vasopressors; increased bowel movements and explosive diarrhea possible; interaction with tricyclic antidepressants reduces the effectiveness of guanethidine.

Guanfacine (Tenex)

COMMON USES: Hypertension.
DOSAGE: 1 mg qhs initially, increase by 1 mg/24h to maximum dose of 3 mg/24h; split dose bid if BP increases at the end of the dosing interval.
NOTES: Use with thiazide diuretic is recommended; sedation, drowsiness common; rebound hypertension may occur with abrupt cessation of therapy.

Haemophilus B Conjugate Vaccine (ProHIBiT)

COMMON USES: Routine immunization between the ages of 18 mo and 5 y against diseases caused by *Haemophilus influenzae* type B.

DOSAGE: *Peds:* 0.5 mL (25 mg) IM in deltoid or vastus lateralis.

NOTES: Booster not required; observe for anaphylaxis.

Haloperidol (Haldol)

COMMON USES: Management of psychotic disorders; schizophrenia; agitation; Tourette's disorders; hyperactivity in children.

DOSAGE: *Adults:* Moderate symptoms: 0.5–2.0 mg PO bid–tid. Severe symptoms or agitation: 3–5 mg PO bid–tid or 1–5 mg IM q4h prn (max 100 mg/d). *Peds:* 3–6 y: 0.01–0.03 mg/kg/24h PO qd; 6–12 y: initially, 0.5–1.5 mg/24h PO, increase by 0.5 mg/24h to maintenance of 2–4 mg/24h (0.05–0.1 mg/kg/24h) or 1–3 mg/dose IM q4–8h to a max of 0.1 mg/kg/24h. Tourette's up to 15 mg/24h PO.

NOTES: Can cause extrapyramidal symptoms, hypotension; reduce dose in elderly patients.

Heparin Sodium

COMMON USES: Treatment and prevention of venous thrombosis and pulmonary emboli, atrial fibrillation with emboli formation, acute arterial occlusion.

DOSAGE: *Adults:* Prophylaxis: 3000–5000 U SC q8–12h. Treatment of thrombosis: Loading dose of 50–75 U/kg IV, then 10–20 U/kg IV qh (adjust based on PTT). *Peds:* Infants: Load 50 U/kg IV bolus then 20 U/kg/h IV infusion. Children: Load 50 U/kg IV then 15–25 U/kg/h continuous infusion or 100 U/kg/dose q4h IV intermittent bolus.

NOTES: Monitor PTT, thrombin time, or activated clotting time to assess effectiveness; heparin has little effect on the prothrombin time; with proper dose PTT is about 1 ½–2 times the control; can cause thrombocytopenia, monitor platelet counts.

Hepatitis A Vaccine (Havrix)

COMMON USES: High-risk exposure to hepatitis A (travelers, health care workers, etc).

DOSAGE: *Adults:* 1 mL IM, booster 6–12 mo. *Peds:* 0.5 mL IM day 1 and 30, booster 6–12 mo.

Hepatitis B Immune Globulin (HyperHep, H-BIG)

COMMON USES: Exposure to HBsAg-positive materials: blood, plasma, or serum (accidental needle-stick, mucous membrane contact, oral ingestion).

DOSAGE: *Adults* and *Peds:* 0.06 mL/kg IM, 5 mL maximum; within 24 h of needle stick or percutaneous exposure; within 14 d of sexual contact; repeat at 1 and 6 mo after exposure.

NOTES: Administered in gluteal or deltoid muscle; if exposure continues should receive hepatitis B vaccine.

Hepatitis B Vaccine (Engerix-B, Recombivax HB)

COMMON USES: Prevention of type B hepatitis in high-risk individuals.

DOSAGE: *Adults:* 3 IM doses of 1 mL each, the first 2 given 1 month apart, the third, 6 mo after the first. *Peds:* 0.5 mL IM dose given on the same schedule as adults.

NOTES: IM injections for adults and older peds to be administered in the deltoid; other peds to be administered in anterolateral thigh; may cause fever, injection site soreness; derived from recombinant DNA technology.

Hetastarch (Hespan)

COMMON USES: Plasma volume expansion as an adjunct in treatment of shock due to hemorrhage, surgery, burns, and other trauma.

DOSAGE: 500–1000 mL (do NOT exceed 1500 mL/d) IV at a rate NOT to exceed 20 mL/kg/h.

NOTES: Not a substitute for blood or plasma; contraindicated in patients with severe bleeding disorders, severe CHF, or renal failure with oliguria or anuria.

Hydralazine (Apresoline)

COMMON USES: Moderate-to-severe hypertension.

DOSAGE: *Adults:* 10 mg PO qid, increase to 25 mg qid to a maximum of 300 mg/d. *Peds:* 0.75–3 mg/kg/24h PO divided q12–6h.

NOTES: Use caution in patients with impaired hepatic function, coronary artery disease; compensatory sinus tachycardia can be eliminated with the addition of propranolol; chronically high doses can cause SLE-like syndrome; SVT can occur after IM administration.

Hydrochlorothiazide (HydroDIURIL, Esidrix, others)

COMMON USES: Edema, hypertension, CHF.
DOSAGE: *Adults:* 25–100 mg PO qd in single or divided doses. *Peds:* 2–3 mg/kg/24h PO divided bid.
NOTES: Hypokalemia is frequent; hyperglycemia, hyperuricemia, hyperlipidemia, and hyponatremia are common side effects.

Hydrochlorothiazide and Amiloride (Moduretic)

COMMON USES: Hypertension, adjunctive therapy for congestive heart failure.
DOSAGE: 1–2 tablets PO qd.
NOTES: Should NOT be given to diabetic patients or patients with renal failure.

Hydrochlorothiazide and Spironolactone (Aldactazide)

COMMON USES: Edema (CHF, cirrhosis), hypertension.
DOSAGE: 1–8 tablets (25–200 mg each component per day) 1–2 divided doses.

Hydrochlorothiazide and Triamterene (Dyazide, Maxzide)

COMMON USES: Edema, hypertension.
DOSAGE: Dyazide: 1–2 capsules PO qd–bid. Maxzide: 1 tablet PO qd.
NOTES: Can cause hyperkalemia and hypokalemia; monitor serum potassium.

Hydrocortisone

See Steroids, page 509.

Hydrocodone and acetaminophen (Lorcet, Vicodin, others) [C]

COMMON USES: Moderate-to-severe pain; hydrocodone has antitussive properties.
DOSAGE: 1–2 PO q4–6h prn.
NOTES: Many different combinations; specify hydrocodone/acetaminophen dose: 2.5/500, 5/400, 5/500, 7.5/400, 10/400, 7.5/500, 7.5/650, 7.5/750, 10/325, 10/400, 10/500, 10/650, Elixir and solution 2.5 mg hydrocodone/167 mg acetaminophen per 5 mL.

Hydrocodone and aspirin (Lortab ASA, others) [C]

COMMON USES: Moderate-to-severe pain.
DOSAGE: 1–2 PO q4–6h prn.
NOTE: 5-mg hydrocodone per 500 mg aspirin per tablet.

Hydrocodone and guaifenesin (Hycotuss expectorant, others) [C]

COMMON USES: Nonproductive cough associated with respiratory infection.
DOSAGE: *Adults* and *Peds > 12 y:* 5 mL q4h, PC and hs. *Peds:* < 2 y, 0.3 mg/kg/d divided qid; 2–12 y, 2.5 mL q4h PC and hs.

Hydrocodone and homatropine (Hycodan, others) [C]

COMMON USES: Relief of cough.
DOSAGE: *Adults:* 5–10 mg q4–6h. *Peds:* 0.6 mg/kg/d divided tid–qid.
NOTES: Dose based on hydrocodone; syrup, 5-mg hydrocodone/5 mL; tablet, 5-mg hydrocodone.

Hydrocodone and ibuprofen (Vicoprofen) [C]

COMMON USES: Moderate-to-severe pain (less than 10 d)
DOSAGE: 1–2 tablets q4–6h prn.
NOTES: 7.5 mg-hydrocodone per 200-mg ibuprofen per tab.

Hydrocodone and pseudoephedrine (Entuss-D, Histussin-D, others) [C]

COMMON USES: Cough and nasal congestion.
DOSAGE: 5 mL qid, prn.

NOTES: 5-mg hydrocodone per 5 mL.

Hydrocodone, chlorpheniramine, phenylephrine, acetaminophen, and caffeine (Hycomine)

COMMON USES: Cough and symptoms of upper respiratory infections.
DOSAGE: 1 PO, q4h, prn.
NOTES: 5-mg hydrocodone per tab.

Hydromorphone (Dilaudid) [C]

COMMON USES: Moderate-to-severe pain.
DOSAGE: 1–4 mg PO, IM, IV, SC, or PR q4–6h prn.
NOTES: 1.5 mg IM equivalent to 10-mg morphine IM.

Hydroxyurea (Hydrea)

COMMON USES: Treatment of cervical and ovarian cancer, melanoma, and leukemia adjunct in sickle cell anemia.
DOSAGE: Continuous therapy: 20–30 mg/kg PO qd; intermittent therapy: 80 mg/kg every 3 d.

Hydroxyzine (Atarax, Vistaril)

COMMON USES: Anxiety, tension, sedation, itching.
DOSAGE: *Adults:* Anxiety or sedation: 50–100 mg PO or IM qid or prn (maximum of 600 mg/d); itching: 25–50 mg PO or IM tid–qid. *Peds:* 0.6–1.0 mg/kg/24h PO or IM q6h.
NOTES: Useful in potentiating the effects of narcotics; NOT for IV use; drowsiness, anticholinergic effects are common.

Hyoscyamine (Anaspaz, Cystospaz, Levsin, others)

COMMON USES: Spasm associated with GI and bladder disorders.
DOSAGE: *Adults:* 0.125–0.25 mg (1–2 tabs) SL 3–4 times a day, pc and hs; 1 capsule q12h (sustained release [Cystospaz-M, Levsinex]).

Hyoscyamine, Atropine, Scopolamine, and Phenobarbital (Donnatal, others)

COMMON USES: Irritable bowel, spastic colitis, peptic ulcer, spastic bladder.
DOSAGE: 0.125–0.25 mg (1–2 tabs) 3–4 times a day, 1 capsule q12h (sustained release), 5–10 mL elixir 3–4 times/d or q8h.

Ibuprofen (Motrin, Rufen, Advil, others)

COMMON USES: Treatment of inflammatory conditions (rheumatoid arthritis, others) arthritis and pain, fever, gout, dysmenorrhea.
DOSAGE: *Adults:* pain, fever, dysmenorrhea 200–400 mg PO q4–6h, maximum 1.2 g/d, inflammatory conditions 400–800 mg ID-qid, max 3.2 g/d. *Peds:* 4–10 mg/kg/dose in 3–4 divided doses; rheumatoid arthritis 30–50 mg/kg/d divided qid, maximum, 2.4 g/d.

Ibutilide (Covert)

COMMON USES: Rapid conversion of atrial fibrillation or flutter.
DOSAGE: < 60 kg, 0.01 mg/kg (maximum 1 mg); > 60 kg, 1 mg IV over 10 min. May be repeated once if needed 10 min later.
NOTES: Do NOT administer Class I or III antiarrhythmics concurrently or within 4 h of ibutilide infusion.

Idarubicin (Idamycin)

COMMON USES: Treatment of leukemia.
DOSAGE: 12 mg/m² daily for 3 d.
NOTES: Do NOT administer if bilirubin is > 5 mg/dL.

Ifosfamide (Ifex)

COMMON USES: Testicular, breast, sarcoma, and ovarian cancer.
DOSAGE: 1.2 g/m²/d for 5 consecutive days. Repeat course every 3 wk.
NOTES: Causes hemorrhagic cystitis; hydrate patients well and administer with MESNA.

Imipenem/Cilastatin (Primaxin)

COMMON USES: Serious infections caused by a wide variety of susceptible bacteria; multiresistant infections, inactive against *S aureus,* group A and B streptococci, and others; empiric therapy of gram-negative sepsis in immunocompromised host.

DOSAGE: *Adults:* 250–500 mg (Imipenem) IV q6h. *Peds:* Children < 3 y: 100 mg/kg/24h IV divided q6h; children > 3 y: 60 mg/kg/24h IV divided q6h.

NOTES: Seizures may occur if drug accumulates; adjust dose for renal insufficiency to avoid drug accumulation if creatinine clearance < 70 mL/min.

Imipramine (Tofranil)

COMMON USES: Depression, enuresis.

DOSAGE: *Adults:* Hospitalized for severe depression: Start at 100 mg/24h PO or IV in divided doses, increase over several wk to 250–300 mg/24h. Outpatient: 50–150 mg PO qhs NOT to exceed 200 mg/24h. *Peds:* antidepressant: 1.5–5.0 mg/kg/24h divided tid; enuresis: 10–25 mg PO qhs; increase by 10–25 mg at 1–2-wk intervals, treat for 2–3 mo, then taper.

NOTES: Do NOT use with MAO inhibitors; less sedation than amitriptyline.

Immune Globulin Intravenous (Gamimune N, Sandoglobulin, Gammar IV)

COMMON USES: IgG antibody deficiency diseases (congenital agammaglobulinemia, common variable hypogammaglobulinemia; idiopathic thrombocytopenic purpura (ITP).

DOSAGE: *Adults* and *Peds:* Immunodeficiency: 100–200 mg/kg IV monthly rate of 0.01–0.04 mL/kg/min to a maximum of 400 mg/kg/dose. ITP: 400 mg/kg/dose IV qd for 5 d. BMT: 500 mg/kg/wk.

NOTES: Adverse effects associated mostly with rate of infusion.

Indapamide (Lozol)

COMMON USES: Hypertension, congestive heart failure.

DOSAGE: 2.5–5.0 mg PO qd.

NOTES: Doses > 5 mg do not have additional effects on decreasing blood pressure.

Indinavir (Crixivan)

COMMON USES: HIV infection as part of a two-drug (nucleosidase plus protease inhibitor) or three-drug (two nucleosidases plus protease inhibitor) treatment program.

DOSAGE: 800 mg PO q8h.

Indomethacin (Indocin)

COMMON USES: Arthritis and closure of the ductus arteriosus.

DOSAGE: *Adults:* 25–50 mg PO bid–tid, 200 mg/d maximum. Infants: 0.2–0.25 mg/kg/dose IV; may be repeated in 12–24 h for up to 3 doses.

NOTES: Monitor renal function.

Infliximab (Remicade)

COMMON USES: Treatment of moderate-to severe-Crohn's disease.

DOSAGE: 5 mg/kg IV infusion, subsequent doses 2 and 6 wk after initial infusion.

NOTES: May cause hypersensitivity reaction, made up of human constant and murine variable regions.

Insulins

COMMON USES: Diabetes mellitus that cannot be controlled by diet and/or oral hypoglycemic agents.

DOSAGE: Based on serum glucose levels; usually given SC can also be given IV or IM (only regular insulin can be given IV). See Table VIII–5, page 522. General guidelines: 0.5–1U/kg/d, 2/3 dose before breakfast, 1/3 before supper; adjust based on blood sugars over several days. Regular/rapid insulin should be dosed q4–6h, NPH/intermediate q8–12h. Keto Acidosis: hydrate patient well with NS, 10 U regular insulin IV followed by infusion 0.1 U/kg/h; optimum serum glucose decline: 50–100 mg/dL/h.

NOTES: The highly purified insulins provide an increase in free insulin; monitor these patients closely for several wk when changing doses; most standard insulins 100 U/mL.

Interferon Alpha (Roferon-A, Intron A)

COMMON USES: Hairy cell leukemia, Kaposi's sarcoma, multiple myeloma, chronic myeloge-nous leukemia, renal cell carcinoma, bladder cancer, melanoma, and chronic hepatitis C.
DOSAGE: Alfa-2a (Roferon): 3 million IU daily for 16–24 wk SQ or IM. Alfa-2b (Intron): 2 mil-lion IU/m^2 IM or SQ 3 times a week for 2–6 mo; intravesical 50–100 million IU in 50 mL NS weekly × 6.
NOTES: Systemic use may cause flulike symptoms; fatigue is common; anorexia occurs in 20–30% of patients; neurotoxicity may occur at high doses; neutralizing antibodies can occur in up to 40% of patients receiving prolonged systemic therapy.

Interferon Alpha and ribavirin (Rebetron, Intron A)

COMMON USES: Chronic hepatitis C.
DOSAGE: Intron A: 3 million IU SQ 3 times with Rebetrol 1000–1200 mg divided PO bid for 24 wk.
NOTES: Supplied in combination with multidose pen injector for Intron A.

Interferon Alfacon-1 (Infergen)

COMMON USES: Management of chronic hepatitis C.
DOSAGE: 9 μg SC 3 times per week.
NOTES: At least 48 h should elapse between injections.

Ipecac Syrup

COMMON USES: Treatment of drug overdose and certain cases of poisoning.
DOSAGE: *Adults:* 15–30 mL PO followed by 200–300 mL water; if no emesis occurs in 20 min, may repeat × 1. *Peds:* 6–12 mo: 5–10 mL PO followed by water. 1–12 y: 15 mL PO followed by water.
NOTES: Do NOT use for ingestion of petroleum distillates, strong acid, base, or other corro-sive or caustic agents; NOT for use in comatose or unconscious patients; caution in CNS de-pressant overdose.

Ipratropium Bromide Inhalant (Atrovent)

COMMON USES: Bronchospasm associated with COPD.
DOSAGE: *Adults* and *children > 12 y:* 2–4 puffs qid.
NOTES: Not for initial treatment of acute episodes of bronchospasm.

Irbesartan (Avapro)

COMMON USES: Treatment of hypertension.
DOSAGE: 150 mg PO daily, may be increased to 300 mg daily.

Iron Dextran (Dexferrum)

COMMON USES: Iron deficiency when oral supplementation is not possible.
DOSAGE: Based on estimate of iron deficiency (see package insert).
NOTES: Must give a test dose since anaphylaxis is common (adult 0.5 mL, infants 0.25 mL; may be given deep IM using "Z-track" technique, although IV route is most preferred.

Isoetharine (Bronkosol, Bronkometer)

COMMON USES: Bronchial asthma and reversible bronchospasm.
DOSAGE: *Adults* and *Peds:* Nebulization: 0.25–1.0 mL diluted 1:3 with saline q4–6h; Metered dose inhaler: 1 2 inhalations q4h.

Isoniazid (INH)

COMMON USES: Treatment of *Mycobacterium* spp. infections.
DOSAGE: *Adults:* Active TB: 5 mg/kg/24h PO or IM qd (usually 300 mg/d). Prophylaxis: 300 mg PO qd for 6–12 mo. *Peds:* Active TB: 10–20 mg/kg/24h PO or IM qd to a maximum of 300 mg/d. Prophylaxis: 10 mg/kg/24h PO qd.
NOTES: Can cause severe hepatitis; given with other antituberculous drugs for active tuber-culosis; IM route rarely used; to prevent peripheral neuropathy, can give pyridoxine 50–100 mg/d.

Isoproterenol (Isuprel, Medihaler-Iso)

COMMON USES: Shock, cardiac arrest, AV nodal block, antiasthmatic.
DOSAGE: *Adults:* Emergency cardiac care: 2–20 mg/min IV infusion, titrated to effect (see Table VIII–8, page 526). Shock: 1–4 mg/min IV infusion, titrated to effect. AV nodal block: 20–60 mg IV push; may repeat q3–5min; 1–5 mg/min IV infusion maintenance. Inhalation: 1–2 inhalations 4–6 times daily. *Peds:* Emergency cardiac care: 0.1–1.5 mg/kg/min IV infusion, titrated to effect. Inhalation: 1–2 inhalations 4–6 times daily.
NOTES: Contraindications include tachycardia; pulse > 130 bpm; may induce ventricular arrhythmias.

Isosorbide Dinitrate (Isordil)

COMMON USES: Angina pectoris.
DOSAGE: Acute angina: 2.5–10.0 mg PO (chewable tablet) or SL prn q5–10min; > 3 doses should NOT be given in 15–30 min period. Angina prophylaxis: 5–60 mg PO tid.
NOTES: Nitrates should NOT be given on chronic q6h or qid basis due to development of tolerance; can cause headaches; usually need to give a higher oral dose to achieve same results as with sublingual forms.

Isosorbide Monohydrate (ISMO)

COMMON USES: Prevention of angina pectoris.
DOSAGE: 20 mg PO bid, with the 2 doses given 7 h apart or extended release 30–120 mg PO qd.

Isradipine (DynaCirc)

COMMON USES: Hypertension.
DOSAGE: 2.5–5.0 mg PO bid.

Itraconazole (Sporanox)

COMMON USES: Treatment of systemic fungal infections caused by *Aspergillus, Blastomycosis,* and *Histoplasma.*
DOSAGE: 200 mg PO or IV qd–bid.
NOTES: Administer with meals or cola; should NOT be used concurrently with H_2-antagonists, proton-pump inhibitors, antacids.

Kaolin-Pectin

COMMON USES: Treatment of diarrhea.
DOSAGE: *Adults:* 60–120 mL PO after each loose stool or q3–4h prn. *Peds:* 3–6 y: 15–30 mL/dose PO prn. 6–12 y: 30–60 mL/dose PO prn.

Ketoconazole (Nizoral)

COMMON USES: Systemic fungal infections: candidiasis, chronic mucocutaneous candidiasis, blastomycosis, coccidioidomycosis, histoplasmosis, and paracoccidioidomycosis; topical cream for localized fungal infections due to dermatophytes and yeast; rapid short treatment of prostate cancer where rapid reduction of testosterone is needed (ie, spinal cord compression).
DOSAGE: *Adults:* Oral: 200 mg PO qd; increase to 400 mg PO qd for very serious infections; prostate cancer 400 mg PO tid (short term). Topical: Apply to affected area once daily. *Peds:* 3.3–6.6 mg/kg/24h PO qd.
NOTES: Associated with severe hepatotoxicity; monitor LFTs closely throughout course of therapy; drug interaction with any agent increasing gastric pH preventing absorption of ketoconazole; may enhance oral anticoagulants; may react with alcohol to produce disulfiram-like reaction.

Ketoprofen (Orudis)

COMMON USES: Treatment of arthritis and pain.
DOSAGE: 25–75 mg PO tid–qid, to a maximum of 300 mg/d.

Ketorolac (Toradol)

COMMON USES: Treatment of arthritis and pain.

DOSAGE: 15–30 mg IV/IM q6h or 10 mg PO qid.
NOTES: Do NOT use for longer than 5 d.

Ketorolac (Acular Ophthalmic)

COMMON USES: Itching associated with seasonal allergic conjunctivitis.
DOSAGE: 1 drop in eye(s) qid.

Labetalol (Trandate, Normodyne)

COMMON USES: Hypertension, hypertensive emergencies.
DOSAGE: *Adults:* Hypertension: initially, 100 mg PO bid; then 200–400 mg PO bid. Hypertensive emergency: 20–80 mg IV bolus, then 2 mg/min IV infusion, titrated to effect. *Peds:* Oral: 3–20 mg/kg/d in divided doses. Hypertensive emergency: 0.4–3 mg/kg/h IV continuous infusion.

Lactobacillus (Lactinex Granules)

COMMON USES: Control of diarrhea, especially after antibiotic therapy.
DOSAGE: *Adults* and *Peds > than 3 y:* 1 packet, 2 capsules, or 4 tablets with meals or liquids tid.

Lactulose (Chronulac, Cephulac)

COMMON USES: Hepatic encephalopathy; laxative; constipation.
DOSAGE: *Adults:* Acute hepatic encephalopathy: 30–45 mL PO q1h until soft stools are observed, then tid–qid. Chronic laxative therapy: 30–45 mL PO tid–qid; adjust the dose every 1–2 d to produce 2–3 soft stools qd. Rectally: 200 g diluted with 700 mL of water instilled into the rectum. *Peds:* Infants: 2.5–10 mL/24h divided tid–qid. Children: 40–90 mL/24 h divided tid–qid.
NOTES: Can cause severe diarrhea.

Lamivudine (Epivir, Epivir-HBV)

COMMON USES: Treatment of HIV infection when therapy is warranted based on clinical and/or immunologic evidence of disease progression, and chronic hepatitis B.
DOSAGE: HIV: *Adults* and *Peds > 12 y:* 150 mg PO bid. *Peds < 12 y:* 4 mg/kg twice daily. HBV: 100 mg once daily.
NOTES: Used in combination with zidovudine; use with caution in pediatric patients because of an increased incidence of pancreatitis.

Lamotrigine (Lamictal)

COMMON USES: Treatment of partial seizures.
DOSAGE: *Adults:* Initially, 50 mg PO qd, then 50 mg PO bid for 2 wk, then maintenance 300–500 mg/d divided bid. *Peds:* 0.15 mg/kg in 1–2 divided doses for week 1 and 2, then 0.3 mg/kg for wk 3 and 4, then maintenance dose of 1 mg/kg/d in 1–2 divided doses.
NOTES: May cause rash and photosensitivity; the value of therapeutic monitoring has not been established.

Lansoprazole (Prevacid)

COMMON USES: Treatment of duodenal ulcers, *H pylori* infection, erosive esophagitis, and hypersecretory conditions.
DOSAGE: 15–30 mg PO once daily.

Latanoprost (Xalatan)

COMMON USES: Glaucoma that does not respond to standard therapies.
DOSAGE: 1 drop in eye(s) qhs.
NOTES: May darken light irides.

Leflunomide (Arava)

COMMON USES: Treatment of active rheumatoid arthritis.
DOSAGE: 100 mg PO once daily for 3 d, followed by 10–20 mg once daily.
NOTES: Pregnancy category X DO NOT USE; monitor ALT.

Lepirudin (Refludan)

COMMON USES: Management of heparin-induced thrombocytopenia.
DOSAGE: Bolus of 0.4 mg/kg IV, followed by 0.15 mg/kg continuous infusion.
NOTES: Monitor aPTT 4 h into initial infusion and at least daily; adjust dose based on aPTT ratio; maintain aPTT ratio of 1.5–2.0.

Leucovorin Calcium (Wellcovorin)

COMMON USES: Overdoses of folic acid antagonist.
DOSAGE: *Adults* and *Peds:* Methotrexate rescue: 10–100 mg/m^2/dose IV or PO q3–6h. Adjunct to antimicrobials: 5–10 mg PO qd.
NOTES: Many different dosing schedules exist for Leucovorin rescue following methotrexate therapy.

Leuprolide (Lupron)

COMMON USES: Treatment of prostate cancer, endometriosis, and central precocious puberty (CPP).
DOSAGE: *Adults:* Prostate: 7.5 mg IM monthly of depot, 22.5 mg 3-month depot or 30 mg 4-month depot. Endometriosis (depot only): 3.75 mg IM as a single monthly dose. *Peds:* CPP: 50 mg/kg/d daily SC injection; titrate upward by 10 mg/kg/d until total down regulation is achieved. Depot: < 25 kg: 7.5 mg IM every 4 wk. 25–37.5 kg: 11.25 mg IM every 4 wk. > 37.5 kg: 15 mg IM every 4 wk.

Levalbuterol (Xopenex)

COMMON USES: Treatment and prevention of bronchospasm.
DOSAGE: 0.63 mg nebulized every 6–8 h.
NOTES: Therapeutically active R-isomer of albuterol.

Levamisole (Ergamisol)

COMMON USES: Adjuvant therapy of Dukes C colon cancer (in combination with 5-FU).
DOSAGE: 50 mg PO q8h for 3 d every 14 d during 5-FU therapy.
NOTES: Toxicity includes nausea and vomiting, diarrhea, abdominal pain, taste disturbance, anorexia, hyperbilirubinemia, disulfiram-like reaction on alcohol ingestion, minimal bone marrow depression, fatigue, fever, and conjunctivitis.

Levetiracetam (Kappra)

COMMON USES: Treatment of partial-onset seizures.
DOSAGE: 500 mg PO bid, may be increased to a maximum of 3000 mg/d.
NOTES: May cause dizziness and somnolence; may impair coordination.

Levobunol (Betagan Liquifilm Opthalmic, others)

COMMON USES: Glaucoma.
DOSAGE: 1–2 drops in eye(s) bid.

Levocabastine (Livostin)

COMMON USES: Allergic seasonal conjunctivitis.
DOSAGE: 1 drop in eye(s) qid up to 4 wk.

Levofloxacin (Levaquin)

COMMON USES: Treatment of lower respiratory tract infections, sinusitis, and urinary tract infections.
DOSAGE: 250–500 mg PO or IV once daily.
NOTES: Reliable activity against *S pneumoniae,* drug interactions with cation-containing products.

Levonorgestrel Implants (Norplant)

COMMON USES: Prevention of pregnancy.
DOSAGE: Implant 6 capsules in the mid-forearm.
NOTES: Prevents pregnancy for up to 5 y; capsules may be removed if pregnancy is desired.

Levorphanol (Levo-Dromoran) [C]

COMMON USES: Moderate-to-severe pain.
DOSAGE: 2 mg PO or SC prn.

Levothyroxine (Synthroid)

COMMON USES: Hypothyroidism.
DOSAGE: *Adults:* 25–50 mg/d PO or IV initially; increase by 25–50 mg/d every month; usual dose 100–200 mg/d. *Peds:* 0–1 y: 8–10 mg/kg/24h PO or IV qd; 1–5 y: 4–6 mg/kg/24h PO or IV qd; > 5 y: 3–4 mg/kg/24h PO or IV qd.
NOTES: Titrate dose based on clinical response and thyroid function tests; dose can be increased more rapidly in young to middle-aged patients.

Lidocaine (Xylocaine)

COMMON USES: Local anesthesia; treatment of cardiac arrhythmias.
DOSAGE: *Adults:* Arrhythmias: 1 mg/kg (50–100 mg) IV bolus, then 2–4 mg/min IV infusion, should repeat bolus after 5 min. Local anesthesia: Infiltrate a few milliliters of a 0.5–1.0% solution with a maximum of 3 mg/kg/dose. *Peds:* Arrhythmias: 1 mg/kg dose IV bolus, then 20–50 mg/kg/min IV infusion. Local anesthetic: Infiltrate a few milliliters of a 0.5–1.0% solution, with a maximum of 3 mg/kg/dose.
NOTES: Epinephrine may be added for local anesthesia to prolong effect and help decrease bleeding; for IV forms, dose reduction is required with liver disease, CHF; dizziness, paresthesias, and convulsions are associated with toxicity.

Lidocaine/Prilocaine (EMLA)

COMMON USES: Topical anesthetic; adjunct to phlebotomy or invasive dermal procedures.
DOSAGE: *Adults:* EMLA Cream and Anesthetic Disc (1 g/10 cm^2): thick layer of cream 2–2.5 g applied to intact skin and covered with an occlusive dressing (Tegaderm) for at least 1 h; Anesthetic Disc : 1 g/10 cm^2 for at least 1 h; *Peds:* Max Dose: up to 3 mo or < 5 kg: 1 g/10 cm^2 for 1 h; 3–12 mo and > 5 kg. 2 g/20 cm^2 for 4 h; 1–6 y and > 10 kg: 10 g/ 100 cm^2 for 4 h; 7–12 y and > 20 kg: 20 g/200 cm^2 for 4 h.
NOTES: Longer contact time gives greater effect.

Linezolid (Zyvox)

COMMON USES: Resistant infections caused by gram-positive bacteria, including vancomycin resistant and methicillin resistant strains.
DOSAGE: 600 mg IV or PO q12h.
NOTES: A reversible, inhibitor of MAO; therefore avoid foods which contain tyramine; avoid cough and cold products containing pseudoephedrine or phenylpropanolamine.

Liothyronine (Cytomel)

COMMON USES: Hypothyroidism.
DOSAGE: *Adults:* Initially, 25 mg/24h, then titration q1–2wk according to clinical response and thyroid function tests to maintenance of 25–75 mg PO qd. *Peds:* Initially, 5 mg/24h, then titration by 5 mg/24h increments at 1–2-wk intervals; maintenance, 25–75 mg/24h PO qd.
NOTES: Reduce dose in elderly patients; monitor thyroid function test.

Lisinopril (Prinivil, Zestril)

COMMON USES: Treatment of hypertension, heart failure, and acute myocardial infarction.
DOSAGE: 5–40 mg/24h PO qd–bid. AMI: 5 mg within 24h of MI, then 5 mg after 24h, 10 mg after 48h, then 10 mg qd.
NOTES: Dizziness, headache, and cough are common side effects; DO NOT use in pregnancy.

Lithium Carbonate (Eskalith, others)

COMMON USES: Manic episodes of manic-depressive illness; maintenance therapy in recurrent disease.
DOSAGE: Acute mania: 600 mg PO tid or 900 mg slow release bid. Maintenance: 300 mg PO tid–qid.

NOTES: Dosage must be titrated; follow serum levels (Table VIII–3, page 520); common side effects are polyuria, tremor; contraindicated in patients with severe renal impairment; sodium retention or diuretic use may potentiate toxicity.

Lodoxamide (Alomide Ophthalmic)

COMMON USES: Seasonal allergic conjunctivitis.
DOSAGE: *Adults* and *Peds > 2 y:* 1–2 drops in eye(s) qid up to 3 mo.

Lomefloxacin (Maxaquin)

COMMON USES: Treatment of UTI and lower respiratory tract infections caused by gram-negative bacteria; prophylaxis in transurethral procedures.
DOSAGE: 400 mg PO qd.
NOTES: May cause severe photosensitivity.

Loperamide (Imodium)

COMMON USES: Diarrhea.
DOSAGE: *Adults:* 4 mg PO initially, then 2 mg after each loose stool, up to 16 mg/d. *Peds:* 0.40.8 mg/kg/24h PO divided q6–12h until diarrhea resolves or for 7 d maximum.
NOTES: Do NOT use in acute diarrhea caused by *Salmonella, Shigella,* or *Clostridium difficile.*

Loracarbef (Lorabid)

COMMON USES: Treatment of infections caused by susceptible bacteria involving the upper and lower respiratory tract, skin, bone, urinary tract, abdomen, and gynecologic system.
DOSAGE: *Adults:* 200–400 mg PO bid. *Peds:* 7.5–15 mg/kg/d PO divided bid.
NOTES: Has more gram-negative activity then first generation cephalosporins.

Loratadine (Claritin)

COMMON USES: Treatment of allergic rhinitis.
DOSAGE: 10 mg PO once daily.
NOTES: Take on empty stomach.

Lorazepam (Ativan, Alzapam) [C]

COMMON USES: Anxiety and anxiety mixed with depression; preoperative sedation; control of status epilepticus.
DOSAGE: *Adults:* Anxiety: 0.5–1.0 mg PO bid–tid. Preoperative: 0.05 mg/kg up to maximum of 4 mg IM 2 h before surgery. Insomnia: 2–4 mg PO qhs. Status epilepticus: 2.5–10 mg/dose IV repeated at 15–20 min interval prn. *Peds:* Status epilepticus: 0.05 mg/kg/dose IV repeated at 15–20 min interval prn.
NOTES: Decrease dose in elderly patients; may take up to 10 min to see effect when given IV.

Losartan (Cozaar)

COMMON USES: Treatment of hypertension.
DOSAGE: 25–50 mg PO qd–bid.
NOTES: Do NOT use in pregnancy; symptomatic hypotension may occur in patients on diuretics.

Lovastatin (Mevacor)

COMMON USES: Adjunct to diet for the reduction of elevated total and LDL cholesterol levels in patients with primary hypercholesterolemia (types IIa and IIb).
DOSAGE: 20 mg PO daily with evening meal; increase at 4-wk intervals to maximum 80 mg/d.
NOTES: Patient should be maintained on standard cholesterol-lowering diet throughout treatment; monitor LFTs every 6 wk during first year of therapy; headache and gastrointestinal intolerance common.

Magaldrate (Riopan, Lowsium)

COMMON USES: Hyperacidity associated with peptic ulcer; gastritis, and hiatal hernia.
DOSAGE: 1–2 tablets PO or 5–10 mL PO between meals and hs.

NOTES: Less than 0.3 mg sodium per tablet or teaspoon; do NOT use in renal insufficiency.

Magnesium Citrate

COMMON USES: Vigorous bowel preparation; constipation.
DOSAGE: *Adults:* 120–240 mL PO prn. *Peds:* 0.5 mL/kg/dose, up to maximum 200 mL PO.
NOTES: Do NOT use in renal insufficiency, intestinal obstruction.

Magnesium Hydroxide (Milk of Magnesia)

COMMON USES: Constipation.
DOSAGE: *Adults:* 15–30 mL PO prn. *Peds:* 0.5 mL/kg/dose PO prn.
NOTES: Do NOT use in renal insufficiency or intestinal obstruction.

Magnesium Oxide (Uro-Mag, Mag-Ox 400, Maox)

COMMON USES: Replacement for low plasma levels.
DOSAGE: 400–800 mg/d divided qd–qid.
NOTES: May cause diarrhea.

Magnesium Sulfate

COMMON USES: Replacement for low plasma levels; refractory hypokalemia and hypocalcemia; preeclampsia and premature labor.
DOSAGE: *Adults:* Supplement: 1–2 g IM or IV; repeat dosing based on response and continued hypomagnesemia. Preeclampsia, premature labor: 1–4 g/h IV infusion. *Peds:* 25–50 mg/kg/dose IM or IV q4–6h for 3–4 doses; may repeat if hypomagnesemia persists.
NOTES: Reduce dose with low urine output or renal insufficiency.

Mannitol

COMMON USES: Osmotic diuresis (cerebral edema, oliguria, anuria, myoglobinuria, etc), bowel preparation.
DOSAGE: *Adults:* Diuresis: 0.2 g/kg/dose IV over 3–5 min; if no diuresis within 2 h, discontinue. *Peds:* Diuresis: 0.75 g/kg/dose IV over 3–5 min; if no diuresis within 2 h, discontinue. *Adults* and *Peds:* Cerebral edema: 0.25 g/kg/dose IV push repeated at 5-min intervals prn; increase incrementally to 1 g/kg/dose prn for intracranial hypertension.
NOTES: Use caution with CHF or volume overload.

Maprotiline (Ludiomil)

COMMON USES: Depressive neurosis; manic-depressive illness; major depressive disorder; anxiety associated with depression.
DOSAGE: 75–150 mg/d qhs, maximum of 300 mg/d.
NOTES: Contraindicated with MAO inhibitors or seizure history; for patients > 60 y, give only 50–75 mg/d; anticholinergic side effects.

Meclizine (Antivert)

COMMON USES: Motion sickness, vertigo associated with diseases of the vestibular system.
DOSAGE: *Adults* and *Peds > 12 y:* 25 mg PO tid–qid prn.
NOTES: Drowsiness, dry mouth, blurred vision are common.

Medroxyprogesterone (Provera, Depot Provera, others)

COMMON USES: Secondary amenorrhea and abnormal uterine bleeding because of hormonal imbalance, endometrial cancer, contraceptive.
DOSAGE: Secondary amenorrhea: 5–10 mg PO qd for 5–10 d. Abnormal uterine bleeding: 5–10 mg PO qd for 5–10 d beginning on the 16th or 21st day of menstrual cycle. Endometrial cancer: 400–1000 mg IM/wk.
NOTES: Contraindicated with past thromboembolic disorders or with hepatic disease.

Megestrol Acetate (Megace)

COMMON USES: Treatment of breast and endometrial cancer; appetite stimulation in cancer and HIV-related cachexia.
DOSAGE: Cancer: 40–320 mg/d PO in divided doses. Appetite: 800 mg/d (100–400mg daily has also been effective).

Meloxicam (Mobic)

COMMON USES: Treatment of osteoarthritis.
DOSAGE: 7.5–15 mg PO once daily.

Melphalan (Alkeran)

COMMON USES: Treatment of breast and ovarian cancer, and multiple myeloma.
DOSAGE: 6 mg/d PO as single dose or 16 mg/m^2 IV every 2 wk for 4 doses.
NOTES: Monitor blood counts closely.

Meperidine (Demerol) [C]

COMMON USES: Relief of moderate-to-severe pain.
DOSAGE: *Adults:* 50–100 mg PO or IM q3–4h prn. *Peds:* 1–1.5 mg/kg/dose PO or IM q3–4h prn.
NOTES: 75 mg IM equivalent to 10 mg morphine IM; beware of respiratory depression; a useful preprocedure sedative, particularly in children, is a so-called cardiac cocktail, consisting of (per 30-lb body weight) 30-mg Demerol, 6.25-mg Thorazine, and 6.25-mg Phenergan given IM.

Meprobamate (Equanil, Miltown) [C]

COMMON USES: Short-term relief of anxiety.
DOSAGE: 200–400 mg PO tid–qid; sustained release 400–800 mg PO bid.
NOTES: May cause drowsiness.

Mercaptopurine (Purinethol)

COMMON USES: Treatment of leukemia.
DOSAGE: *Adults* and *Peds:* 2.5 mg/kg/d PO.

Meropenem (Merrem)

COMMON USES: Serious infections caused by a wide variety of bacteria including intra-abdominal and polymicrobic; bacterial meningitis.
DOSAGE: *Adults:* 1 g IV q8h. *Peds:* 20–40 mg/kg IV q8h.
NOTES: Adjust dose for renal function; less seizure potential than imipenem.

Mesalamine (Rowasa, Asacol, Pentasa)

COMMON USES: Treatment of mild-to-moderate distal ulcerative colitis, proctosigmoiditis, or proctitis.
DOSAGE: Retention enema at bedtime daily or insert 1 suppository bid. Oral: 800–1000 mg PO 3–4 times a day.

Mesna (Mesnex)

COMMON USES: Reduce the incidence of ifosfamide-induced hemorrhagic cystitis.
DOSAGE: 20% of the ifosfamide dose (w/w) IV at the time of ifosfamide infusion and 4 and 8 h after, for a total dose equal to 60% of the ifosfamide dose.

Mesoridazine (Serentil)

COMMON USES: Schizophrenia; acute and chronic alcoholism; chronic brain syndrome.
DOSAGE: 25–50 mg PO or IV tid initially; titrate to maximum of 300–400 mg/d.
NOTES: Low incidence of extrapyramidal side effects.

Metaproterenol (Alupent, Metaprel)

COMMON USES: Bronchodilator for asthma and reversible bronchospasm.
DOSAGE: *Adults:* Inhalation: 1–3 inhalations q3–4h to maximum of inhalations 12 per 24 h; allow at least 2 min between inhalations. Oral: 20 mg q6–8h. *Peds:* Inhalation: 0.5 mg/kg/dose up to maximum of 15 mg/dose inhaled q4–6h by nebulizer or 1–2 puffs q4-6h. Oral: 0.3–0.5 mg/kg/dose q6–8h.
NOTES: Fewer beta-1 effects than isoproterenol and longer acting.

Metaraminol (Aramine)

COMMON USES: Prevention and treatment of hypotension due to spinal anesthesia.

DOSAGE: *Adults:* Prevention: 2–10 mg IM q10–15min prn. Treatment: 0.5–5 mg IV bolus followed by IV infusion of 1–4 mg/kg/min titrated to effect. *Peds:* Prevention: 0.1 mg/kg/dose IM prn. Treatment: 0.01 mg/kg IV bolus followed by IV infusion of 5 mg/kg/min titrated to effect.
NOTES: Allow 10 min for maximal effect; employ other shock management techniques, such as fluid resuscitation as needed; may cause cardiac arrhythmias.

Metaxalone (Skelaxin)

COMMON USES: Relief of painful musculoskeletal conditions.
DOSAGE: 800 mg PO 3–4 times a day.

Metformin (Glucophage)

COMMON USES: Treatment of non-insulin-dependent diabetes mellitus.
DOSAGE: Initial dose of 500 mg PO bid; may be increased to a maximum daily dose of 2500 mg.
NOTES: Administer with the morning and evening meals; may cause lactic acidosis; contraindicated in patients with creatinine > 1.4 in females or > 1.5 in males, in patients with heart failure on pharmacologic therapy.

Methadone (Dolophine) [C]

COMMON USES: Relief of severe pain; detoxification and maintenance of narcotic addiction.
DOSAGE: *Adults:* 2.5–10 mg IM q8h or 5–15 mg PO q8h (titrate as needed). *Peds:* 0.7 mg/kg/24h PO or IM divided q8h.
NOTES: Equianalgesic with parenteral morphine; long half-life; increase dose slowly to avoid respiratory depression.

Methenamine (Hiprex, Urex, others)

COMMON USES: Suppression or elimination of bacteriuria associated with chronic and recurrent infections of the urinary tract.
DOSAGE: Initially, 2 tablets 4 times a day; maintenance, 2–4 tablets daily in divided doses.
NOTES: Contraindicated in patients with renal insufficiency, severe hepatic disease, and severe dehydration.

Methimazole (Tapazole)

COMMON USES: Hyperthyroidism; preparation for thyroid surgery or radiation.
DOSAGE: *Adults:* Initially, 15–60 mg/d PO divided tid; maintenance of 5–15 mg PO qd. *Peds:* Initially, 0.4–0.7 mg/kg/24h PO divided tid; maintenance of 0.2 mg/kg/d divided tid.
NOTES: Monitor patient clinically and with thyroid function tests.

Methocarbamol (Robaxin)

COMMON USES: Relief of discomfort associated with painful musculoskeletal conditions.
DOSAGE: *Adults:* 1.5 g PO qid for 2–3 d, then 1 g PO qid maintenance therapy; IV form rarely indicated. *Peds:* 60 mg/kg/24h PO divided qid.
NOTES: Can discolor urine; may cause drowsiness or gastrointestinal upset; contraindicated with myasthenia gravis.

Methotrexate (Folex)

COMMON USES: ALL, AML, leukemic meningitis, trophoblastic tumors (chorioepithelioma, choriocarcinoma, chorioadenoma destruens, hydatidiform mole), breast cancer, Burkitt's lymphoma, mycosis fungoides, osteosarcoma, head and neck cancer, Hodgkin's and non-Hodgkin's lymphoma, lung cancer; psoriasis; and rheumatoid arthritis.
DOSAGE: Cancer: "conventional dose": 15–30 mg PO or IV 1–2 times a week every 1–3 wk; intermediate dose: 50–240 mg or 0.5–1 g/m^2 IV once every 4 d to 3 wk, high dose: 1–12 g/m^2 IV once every 1–3 wk; 12 mg/m^2 (maximum 15 mg) intrathecally, weekly until the CSF cell count returns to normal. Rheumatoid arthritis: 7.5 mg/wk PO as a single dose or 2.5 mg q12h PO for 3 doses each week.
NOTES: Toxicity includes myelosuppression, nausea and vomiting, anorexia, mucositis, diarrhea, hepatotoxicity (transient and reversible; may progress to atrophy, necrosis, fibrosis, cirrhosis), rashes, dizziness, malaise, blurred vision, renal failure, pneumonitis, and, rarely,

pulmonary fibrosis. Chemical arachnoiditis and headache may occur with intrathecal delivery. High-dose therapy requires leucovorin rescue to prevent severe hematologic and mucosal toxicity (see page 482); monitor blood counts and methotrexate levels carefully.

Methoxamine (Vasoxyl)

COMMON USES: Support, restoration, or maintenance of blood pressure during anesthesia; for termination of some episodes of paroxysmal supraventricular tachycardia.
DOSAGE: *Adults:* Anesthesia: 10–15 mg IM; if emergency exists, 3–5 mg slow IV push. Paroxysmal SVT: 10 mg by slow IV push. *Peds:* 0.25 mg/kg/dose IM or 0.08 mg/kg/dose slow IV push.
NOTES: IM dose requires 15 min to act; use 5–10 mg phentolamine locally in case of extravasation; interaction with MAO inhibitors and tricyclic antidepressants to potentiate methoxamine effect.

Methyldopa (Aldomet)

COMMON USES: Essential hypertension.
DOSAGE: *Adults:* 250–500 mg PO bid–tid (max 2–3 g/d) or 250 mg to 1 g IV q4–8h. *Peds:* 10 mg/kg/24h PO in 2–3 divided doses (max 40 mg/kg/24h divided q6–12h) or 5–10 mg/kg/dose IV q6–8h to a total dose of 20–40 mg/kg/24h.
NOTES: Do NOT use in patient with liver disease; can discolor urine; initial transient sedation or drowsiness occurs frequently.

Methylene Blue

COMMON USES: Methemoglobinemia (except in patients with glucose-6 phosphate dehydrogenase), urolithiase.
DOSAGE: *Adults* and *Peds:* 1–2 mg/kg IV over several minutes.

Methylergonovine (Methergine)

COMMON USES: Prevention and treatment of postpartum hemorrhage caused by uterine atony.
DOSAGE: 0.2 mg IM after delivery of placenta, may repeat at 2–4-hour intervals or 0.2–0.4 mg PO q6–12h for 2–7 d.
NOTES: IV doses should be given over NOT less than 1 min with frequent BP monitoring.

Methylprednisolone (Solu-Medrol)

See Steroids, page 509.

Metoclopramide (Reglan, Clopra, Octamide)

COMMON USES: Relief of diabetic gastroparesis; symptomatic gastroesophageal reflux; relief of cancer chemotherapy-induced nausea and vomiting.
DOSAGE: *Adults:* Diabetic gastroparesis: 10 mg PO 30 min ac and hs for 2–8 wk prn; or same dose given IV for 10 d, then switch to PO. Reflux: 10–15 mg PO 30 min ac and hs. Antiemetic: 1–3 mg/kg/dose IV 30 min before antineoplastic agent, then q2h for 2 doses, then q3h for 3 doses. *Peds:* Reflux: 0.1 mg/kg/dose PO qid. Antiemetic: 2 mg/kg/dose IV on same schedule as adults.
NOTES: Dystonic reactions common with high doses that can be treated with IV diphenhydramine; can also be used to facilitate small-bowel intubation and radiologic evaluation of the upper gastrointestinal tract.

Metolazone (Mykrox, Zaroxolyn)

COMMON USES: Treatment of mild-to-moderate essential hypertension; edema of renal disease or cardiac failure.
DOSAGE: *Adults:* Hypertension: 2.5–5 mg PO daily. Edema: 5–20 mg PO daily. *Peds:* 0.2–0.4 mg/kg/d PO divided q12h–qd.
NOTES: Monitor fluid and electrolyte status of patient during treatment.

Metoprolol (Lopressor, Toprol XL)

Used for emergency cardiac care.
COMMON USES: Treatment of hypertension, angina, and myocardial infarction.
DOSAGE: Angina: 50–100 mg PO bid. HTN: 100–450 mg PO qd. AMI: 5 mg IV × 3 doses, then 50 mg PO q6h × 48 h, then 100 mg PO bid.

Metronidazole (Flagyl)

COMMON USES: Amebiasis, trichomoniasis, *C difficile,* and anaerobic infections.
DOSAGE: *Adults:* Anaerobic infections: 500 mg IV q6–8h. Amebic dysentery: 750 mg PO qd for 5–10 d. Trichomoniasis: 250 mg PO tid for 7 d or 2 g PO in 1 dose.
C difficile: 500 mg PO or IV q8h for 7–10 d. *Peds:* Anaerobic infections: 30 mg/kg/24h PO or IV divided q6h. Amebic dysentery: 35–50 mg/kg/24h PO in 3 divided doses for 5–10 d.
NOTES: For *Trichomonas* infections, also treat partner; reduce dose in hepatic failure; no activity against aerobic bacteria; use in combination in serious mixed infections; may cause disulfiram-like reaction.

Metyrapone (Metopirone)

COMMON USES: Diagnostic test for hypothalamic-pituitary ACTH function.
DOSAGE: Metyrapone test: Day 1: Control period: collect 24-h urine to measure 17-hydroxy-corticosteroids (17-OHCS) or 17-ketogenic steroids (17-KSG). Day 2: ACTH test: 50 U ACTH infused over 8 h and measure 24-h urinary steroids. Days 3–4: Rest period. Day 5: Administer metyrapone with milk or snack. *Peds:* 15 mg/kg q4h for 6 doses (min 250-mg dose). Day 6: Determine 24-hour urinary steroids.
NOTES: Normal 24-hour urine 17-OHCS is 3–12 mg; following ACTH, it increases to 15–45 mg/24h; normal response to metyrapone is between a two- and fourfold increase in 17-OHCS excretion; drug interactions with phenytoin, cyproheptadine, and estrogens may lead to subnormal response.

Metyrosine (Demser)

COMMON USES: Pheochromocytoma; short-term preoperative and long term when surgery is contraindicated.
DOSAGE: *Adults* and *Peds > 12 y:* 250 mg PO qid, increase by 250–500 mg/d up to 4 g/d; maintenance dose, 2–3 g/d divided qid.
NOTES: Administer at least 5–7 d preoperatively.

Mexiletine (Mexitil)

COMMON USES: Suppression of symptomatic ventricular arrhythmias.
DOSAGE: Administer with food or antacids; 200–300 mg PO q8h, max 1200 mg/d.
NOTES: Not to be used in cardiogenic shock, second- or third-degree AV block if no pacemaker; may worsen severe arrhythmias; monitor liver function during therapy; drug interactions with hepatic enzyme inducers and suppressors requiring dosing changes.

Mezlocillin (Mezlin)

COMMON USES: Infections caused by susceptible strains of gram-negative bacteria including *Klebsiella, Proteus, E coli, Enterobacter, P aeruginosa,* and *Serratia,* involving the skin, bone, respiratory tract, urinary tract, abdomen, and septicemia.
DOSAGE: *Adults:* 3 mg IV q4–6h. *Peds:* 200–300 mg/kg/d divided q4–6h.
NOTES: Often used in combination with aminoglycosides.

Miconazole (Monistat)

COMMON USES: Severe systemic fungal infections including coccidioidomycosis, candidiasis, *Cryptococcus,* and others; various tinea forms; cutaneous candidiasis; vulvovaginal candidiasis; tinea versicolor.
DOSAGE: *Adults:* Systemic: from 200–3600 mg/24h IV based on diagnosis divided into 3 doses. Topical: Apply to affected area twice daily for 2–4 wk. Intravaginally: Insert 1 full applicator or suppository at bedtime for 7 d. *Peds:* 20–40 mg/kg/24h IV divided q8h.
NOTES: Antagonistic to amphotericin-B in vivo; rapid IV infusion may cause tachycardia or arrhythmias; may potentiate warfarin drug activity.

Midazolam (Versed) [C]

COMMON USES: Preoperative sedation; conscious sedation for short procedures; induction of general anesthesia.

DOSAGE: *Adults:* 1–5 mg IV or IM, titrate dose to effect (see Table VIII–10, page 528). *Peds:* Conscious sedation: 0.08 mg/kg IM × 1. General anesthesia: 0.15 mg/kg IV followed by 0.05 mg/kg/dose q2 min for 1–3 doses as needed to induce anesthesia.
NOTES: Monitor patient for respiratory depression; may produce hypotension in conscious sedation.

Miglitol (Glyset)

COMMON USES: Treatment of Type 2 diabetes mellitus
DOSAGE: Initial 25 mg PO three times daily taken at the first bite of each meal; maintenance 50–100 mg three times daily with meals.
NOTES: May be used alone or in combination with sulfonylureas; can cause GI disturbances.

Milrinone (Primacor)

COMMON USES: Treatment of congestive heart failure.
DOSAGE: Loading dose of 50 µg/kg, followed by a continuous infusion of 0.375–0.75 µg/kg/min (see Table VIII–8, page 526}.
NOTES: Carefully monitor fluid and electrolyte status.

Mineral Oil

COMMON USES: Constipation.
DOSAGE: *Adults:* 15–45 mL PO prn. *Peds > 6 y:* 10–20 mL PO bid.

Minoxidil (Loniten, Rogaine)

COMMON USES: Severe hypertension; treatment of male and female pattern baldness.
DOSAGE: *Adults:* Oral: 2.5–10 mg PO bid–qid. Topical Rogaine: Apply twice daily to affected area. *Peds:* 0.2–1 mg/kg/24h divided PO q12–24h.
NOTES: Pericardial effusion and volume overload may occur; hypertrichosis after chronic use.

Mirtazapine (Remeron)

COMMON USES: Treatment of depression.
DOSAGE: 15 mg PO qhs, up to 45 mg qhs.
NOTES: Do NOT increase dose at intervals of less than 1–2 wk.

Misoprostol (Cytotec)

COMMON USES: Prevention of NSAID-induced gastric ulcers.
DOSAGE: 200 mg PO qid with food.
NOTES: Do NOT take if pregnant, can cause miscarriage with potentially dangerous bleeding; gastrointestinal side effects are common.

Mitomycin (Mutamycin)

COMMON USES: Treatment of breast, cervical, ovarian cancer, and GI adenocarcinomas; intravesical for bladder cancer.
DOSAGE: 20 mg/m^2 IV as a single dose every 6–8 wk; bladder cancer: 20–40 mg in 40 mL of NSS via a urethral catheter once a week for 8 wk followed by monthly treatments for 1 y.
NOTES: May cause cumulative myelosuppression.

Mitoxantrone (Novantrone)

COMMON USES: Treatment of leukemia, lymphoma, prostate, and breast cancer.
DOSAGE: 12 mg/m^2/d IV infusion for 2–3 d of each chemotherapy cycle.
NOTES: Causes severe myelosuppression.

Mivacurium (Mivacron)

COMMON USES: Adjunct to general anesthesia or mechanical ventilation.
DOSAGE: *Adults:* 0.15 mg/kg/dose IV, may need to repeat at 15-min intervals. *Peds:* 0.2 mg/kg/dose IV, may need to repeat at 10-min intervals.

Moexipril (Univasc)

COMMON USES: Treatment of hypertension.

DOSAGE: 7.5–30 mg in 1–2 divided doses administered 1 h before meals.

Molindone (Moban)

COMMON USES: Management of psychotic disorders.
DOSAGE: 5–100 mg PO tid–qid.

Montelukast (Singulair)

COMMON USES: Prophylaxis and treatment of chronic asthma.
DOSAGE: *Adults > 15 y:* 10 mg PO daily taken in the evening. *Peds 6–14 y:* 5 mg PO daily taken in the evening.
   Peds 2–5 y: 4 mg PO daily taken in the evening.
NOTES: NOT for acute asthma attacks.

Moricizine (Ethmozine)

COMMON USES: Treatment of ventricular arrhythmias.
DOSAGE: 200–300 mg PO tid.

Morphine Sulfate [C]

COMMON USES: Relief of severe pain.
DOSAGE: *Adults:* Oral: 10–30 mg q4h prn; sustained release tablets 30–60 mg q8–12h. IV/IM: 2.5–15 mg q4h prn (see Table VIII–10, page 528).
   Peds: 0.1–0.2 mg/kg/dose IM/IV q2–4h prn up to maximum 15 mg/dose.
NOTES: Large number of narcotic side effects; may require scheduled dosing to relieve severe chronic pain.

Moxifloxacin (Avelox)

COMMON USES: Treatment of acute sinusitis, acute bronchitis, and community-acquired pneumonia.
DOSAGE: 400 mg once daily.
NOTES: Active against gram-negative bacteria and *Streptococcus pneumoniae;* interactions with Mg-, Ca-, Al-, and Fe-containing products and Class IA and III antiarrhythmic agents.

Mupirocin (Bactroban)

COMMON USES: Treatment of impetigo; eradication of MRSA nasal carrier state.
DOSAGE: Topical: apply small amount to affected area. Nasal: apply twice daily in the nostrils.
NOTES: Do NOT use concurrently with other nasal products.

Muromonab-CD3 (Orthoclone OKT3)

COMMON USES: Treatment of acute rejection following organ transplantation.
DOSAGE: 5 mg IV qd for 10–14 d.
NOTES: This is a murine antibody; may cause significant fever and chills after the first dose.

Mycophenolate mofetil (CellCept)

COMMON USES: Prevention of organ rejection following transplantation.
DOSAGE: 1 g PO bid.
NOTES: Used in conjunction with corticosteroids and cyclosporine.

Nabumetone (Relafen)

COMMON USES: Arthritis and pain.
DOSAGE: 1000–2000 mg/d divided qd–bid.

Nadolol (Corgard)

COMMON USES: Hypertension and angina, prevention of migraines.
DOSAGE: 40–80 mg qd; 160 mg/d maximum.

Nafcillin (Nallpen)

COMMON USES: Treatment of infections caused by susceptible strains of *S aureus* and *Streptococcus.*

DOSAGE: *Adults:* 250–500 mg (1 g max) PO q4–6h; 1–2 g IV q4–6h; 500 mg IM q4–6h. *Peds:* 50–200 mg/kg/d divided q4–6h (max 12 g/d); 50–100 mg/kg/d divided q6h.
NOTES: No adjustments for renal function.

Nalbuphine (Nubain)

COMMON USES: Relief of moderate-to-severe pain.
DOSAGE: 10–20 mg IM, IV, SC q4–6h prn.
NOTES: Causes CNS depression and drowsiness; use with caution in patients receiving opiate drugs.

Nalidixic Acid (NegGram)

COMMON USES: Urinary tract infections caused by susceptible strains of *Proteus, Klebsiella, Enterobacter,* and *E coli* but NOT *Pseudomonas.*
DOSAGE: *Adults:* 1 g PO qid for 7–14 d. *Peds:* 55 mg/kg/24h in 4 divided doses.
NOTES: Resistance emerges within 48 h in significant percentage of trials; may enhance effect of oral anticoagulants; may cause CNS adverse effects which reverse on discontinuation of the drug.

Naloxone (Narcan)

COMMON USES: Reversal of narcotic effect.
DOSAGE: *Adults:* 0.4–2.0 mg IV, IM, or SC every 5 min, maximum total dose of 10 mg. *Peds:* 0.01 mg/kg/dose IV, IM, or SC; may repeat IV every 3 min for 3 doses prn.
NOTES: May precipitate acute withdrawal in addicts; if no response after 10 mg, suspect a non-narcotic cause.

Naltrexone (ReVia)

COMMON USES: Treatment of alcoholism and narcotic addiction.
DOSAGE: 50 mg PO qd.
NOTES: May cause hepatotoxicity; do NOT give until opioid free for 7–10 d.

Naphazoline and antazoline (Albalon-A Ophthalmic, others)

Naphazoline and pheniramine (Naphcon-A Opthalmic, others)

COMMON USES: Ocular congestion and itching.
DOSAGE: 1–2 drops in eye(s) every 3–4 h.

Naproxen (Naprosyn, Anaprox)

COMMON USES: Treatment of arthritis and pain.
DOSAGE: *Adults* and *Peds* > *12 y:* 200–500 mg bid–tid, to a maximum of 1500 mg per day.

Nedocromil (Tilade)

COMMON USES: Management of patients with mild-to-moderate asthma.
DOSAGE: 2 inhalations 4 times a day.

Nefazodone (Serzone)

COMMON USES: Treatment of depression.
DOSAGE: Initially, 100 mg PO bid; usual effective range is 300–600 mg/d in 2 divided doses.
NOTES: May cause postural hypotension and allergic reactions.

Nelfinavir (Viracept)

COMMON USES: Treatment of HIV infection in combination with other agents.
DOSAGE: *Adults:* 750 mg po tid. *Peds:* 2–13 y: 20–30 mg/kg (maximum dose, 1500 mg) tid.

Neomycin

COMMON USES: Hepatic coma; preoperative bowel preparation; minor skin infections.
DOSAGE: *Adults:* 3–12 g/24h PO in 3–4 divided doses. *Peds:* 50–100 mg/kg/24h PO in 3–4 divided doses.
NOTES: Part of Condon bowel preparation.

Neomycin, polymyxin-B bladder Irrigant Solution

COMMON USES: Continuous irrigant for prophylaxis against bacteriuria and gram-negative bacteremia associated with in-dwelling catheter use.
DOSAGE: 1-mL irrigant added to 1-L 0.9% NaCl; continuous irrigation of the bladder with 1–2 L of solution per 24 h.
NOTES: Potential for bacterial or fungal superinfection; possibility for neomycin-induced ototoxicity or nephrotoxicity.

Neomycin, polymyxin-B and dexamethasone (Maxitrol)

COMMON USES: Steroid-responsive ocular conditions with bacterial infection.
DOSAGE: 1–2 drops in eye(s) q4–6h; apply ointment in eye 3–4 times per day.
NOTES: Should be used under supervision of ophthalmologist.

Neomycin, polymyxln-B, and hydrocortisone (Cortisporin Opthalmic and Otic, others)

COMMON USES: Superficial bacterial infections of the eye or external auditory canal by organisms sensitive to neomycin or polymyxin and associated with inflammation; suspension used in the treatment of infections in mastoidectomy and fenestration cavities.
DOSAGE: *Adults* and *Peds:* Ophthalmic: ointment, apply every 3–4 h; suspension 1 drop q3–4h. Otic: 3–4 drops into external auditory canal tid–qid.
NOTES: Use suspension in cases of ruptured ear drum. Limit use to < 10 d; ocular use should be used under supervision of ophthalmologist

Neomycin, polymixin-B, and prednisolone (Poly-Pred)

COMMON USES: Steroid-responsive ocular conditions with bacterial infection.
DOSAGE: 1–2 drops in eye(s) q4–6h; apply ointment in eye 3–4 times per day.
NOTES: Should be used under supervision of ophthalmologist.

Nevirapine (Viramune)

COMMON USES: Treatment of HIV infection in combination with other agents.
DOSAGE: 200 mg/d for 14 d, then 200 mg bid.

Niacin (Nicolar)

COMMON USES: Adjunctive therapy in patients with significant hyperlipidemia who do not respond adequately to diet and weight loss.
DOSAGE: 1–2 g PO tid with meals; up to 8 g/d.
NOTES: Upper body and facial flushing and warmth following dose; may cause gastrointestinal upset and pruritus.

Nicardipine (Cardene)

COMMON USES: Chronic stable angina, hypertension.
DOSAGE: Oral: 20–40 mg PO tid. Sustained release: 30–60 mg PO bid. Intravenous: 0.5–15 mg/h continuous infusion. Titrate to desired blood pressure.
NOTES: Oral to IV conversion: 20 mg tid = 0.5 mg/h; 30 mg tid = 1.2 mg/h; 40 mg tid = 2.2 mg/h.

Nifedipine (Procardia, Procardia XL, Adalat, Adalat CC)

COMMON USES: Vasospastic or chronic stable angina; hypertension.
DOSAGE: *Adults:* 10–30 mg PO q8h, maximum 180 mg/d, or sustained-release tablets 30–90 mg once daily. *Peds:* 0.6–0.9 mg/kg/24h divided tid–qid.
NOTES: Headaches common on initial treatment; reflex tachycardia may occur; Adalat CC and Procardia XL are NOT interchangeable dosing forms.

Nilutamide (Nilandron)

COMMON USES: Combination with surgical castration for the treatment of metastatic prostate cancer.
DOSAGE: 300 mg/d in divided doses for the first 30 d, then 150 mg/d.

NOTES: Toxicity can include hot flashes, loss of libido, impotence, diarrhea, nausea, vomiting, gynecomastia, hepatic dysfunction (Monitor LFTs), and interstitial pneumonitis.

Nimodipine (Nimotop)

COMMON USES: Prevention of vasospasms following subarachnoid hemorrhage.
DOSAGE: 60 mg PO q4h for 21 d.
NOTES: Contents of capsule may be extracted and administered down an NG tube if the capsule cannot be swallowed whole.

Nisoldipine (Sular)

COMMON USES: Treatment of hypertension.
DOSAGE: 10–60 mg PO once daily.
NOTES: Do NOT take with grapefruit juice or high-fat meal.

Nitrofurantoin (Macrodantin, Furadantin)

COMMON USES: Urinary tract infections.
DOSAGE: *Adults:* Suppression: 50–100 mg PO qd. Treatment: 50–100 mg PO qid. *Peds:* 5–7 mg/kg/24h in 4 divided doses.
NOTES: Gastrointestinal side effects common; should be taken with food, milk, or antacid; macrocrystals (Macrodantin) cause less nausea than other forms of drug, may cause pulmonary fibrosis.

Nitroglycerin (Nitrostat, Nitrolingual, Nitro-Bid Ointment, Nitro-Bid IV, Nitrodisc, Transderm-Nitro)

COMMON USES: Angina pectoris; acute and prophylactic therapy; congestive heart failure, blood pressure control, pulmonary hypertension in children.
DOSAGE: *Adults:* Sublingual: 1 tablet (0.3, 0.4, 0.6 mg) SL. q5min prn × 3 doses. Translingual: 1–2 doses sprayed under tongue q5min prn × 3 doses. Oral: 2.5-, 6.5-, or 9-mg sustained-release capsule or tablet PO tid. Intravenous: 5–20 µg/min titrated to effect 200 µg/min maximum. Topical: 1–2 inches ointment to chest wall q6h, then wipe off at night. Transdermal: 0.2–0.4 mg/h, titrated to 0.4–0.8 mg/h; patches deliver in 24 h: 2.5, 5, 7.5, 10, or 15 mg; keep patch off 10–12 h each day. *Peds:* 1 µg/kg/min IV titrated to effect, maximum, 5 µg/kg/min.
NOTES: Tolerance to nitrates develops with chronic use after 1–2 wk; this can be avoided by providing a nitrate-free period each day; shorter acting nitrates should be used on a tid basis, and long-acting patches and ointment should be removed before bedtime to prevent the development of tolerance.

Nitroprusside (Nipride, Nitropress)

COMMON USES: Hypertensive emergency, aortic dissection, pulmonary edema.
DOSAGE: *Adults* and *Peds:* 0.5–10 µg/kg/min IV infusion titrated to desired effect.
NOTES: Thiocyanate, the metabolite, is excreted by the kidney; thiocyanate toxicity occurs at plasma levels of 5–10 mg/dL; if used to treat aortic dissection, a beta-blocker must be used concomitantly.

Nizatidine (Axid)

COMMON USES: Treatment of duodenal ulcers.
DOSAGE: Active ulcer: 150 mg PO bid or 300 mg PO qhs. Maintenance: 150 mg PO qhs.

Norepinephrine (Levophed)

COMMON USES: Acute hypotensive states.
DOSAGE: *Adults:* 8–12 µg/kg/min IV titrated to desired effect (see Table VIII–8, page 526). *Peds:* 0.1 µg/kg/min IV titrated to desired effect.
NOTES: Correct blood volume depletion as much as possible before initiation of vasopressor therapy; drug interaction with tricyclic antidepressants leading to severe profound hypertension; infuse into large vein to avoid extravasation; phentolamine 5–10 mg/10 mL NSS injected locally is antidote to extravasation.

Norfloxacin (Noroxin, Chibroxin Ophthalmic)

COMMON USES: Complicated and uncomplicated urinary tract infections resulting from a wide variety of gram-negative bacteria, and prostatitis; topical for ocular infections.
DOSAGE: *Adults:* 400 mg PO bid; ophthalmic: 1–2 drops qid; if severe, use up to q2h. *Peds:* Not recommended for use in patients < 18 y.
NOTES: Not for use in pregnancy; drug interactions with antacids, theophylline, and caffeine.

Nortriptyline (Aventyl, Pamelor)

COMMON USES: Endogenous depression.
DOSAGE: 25 mg PO tid–qid; doses greater than 100 mg/d are not recommended.
NOTES: Many anticholinergic side effects, including blurred vision, urinary retention, and dry mouth.

Nystatin (Mycostatin, Nilstat)

COMMON USES: Treatment of mucocutaneous *Candida* infections (thrush, vaginitis).
DOSAGE: *Adults:* Oral: 400,000–600,000 U PO "swish and swallow" qid or troche 200,000 U 1–2 dissolved in mouth. Vaginal: 1 tablet inserted into vagina qhs. Topical: Apply 2–3 times daily to affected area (cream, ointment, or powder). *Peds:* Infants: 200,000 units PO q6h. Children: See adult.
NOTES: Not absorbed orally, therefore not effective for systemic infections.

Octreotide Acetate (Sandostatin)

COMMON USES: Suppresses or inhibits severe diarrhea associated with carcinoid and vasoactive intestinal tumors.
DOSAGE: *Adults:* 100–600 mg/d SC in 2–4 divided doses. *Peds:* 1–10 mg/kg/24h SC in 2–4 divided doses.
NOTES: May cause nausea, vomiting, and abdominal discomfort.

Ofloxacin (Floxin, Ocuflox Ophthalmic)

COMMON USES: Infections of the lower respiratory tract, skin and skin structure, and urinary tract; prostatitis, uncomplicated gonorrhea, and chlamydia infections; topical for bacterial conjunctivitis and otitis externa.
DOSAGE: *Adults:* 200–400 mg PO bid or IV q12h. *Adults* and *Peds > 1 y:* ophthalmic: 1–2 drops in eye(s) q2–4h for 2 d, then qid for 5 additional days. *Peds:* Systemic administration should NOT be used in children < 18 y. *Peds 1–12 y:* otic: 5 drops in ear bid for 10 d. *Peds > 12 y* and *Adults:* otic: 10 drops in ear bid for 10 d.
NOTES: May cause nausea, vomiting, diarrhea, insomnia, and headache; drug interactions with antacids, sucralfate, and iron- and zinc-containing products that decrease the absorption of ofloxacin; may increase theophylline levels.

Olanzapine (Zyprexa)

COMMON USES: Treatment of psychotic disorders.
DOSAGE: Titrate up to maximum of 20 mg/d.
NOTES: May take many wk to titrate to therapeutic dose; cigarette smoking will decease levels.

Olsalazine (Dipentum)

COMMON USES: Maintenance of remission of ulcerative colitis.
DOSAGE: 500 mg PO bid.
NOTES: Take with food; may cause diarrhea.

Omeprazole (Prilosec)

COMMON USES: Treatment of duodenal and gastric ulcers, Zollinger-Ellison syndrome, GERD, and *H pylori* infections.
DOSAGE: 20–40 mg PO qd–bid.
NOTES: Combination therapy necessary for *H pylori*.

Ondansetron (Zofran)

COMMON USES: Prevention of nausea and vomiting associated with cancer chemotherapy and postoperative nausea and vomiting.

DOSAGE: *Adults* and *Peds:* Chemotherapy: 0.15 mg/kg/dose IV before chemotherapy, then repeated 4 and 8 h after the first dose or 4–8 mg PO tid; administer first dose 30 min before chemotherapy. *Adults:* Postoperative: 4 mg IV immediately before induction or postoperatively.
NOTES: May cause diarrhea and headache.

Orphenadrine (Norflex)
COMMON USES: Treatment of muscle spasms.
DOSAGE: 60–100 mg bid.
NOTES: Dose is dependent on route of administration.

Oseltamivir (Tamiflu)
COMMON USES: Prevention and treatment of influenza types A and B.
DOSAGE: 75 mg twice daily for 5 d.
NOTES: Must be taken within 48 h of onset of symptoms, otherwise oseltamivir is NOT effective.

Oxacillin (Bactocill, Prostaphlin)
COMMON USES: Treatment of infections caused by susceptible strains of *S aureus* and *Streptococcus.*
DOSAGE: *Adults:* 1–2 mg IV q4–6h. *Peds:* 150–200 mg/kg/d IV q4–6h.

Oxaprozin (Daypro)
COMMON USES: Treatment of arthritis and pain.
DOSAGE: 600–1200 mg qd.

Oxazepam (Serax) [C]
COMMON USES: Anxiety; acute alcohol withdrawal; anxiety with depressive symptoms.
DOSAGE: 10–15 mg PO tid–qid; severe anxiety and alcohol withdrawal may require up to 30 mg qid.
NOTES: Oxazepam is one of the metabolites of diazepam (Valium).

Oxcarbazepine (Trileptal)
COMMON USES: Treatment of partial seizures.
DOSAGE: *Adults:* 300 mg, increase dose weekly to a usual dose of 1200–2400 mg/d. *Peds:* 8–10 mg/kg PO bid, 600 mg/d maximum; increase dose weekly to target maintenance dose.
NOTES: May cause hyponatremia.

Oxybutynin (Ditropan, Ditropan XL)
COMMON USES: Symptomatic relief of urgency, nocturia, and incontinence associated with neurogenic or reflex neurogenic bladder.
DOSAGE: *Adults* and *Peds > 5 y:* 5 mg PO tid–qid. *Adults:* extended-release 5 mg PO qd; can titrate to 30 mg PO, qd (5 and 10 mg/tab). *Peds 1–5 y:* 0.02 mg/kg/dose 2–4 times a day (syrup, 5 mg per 5 mL).
NOTES: Anticholinergic side effects (dry mouth, constipation, dry eyes, somnolence, others).

Oxycodone (OxyContin, Roxicodone, others) [C]
COMMON USES: Relief of moderate-to-severe pain usually in combination with other analgesics.
DOSAGE: *Adults:* 5 mg PO q4–6h prn; 10–40 mg PO q12h sustained release. *Peds:* 6–12 y: 1.25 mg PO q6h prn. Children > 12 y: 2.5 mg PO q6h prn.
NOTES: Sustained release (OxyContin)10, 20, 40, 80 mg; liquid, 5 mg per 5 mL; solution, 20 mg/mL.

Oxycodone and Acetaminophen (Percocet, Tylox) [C]
COMMON USES: Relief of moderate-to-severe pain.
DOSAGE: *Adults:* 1–2 tablets/capsules PO q4–6h prn (specify oxycodone/acetaminophen dose). *Peds:* 0.05–0.15 mg/kg/dose q4–6h, maximum 5 mg/dose (based on oxycodone).

NOTES: Supplied as (Percocet: oxycodone/acetaminophen, 2.5 mg/325 mg, 5 mg/325 mg, 7.5 mg/500 mg, 10 mg/500 mg; Tylox: 5-mg oxycodone, 500-mg acetaminophen) solution, 5-mg oxycodone/325-mg acetaminophen/5 mL.

Oxycodone and Aspirin (Percodan, Percodan-Demi) [C]

COMMON USES: Relief of moderate to moderately severe pain.
DOSAGE: *Adults:* 1–2 tablets/capsules PO q4–6h prn. *Peds:* 0.05–0.15 mg/kg/dose q4–6h, maximum 5 mg/dose (based on oxycodone).
NOTES: (Percodan: 4.5-mg oxycodone hydrochloride 0.38-mg oxycodone terephthalate, 325-mg aspirin; Percodan-Demi: 2.25-mg oxycodone hydrochloride, 0.19-mg oxycodone terephthalate, 325 mg aspirin).

Oxymorphone (Numorphan) [C]

COMMON USES: Treatment of moderate–severe pain, sedative.
DOSAGE: 0.5 mg IM, SC, IV initially, 1–1.5 mg q4–6h prn. Rectal: 5 mg q4–6h prn.
NOTES: Chemically related to hydromorphone.

Oxytocin (Pitocin, Syntocinon)

COMMON USES: Induction of labor; control of postpartum hemorrhage.
DOSAGE: 0.001–0.002 U/min IV titrate to effect, maximum, 0.02 U/min.
NOTES: Can cause uterine rupture and fetal death; monitor vital signs closely.

Paclitaxel (Taxol)

COMMON USES: Treatment of ovarian cancer.
DOSAGE: 135 mg/m^2 IV every 3 wk.
NOTES: May cause severe neutropenia.

Pancreatin

Pancrelipase (Pancrease, Cotazym)

COMMON USES: For patients deficient in exocrine pancreatic secretions (cystic fibrosis, chronic pancreatitis, other pancreatic insufficiency), and for steatorrhea of malabsorption syndrome.
DOSAGE: *Adults* and *Peds:* 1–3 capsules (tablets) with meals and snacks may be increased up to 8 capsules (tablets).
NOTES: Avoid antacids; may cause nausea, abdominal cramps, or diarrhea; do NOT crush or chew enteric-coated products.

Pancuronium (Pavulon)

COMMON USES: Aid in the management of patients on mechanical ventilator.
DOSAGE: *Adults:* 2–4 mg IV q2–4h prn. *Peds:* 0.02–0.10 mg/kg/dose q2–4h prn.
NOTES: Patient must be intubated and on controlled ventilation; use adequate amount of sedation or analgesia.

Pantoprazole (Protonix)

COMMON USES: GERD.
DOSAGE: 40 mg PO/IV once daily.
NOTES: Delayed-release medication, therefore do NOT crush or chew tablet.

Paregoric [C]

COMMON USES: Diarrhea, pain and neonatal withdrawal syndrome.
DOSAGE: *Adults:* 5–10 mL qd–qid prn.
NOTES: Contains opium.

Paroxetine (Paxil)

COMMON USES: Depression.
DOSAGE: 20–50 mg PO as a single daily dose.

Penbutolol (Levatol)

COMMON USES: Hypertension.

DOSAGE: 20–40 mg qd.

Penicillin G Aqueous (Potassium or Sodium) (Pfizerpen, Pentids)

COMMON USES: Most gram-positive infections (except penicillin-resistant staphylococci) including streptococci, *Neisseria meningitidis,* syphilis, clostridia, corynebacteria, and some coliforms.

DOSAGE: *Adults:* 400,000–800,000 U PO qid; IV doses vary greatly depending on indications: range, 1.2–24 million U/d. *Peds:* Newborns < 1 wk: 25,000–50,000 U/kg/dose IV q12h. Infants 1 wk–1 mo: 25,000–50,000 U/kg/dose IV q8h. Children: 100,000–300,000 U/kg/24h IV divided q4h.

NOTES: Beware of hypersensitivity reactions; drug of choice for group A streptococcal infections and syphilis.

Penicillin G Benzathine (Bicillin)

COMMON USES: Useful as a single-dose treatment regimen for streptococcal pharyngitis, rheumatic fever and glomerulonephritis prophylaxis, and syphilis.

DOSAGE: *Adults:* 1.2–2.4 million U deep IM injection q2–4wk. *Peds:* 50,000 U/kg/dose to a maximum of 2.4 million U/dose deep IM injection q2–4wk.

NOTES: Sustained action with detectable levels up to 4 wk; considered drug of choice for treatment of non-congenital syphilis; Bicillin L-A contains the benzathine salt only; Bicillin C-R contains a combination of the benzathine and procaine salts and is used for most acute streptococcus infections (300,000 U procaine with 300,000 U benzathine/mL or 900,000 U benzathine with 300,000 U procaine per 2 mL).

Penicillin G Procaine (Wycillin, others)

COMMON USES: Moderately severe infections caused by penicillin G-sensitive organisms that respond to low persistent serum levels (syphilis, uncomplicated pneumococcal pneumonia).

DOSAGE: *Adults:* 300,000–1.2 million U/d IM divided qd–bid. *Peds:* 25,000–50,000 U/kg/d IM divided qd–bid.

NOTES: A long-acting parenteral penicillin; blood levels up to 15 h; give probenecid at least 30 min before administration of penicillin to prolong action.

Penicillin V (Pen-Vee K, Veetids, others)

COMMON USES: Most gram-positive infections (except penicillin-resistant staphylococci) including streptococci, *N meningitidis,* syphilis, clostridia, corynebacteria, and some coliforms.

DOSAGE: *Adults:* 250–500 mg PO q6h. *Peds:* 25–50 mg/kg/24h PO in 4 divided doses.

NOTES: A well-tolerated oral penicillin; 250 mg = 400,000 U Penicillin G.

Pentamidine Isethionate (Pentam 300, NebuPent)

COMMON USES: Treatment and prevention of *Pneumocystis carinii* pneumonia.

DOSAGE: *Adults* and *Peds:* 4 mg/kg/24h IV daily for 14–21 d. *Adults:* Prevention: 300 mg once every 4 wk, administered via Respirgard II nebulizer.

NOTES: Monitor patient for severe hypotension following IV administration; associated with pancreatic islet-cell necrosis, leading to hypoglycemia and hyperglycemia; monitor hematology labs for leukopenia and thrombocytopenia.

Pentazocine (Talwin) [C]

COMMON USES: Relief of moderate-to-severe pain.

DOSAGE: 30 mg IM or IV; 50–100 mg PO q3–4h prn.

NOTES: 30–60 mg IM equianalgesic to 10-mg morphine IM; associated with considerable dysphoria.

Pentobarbital (Nembutal, others) [C]

COMMON USES: Insomnia, convulsions, induced coma following severe head injury.

DOSAGE: *Adults:* Sedative: 20–40 mg PO or PR q6–12h. Hypnotic: 100–200 mg PO or PR qhs prn. Induced coma: load 3–5 mg/kg IV × 1, then maintenance 2–3.5 mg/kg/dose IV q1h

prn to keep level between 25–40 mg/mL. **Peds:** Hypnotic: 2–6 mg/kg/dose PO qhs prn. Induced coma: See adult.
NOTES: Can cause respiratory depression; may produce hypotension when used IV for cerebral edema; tolerance to sedative-hypnotic effect acquired within 1–2 wk.

Pentosan Polysulfate Sodium (Elmiron)

COMMON USES: Bladder pain and discomfort associated with interstitial cystitis.
DOSAGE: 100 mg PO three times a day.
NOTES: Alopecia, diarrhea, nausea, and headaches have been reported.

Pentoxifylline (Trental)

COMMON USES: Intermittent claudication.
DOSAGE: 400 mg PO tid with meals.
NOTES: Treat for at least 8 wk to see full effect.

Pergolide (Permax)

COMMON USES: Parkinson's disease.
DOSAGE: Initially, 0.05 mg PO tid, titrated every 2–3 d to desired effect.
NOTES: May cause hypotension during initiation of therapy.

Perindopril (Aceon)

COMMON USES: Treatment of hypertension and CHF.
DOSAGE: 4–8 mg daily.
NOTES: Avoid taking with food.

Permethrin (Elimite, Nix)

COMMON USES: Eradication of lice.
DOSAGE: **Adults** and **Peds:** Lice: Saturate hair and scalp with cream rinse; allow to remain in hair for 10 min before rinsing out. Scabies: apply cream over entire body; rinse after 8–14 h.

Perphenazine (Trilafon)

COMMON USES: Psychotic disorders, intractable hiccups, severe nausea.
DOSAGE: Antipsychotic: 4–8 mg PO tid, maximum 64 mg/d. Hiccups: 5 mg IM q6h prn or 1 mg IV at NOT less than 1–2- mg/min intervals up to 5 mg.

Phenazopyridine (Pyridium)

COMMON USES: Symptomatic relief of discomfort from lower urinary tract irritation.
DOSAGE: **Adults:** 200 mg PO tid. **Peds 6–12 y:** 12 mg/kg/24h PO in 3 divided doses.
NOTES: Gastrointestinal disturbances; causes red-orange urine color, which can stain clothing.

Phenobarbital [C]

COMMON USES: Seizure disorders, insomnia, anxiety.
DOSAGE: **Adults:** Sedative-hypnotic: 30–120 mg PO or IM qd prn. Anticonvulsant: Load 10–12 mg/kg in 3 divided doses, then 1–3 mg/kg/24h PO, IM, or IV (see Tables VIII–3 and VIII–9, pages 520 and 527). **Peds:** Sedative-hypnotic: 2–3 mg/kg/24h PO or IM qhs prn. Anticonvulsant: Load 15–20 mg/kg divided into 2 equal doses 4 h apart, then 3–5 mg/kg/24h PO divided in 2–3 doses.
NOTES: Tolerance develops to sedation; paradoxical hyperactivity seen in pediatric patients; long half-life allows single daily dosing.

Phenylephrine (Neo-Synephrine)

COMMON USES: Treatment of vascular failure in shock, hypersensitivity, or drug-induced hypotension; nasal congestion; mydriatic.
DOSAGE: **Adults:** Relief of mild-to-moderate hypotension: 2–5 mg IM or SC increases BP for 2 h; 0.1–0.5 mg IV increases BP for 15 min. Severe hypotension/shock: Infusion at 100–180 µg/min; after BP is stabilized, maintenance rate of 40–60 µg/min (see Table VIII–8, page 526). Nasal congestion: 1–2 sprays into each nostril prn. **Adults** and **Peds > 1 y:** Mydriasis: 1 drop 2.5–10% solution in eye(s) 30 min before procedure; may repeat in 10–60 min if

needed. *Peds:* Hypotension: 5–20 mg/kg/dose IV q10–15min or 0.1–0.5 mg/kg/min IV infusion titrated to desired effect. Nasal congestion: 1 spray into each nostril q3–4h prn. *Peds < 1 y:* Mydriasis: 1 drop 2.5% solution in eye(s) 30 min before procedure.

NOTES: Promptly restore blood volume if loss has occurred; use caution in patients with hyperthyroidism, bradycardia, partial heart block, myocardial disease, or severe arteriosclerosis; use large veins for infusion to avoid extravasation; phentolamine 10 mg in 10–15-mL saline for local injection as antidote for extravasation; activity potentiated by oxytocin, MAOIs, and tricyclic antidepressants.

Phenytoin (Dilantin)

COMMON USES: Tonic-clonic and partial seizures.

DOSAGE: *Adults* and *Peds,* IV at a maximum infusion rate of 25 mg/min or orally in 400-mg doses at 4 h-intervals. *Adults:* Maintenance: 200 mg PO or IV bid or 300 mg qhs initially, then monitor serum level (see Tables VIII–3 and VIII–9, pages 520 and 527). *Peds:* Maintenance: 4–7 mg/kg/24h PO or IV divided qd–bid.

NOTES: Use caution with cardiac depressant side effects, especially with IV administration; monitor levels as needed (see Tables VIII–3 and VIII–9); nystagmus and ataxia are early signs of toxicity; gum hyperplasia occurs with long-term use; avoid use of oral suspension if possible due to erratic absorption; avoid use in pregnancy.

Physostigmine (Antilirium)

COMMON USES: Antidote for tricyclic antidepressant, atropine, and scopolamine overdose.

DOSAGE: *Adults:* 2 mg IV/IM q15min. *Peds:* 0.01–0.03 mg/kg/dose IV q15-30min.

NOTES: Rapid IV administration associated with convulsions; cholinergic side effects; may cause asystole.

Phytonadione [Vitamin K] (AquaMEPHYTON, others)

COMMON USES: Coagulation disorders caused by faulty formation of factors II, VII, IX, and X, hyperalimentation.

DOSAGE: *Adults* and *Peds:* Anticoagulant-induced prothrombin deficiency: 2.5–10.0 mg PO or IV slowly. Hyperalimentation: 10 mg IM or IV every week. Infants: 0.5–1.0 mg/dose IM, SC, or PO.

NOTES: With parenteral treatment, usually see first change in prothrombin in 12–24 h; anaphylaxis can result from IV dosing; should be administered slowly IV.

Pilocarpine (Salagen Oral, Ocusert Pilo-20, Ocusert Pilo-40, others)

COMMON USES: Glaucoma and reversal of cycloplegia; radiation-induced xerostomia.

DOSAGE: Reversal of mydriasis: 1 drop 1% solution to eye. Glaucoma: 1–2 drops hydrochloride solution up to 6 times a day; titrate based on pressures; 0.5″ ribbon into eye qhs; Ocusert: 1 in eye weekly.

NOTES: Ocusert implant system releases 20 or 40 μg/h over 1 wk.

Pindolol (Visken)

COMMON USES: Treatment of hypertension.

DOSAGE: 5–10 mg bid.

Pioglitazone (Actos)

COMMON USES: Management of Type 2 diabetes.

DOSAGE: 15–45 mg once daily.

Pipecuronium (Arduan)

COMMON USES: Adjunct to general anesthesia.

DOSAGE: *Adults:* 50–100 mg/kg IV. *Peds:* 40–57 mg/kg IV.

Piperacillin (Pipracil)

COMMON USES: Infections caused by susceptible strains of gram-negative bacteria including *Klebsiella, Proteus, E coli, Enterobacter, P aeruginosa,* and *Serratia* involving the skin, bone, respiratory tract, urinary tract, abdomen, and septicemia.

DOSAGE: *Adults:* 3 g IV q4–6h. *Peds:* 200–300 mg/kg/d IV divided q4–6h.

NOTES: Often used in combination with aminoglycosides.

Piperacillin/Tazobactam (Zosyn)

COMMON USES: Treatment of infections caused by susceptible strains of gram-negative bacteria including *Klebsiella*, *Proteus*, *E coli*, *Enterobacter*, *P aeruginosa*, and *Serratia* involving the skin, bone, respiratory tract, urinary tract, abdomen, and septicemia.
DOSAGE: *Adults:* 3.375–4.5 g IV q6h.
NOTES: Often used in combination with aminoglycosides.

Pirbuterol (Maxair)

COMMON USES: Prevention and reversal of bronchospasm.
DOSAGE: *Adults* and *Peds > 12 y:* 2 inhalations q4–6h, maximum of 12 inhalations per day.

Piroxicam (Feldene)

COMMON USES: Treatment of arthritis and pain.
DOSAGE: 10–20 mg qd.

Plasma Protein Fraction (Plasmanate, others)

COMMON USES: Shock and hypotension.
DOSAGE: *Adults:* 250–500 mL IV initially (NOT 0.10 mL/min); subsequent infusions should depend on clinical response. *Peds:* 10–15 mL/kg/dose IV; subsequent infusions should depend on clinical response.
NOTES: Hypotension associated with rapid infusion; 130–160-mEq sodium per liter; NOT a substitute for red cells.

Plicamycin (Mithracin)

COMMON USES: Hypercalcemia of malignancy.
DOSAGE: 25 mg/kg/d IV for 3–4 d.

Pneumococcal Vaccine, Polyvalent (Pneumovax-23)

COMMON USES: Immunization against pneumococcal infections in patients predisposed to or at high risk of acquiring these infections (ie, before elective splenectomy).
DOSAGE: *Adults* and *Peds > 2 y:* 0.5 mL IM.
NOTES: Do NOT vaccinate during immunosuppressive therapy.

Pneumococcal 7-Valent Conjugate Vaccine (Prevnar)

COMMON USES: Immunization against pneumococcal infections in infants and children.
DOSAGE: 0.5 mL IM per dose; series consists of 3 doses; first dose at 2 mo of age with subsequent doses every 2 mo.

Polyethylene glycol-electrolyte solution (Go-LYTLEY, Colyte)

COMMON USES: Bowel cleansing before examination or surgery.
DOSAGE: *Adults:* Following 3–4 h-fast, the patient must drink 240 mL of solution every 10 min until 4 L is consumed. *Peds:* 25–40 mL/kg/h over 4–10 h.
NOTES: First bowel movement should occur in approximately 1 h; may cause some cramping or nausea.

Porfimer (Photofrin)

COMMON USES: Photodynamic therapy of early endobronchial non-small-cell cancer; and palliation of esophageal cancer.
DOSAGE: 2 mg/kg IV over 3–5 min (follow up with photodynamic therapy 40–50 h later).

Potassium Citrate (Urocit-K)

COMMON USES: Alkalinize urine, prevention of urinary stones (uric acid, calcium stones if hypocitraturic; urinary alkalinizer.
DOSAGE: 10–20 mEq PO tid with meals, maximum, 100 mEq/d.
NOTES: Tablets: 540 mg = 5 mEq, 1080 mg = 10 mEq.

Potassium Citrate and Citric Acid (Polycitra-K)

COMMON USES: Alkalinize urine, prevention of urinary stones (uric acid, calcium stones if hypocitraturic; urinary alkalinizer.
DOSAGE: 10–20 mEq PO tid with meals, maximum, 100 mEq/d.
NOTES: Solution: 10 mEq per 5 mL; powder 30 mEq/packet.

Potassium Iodide [Lugol's solution] (SSKI, Thyro-Block)

COMMON USES: Thyroid crisis, reduction of vascularity prior to thyroid surgery, thin bronchial secretions.
DOSAGE: Preoperative thyroidectomy: **Adults** and **Peds:** 50–250 mg PO tid 3 times per day (2–6 drops strong iodine solution); administer for 10 d before surgery. Thyroid crisis: **Adults** and **Peds > 1 y:** 300 mg (6 drops SSKI q8h); Infants < 1 y, 1/2 dose.
NOTES: SSKI = 1 g/mL, Lugol's = 100 mg/mL.

Potassium Supplements

COMMON USES: Prevention or treatment of hypokalemia.
DOSAGE: **Adults:** 20–100 mEq/d PO divided qd–bid; IV, 10–20 mEq/h, maximum, 40 mEq/h and 150 mEq/d (monitor frequent potassium levels when using high-dose IV infusions). **Peds:** Calculate potassium deficit; 1–3 mEq/kg/d PO divided qd–qid; IV max dose 0.5–1 mEq/kg/h.
NOTES: Dosing ranges based on clinical conditions. See Table VIII–6 on page 523 for oral agents. Can cause gastrointestinal irritation; powder and liquids must be mixed with beverage (unsalted tomato juice, etc); use cautiously in renal insufficiency, and along with NSAIDs and ACE inhibitors; chloride salt recommended in coexisting alkalosis; for coexisting acidosis use acetate, bicarbonate, citrate, or gluconate salt.

Pramipexole (Mirapex)

COMMON USES: Treatment of Parkinson's disease.
DOSAGE: 1.5–4.5 mg/d in 3 equally divided doses titrated slowly.

Pramoxine (Anusol, Proctofoam-NS, others)
Pramoxine with hydrocortisone (Proctofoam-HC, Anusol-HC, others)

COMMON USES: Relief of pain and itching from external and internal hemorrhoids and anorectal surgery.
DOSAGE: 1 suppository every morning and bedtime and following each bowel movement; apply cream, ointment, gel, or spray freely to anal area q6–12h.
NOTES: Anusol-HC/Proctofoam HA contains 1% hydrocortisone.

Pravastatin (Pravachol)

COMMON USES: Reduction of increased cholesterol levels.
DOSAGE: 10–40 mg PO qhs.

Prazosin (Minipress)

COMMON USES: Hypertension and CHF.
DOSAGE: **Adults:** 1 mg PO tid to total daily dose of 20 mg/d prn. **Peds:** 5–25 mg/kg/dose q6h.
NOTES: Can cause orthostatic hypotension, so the patient should take the first dose at bedtime; tolerance develops to this effect; tachyphylaxis may result.

Prednisone

See Steroids, page 509.

Prednisolone

See Steroids, page 509.

Prednisolone, Ophthalmic (AK-Pred Ophthalmic, Pred-Forte Ophthalmic, others)

COMMON USES: Iritis, postoperative inflammation, palpebral and bulbar conjunctivitis, chemical, radiation, or thermal injury, corneal abrasion.
DOSAGE: 1–2 drops in eye(s) q1h during day and q2h at night until inflammation subsides, then 1 drop q4h.

NOTES: Can increase intraocular pressure, cause cataracts, and worsen herpes keratitis.

Probenecid (Benemid)

COMMON USES: Gout, maintenance of serum levels of penicillins or cephalosporins.
DOSAGE: *Adults:* Gout: 0.25 g bid for 1 wk; then 0.5 g PO bid. Antibiotic effect: 1–2 g PO 30 min before dose of antibiotic. *Peds:* 25 mg/kg, then 40 mg/kg/d PO divided qid.

Procainamide (Pronestyl, Procan)

COMMON USES: Treatment of supraventricular and ventricular arrhythmias.
DOSAGE: *Adults:* Emergency cardiac care: 100–200 mg/dose IV q5min until dysrhythmia resolves, hypotension ensues, or dose totals 1 g; then maintenance of 1–4 mg/min IV infusion. Chronic dosing: 50 mg/kg/d PO in divided doses q4–6h. *Peds:* Emergency cardiac care: 3–6 mg/kg/dose IV over 5 min, then 20–80 mg/kg/min IV infusion. Maintenance: 15–50 mg/kg/24h PO divided q3–6h.
NOTES: Can cause hypotension and a lupus-like syndrome; dose adjustment renal impairment; see Table VIII–3, page 520.

Prochlorperazine (Compazine)

COMMON USES: Nausea, vomiting, agitation, psychotic disorders.
DOSAGE: *Adults:* Antiemetic: 5–10 mg PO tid–qid or 25 mg PR bid or 5–10 mg IM q4–6h. Antipsychotic: 10–20 mg IM acutely or 5–10 mg PO tid–qid for maintenance. *Peds:* 0.1–0.15 mg/kg/dose IM q4–6h or 0.4 mg/kg/24h PO divided tid–qid.
NOTES: Much larger dose may be required for antipsychotic effect; extrapyramidal side effects common; treat acute extrapyramidal reactions with diphenhydramine.

Procyclidine (Kemadrin)

COMMON USES: Treatment of Parkinson's syndrome.
DOSAGE: 2.5 mg PO tid.
NOTES: Contraindicated for glaucoma patients.

Promethazine (Phenergan)

COMMON USES: Nausea, vomiting, motion sickness.
DOSAGE: *Adults:* 12.5–50 mg PO, PR, or IM bid–qid prn. *Peds:* 0.1–0.5 mg/kg/dose PO or IM q4–6h prn.
NOTES: High incidence of drowsiness.

Propafenone (Rythmol)

COMMON USES: Treatment of life-threatening ventricular arrhythmias.
DOSAGE: 150–300 mg PO q8h.
NOTES: May cause dizziness, unusual taste, and first-degree heart block.

Propantheline (Pro-Banthine)

COMMON USES: Symptomatic treatment of small-intestine hypermotility, spastic colon, ureteral spasm, bladder spasm, pylorospasm.
DOSAGE: *Adults:* 15 mg PO ac and 30 mg PO hs. *Peds:* 1.5–3.0 mg/kg/24h PO divided tid–qid.
NOTES: Anticholinergic side effects, such as dry mouth and blurred vision are common.

Propofol (Diprivan)

COMMON USES: Induction or maintenance of anesthesia; continuous sedation in intubated patients.
DOSAGE: Anesthesia: 20–40 mg every 10 min until induction onset, then 50–200 µg/kg/min continuous infusion. ICU sedation: 5–50 µg/kg/min continuous infusion (see Table VIII–10, page 528).
NOTES: 1 mL of propofol contains 0.1 g of fat; may increase serum triglycerides when administered for extended periods.

Propoxyphene (Darvon) [C]
Propoxyphene and acetaminophen (Darvocet) [C]
Propoxyphene and aspirin (Darvon Compound-65, Darvon-N with Aspirin) [C]

COMMON USES: Relief of mild-to-moderate pain.

DOSAGE: 1–2 PO q4h prn.

NOTES: Darvon: propoxyphene HCl capsule, 65 mg; Darvon-N: propoxyphene napsylate, 100-mg tablet. Darvocet-N: propoxyphene napsylate, 50 mg/acetaminophen, 325 mg. Darvocet-N 100: propoxyphene napsylate, 100 mg/acetaminophen, 650 mg. Darvon Compound-65: propoxyphene HCl, 65 mg/aspirin, 389 mg/caffeine, 32-mg capsules. Darvon-N with aspirin: propoxyphene napsylate, 100 mg/aspirin, 325 mg.

Propranolol (Inderal)

COMMON USES: Treatment of hypertension, angina, myocardial infarction prophylaxis, arrhythmias (a-fib, a-flutter, others) essential tremor, pheochromocytoma, thyrotoxicosis, migraine prevention.

DOSAGE: *Adults:* Angina: 80–320 mg PO qd divided bid–qid or 80–160 mg SR qd. Arrhythmia: 10–80 mg PO tid–qid or 1 mg IV slowly, repeat q5min up to 5 mg. HTN: 40 mg PO bid or 60–80 mg SR qd, increase weekly to maximum 640 mg/d. Hypertropic Sub Aortic Stenosis: 20–40 mg PO tid–qid. MI: 180–240 mg PO divided tid–qid. Migraine Prophylaxis: 80 mg/d divided qid–tid, increase weekly to maximum 160–240 mg/d divided tid–qid; wean off if no response in 6 wk. Pheochromocytoma: 30–60 mg/d divided tid–qid. Thyrotoxicosis: 1–3 mg IV single dose; 10–40 mg PO q6h. Tremor: 40 mg PO bid, increase as needed to maximum 320 mg/d. *Peds:* Arrhythmia 0.5–1.0 mg/kg/d divided tid–qid, increase as needed q3–7d to maximum 60 mg/d; 0.01–0.1 mg/kg IV over 10 min, maximum dose, 1 mg. Hypertension: 0.5–1.0 mg/kg divided bid–qid, increase as needed q3–7d to 2 mg/kg/d maximum.

Propylthiouracil [PTU]

COMMON USES: Hyperthyroidism.

DOSAGE: *Adults:* 100 mg PO q8h, increase up to 1200 mg/d after euthyroid (6–8 wk), taper dose by 1/3 every 4–6 wk to a maintenance dose of 50–150 mg/24h; treatment is often discontinued in 2–3 y. *Peds:* Initial 5–7 mg/kg/24h PO divided q8h, then maintenance of 1/3–2/3 of initial dose.

NOTES: Monitor patient clinically; monitor thyroid function tests.

Protamine Sulfate

COMMON USES: Reversal of heparin effect.

DOSAGE: *Adults* and *Peds:* Based on amount of heparin reversal desired; given slow IV, 1 mg will reverse approximately 100 U of heparin given in the preceding 3–4h to maximum dose of 50 mg.

NOTES: Monitor coagulation studies; may have anticoagulant effect if given without heparin.

Pseudoephedrine (Sudafed, Novafed, Afrinol)

COMMON USES: Decongestant.

DOSAGE: *Adults:* 30–60 mg PO q6–8h; sustained release capsules 120 mg PO q12h. *Peds:* 4 mg/kg/24h PO divided qid.

NOTES: Contraindicated for patients with hypertension or coronary artery disease, and for patients taking MAO inhibitors; an ingredient in many cough and cold preparations.

Psyllium (Metamucil, Serutan, Effer-Syllium)

COMMON USES: Constipation, diverticular disease of the colon.

DOSAGE: 1 teaspoon (7 g) in a glass of water qd–tid.

NOTES: Do NOT use if bowel obstruction is suspected; one of the safest laxatives; psyllium in effervescent (Effer-Syllium) form usually contains potassium and should be used with caution for patients with renal failure.

Pyrazinamide

COMMON USES: Treatment of active tuberculosis.
DOSAGE: *Adults:* 20–35 mg/kg/24h PO divided tid–qid, maximum dose is 3 g/d. *Peds:* 15–30 mg/kg/d PO divided bid or qd.
NOTES: May cause hepatotoxicity; use in combination with other antituberculosis drugs.

Pyridoxine (Vitamin B$_6$)

COMMON USES: Treatment and prevention of vitamin B$_6$ deficiency.
DOSAGE: Deficiency: 2.5–10.0 mg PO qd. Drug-induced neuritis: 50 mg PO qd.

Quazepam (Doral) [C]

COMMON USES: Insomnia.
DOSAGE: 7.5–15 mg PO qhs prn.
NOTES: Reduce dose in elderly patients.

Quinapril (Accupril)

COMMON USES: Treatment of hypertension.
DOSAGE: 10–80 mg PO qd in single dose.

Quinidine (Quinidex, Quinaglute)

COMMON USES: Prevention of tachydysrhythmias.
DOSAGE: PAC, PVCs: 200–300 mg PO tid–qid. Conversion of atrial fibrillation or flutter: Use after digitalization, 200 mg q2–3h for 8 doses; then increase daily dose to maximum of 3–4 g or until normal rhythm is present. *Peds:* 30 mg/kg/24h PO 4–5 divided doses.
NOTES: Contraindicated in digitalis toxicity, AV block; monitor serum levels if available (see Table VIII–3 page 520); extreme hypotension seen with IV administration. Sulfate salt contains 83% quinidine, gluconate salt is 62% quinidine.

Quinupristin/Dalfopristin (Synercid)

COMMON USES: Infections caused by vancomycin-resistant *Entercoccus faecium,* and other gram-positive organisms.
DOSAGE: *Adults* and *Peds:* 7.5 mg/kg IV q8–12h.
NOTES: Administer through central line if possible; NOT compatible with saline or heparin, therefore flush IV lines with dextrose.

Rabeprazole (Aciphex)

COMMON USES: Peptic ulcers, GERD, and hypersecretory conditions
DOSAGE: 20 mg once daily; may be increased to 60 mg daily.
NOTES: Do NOT crush tablets.

Raloxifene (Evista)

COMMON USES: Prevention of osteoporosis.
DOSAGE: 60 mg/d.

Ramipril (Altace)

COMMON USES: Hypertension and heart failure.
DOSAGE: 2.5–20 mg/d PO divided qd–bid.
NOTES: May use in combination with diuretics; may cause a nonproductive cough.

Ranitidine (Zantac)

COMMON USES: Duodenal ulcer, active benign ulcers, hypersecretory conditions, gastroesophageal reflux.
DOSAGE: *Adults:* Ulcer: 150 mg PO bid, 300 mg PO qhs, or 50 mg IV q6–8h; or 400 mg IV/d continuous infusion. Maintenance: 150 mg PO qhs. Hypersecretion: 150 mg PO bid. *Peds:* 0.1–0.8 mg/kg/dose IV q6–8h or 1.25–2.0 mg/kg/dose PO q12h.
NOTES: Reduce dose with renal failure; note oral and parenteral doses are different.

Rimexolone (Vexol Ophthalmic)

COMMON USES: Postoperative inflammation and uveitis.

DOSAGE: *Adults* and *Peds > 2 y:* Uveitis: 1–2 drops q1h daytime and q2h at night, can taper to 1 drop q4h; postoperative 1–2 drops qid for up to 2 wk.
NOTES: Should taper off dose.

Repaglinide (Prandin)

COMMON USES: Management of Type 2 diabetes.
DOSAGE: 0.5–4 mg ac.

Reteplase (Retavase)

COMMON USES: Thrombolytic after acute myocardial infarction.
DOSAGE: 10 U IV over 2 min, 2nd dose 30 min later of 10 U IV over 2 min.

Ribavirin (Virazole, Rebetron)

COMMON USES: Treatment of infants and children with respiratory syncytial virus infection; treatment of Hepatitis C.
DOSAGE: RSV: 6 g in 300 mL of sterile water inhaled over 12–18 h. Hepatitis C: 600 mg PO bid in combination with interferon alfa-2b.
NOTES: Aerosolized by a SPAG generator; may accumulate on soft contact lenses; monitor H&H frequently; pregnancy test every month.

Rifampin (Rifadin)

COMMON USES: Tuberculosis, treatment, and prophylaxis of *N meningitidis, H influenzae, or S aureus* carriers.
DOSAGE: *Adults:* N meningitidis and H influenzae carrier: 600 mg PO qd 3–4 d. Tuberculosis: 600 mg PO or IV qd or twice weekly with combination therapy regimen. *Peds:* 10–20 mg/kg/dose PO or IV qd–bid.
NOTES: Multiple side effects; causes orange-red discoloration of bodily secretions including tears; never used as a single agent to treat active tuberculosis infections.

Rifapentine (Priftin)

COMMON USES: Treatment of tuberculosis.
DOSAGE: Intensive phase: 600 mg PO twice weekly for 2 mo; separate doses by 3 or more days; continuation phase: 600 mg once weekly.
NOTES: Has similar adverse effects and drug interactions as rifampin.

Rimantadine (Flumadine)

COMMON USES: Prophylaxis and treatment of influenza A virus infections.
DOSAGE: *Adults:* 100 mg PO bid. *Peds:* 5 mg/kg PO qd, NOT to exceed 150 mg/d.

Risedronate (Actonel)

COMMON USES: Prevention and treatment of postmenopausal osteoporosis.
DOSAGE: 5 mg PO once daily with 6–8 oz of water.
NOTES: Take 30 min before first food or drink of the day; interaction with calcium supplements; may cause GI distress and arthralgia.

Risperidone (Risperdal)

COMMON USES: Management of psychotic disorders.
DOSAGE: 1–8 mg PO bid.

Ritonavir (Norvir)

COMMON USES: HIV in combination with two or three other agents.
DOSAGE: 600 mg PO bid with food.

Rofecoxib (Vioxx)

COMMON USES: Osteoarthritis, acute pain, and primary dysmenorrhea.
DOSAGE: 12.5–50 mg/d.
NOTES: Alert patients to be aware of GI ulceration or bleeding.

Rosiglitazone (Avandia)

COMMON USES: Treatment of Type 2 diabetes mellitus.

DOSAGE: 4–8 mg PO once daily or in 2 divided doses.
NOTES: May be taken with or without meals.

Salmeterol (Serevent)

COMMON USES: Treatment of asthma and exercise-induced bronchospasm.
DOSAGE: 2 inhalations twice daily.

Saquinavir (Fortovase, Invirase)

COMMON USES: HIV in combination with two or three other agents.
DOSAGE: Fortovase: 1200 mg tid after meals; Invirase: 600 mg PO tid after meals.

Sargramostim [GM-CSF] (Prokine, Leukine)

COMMON USES: Treatment of myeloid recovery following bone marrow transplantation.
DOSAGE: *Adults* and *Peds:* 250 mg/m^2/d IV for 21 d.
NOTES: May cause bone pain.

Scopolamine

Scopolamine, Transdermal (Transderm-Scop)

COMMON USES: Prevention of nausea and vomiting associated with motion sickness; preoperative control of secretions.
DOSAGE: Transderm-Scop: Apply 1 patch behind the ear every 3 d; 0.3–0.65 IM/IV/SC; repeat prn q4–6h.
NOTES: May cause dry mouth, drowsiness, and blurred vision.

Secobarbital (Seconal) [C]

COMMON USES: Insomnia.
DOSAGE: *Adults:* 100 mg PO, or IM qhs prn. *Peds:* 3–5 mg/kg/dose PO or IM qhs prn.
NOTES: Beware of respiratory depression; tolerance acquired within 1–2 wk.

Selegiline (Eldepryl)

COMMON USES: Parkinson's disease.
DOSAGE: 5 mg PO bid.
NOTES: May cause nausea and dizziness.

Sertraline (Zoloft)

COMMON USES: Treatment of depression.
DOSAGE: 50–200 mg PO qd.
NOTES: Can activate manic/hypomanic state; has caused weight loss in clinical trials.

Silver nitrate

COMMON USES: Prevention of ophthalmia neonatorium due to GC; removal of granulation tissue; cauterization of wounds.
DOSAGE: *Adults* and *Peds:* Apply to moist surface 2–3 times a week for several wk or until desired effect. *Peds:* Newborns: apply 2 drops immediately after birth into conjunctival sac.

Silver Sulfadiazine (Silvadene)

COMMON USES: Prevention of sepsis in second-degree and third-degree burns.
DOSAGE: *Adults* and *Peds:* Aseptically cover affected area with ¼-inch coating bid.
NOTES: Can have systemic absorption with extensive application.

Simethicone (Mylicon)

COMMON USES: Symptomatic treatment of flatulence.
DOSAGE: *Adults* and *Peds:* 40–125 mg PO pc and hs prn.

Simvastatin (Zocor)

COMMON USES: Reduction of increased cholesterol levels.
DOSAGE: 5–40 mg PO qhs.
NOTES: May cause myopathy, monitor LFTs.

Sirolimus (Rapamune)

COMMON USES: Prophylaxis of organ rejection.
DOSAGE: 2 mg PO per day.
NOTES: Dilute in water or orange juice; do NOT drink grapefruit juice while on sirolimus; take 4 h after cyclosporin.

Sodium Bicarbonate

COMMON USES: Alkalinization of urine, renal tubular acidosis (RTA), treatment of metabolic acidosis.
DOSAGE: *Adults:* Emergency cardiac care: initiate adequate ventilation, 1 mEq/kg/dose IV ; can repeat 0.5 mEq/kg in 10 min one time or based on acid/base status. Metabolic acidosis: 2–5 mEq/kg IV over 8 h and prn, based on acid/base status. Alkalinize urine: 4 g (48 mEq) PO, then 1–2 g q4h, adjust based on urine pH. Chronic renal failure: 1–3 mEq/kg/d. Distal RTA: 1 mEq/kg/d PO. *Peds > 1 y:* Emergency cardiac care: see adult. *Peds < 1 y:* Emergency cardiac care: initiate adequate ventilation, 1:1 dilution 1 mEq/mL dosed 1 mEq/kg IV ; can repeat with 0.5 mEq/kg in 10 min one time or based on acid/base status. Chronic renal failure: see *Adults.* Distal RTA: 2–3 mEq/kg/d PO; Proximal RTA: 5–10 mEq/kg/d, titrate based on serum bicarbonate levels. Urine alkalinization: 84–840 mg/kg/d (1–10 mEq/kg/d) divided doses; adjust based on urine pH.
NOTES: 1 g neutralizes 12 mEq of acid; in infants do NOT exceed 10 mEq/min infusion; supplied as IV infusion, powder and tablets: 300 mg = 3.6 mEq; 325 mg = 3.8 mEq; 520 mg = 6.3 mEq; 600 mg = 7.3 mEq; 650 mg = 7.6 mEq.

Sodium Citrate (Bicitra)

COMMON USES: Alkalinization of urine; dissolve uric acid and cysteine stones.
DOSAGE: *Adults:* 2–6 teaspoonfuls (10–30 mL) diluted in 1–3 oz of water pc and hs. *Peds:* 1–3 teaspoonfuls (5–15 mL) diluted in 1–3 oz of water pc and hs. Supplied:15-, 30-mL unit dose of 16 (473 mL) or 4 (118 mL) fluid ounces.
NOTES: Should NOT be given to patients on aluminum-based antacids. Contraindicated for patients with severe renal impairment or on sodium-restricted diets.

Sodium Ferric Gluconate (Ferrlecit)

COMMON USES: Treatment of iron-deficiency anemia.
DOSAGE: Dependent on how much iron replacement is needed, usual dosage is 125 mg IV infusion over 1 h × 8 sessions.
NOTES: May cause severe sensitivity reactions.

Sodium Polystyrene Sulfonate (Kayexalate)

COMMON USES: Treatment of hyperkalemia.
DOSAGE: *Adults:* 15–60 g PO or 30–60 g PR q6h based on serum potassium. *Peds:* 1 g/kg/dose PO or PR q6h based on serum potassium.
NOTES: Can cause hypernatremia; given with agent such as sorbitol (mixed in 20–100 mL of 70% solution) to promote movement through bowel.

Sorbitol

COMMON USES: Constipation.
DOSAGE: *Adults* and *Peds >12 y:* 30–150 mL of a 20–70% solution prn.

Sotalol (Betapace)

COMMON USES: Treatment of ventricular arrhythmias.
DOSAGE: 80 mg PO bid; may be increased to 240–320 mg/d.
NOTES: Dose should be adjusted for renal insufficiency.

Spironolactone (Aldactone)

COMMON USES: Treatment of hyperaldosteronism, essential hypertension, edematous states (CHF, cirrhosis), polycystic ovary.
DOSAGE: *Adults:* 25–100 mg PO qid. *Peds:* 1–3.3 mg/kg/24h PO divided bid–qid.

NOTES: Can cause hyperkalemia and gynecomastia; avoid prolonged use; diuretic of choice for cirrhotic edema and ascites.

Steroids, Systemic

The following relates only to the commonly used systemic glucocorticoids.

COMMON USES: Endocrine disorders (adrenal insufficiency), rheumatoid disorders, collagen-vascular diseases, dermatologic diseases, allergic states, edematous states (cerebral, nephrotic syndrome), immunosuppression for transplantation, hypercalcemia, malignancies (breast, lymphomas), preoperatively (in any patient who has been on steroids in the previous year, known hypoadrenalism, preoperative for adrenalectomy); injection into joints/tissue.

DOSAGE: Varies with use and institutional protocols. Some commonly used doses are: Adrenal insufficiency, Acute (Addisonian crisis): **Adults:** hydrocortisone 100 mg IV q8h; then 300 mg/d divided Q8h; convert to 50 mg PO q8h × 6 doses, taper to 30–50 mg/d divided bid. **Peds:** hydrocortisone: 1–2 mg/kg IV; then 150–250 mg/d divided tid. Adrenal insufficiency, chronic (physiologic replacement): May also need mineralocorticoid supplementation such as DOCA. **Adults:** hydrocortisone 20 mg PO qAM, 10 mg PO qPM; cortisone: 0.5–0.75 mg/kg/d divided bid; cortisone: 0.25–0.35 mg/kg IM qd; dexamethasone: 0.03–0.15 mg/kg/d or 0.6-0.75 mg/m^2/d in divided q6–12h PO, IM, IV. **Peds:** hydrocortisone 0.5–0.75 mg/kg/d PO tid; hydrocortisone succinate 0.25–0.35 mg/kg/d IM. Asthma, Acute: **Peds:** prednisolone 1–2 mg/kg/d or prednisone 1–2 mg/kg/d divided qd–bid for up to 5 d; prednisolone 2–4 mg/kg/d IV divided tid. Congenital Adrenal Hyperplasia: **Peds:** Initially, hydrocortisone 30–36 mg/m^2/d PO divided 1/3 dose qAM, 2/3 dose qPM; maintenance: 20–25 mg/m^2/d divided bid. Extubation/airway edema: dexamethasone 0.5–1 mg/kg/d IM/IV divided 6h, start beginning 24 h before extubation; continue 4 additional doses. Immunosuppressive/anti-inflammatory: **Adults** and **Older Peds:** Hydrocortisone: 15–240 mg PO, IM, IV q12h; methylprednisolone: 4–48 mg/d PO, taper to lowest effective dose; methylprednisolone sodium succinate: 10–80 mg IM qd. **Adults:** prednisone or prednisolone 5–60 mg/d PO, divided qd–qid. Infants and younger children: 2.5–10 mg/kg/d hydrocortisone PO divided q6–8h; 1–5 mg/kg/d IM/IV divided bid/qd. Nephrotic syndrome: Children: prednisolone or prednisone 2 mg/kg/d PO divided tid–qid until urine is protein free for 5 d, use up to 28 d; for persistent proteinuria, 4 mg/kg/dose PO qod max 120 mg/day for an additional 28 days; maintenance: 2 mg/kg/dose qod for 28 d; taper over 4–6 wk (max 80 mg/d). Septic Shock: **Adults:** hydrocortisone 500 mg – 1 g IM/IV q2–6h. **Peds:** hydrocortisone 50 mg/kg IM/IV, repeat q4–24 h prn. Status Asthmaticus: **Adults** and **Peds:** hydrocortisone: 1–2 mg/kg/dose IV q6h; then 0.5–1 mg/kg q6h. Rheumatic disease: **Adults:** Intra-articular: hydrocortisone acetate 25–37.5 mg, large joint; 10–25 mg, small joint; methylprednisolone acetate: 20–80 mg, large joint; 4–10 mg, small joint. Intra-bursal: hydrocortisone acetate, 25–37.5 mg. Intra-ganglia: hydrocortisone acetate, 25–37.5 mg. Tendon sheath: hydrocortisone acetate, 5–12.5 mg. Perioperative steroid coverage: hydrocortisone 100 mg IV night before surgery, 1 h preoperatively, intraoperatively, and 4, 8, and 12 h postoperatively; POD No. 1, 100 mg IV q6h; POD No. 2, 100 mg IV q8h; POD No. 3, 100 mg IV q12h; POD No. 4, 50 mg IV q12h; POD No. 5, 25 mg IV q12h; then, resume prior oral dosing if chronic use or discontinue if only perioperative coverage required. Cerebral edema: dexamethasone 10 mg IV; then 4 mg IV q6h.

NOTES: See Table VIII–4, page 521. All can cause hyperglycemia, "steroid psychosis," adrenal suppression; never acutely stop steroids, especially if chronic treatment; taper dose. Hydrocortisone succinate administered systemically, acetate form, intra-articular.

Steroids, Topical

COMMON USES: Topical therapy of a variety of inflammatory and pruritic dermatologic conditions that respond to corticosteroid therapy.

DOSAGE: Application based on individual agent (See Table VIII–7, page 523).

Streptokinase (Streptase, Kabikinase)

COMMON USES: Coronary artery thrombosis; acute massive pulmonary embolism; deep vein thrombosis; some occluded vascular grafts.

DOSAGE: Pulmonary embolus: Loading dose of 250,000 IU IV through a peripheral vein over 30 min, then 100,000 IU/h IV for 24–72 h. Deep vein thrombosis or arterial embolism: Load as with pulmonary embolus, then 100,000 IU/h for 72 h.

NOTES: If maintenance infusion not adequate to maintain thrombin clotting time 2–5 times control, refer to package insert, PDR, or Hospital Formulary Service for adjustments.

Succinylcholine (Anectine, Quelicin, Sucostrin)

COMMON USES: Adjunct to general anesthesia to facilitate endotracheal intubation and to induce skeletal muscle relaxation during surgery or mechanically supported ventilation.
DOSAGE: *Adults:* 0.6 mg/kg IV over 10–30 s followed by 0.04–0.07 mg/kg as needed to maintain muscle relaxation. *Peds:* 1–2 mg/kg/dose IV followed by 0.03–0.06 mg/kg/dose at intervals of 10–20 min.
NOTES: May precipitate malignant hyperthermia; respiratory depression or prolonged apnea may occur; many drug interactions potentiating activity of succinylcholine; observe for cardiovascular effects; use only freshly prepared solutions.

Sucralfate (Carafate)

COMMON USES: Treatment of duodenal ulcers, gastric ulcers.
DOSAGE: *Adults:* 1 g PO qid, 1 h before meals and hs. *Peds:* 40–80 mg/kg/d divided q6h.
NOTES: Treatment should be continued for 4–8 wk unless healing is demonstrated by radiograph or endoscopy; constipation is the most frequent side effect.

Sufentanil (Sufenta) [C]

COMMON USES: Analgesic adjunct to maintain balanced general anesthesia.
DOSAGE: Adjunctive: 1–8 mg/kg with nitrous oxide/oxygen; maintenance of 10–50 mg as needed. General anesthesia: 8–30 mg/kg with oxygen and a skeletal muscle relaxant; maintenance of 25–50 mg as needed.
NOTES: Respiratory depressant effects persisting longer than the analgesic effects; 80 times more potent than morphine.

Sulfacetamide

COMMON USES: Conjunctival infections.
DOSAGE: 10% ointment: apply qid and qhs; 10, 15, 30% solution for keratitis: apply q2–3h depending on severity.

Sulfasalazine (Azulfidine)

COMMON USES: Ulcerative colitis.
DOSAGE: *Adults:* 1–2 g PO initially, increase to maximum of 8 g/d in 3–4 divided doses; maintenance, 500 mg PO qid. *Peds:* 40–60 mg/kg/24h PO divided q4–6h initially; maintenance 20–30 mg/kg/24h PO divided q6h.
NOTES: Can cause severe gastrointestinal upset; discolors urine.

Sulfinpyrazone (Anturane)

COMMON USES: Acute and chronic gout.
DOSAGE: 100–200 mg PO bid for 1 wk, then increase as needed to maintenance of 200–400 mg bid.

Sulindac (Clinoril)

COMMON USES: Treatment of arthritis and pain.
DOSAGE: 150–200 mg bid.

Sulfisoxazole (Gantrisin, others)

COMMON USES: Acute uncomplicated urinary tract infections.
DOSAGE: *Adults:* Between 500 mg and 1 g PO qid. *Peds > 2 mo:* 120–150 mg/kg/24h PO divided q4–6h.
NOTES: Avoid use in last half of pregnancy (causes fetal hyperbilirubinemia).

Tacrine (Cognex)

COMMON USES: Treatment of mild-to-moderate dementia.
DOSAGE: 10–40 mg PO qid.
NOTES: May cause elevations in transaminases; LFTs should be monitored regularly.

Tacrolimus [FK 506] (Prograf)
COMMON USES: Prophylaxis of organ rejection.
DOSAGE: IV: 0.05–0.1 mg/kg/d as continuous infusion. PO: 0.15–0.3 mg/kg/d divided into 2 doses.
NOTES: May cause neurotoxicity and nephrotoxicity.

Tamoxifen (Nolvadex)
COMMON USES: Adjuvant treatment of breast cancer.
DOSAGE: 10–20 mg PO bid.
NOTES: May increase the risk of secondary uterine cancer.

Tamsulosin (Flomax)
COMMON USES: Treatment of benign prostatic hyperplasia.
DOSAGE: 0.4–0.8 mg qd.

Telmisartan (Micardis)
COMMON USES: Treatment of hypertension.
DOSAGE: 40–80 mg once daily.
NOTES: Avoid use during pregnancy.

Temazepam (Restoril) [C]
COMMON USES: Insomnia.
DOSAGE: 15–30 mg PO qhs prn.
NOTES: Reduce dose in elderly patients.

Tenecteplase (TNKase)
COMMON USES: Reduction of mortality associated with acute myocardial infarction.
DOSAGE: 30–50 mg IV (50 mg max); see product information for weight-based dosing.

Teniposide (Vumon)
COMMON USES: Treatment of leukemia.
DOSAGE: 165 mg/m^2 IV twice weekly for 8–9 doses.

Terazosin (Hytrin)
COMMON USES: Treatment of hypertension and benign prostatic hyperplasia.
DOSAGE: Initially, 1 mg PO hs; titrate up to maximum of 20 mg PO qhs.
NOTES: Hypotension and syncope following first dose; dizziness, weakness, nasal congestion, peripheral edema common; often used with thiazide diuretic.

Terbutaline (Brethine, Bricanyl)
COMMON USES: Reversible bronchospasm (asthma, COPD); inhibition of labor.
DOSAGE: *Adults:* Bronchodilator: 2.5–5 mg PO qid or 0.25 mg SC, may repeat in 15 min (maximum 0.5 mg in 4 h). Metered dose inhaler: 2 inhalations q4–6h. Premature labor: 10–80 mg/min IV infusion for 4 h, then 2.5 mg PO q4–6h until term. *Peds:* Oral: 0.05–0.15 mg/kg/dose PO tid; maximum 5 mg per 24 h.
NOTES: Use caution for patients with diabetes, hypertension, hyperthyroidism; high doses may precipitate β-1-adrenergic effects.

Terconazole (Terazol 7)
COMMON USES: Vaginal fungal infections.
DOSAGE: 1 applicator intravaginally qhs for 7 d.

Tetanus Immune Globulin
COMMON USES: Passive immunization against tetanus for any person with a suspect contaminated wound and unknown immunization status (see Appendix).
DOSAGE: *Adults* and *Peds:* 250–500 U IM (higher doses if delay in initiation of therapy).
NOTES: May begin active immunization series at different injection site if required.

Tetanus Toxoid

COMMON USES: Protection against tetanus.
DOSAGE: See Appendix for tetanus prophylaxis.

Tetracycline (Achromycin V, Sumycin)

COMMON USES: Broad-spectrum antibiotic treatment against *Staphylococcus, Streptococcus, Chlamydia, Rickettsia,* and *Mycoplasma.*
DOSAGE: *Adults:* 250–500 mg PO bid–qid. *Peds > 8 y:* 25–50 mg/kg/24h PO q6–12h. Do NOT use in children < 8 y.
NOTES: Can stain enamel and depress bone formation in children; caution with use in pregnancy; do NOT use in presence of impaired renal function (see Doxycycline, page 465).

Theophylline (Theolair, Theo-Dur, Somophyllin, others)

COMMON USES: Asthma, bronchospasm.
DOSAGE: *Adults:* 24 mg/kg/24h PO divided q6h; sustained release products may be divided q8–12h. *Peds:* 16 mg/kg/24h PO divided q6h; SR products may be divided q8–12h.
NOTES: See drug levels in Table VIII–3 on page 520; many drug interactions; side effects include nausea, vomiting, tachycardia, and seizures.

Thiamine (Vitamin B$_1$)

COMMON USES: Thiamine deficiency (beriberi); alcoholic neuritis; Wernicke's encephalopathy.
DOSAGE: *Adults:* Deficiency: 100 mg IM qd for 2 wk, then 5–10 mg PO qd for 1 mo. Wernicke's encephalopathy: 100 mg IV × 1 dose, then 100 mg IM qd for 2 wk. *Peds:*10–25 mg IM qd for 2 wk, then 5–10 mg/24h PO qd for 1 mo.
NOTES: IV thiamine administration associated with anaphylactic reaction; must be given slowly IV.

Thiethylperazine (Torecan)

COMMON USES: Nausea and vomiting.
DOSAGE: 10 mg PO, PR, or IM qd–tid.
NOTES: Extrapyramidal reactions may occur.

Thioridazine (Mellaril)

COMMON USES: Psychotic disorders; short-term treatment of depression, agitation, organic brain syndrome.
DOSAGE: *Adults:* Initially, 50–100 mg PO tid; maintenance, 200–800 mg/24h PO in 2–4 divided doses. *Peds > 2 y:* 1–2.5 mg/kg/24h PO divided bid–tid.
NOTES: Low incidence of extrapyramidal effects.

Thiotepa /Triethylenethiophosphoramide (Thio-TEPA, TESPA, TSPA, Thioplex)

COMMON USES: Breast, ovarian cancer; intracavitary for serosal malignant implants; intravesical for superficial papillary bladder cancer.
DOSAGE: 0.3–0.4 mg/kg IV at 1–4-wk intervals. Intravesical: 60 mg in 30–60-mL saline, held for 2 h if possible; treat weekly for 4 wk. Additional 4-wk course can be given with caution because myelosuppression can occur.
NOTES: Toxicity includes myelosuppression, nausea, vomiting, dizziness, headache, allergy, paresthesias.

Thiothixene (Navane)

COMMON USES: Psychotic disorders.
DOSAGE: *Adults* and *Peds > 12 y:* Mild-to-moderate psychosis: 2 mg PO tid. Severe psychosis: 5 mg PO bid; increase to maximum dose of 60 mg/24h prn. IM use: 16–20 mg/24h divided bid–qid; maximum 30 mg/d. *Peds < 12 y:* 0.25 mg/kg/24 h PO divided q6–12h.
NOTES: Drowsiness and extrapyramidal side effects most common.

Thyroid

COMMON USES: Replacement in hypothyroidism.

DOSAGE: 30 mg/d PO, titrate 30 mg/d over several wk; maintenance, 60–120 mg/d.

Tiagabine (Gabitril)

COMMON USES: Adjunctive therapy in treatment of partial seizures.
DOSAGE: Initial 4 mg once daily, increase by 4 mg during 2nd week; increase by 4–8 mg/d until clinical response is achieved; maximum dose 32 mg/d.
NOTES: Use gradual withdrawal; used in combination with other anticonvulsants.

Ticarcillin (Ticar)

COMMON USES: Infections caused by susceptible strains of gram-negative bacteria including *Klebsiella, Proteus, E coli, Enterobacter, P aeruginosa,* and *Serratia* involving the skin, bone, respiratory tract, urinary tract, abdomen, and septicemia.
DOSAGE: *Adults:* 3 g IV q4–6h. *Peds:* 200–300 mg/kg/d IV divided q4–6h.
NOTES: Often used in combination with aminoglycosides.

Ticarcillin/Potassium Clavulanate (Timentin)

COMMON USES: Infections due to susceptible strains of gram-negative bacteria (*Klebsiella, Proteus, E coli, Enterobacter, P aeruginosa,* and *Serratia*) involving the skin, bone, respiratory tract, urinary tract, abdomen, and septicemia.
DOSAGE: *Adults:* 3.1 g IV q4–6h. *Peds:* 200–300 mg/kg/d IV divided q4–6h.
NOTES: Often used in combination with aminoglycosides.

Ticlopidine (Ticlid)

COMMON USES: Reduce the risk of thrombotic stroke.
DOSAGE: 250 mg PO bid.
NOTES: Should be administered with food.

Timolol (Blocadren, Timoptic)

COMMON USES: Treatment of hypertension and myocardial infarction; glaucoma.
DOSAGE: HTN: 10–20 mg bid. MI: 10 mg bid. Ophthalmic: 0.25% 1 drop bid; decrease to qd when controlled; use 0.5% if needed; 1 drop gel qd.
NOTES: Timoptic XE (0.25, 0.5%) is a gel-forming solution.

Tioconazole (Vagistat)

COMMON USES: Vaginal fungal infections.
DOSAGE: 1 applicator intravaginally at bedtime (single dose)

Tirofiban (Aggrastat)

COMMON USES: Management of acute coronary syndrome.
DOSAGE: Initial 0.4 µg/kg/min for 30 min, followed by 0.1 µg/kg/min.
NOTES: Adjust dose in renal insufficiency; use in combination with heparin.

Tobramycin (Nebcin)

COMMON USES: Serious gram-negative infections, especially *Pseudomonas.*
DOSAGE: Based on renal function 2 mg/kg IV load followed 1.5 mg/kg IV q8h; refer to Aminoglycoside Dosing on page 518.
NOTES: Nephrotoxic and ototoxic; decrease dose with renal insufficiency; monitor creatinine clearance and serum concentrations for dosing adjustments; see Table VIII–3, page 520.

Tobramycin Ophthalmic (Tobrex)

COMMON USES: Ocular bacterial infections.
DOSAGE: 0.3% ointment, apply q3–8h or solution 0.3%, apply 1–2 drops q1–4h based on severity of infection.

Tobramycin and Dexamethasone Ophthalmic (TobraDex)

COMMON USES: Ocular bacterial infections associated with significant inflammation.
DOSAGE: 0.3% ointment, apply q3–8h or 0.3% solution, apply 1–2 drops q1–4h.

Tocainide (Tonocard)

COMMON USES: Suppression of ventricular arrhythmias including PVCs, and ventricular tachycardia.
DOSAGE: 400–600 mg PO q8h.
NOTES: Properties similar to lidocaine; reduce dose in renal failure; CNS and gastrointestinal side effects are common.

Tolazamide (Tolinase)

COMMON USES: Management of non-insulin-dependent diabetes mellitus.
DOSAGE: 100–500 mg qd.

Tolazoline (Priscoline)

COMMON USES: Persistent pulmonary vasoconstriction and hypertension of the newborn, peripheral vasospastic disorders.
DOSAGE: *Adults:* 10–50 mg IM/IV/SC qid. Neonates: 1–2 mg/kg IV over 10–15 min, followed by 1–2 mg/kg/h.

Tolbutamide (Orinase)

COMMON USES: Management of non-insulin-dependent diabetes mellitus.
DOSAGE: 500–1000 mg bid.

Tolmetin (Tolectin)

COMMON USES: Treatment of arthritis and pain.
DOSAGE: 200–600 mg tid, to a maximum of 2000 mg /d.

Topiramate (Topamax)

COMMON USES: Treatment of partial-onset seizures.
DOSAGE: Total dose, 400 mg/d. See product information of 8-wk titration schedule.
NOTES: May precipitate kidney stones.

Torsemide (Demadex)

COMMON USES: Edema, hypertension, congestive heart failure, and hepatic cirrhosis.
DOSAGE: 5–20 mg PO or IV once daily.

Tramadol (Ultram)

COMMON USES: Management of moderate–severe pain.
DOSAGE: 50–100 mg PO q4–6h prn, NOT to exceed 400 mg/d.

Trandolapril (Mavik)

COMMON USES: Treatment of hypertension, CHF, left-ventricular systolic dysfunction, post acute MI.
DOSAGE: HTN: 2–4 mg/d. CHF/LV dysfunction: 4 mg/d.

Trazodone (Desyrel)

COMMON USES: Major depression.
DOSAGE: 50–150 mg PO qd–qid; maximum, 600 mg/d.
NOTES: May take 1–2 wk for symptomatic improvement; anticholinergic side effects.

Triamterene (Dyrenium)

COMMON USES: Edema associated with CHF, cirrhosis.
DOSAGE: 100–300 mg/24h PO divided qd–bid.
NOTES: Can cause hyperkalemia; blood dyscrasias, liver damage, and other reactions.

Triazolam (Halcion) [C]

COMMON USES: Insomnia.
DOSAGE: 0.125–0.5 mg PO qhs prn.
NOTES: Additive CNS depression with alcohol and other CNS depressants.

Trifluoperazine (Stelazine)

COMMON USES: Psychotic disorders.

DOSAGE: *Adults:* 2–10 mg PO bid. *Peds 6–12 y:* 1 mg PO qd–bid, gradually increase up to 15 mg/d.
NOTES: Decrease dose in elderly and debilitated patients; oral concentrate must be diluted to 60 mL or more before administration.

Trifluridine (Viroptic)

COMMON USES: Herpes simplex keratitis and conjunctivitis.
DOSAGE: 1 drop q2h (max 9 drops/d); decrease to 1 drop q4h after healing begins; treat up to 14 d.

Trihexyphenidyl (Artane)

COMMON USES: Parkinson's disease.
DOSAGE: 2–5 mg PO qd–qid.
NOTES: Contraindicated in narrow-angle glaucoma.

Trimethaphan (Arfonad)

COMMON USES: Controlled hypotension during surgery; treatment of hypertensive crisis; treatment of pulmonary edema with pulmonary hypertension and systemic hypertension; dissecting aortic aneurysm.
DOSAGE: *Adults:* 0.3–6 mg/min IV infusion titrated to effect. *Peds:* 50–150 mg/kg/min IV infusion.
NOTES: Additive effect with other antihypertensive agents; vasopressors may be used to reverse hypotension if required; phenylephrine is vasopressor of choice for reversal of effects.

Trimethobenzamide (Tigan)

COMMON USES: Nausea and vomiting.
DOSAGE: *Adults:* 250 mg PO or 200 mg PR or IM tid–qid prn. *Peds:* 20 mg/kg/24h PO or 15 mg/kg/24h PR or IM in 3–4 divided doses (NOT recommended for infants).
NOTES: In the presence of viral infections, may contribute to Reye's syndrome; may cause parkinsonian-like syndrome.

Trimethoprim (Trimpex, Proloprim)

COMMON USES: Urinary tract infections caused by susceptible gram-positive and gram-negative organisms.
DOSAGE: 100 mg PO bid or 200 mg PO qd.
NOTES: Reduce dose in renal failure.

Trimethoprim-Sulfamethoxazole (Co-trimoxazole Bactrim, Septra)

COMMON USES: Urinary tract infections, otitis media, sinusitis, bronchitis, *Shigella*, *P carinii*, *Nocardia*.
DOSAGE: *Adults:* 1 double-strength (DS) tablet PO bid or 5–10 mg/kg/24h (based on trimethoprim component) IV in 3–4 divided doses. *P carinii:* 15–20 mg/kg/d IV or PO (trimethoprim component) in 4 divided doses. *Peds:* 8–10 mg/kg/24 h (trimethoprim) PO divided into 2 doses or 3–4 doses IV; do NOT use in newborn.
NOTES: Synergistic combination; reduce dose in renal failure.

Trimipramine (Surmontil)

COMMON USES: Treatment of depression.
DOSAGE: 75–300 mg PO qhs.

Tropicamide (Mydriacyl)

COMMON USES: Ocular exam; mydriatic and cycloplegic.
DOSAGE: 1–2 drops of 0.5–1% solution 30 min before exam; repeat q30min prn.
NOTES: Effects last 4–6 h.

Urokinase (Abbokinase)

COMMON USES: Pulmonary embolism, deep venous thrombosis, restore patency to IV catheters, coronary artery thrombosis.

DOSAGE: *Adults* and *Peds:* Systemic effect: 4400 IU/kg IV over 10 min, followed by 4400 IU/kg/h for 12 h. Restore catheter patency: Inject 5000 IU into catheter and gently aspirate.
NOTES: Do NOT use systemically within 10 d of surgery, delivery, or organ biopsy.

Valacyclovir (Valtrex)

COMMON USES: Treatment of herpes zoster.
DOSAGE: 1 g PO tid.

Valproic Acid and Divalproex (Depakene and Depakote)

COMMON USES: Epilepsy, mania, and prophylaxis of migraines.
DOSAGE: *Adults* and *Peds:* Seizures: 30–60 mg/kg/24 h PO divided tid. Mania: 750 mg in three divided doses, increased to a maximum of 60 mg/kg/d. Migraines: 250 mg bid, increased to 1000 mg/d.
NOTES: Monitor liver functions and serum levels (see Table VIII–3, page 520); concurrent use of phenobarbital and phenytoin may alter serum levels of these agents.

Valsartan (Diovan)

COMMON USES: Hypertension.
DOSAGE: 80 mg once daily.
NOTES: Use with caution with potassium-sparing diuretics or potassium supplements.

Vancomycin (Vancocin, Vancoled)

COMMON USES: Serious infections resulting from methicillin-resistant staphylococci and in enterococcal endocarditis in combination with aminoglycosides in penicillin-allergic patients; oral treatment of *C difficile* pseudomembranous colitis.
DOSAGE: *Adults:* 1 g IV q12h; for colitis 250–500 mg PO q6h. *Peds (NOT neonates):* 40 mg/kg/24h IV in divided doses q12–6h.
NOTES: Ototoxic and nephrotoxic; NOT absorbed orally, provides local effect in gut only; IV dose must be given slowly over 1 h to prevent "red-man syndrome"; adjust dose in renal failure; see Table VIII–3, page 520.

Vasopressin (Antidiuretic Hormone) (Pitressin)

COMMON USES: Treatment of diabetes insipidus; gaseous gastrointestinal tract distention; severe gastrointestinal bleeding, and an alternative pressor agent in treatment of adult shock-refractory ventricular fibrillation.
DOSAGE: *Adults* and *Peds:* Diabetes insipidus: 2.5–10 U SC or IM tid–qid or 1.5–5.0 U IM q1–3d of the tannate. Gastrointestinal hemorrhage: 20 U in 50–100-mL D5W or NS given IV over 15–30 min.
NOTES: Should be used with caution with any vascular disease.

Vecuronium (Norcuron)

COMMON USES: Skeletal muscle relaxation during surgery or mechanical ventilation.
DOSAGE: *Adults* and *Peds:* 0.08–0.1 mg/kg IV bolus; maintenance of 0.010–0.015 mg/kg after 25–40 min followed with additional doses every 12–15 min.
NOTES: Drug interactions leading to increased effect of vecuronium include aminoglycosides, tetracycline, and succinylcholine; less cardiac effects then pancuronium.

Venlafaxine (Effexor)

COMMON USES: Treatment of depression.
DOSAGE: 75–225 mg/d divided in 2–3 equal doses.

Verapamil (Calan, Isoptin)

COMMON USES: Supraventricular tachyarrhythmias (PAT, Wolff-Parkinson-White syndrome, atrial flutter or fibrillation); vasospastic (Prinzmetal's) and unstable (crescendo, preinfarction) angina; chronic stable angina (classical effort-associated); hypertension.
DOSAGE: *Adults:* Tachyarrhythmias: 5–10 mg IV over 2 min (may repeat in 30 min). Angina: 240–480 mg/24h divided in 3–4 doses. Hypertension: 80–180 mg PO tid or SR tablet 240 mg PO qd. *Peds:* < 1 y: 0.1–0.2 mg/kg IV over 2 min (may repeat in 30 min). 1–15 y: 0.1–0.3 mg/kg IV over 2 min (may repeat in 30 min); Do NOT exceed 5 mg.

NOTES: Use caution with elderly patients; reduce dose in renal failure; constipation is a common side effect.

Vidarabine (Vira-A)

COMMON USES: Herpes simplex keratitis and conjunctivitis.
DOSAGE: Apply ointment 5 times a day divided q3–4h; after healing begins, decrease to bid for up to 7 d.

Vinblastine (Velban)

COMMON USES: Hodgkin's disease, lymphoma, and testicular and ovarian cancer.
DOSAGE: Based on protocol; typical dosing 4–12 mg/m^2 q7–10d or 5-d continuous infusion 1.4–1.8 mg/m^2/d.
NOTES: May cause neutropenia; reduce dose after radiation exposure.

Vincristine (Oncovin)

COMMON USES: Cervical and ovarian cancer, sarcoma, leukemia, and Hodgkin's disease.
DOSAGE: Varies with protocol; 1.4–2 mg/m^2 IV once a week.
NOTES: May cause severe extravasation.

Vitamin B$_{12}$

See Cyanocobalamin, page 459.

Vitamin K

See Phytonadione, page 500.

Warfarin Sodium (Coumadin)

COMMON USES: Prophylaxis and treatment of pulmonary embolism and venous thrombosis, atrial fibrillation with embolization, other postoperative uses.
DOSAGE: *Adults:* Need to individualize dose to keep INR 2–3; some mechanical heart valves require INR 2.5–3.5; initially, 10 mg PO, IM, or IV qd for 1–3 d; then maintenance, 2–10 mg PO, IV, or IM qd; monitor INR during initial phase to guide dosing. *Peds:* 0.05–0.34 mg/kg/24h PO, IM, or IV qd. Monitor PT closely to adjust dose.
NOTES: Monitor INR while on maintenance dose; beware of bleeding caused by excessive anticoagulation (PT > 3 times control), caution patient on effects of taking Coumadin with other medications, especially aspirin; to rapidly correct excessive dosage, use vitamin K or fresh frozen plasma or both; highly teratogenic, do NOT use in pregnancy.

Witch Hazel (Tucks Pads)

COMMON USES: After bowel movement cleansing to decrease local irritation or relieve hemorrhoids; after anorectal surgery and episiotomy.
DOSAGE: Apply as needed.

Zafirlukast (Accolate)

COMMON USES: Prophylaxis and chronic treatment of asthma.
DOSAGE: 20 mg bid.
NOTES: Not for acute exacerbations of asthma; contraindicated in nursing women.

Zalcitabine (Hivid)

COMMON USES: HIV infection for patients intolerant to zidovudine and didanosine.
DOSAGE: 0.75 mg PO tid.
NOTES: May be used in combination with zidovudine; may cause peripheral neuropathy.

Zaleplon (Sonata)

COMMON USES: Insomnia.
DOSAGE: 5–20 mg qhs prn.

Zanamivir (Relenza)

COMMON USES: Treatment of influenza.
DOSAGE: 2 inhalations (10 mg) twice daily.
NOTES: Uses a Diskhaler for administration.

Zidovudine (Retrovir)

COMMON USES: Management of patients with HIV infections.
DOSAGE: *Adults:* 200 mg PO tid or 300 mg PO bid or 1–2 mg/kg/dose IV q4h. Pregnancy: 100 mg PO 5 times per day until labor; during labor, 2 mg/kg over 1 h followed by 1 mg/kg/h until clamping of the umbilical cord. *Peds:* 720 mg/m^2/24h PO divided 5 times per day.
NOTES: Not a cure for HIV infections.

Zidovudine and lamivudine (Combivir)

COMMON USES: Management of patients with HIV infections.
DOSAGE: *Adults* and *Peds > 12 y:* 1 tablet bid.

Zileuton (Zyflo)

COMMON USES: Prophylaxis and chronic treatment of asthma.
DOSAGE: 600 mg qid.
NOTES: MUST take on a regular basis; does NOT treat acute exacerbation.

Zolpidem (Ambien) [C]

COMMON USES: Short-term treatment of insomnia.
DOSAGE: 5–10 mg PO qhs prn.

Zonisamide (Zonegran)

COMMON USES: Partial seizures.
DOSAGE: Initially, 100 mg once daily; may be increased to 400 mg/d.
NOTES: Contraindicated in persons with hypersensitivity to sulfonamides.

TABLE VIII–1. AMINOGLYCOSIDE DOSING.

See Table VIII–3, page 520, "Common Drug Levels" for the trough and peak levels of the aminoglycosides gentamicin, tobramycin, and amikacin. Peak levels should be drawn 30 min after the dose is completely infused; trough levels should be drawn 30 min before the dose. As a general rule, draw the peak and trough around the fourth maintenance dose.

Therapy can be initiated with the recommended guidelines that follow. The following calculations are not valid for netilmicin.

Procedure (Adult)

1. Calculate the estimated creatinine clearance (CrCl) based on serum creatinine (SCr), age, and body weight, or you can order a formal creatinine clearance, if time permits.

$$\text{CrCl: Male} = \frac{(140 - \text{age [y]}) \times (\text{body wt. [kg]})}{(\text{SCr [mg / dL]}) \times 72}$$

$$\text{CrCl: Female} = 0.85 \times \text{CrCl}$$

2. Select the loading dose:

Gentamicin: 1.5–2.0 mg/kg   Tobramycin: 1.5–2.0 mg/kg
Amikacin: 5.0–7.5 mg/kg

3. By using Table VIII–2, page 519 you can now select the maintenance dose (as a percentage of the chosen loading dose) most appropriate for the renal function of the patient based on CrCl and dosing interval. Bold numbers are the suggested percentages and intervals for any given creatinine clearance.

TABLE VIII–2. PERCENTAGE OF LOADING DOSE REQUIRED FOR DOSAGE INTERVAL SELECTED.[a]

CrCl (mL/min)	Dosing Interval		
	8 h	12 h	24 h
90	**90**[b]	—	—
90	**86**	—	—
70	**84**	—	—
60	**79**	91	—
50	**74**	87	—
40	66	**80**	—
30	57	**72**	92
25	51	**66**	88
20	45	**59**	83
15	37	**50**	75
10	29	40	**64**
7	24	33	**55**
5	20	28	**48**
2	14	20	**35**
0	9	13	**25**

[a]Based on data from Hull JH, Sarubbi FA: Gentamicin serum concentrations: Pharmacokinetic predictions. Ann Intern Med 1976;85:183.
[b]Bold numbers indicate suggested dosage intervals. This is only an empirical dose to begin therapy. Serum levels should be monitored routinely for optimal therapy. Use Table VIII–3, "Common Drug Levels," page 520

TABLE VIII–3. COMMON DRUG LEVELS.[a]

Drug	Therapeutic Level	Toxic Level
Carbamazepine	4.0–12.0 mg/mL	>15.0 mg/mL
Cyclosporine	150–300 ng/mL (variable)	
Digoxin	0.8–2.0 ng/mL	>2.4 ng/mL
Ethanol		100–200 mg/100mL (legally drunk most states, labile behavior)
		150–300 mg/100 mL (confusion)
		250–400 mg/100 mL (stupor)
		350–500 mg/100 mL (coma)
		>450 mg/100 mL (death)
Ethosuximide	40.0–100.0 mg/mL	>150.0 mg/mL
Lidocaine	1.5–6.5 mg/mL	>6.0–8.0 mg/mL
Lithium	0.6–1.2 mmol/L	>2.0 mmol/L
Phenobarbital	15.0–40.0 mg/mL	>45.0 mg/mL
Phenytoin	10.0–20.0 mg/mL	>25.0 mg/mL
Procainamide	4.0–10.0 mg/mL	>16.0 mg/mL
Quinidine	3.0–7.0 mg/mL	>7 mg/mL
Theophylline	10.0–20.0 mg/mL	>20.0 mg/mL
Valproic acid	50–100 mg/mL	>150 mg/mL
Antibiotic (maintain below upper limit)		
	Trough (< mg/mL)	Peak (mg/mL)
Amikacin	5.0–7.5	25–35
Gentamicin	1.5–2.0	5–8
Tobramycin	1.5–2.0	5–8
Netilmicin	0.5–2.0	6–10
Vancomycin	5.0–10.0	20–40

[a]Each lab may have values that differ slightly from those provided. Therapeutic levels are usually determined as a trough just before next dose.

TABLE VIII–4. COMPARISON OF SYSTEMIC GLUCOCORTICOIDS (see page 509).

Drug	Relative Equivalent Dose (mg)	Activity	Mineralocorticoid Duration	Route
Betamethasone	0–0.75	0	36–72 h	PO, IM
Cortisone (Cortone)	25.00	2	8–12 h	PO, IM
Dexamethasone (Decadron)	0.75	0	36–72 h	PO, IV
Hydrocortisone (Solu-Cortef, Hydrocortone)	20.00	2	8–12 h	PO, IM, IV
Methylprednisolone acetate (Depo-Medrol)	4.00	0	36–72 h	PO, IM, IV
Methylprednisolone Succinate (Solu-Medrol)	4.00			PO, IM, IV
Prednisone (Deltasone)	5.00	1	12–36 h	PO
Prednisolone (Delt-Cortef)	5.00	1	12–36 h	PO, IM, IV

PO = by mouth; TM = intramuscular; IV = intravenous.

TABLE VIII–5. COMPARISON OF INSULINS.

Type of Insulin	Onset (h)	Peak (h)	Duration (h)
Ultra Rapid			
Humalog (Lispro)	Immediate	0.5–1.5	3–5
Novolog (Insulin aspart)	Immediate	0.5–1.5	3–5
Rapid			
Regular Iletin II	0.25–0.5	2.0–4.0	5–7
Humulin R	0.5	2.0–4.0	6–8
Novolin R	0.5	2.5–5.0	5–8
Velosulin	0.5	2.0–5.0	6–8
Intermediate			
NPH Iletin II	1.0–2.0	6–12	18–24
Lente Iletin II	1.0–2.0	6–12	18–24
Humulin N	1.0–2.0	6–12	14–24
Novulin L	2.5–5.0	7–15	18–24
Novulin 70/30	0.5	7–12	24
Prolonged			
Ultralente	4.0–6.0	14–24	28–36
Humulin U	4.0–6.0	8–20	24–28
Lantus (Insulin glargine)	4.0–6.0	no peak	24
Combination Insulins			
Humalog Mix (Lispro protamine/Lispro)	0.25–0.5	1–4	24

TABLE VIII–6. SOME COMMON ORAL POTASSIUM SUPPLEMENTS.

Brand Name	Salt	Form	mEq Potassium/ Dosing Unit
Glu-K	Gluconate	Tablet	2 mEq/tablet
Kaochlor 10%	KCl	Liquid	20 mEq/15 mL
Kaochlor S-F10% (sugar-free)	KCl	Liquid	20 mEq/15 mL
Kaochlor Eff	Bicarbonate/KCl/ citrate	Effervescent tablet	20 mEq/tablet
Kaon Elixir	Gluconate	Liquid	20 mEq/15 mL
Kaon	Gluconate	Tablet	5 mEq/tablet
Kaon-Cl	KCl	Tablet, SR	6.67 mEq/tablet
Kaon-Cl 20%	KCl	Liquid	40 mEq/15 mL
KayCiel	KCl	Liquid	20 mEq/15 mL
K-Lor	KCl	Powder	15 or 20 mEq/packet
Klorvess	Bicarbonate/KCl	Liquid	20 mEq/15 mL
Klotrix	KCl	Tablet, SR	10 mEq/tablet
K-Lyte	Bicarbonate/citrate	Effervescent tablet	25 mEq/tablet
K-Tab	KCl	Tablet, SR	10 mEq/tablet
Micro-K	KCl	Capsule, SR	8 mEq/capsule
Slow-K	KCl	Tablet, SR	8 mEq/tablet
Tri-K	Acetate/bicarbonate and citrate	Liquid	45 mEq/15 mL
Twin-K	Citrate/gluconate	Liquid	20 mEq/5 mL

TABLE VIII–7. TOPICAL STEROID PREPARATIONS.

Agent	Common Trade Names	Potency	Apply
Aclometasone dipropionate	Aclovate, cream, ointment 0.05%	Low	bid/tid
Amcinonide	Cyclocort, cream, lotion, ointment 0.1%	High	bid/tid
Betamethasone valerate	Valisone cream, lotion 0.01%	Low	qd/bid
	Valisone cream 0.01, 0.1%, ointment, lotion 0.1%	Intermediate	qd/bid
Betamethasone dipropionate	Diprosone cream, lotion, ointment 0.05%	High	qd/bid
	Diprosone aerosol (0.1%)		
Betamethasone dipropionate, augmented	Diprolene ointment, gel 0.05%	Ultrahigh	qd/bid
Clobetasol propionate	Temovate cream, gel, ointment, scalp, solution 0.05%	Ultrahigh	bid (2 weeks max)
Clocortolone pivalate	Cloderm cream 0.1%	Intermediate	qd–qid
Desonide	DesOwen, cream, ointment, lotion 0.05%	Low	bid–qid
Desoximetasone	Topicort LP cream, gel 0.05%	Intermediate	bid–tid
	Topicort cream, ointment 0.25%	High	
Dexamethasone base	Aeroseb-Dex aerosol 0.01%	Low	bid–qid
	Decadron cream 0.1%		
Diflorasone diacetate	Psorcon cream, ointment 0.05%	Ultrahigh	bid–qid
Fluocinolone acetonide 0.01%	Synalar cream, solution 0.01%	Low	bid–tid
	Synalar ointment, cream 0.025%	Intermediate	bid–tid
	Synalar-HP cream 0.2%	High	bid–tid
Fluocinonide 0.05%	Lidex, anhydrous cream, gel, ointment, solution 0.05%	High	bid–tid
	Lidex-E aqueous cream 0.05%	High	bid–tid

(continued)

TABLE VIII–7. TOPICAL STEROID PREPARATIONS (CONTINUED).

Agent	Common Trade Names	Potency	Apply
Flurandrenolide	Cordran cream, ointment 0.025%	Intermediate	bid/tid
	cream, lotion, ointment 0.05%	Intermediate	bid/tid
	tape, 4 μg/cm²	Intermediate	qd
Fluticasone propionate	Cutivate cream 0.05%, ointment 0.005%	Intermediate	bid
Halobetasol	Ultravate cream, ointment 0.05%	Very High	bid
Halcinonide	Halog cream 0.025%, emollient base 0.1%	High	qd/tid
	Cream, ointment, solution 0.1%		
Hydrocortisone	Cortizone, Caldecort, Hycort, Hytone, others	Low	tid/qid
	Aerosol 1%, cream: 0.5, 1, 2.5%, gel 0.5%		
	ointment 0.5, 1, 2.5%, lotion 0.5, 1, 2.5%		
	paste 0.5% solution 1%		
Hydrocortisone acetate	Corticaine cream, ointment 0.5, 1%	Low	tid/qid
Hydrocortisone butyrate	Locoid ointment solution 0.1%	Intermediate	bid/tid
Hydrocortisone valerate	Westcort cream, ointment 0.2%	Intermediate	bid/tid
Mometasone furoate	Elocon 0.1% cream, ointment, lotion	Intermediate	qd
Prednicarbate	Dermatop 0.1% cream	Intermediate	bid
Triamcinolone acetonide	Aristocort, Kenalog cream, ointment, lotion 0.025%	Low	tid/qid
	Aristocort, Kenalog cream, ointment, lotion 0.1%	Intermediate	tid/qid
	Aerosol 0.2 mg/2sec spray		
Triamcinolone acetonide	Aristocort, Kenalog cream, ointment 0.5%	High	tid/qid

TABLE VIII–8. COMPARISON OF CLINICAL EFFECTS OF VASOPRESSOR AGENTS.

Drug/Therapy	Usual Adult Intravenous Dose	Hemodynamic Effects						
		Vasodilation	Vasoconstriction	Inotropic	Chronotropic	Arrhythmogenic Potential	Renal Perfusion	Cardiac Output
Dobutamine[a]	2–20 µg/kg/min	++	+	++++	+	++	↑	↑
Dopamine[a]	1–20 µg/kg/min	+	+++	+++	+++	+++	↑	↑
Epinephrine[a]	0.01–0.1 µg/kg/min	+	+	+++	++	++	↑	↑
Isoproterenol	2–10 µg/min	+++	0	++++	++++	++	↑	↑
Milrinone	0.375–0.75 µg/kg/min	++	0	+++	+++	++	↑	↑
Norepinephrine	2–20 µg/min	0	++++	+	++	+++	↑↓	↑↓0
Phenylephrine	0.5–5 µg/min	0	+++	0	0	0	↑	↑↓0
Vasopressin[b]	40 units × 1	0	+++	0	0	0	↓	↓

[a]The effects of these drugs are dose dependent, the effects listed are reflective of higher doses.
[b]Vasopressin has recently been added to the ACLS (advanced cardiovascular life support) guidelines in treatment of adult shock-refractory ventricular fibrillation. plus sign (+) = positive effect; up arrow (↑) = increased effect; down arrow (↓) = decreased effect; zero (0) = no effect.

TABLE VIII–9. ANTIEPILEPTIC DRUGS

	Carbamazepine	Phenobarbital	Phenytoin
Route/Adult Dose	Oral: start at 200 mg bid, increase weekly 200 mg/d maintenance dose 800–1200 mg/d in divided doses. Maximum dose: 2.4 g/d	IV/Oral: maintenance dose is 1–3 mg/kg/d	IV/Oral: loading dose is 10–20 mg/kg with a maximum dose of 1500 mg. Maintenance dose is 5–6 mg/kg/d in divided doses.
Usual therapeutic range (mg/mL)[a]	8–12	15–40	10–20
Side effects[a]	Thrombocytopenia, hepatotoxic	Cardiac arrhythmia, agranulocytosis, thrombocytopenia, hepatotoxicity	Thrombocytopenia, neutropenia, anemia, hepatotoxicity, gum hyperplasia, nystamus, ataxia

[a]Monitoring parameters: drug serum concentrations seizure activities, LFTs, CBC.

TABLE VIII–10. SEDATIVE/PAIN AGENTS.

Therapeutic Agents	Classification	Routes	Adult Dosage
Lorazepam	Intermediate-acting benzodiazepine	IM, IV, SQ, PO	IV: 1–2 mg q4–6 h
Midazolam	Benzodiazepine (has an active metabolite)	IM, IV	IV: 0.5–2 mg/dose
Propofol	Short-acting sedative-hypnotic	IV	IV: 5–50 µg/kg/min
Fentanyl	Potent opioid (50–100 × more potent than morphine)	IM, IV, transdermal	IV: 0.5–1 µg/kg/dose
Morphine	Opioid	IM, IV, SQ, PO, PR	IV: 2–15 mg/dose

IV = intravenous; IM = intramuscular; SQ = subcutaneous; PO = by mouth; PR = per rectum.

Appendices

APPENDIX 1: CRITICAL CARE FORMULAS

Parameter (Abbreviation)	Unit	Measured (M) or Derived (D)	Derivation	Normal Range
A-a gradient	mm Hg	D	$[(713) Fio_2 - Paco_2 (1.25)]Pao_2$	Room air: 2–22 mm Hg
Alveolar ventilation	L/min	M	$Vco_2/Paco_2 \times K$	4–6 L/min
Arterial blood O_2 tension (Pao_2)	mm Hg	M	—	70–100
Arterial CO_2 content	mm Hg	M	—	35–45
Arterial hemoglobin O_2 saturation (Sao_2)	(fraction)	M	—	>0.92
Arterial O_2 content (Cao_2)	mL O_2/dL blood	D	$(Hgb \times 1.34) Sao_2 + (Pao_2 \times 0.0031)$	16–22
Cardiac index (CI)	L/min/m^2	D	$CI = CO/BSA$	2.8–4.2
Central venous pressure (CVP)	mm Hg	M	—	0–8
Cerebral perfusion pressure (CPP)	mm Hg	D	$MAP - ICP$	>70 mm Hg
Creatinine clearance		D	$Wt \times (140-age)/(72 \times Pl_{cr})$ males (estimate) $(0.85 \times wt) \times (140-age)/(72 \times Pl_{cr})$ females (estimate)	
Diastolic blood pressure(DBP)	mm Hg	M	—	60–90
Intracranial pressure (ICP)	mm Hg	M	—	0–20 mm Hg
Left ventricular stroke work index (LVSWI)	g·m/m^2	D	$LVSWI = (MAP - PAWP) \times SVI \times 0.0136$	43–61
Mean arterial blood pressure (MAP)	mm Hg	D	$MAP = diast + (sys - diast)/3$	70–105
Mean pulmonary artery pressure (MPAP)	mm Hg	D	$MPAP = diast_p + (sys_p - diast_p)/3$	9–16
Mixed venous blood O_2 tension (Pvo_2)	mm Hg	M	—	33–53
Mixed venous hemoglobin O_2 saturation (Svo_2)	(fraction)	M	—	0.65–0.80

(continued)

Parameter (Abbreviation)	Unit	Measured (M) or Derived (D)	Derivation	Normal Range
Mixed venous O_2 content (Cvo_2)	mL O_2/dL blood	D	$(Hgb \times 1.34)$ $Svo_2 + (Pvo_2 \times 0.0031)$	12–17
O_2 consumption (Vo_2)	mL/min/m²	D	C (a–v) $c_2 \times CO \times 10$	110–160
O_2 delivery (Do_2)	mL/min/m²	D	$Cao_2 \times CO \times 10$	520–720
O_2 extraction [C (a–v) o_2]	mL O_2/dL blood	D	C (a–v) $o_2 = (Hgb \times 1.34)$ $(Sao_2 - Svo_2)$	3.5–5.5
O_2 extraction ratio (O_2 ER)	(fraction)	D	O_2 ER = Vo_2/Do_2	0.22–0.32
Pulmonary artery diastolic pressure (PADP)	mm Hg	M	—	4–12
Pulmonary artery systolic pressure (PASP)	mm Hg	M	—	15–30
Pulmonary artery wedge pressure (PAWP)	mm Hg	M	—	2–12
Pulmonary compliance	ml/cm H_2O	D	$\Delta V/\Delta P$	
Pulmonary vascular resistance index (PVRI)	dyne sec/cm⁵/m²	D	PVRI = (PAP–PAWP) × 80/CI	80–240
Right ventricular end-diastolic pressure (RVEDP)	mm Hg	M	—	0–8
Right ventricular stroke work index (RVSWI)	g m/m²	D	RVSWI = (PAP–CVP) × SVI × 0.0136	7–12
Right ventricular systolic pressure (RVSP)	mm Hg	M	—	15–30
Serum lactate	mmol/l	M	—	0–4
Shunt fraction	—	D	$(Ccc_2 - Cao_2)$/$(Cco_2 - Cvo_2)$	5%
Stroke volume index (SVI)	mL/beat/m²	D	CI/HR × 1000	30–65
Systemic vascular resistance index (SVRI)	dyne sec/cm⁵/m²	D	SVRI = (MAP – CVP) × 80/CI	200–2500
Systolic blood pressure (SBP)	mm Hg	M	—	100–140

531

Step 1: Obtain an Arterial blood gas (for normal values, see page 270).

Step 2: Look at the pH.

1. If pH < 7.35, there is **acidosis.**
2. If pH > 7.45, there is **alkalosis.**
3. If 7.35 < pH < 7.45, there is:

    No acid-base disorder, or

    Compensated disorder, or

    Mixed disorder.

Step 3: Look at the $Paco_2$.

1. If the pH < 7.35 and the $Paco_2$ > 45, it is **respiratory acidosis.**
2. If the pH < 7.35 and the $Paco_2$ < 35, it is **metabolic acidosis.**
3. If the pH > 7.45 and the $Paco_2$ < 35, it is **respiratory alkalosis.**
4. If the pH > 7.45 and the $Paco_2$ > 45, it is **metabolic alkalosis.**

Step 4:

1. If **respiratory acidosis,** look at the increase in Hco_3 for each 10-mm increase in $Paco_2$.

    If 1.0–1.2, it is **acute respiratory acidosis.**

    If 1.3–3.0, it is **partially compensated.**

    If 3.1–4.0, it is **fully compensated.**

2. If **pure metabolic acidosis.**

    $Paco_2$. = $(1.5 \times Hco_3) + 8 \pm 2$.

    $Paco_2$. = $Hco_3 + 15$ if $Hco_3 > 10$.

3. If **respiratory alkalosis,** look at the fall of Hco_3 for each 10-mm fall of $Paco_2$.

    If 2.5, it is acute **respiratory alkalosis.**

    If 5.0, it is **chronic respiratory alkalosis.**

4. If **respiratory alkalosis,** look at the rise in pH for 10-mm fall of $Paco_2$.

    If 0.08, it is **acute respiratory alkalosis.**

    If 0.03, **chronic respiratory alkalosis.**

5. If **metabolic alkalosis.**

    $Paco_2 = 0.7 \times Hco_3 + 20 \pm 1.5$.

Limits of compensation.

1. In acute respiratory acidosis Hco_3 cannot rise above 30.
2. In chronic respiratory acidosis Hco_3 can rise above 55.
3. In respiratory alkalosis $Paco_2$ cannot fall below 16 mmHg.
4. In metabolic acidosis the $Paco_2$ cannot fall below 10 mmHg.
5. In metabolic alkalosis $Paco_2$ cannot rise above 55.
6. If the values deviate from the above it is a mixed disorder.
7. There is never overcompensation.

Response	Score
Eye Opening (E)	
Spontaneous	4
To Call	3
To name	2
None	1
Motor (M)	
Obeys Commands	6
Localizes Pain	5
Normal Flexion (withdrawal)	4
Abnormal flexion (decorticate)	3
Extension (decerebrate)	2
None (flaccid)	1
Verbal Response (V)	
Oriented	5
Confused Conversation	4
Inappropriate words	3
Incomprehensible sounds	2
None	1
Total Score = E + M + V (Minimum = 3, Maximum = 15)	

BODY SURFACE AREA: ADULT

Subject Index